Health Informatics

Marion J. Ball • Judith V. Douglas
Patricia Hinton Walker • Donna DuLong • Brian Gugerty
Kathryn J. Hannah • Joan M. Kiel • Susan K. Newbold
Joyce Sensmeier • Diane J. Skiba • Michelle R. Troseth
(Editors)

Marion J. Ball • Kathryn J. Hannah
(Series Editors)

Nursing Informatics

Where Technology and Caring Meet

Fourth Edition

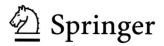 Springer

Editors

Marion J. Ball
IBM Research
Center for Healthcare Management
Baltimore, MD 21239, USA

Judith V. Douglas
Reisterstown, Maryland 21136, USA

Patricia Hinton Walker
Uniformed Services
University of the Health Sciences
4301 Jones Bridge Road
Bethesda, MD 20814, USA

Donna DuLong
The Tiger Initiative
Denver, CO 80045, USA

Brian Gugerty
Gugerty Consulting LLC
1038 Bayberry Drive
Arnold, MD 21012, USA

Kathryn J. Hannah
HECS Inc.
Calgary, Alb, Canada

Joan M. Kiel
Duquesne University
600 Forbes Avenue
Pittsburgh, PA 15282, USA

Susan K. Newbold
Franklin, TN, USA

Joyce Sensmeier
Healthcare Information and
Management Systems Informatics
230 East Ohio St, Suite 500
Chicago, IL 60611, USA

Diane J. Skiba
University of Colorado Denver
College of Nursing
13120 E. 19th Ave.
Aurora, CO 80045, USA

Michelle R. Troseth
CPM Resource Center
3196 Kraft Ave SE
Grand Rapids, MI 49512, USA

ISBN 978-1-84996-277-3   e-ISBN 978-1-84996-278-0
DOI 10.1007/978-1-84996-278-0
Springer London Dordrecht Heidelberg New York

British Library Cataloguing in Publication Data
A catalogue record for this book is available from the British Library

Library of Congress Control Number: 2010937960

Cover design: eStudioCalamar, Figueres/Berlin

Printed on acid-free paper

Springer is part of Springer Science+Business Media (www.springer.com)

This is the fourth edition of *Nursing Informatics*, catchily subtitled *Where Technology and Caring Meet*. In the two decades since the first edition debuted, the juxtaposition between technology and caring has moved from an uncomfortable tension felt by individuals to a creative force seeking to transform all aspects of the nursing profession, from staff development to the design of overarching process improvements. What began as the opposition of two world views – caring vs. technology – has evolved to become the driving force in articulating a twenty-first century view of nursing as a field able to change the health care system by strategically using technology to realize quality care. In this case, point and counter-point have syllogistically led to a synthesis not unlike the one proposed by the Institute of Medicine[1] urging all health professionals to use informatics to make care more patient-centered.

This fourth edition is dramatically different from preceding editions because it builds on the extensive work of the *TIGER* Initiative, an acronym for Technology Informatics Guiding Education Reform,[2] which began in 2004 when a few nurse/informatics activists attending the first national health information technology summit decided that something comprehensive needed to be launched to transform nursing practice, education, scholarship, and leadership through information technology (IT). Believing that IT was not merely an add-on but the key to a paradigm shift in how future health care would be provided, they eventually convened their own summit of stakeholders that crossed clinical specialties, functional areas, and professional organizations ($n = \geq 70$).

The 2006 summit gave birth to an action agenda that led to the formation of nine collaboratives that collectively addressed workforce advancement (competencies, faculty development, staff preparation, leadership for change, virtual-demonstration education), development of an IT infrastructure (standards and interoperability, a National Health IT Agenda), and improved technologic solutions (standards and interoperability, usability and clinical-application design, consumer empowerment, and health records) (TIGER 2007). By the end of 2008, over 1,400 people had been involved in this boundary-spanning effort that worked to change matters both through existing organizational structures – National League for Nursing's Informatics Agenda[3]; American Association of Colleges of Nursing's competencies for Doctor of Nursing Practice[4] – and new initiatives – statewide Minnesota TIGER.[5]

Because the editors of this edition were also leaders in the TIGER Initiative, they had access to the wealth of information generated by that multiphase initiative, and that richness is evident in the selection of the chapter authors and in the range of topics covered.

For example, the section on future directions provides insights into subjects often not discussed in any depth, e.g., the interface between comparative effectiveness research and personalized health care. Because the TIGER Initiative has attracted international attention, a global perspective prevails.

Though nurse informaticists will find this edition must reading, this is a book that will be invaluable to any clinician, educator, manager, or executive interested in one-stop shopping for a comprehensive statement on the subject. Chief Nurse Officers will want to share this book with Chief Informatics Officers at their institutions; faculty will want to adopt the book for DNP courses. Administrators wishing to understand user interface and clinical design issues will want to read this edition to frame discussions in their home settings; researchers will look to this book for insights on how the informatics revolution is accelerating the demand for comparative effectiveness research. The fact that this edition was peer reviewed, therefore subject beforehand to scientific scrutiny, adds to the confidence one has in using the volume as a major reference.

The increased sophistication of nursing informatics is visible in this fourth edition, reflecting in part the policy-oriented perspective of the Alliance for Nursing Informatics, which came into existence after the third edition to provide a coordinated voice for nursing in various informatics debates. As in the past, mention is made of needed development in workforce competencies and of enabling technologies, but the day-to-day concerns of the individual are couched in larger contextual issues too, for example, how practice is being shaped by reform efforts requiring standardized clinical performance measures and clinical decision support to manage chronic conditions. Hinton Walker's chapter on culture change provides a framework for examining the transformations taking place locally, regionally, nationally, and internationally as nurses play a leadership role in designing and using information systems that were once thought to be only the province of physicians.

There used to be a time when one book could be the bible for nursing – I'm thinking of Harmer and Henderson's *The Principles and Practice of Nursing*. Given the scope of twenty-first century nursing, that is increasingly impossible, but this book approaches that status because the content is relevant to all aspects of nursing. Writing about her specialty of psychiatric nursing, Haber[6] noted that even the legendary Hildegard Peplau would be embracing information technology and evidence-based practice if she were alive today. And I suspect this fourth edition would be in her library.

Angela Barron McBride
Distinguished Professor-University Dean Emerita
Indiana University School of Nursing

References

1. Institute of Medicine. *Health Professions Education: A Bridge to Quality.* Washington, DC: The National Academies Press; 2003.
2. Technology Informatics Guiding Education Reform. The TIGER Initiative. Collaborating to integrate evidence and informatics into nursing practice and education: an executive summary.

http://www.tigersummit.com/uploads/TIGER_Collaborative_Exec_Summary_040509.pdf 2007 Accessed 20.09.09.

3. National League for Nursing. Preparing the next generation of nurses to practice in a technology-rich environment: an informatics agenda. http://www.nln.org/aboutnln/PositionStatements/informatics_052808.pdf; 2008 Accessed 20.09.09.

4. American Association of Colleges of Nursing. The essentials of doctoral education for advanced nursing practice. http://www.aacn.nche.edu/DNP/pdf/Essentials.pdf; 2006 Accessed 20.09.09.

5. University of Minnesota School of Nursing. Minnesota TIGER Summit: springing into action. http://www.nursing.umn.edu/MNTiger; 2009 Accessed 20.09.09.

6. Haber J. Hildegard E. Peplau: the psychiatric nursing legacy of a legend. *J Am Psych Nurs Assoc.* 2000;6:56-62.

There are several, significant challenges facing healthcare delivery in the United States. The quality, safety, efficiency, and accessibility of care are not at levels that we would regard as satisfactory. These challenges will be exacerbated by inexorable movements to deliver care that is more patient-centric, widen access to care, increase the emphasis on wellness and preventive care, improve the accountability for care, reduce the costs of care, and incorporate advances such as personalized medicine.

While the term "transformation" is overused, it is nonetheless the correct description of what we must do to our system of providing care to those who need it.

Information Technology as a Tool

Improving care through electronic health records (EHRs) requires that we understand the nature of EHRs as tools.

There is no question that information technology can be a very potent tool in our efforts to address the challenges that confront our health care system. There is also no question that information technology is a tool and as a tool does not, in and of itself, have magic care improvement properties.

For the EHR to achieve any objectives, not only does the organization need the technology, but also needs leadership, an ability to effectively change processes, means to provide training and ongoing support to clinicians, and approaches to measure objectives and engage in ongoing tuning of the application and care processes.

The EHR is a specific kind of tool. At times, we view EHRs as systems that must be implemented and our task as done once they are implemented. We view EHRs as interventions. They are not. They are foundations.

A foundation provides the broad ability to perform a "never-ending" series of application-leveraged small, medium-sized, and occasionally large advances and improvements in processes.

For example, provider order entry systems can be used as a foundation to improve provider decision making. Once implemented, the organization can, on an ongoing basis, introduce a series of decision support rules and guides. These rules can address medication safety issues, improve the appropriateness of test and procedure orders, and assure that data relevant to an order are displayed to the clinician.

These rules and guides can be implemented over the course of many years. No single rule may turn the tide in an organization's efforts to improve care. But in aggregate they can be leveraged to effect significant improvements. A view of EHRs as foundations means that implementation never ends.

Factors

If we are to be successful in our efforts to apply electronic health records to effect material gains in care delivery, we must create and evolve many interdependent factors.

Incentives must exist that provide compelling motivation for providers and provider organizations to acquire, implement, and manage the necessary information technology. These incentives can be diverse; financial rewards, avoidance of penalties, competitive position, professional recognition, and leverage of mission. These incentives must also focus on improvements in care rather than simply "adoption" of the technology.

Information technology tools, such as the EHR, must be available for all segments of health care, ranging from a large academic medical center to a solo practitioner. These tools must have a robust set of features and functions, accommodate differences in workflow, able to deliver knowledge to the provider, and exhibit high degrees of reliability and security. The tools need to be flexible, able to accommodate changes in practice. And these tools must have the ability to capture, share, and analyze data to support efforts to manage populations of patients.

Support resources must be available to assist the provider in acquiring, installing, and managing the needed information technology. There must be resources that can guide efforts to redesign care processes and support the use of information technology to facilitate ongoing care improvement initiatives.

An *exchange infrastructure* must be developed that enables the sharing of patient information across providers. This sharing is a predicate to any effort to coordinate the care of patient with a chronic disease or manage the care of a trauma patient as she moves through a continuum of providers. This infrastructure is a composite of transaction standards, technical infrastructure, privacy and security policies, and standards and data sharing, and it uses agreements between and across providers.

The development of *evidence and best practices* must continue to be undertaken. We will have to ensure that our providers are able to access knowledge that reflects the best evidence of care practices. The systems should, based on this evidence, provide reminders, alerts, and suggestions at appropriate points in the workflow and in the context of decisions that should be made. In addition, the experiences of many organizations and professions have taught us about how best to ensure that the systems we implement help lead to the desired outcomes in care delivery and operational performance.

A *committed and educated workforce of professionals* must be trained in how to best leverage the potential of information technology. The types of training will be diverse, ranging from using the technology to deliver care to managing information technology projects to performing systems analysis to advancing the field of informatics.

We must develop and evolve all of these factors. And since these factors are interdependent, we must define and manage that interdependence.

Collaboration

Patient care is a collaborative undertaking. This collaboration involves the patient, a wide range of healthcare professionals, government, purchasers of care, researchers, and organizations that provide products and services to the care team.

It is incumbent upon each profession and stakeholder to develop the factors in a way that serves their profession and constituency. It is incumbent that each profession develops the factors in a way that is responsive to and supports the needs of other stakeholders. It is also incumbent that each profession shares its plans, progress, and learnings with others that are pursuing similar goals; while there are differences across professions and stakeholders, the commonalties are substantial.

Collaboration is most effective when the individual components are strong and when the collective is strong.

Context

If we are to leverage information technology, it is critical that we understand the nature of the electronic health record as a tool, address multiple interdependent factors, and engage in multidisciplinary collaboration. However, our most important consideration is that we treasure and enrich the context of care.

Patient care is a very human undertaking. Patients are not abstractions; they are parents, spouses, brothers, sisters, and friends. They could be, at times they are, someone we love. And they are scared, in pain and, at times, dying. They require caring in the sense of delivering skilled nursing and medical care. They require caring in the sense that human beings reach out to other human beings who need help.

This context must always govern the delivery of treatments and therapies. This context is the reason that most of us have committed our professional lives to this field. This context is fundamental.

Our efforts to apply the technology should seek to reduce patient care errors and costs and improve quality. And our efforts must strengthen the ability of those who are practitioners to deliver human care.

It is an honor to acknowledge the authors whose superb contributions make up this book, the 4th edition of *Nursing Informatics: Where Technology and Caring Meet*. Their work covers key issues such as workforce development, interoperability, usability, and evidence-based decision support. It stresses the need for collaboration within and across disciplines and illuminates the contexts within which change must occur. Their analysis and insights provide the framework that is needed to maximize the use of information technology tools in order to improve patient safety and the quality of care.

It is also an honor to salute those who have committed to advancing our ability to apply information technology to improve care delivery.

And most of all, it is an honor to pay tribute to those who deliver care.

John P. Glaser
chief executive officer
Siemens Health Services Business Unit
Boston, MA

Series Preface

This series is directed to healthcare professionals leading the transformation of health care by using information and knowledge. For over 20 years, Health Informatics has offered a broad range of titles: some address specific professions such as nursing, medicine, and health administration; others cover special areas of practice such as trauma and radiology; still other books in the series focus on interdisciplinary issues, such as the computer-based patient record, electronic health records, and networked health care systems. Editors and authors, eminent experts in their fields, offer their accounts of innovations in health informatics. Increasingly, these accounts go beyond hardware and software to address the role of information in influencing the transformation of healthcare delivery systems around the world. The series also increasingly focuses on the users of the information and systems: the organizational, behavioral, and societal changes that accompany the diffusion of information technology in health services environments.

Developments in health care delivery are constant; in recent years, bioinformatics has emerged as a new field in health informatics to support emerging and ongoing developments in molecular biology. At the same time, further evolution of the field of health informatics is reflected in the introduction of concepts at the macro or health systems delivery level with major national initiatives related to electronic health records (EHR), data standards, and public health informatics.

These changes will continue to shape health services in the twenty-first century. By making full and creative use of the technology to tame data and to transform information, Health Informatics will foster the development and use of new knowledge in health care.

Marion J. Ball
Kathryn J. Hannah

Preface

Around the globe, the challenges facing health care are daunting, and the United States is not exempt from the pressures posed by demographic and economic trends. Obesity and diabetes are reaching epidemic proportions across the US, and our aging population has growing need of medical services. These services are in turn increasing in cost and complexity, as new treatments become available and new delivery approaches are introduced.

The problems are particularly acute in the United States. Despite paying more for health care than any other country in the world, the U.S. ranks below 41 other countries in life expectancy – down from 11th place two decades earlier. The question is why? As a recent report queried, "With growth in health care costs continually exceeding GDP [editors: Gross Domestic Product] growth, it begs the question: are we receiving commensurate value for the money that is spent?".[1]

Whatever the reasons for high costs and poor outcomes may be, the message is clear. As the Institute of Medicine (IOM) advises in *Crossing the Quality Chasm*,[2] "The current care systems cannot do the job. Trying harder will not work. Changing systems will." What we need is a new system that is, as defined by the IOM, "safe, effective, patient-centered, timely, efficient, and equitable." According to Angela McBride, who spent a year as an IOM Scholar while the Institute was pursuing its quality agenda, information technology is more than an "enabler" for nurses: it is a critical component to efforts to transform nursing practice and education. "There is no aspect of our profession that will be untouched by the informatics revolution in progress."[3]

As the health care industry joins with policy makers in creating a new system, what will this mean for nurses? In the past, healthcare analysts and activists alike often overlooked the role of nurses in delivering care and the need to involve them in transforming the health care system. Nurses were not given high visibility at the 2004 summit held in Washington, DC, to launch the 10-year drive toward electronic health records. Unlike the terms "physicians" and "doctors," the terms "nurses" or "nursing" did not even appear in the indexes for two recent mainstream critiques, *Redefining Health Care*[4] or *Who Killed Health Care?*[5] Discussions of information technology adoption have tended to focus on doctors, "physician resistance," and "physician buy-in" rather than on nurses who comprise more than half of the healthcare workforce. Yet, for decades, it has been nurses who have been held responsible for making computerized hospital information systems work – systems they rarely were given a voice in selecting. When systems are installed, "the workflow process often pays too much attention to physicians, who order medicine from the system and not enough on nurses, whose workflow can be more drastically changed by the system."[6]

In July 2004, David Brailer convened the first national health information technology summit, to launch the national initiative to transform health care by giving every American an electronic health record by 2014. Nurse leaders were there, eager to join in. Yet nurses were not on the speakers' platform, and the role of nursing in achieving this bold vision was given short shrift. Following the summit, a small band of nursing leaders and advocates (many of whom are editors and chapter authors in this new edition of *Nursing Informatics*) met and determined that the situation as it was could not stand. Their determination gave birth to the initiative known as Technology Informatics Guiding Education Reform (TIGER), which is one of the most significant responses to this critical need for change in the nursing profession.

Since TIGER held its first invitational conference in 2006, it has proven to be a TIGER indeed. The results of their work, work they all know is critical and still ongoing, are in the pages of this book. More than 70 organizations participated in the TIGER Summit, and each agreed that nursing must integrate informatics technology into education and practice. Each has pledged to incorporate the TIGER vision and action steps into their organization's strategic plans. Each fulfilled a critical role by distributing the TIGER Summit Summary Report within their network to engage additional support for this agenda. A list of the participating organizations is available on the TIGER website at www.tigersummit.com/participants.

After the initial summit, members of this important initiative moved into TIGER Phase II. Nurses across the nation and from differing aspects of the profession joined in the work of nine collaboratives to develop recommendations for change in nine critical areas:

- Education and faculty development
- Staff development
- Informatics competencies
- Standards and interoperability
- Usability and clinical application design
- Leadership development
- National Health Information Technology Agenda
- Virtual demonstration center
- Consumer and personal health record

Chapters authored by leaders of these collaboratives reflect the work of the groups they chaired, as does the TIGER Executive Summary included in the back of the book as Appendix A. Other chapters provide content needed to provide a comprehensive view of where nursing informatics is today and where it needs to go in the future. Continuing a theme that ran throughout TIGER from its beginning, chapters address issues related to change, through emerging technologies and innovative approaches to practice and policy.

Each section introduction provides an overview of core concepts, summarizes the chapters in that section, and cross-references related chapters in other sections to guide readers with focused interests.

Sections and Chapters

This book is divided into five sections. Section 1 sets the stage for the book in three chapters. The first chapter provides the context that makes a new emphasis related to nursing informatics critical at this time in significant change in health and in health informatics. An important chapter on culture change also frames much of the chapters for the rest of the book and provides four approaches to cultural change. In addition to highlighting the context, history, process, and contributions of the collaborative efforts of TIGER Phase II, the investment of intellectual and social capital is addressed in the third chapter in this section.

The next section addresses important issues related to nursing informatics such as workforce imperatives (including education, competencies, staff development, and leadership). Also, in Section 2 related to workforce issues, an updated chapter on academic programming from the 3rd edition is included and an exemplar of collaboration between academe and industry that enhances learning of future nurses is also included. Anchoring Section 3 is a comprehensive picture of the national health information technology structure and a timely synopsis of the funding options for Health IT in The American Recovery and Reinvestment Act of 2009 (ARRA). In addition, critical infrastructure issues related to standards, interoperability, usability, clinical design, and evidence-based clinical decision support are highlighted in this section.

The fourth section provides a wide range of perspectives on the future. This section has a compilation of chapters that are seemingly unrelated, but provide a context for where health care, informatics, interdisciplinary practice, and organizational development are headed in the future. The first chapter in Section 4 is focused on the Personal Health Record (PHR) and consumer health. Innovation is the key word describing the next three chapters that discuss future technology and informatics contributions to nursing and health. These chapters include: a new perspective on point-of-care innovation; voice-assisted technology which holds promise for extending professional practice in context of nursing workforce shortages; and description of a futuristic virtual learning environment which will help bridge the digital divide between and among interdisciplinary groups, as well as minority and rural care providers. By design, in this spirit several of the chapters in this section are authored or coauthored by interdisciplinary colleagues and bring a broadened and fresh perspective regarding the future of health IT and nursing informatics. The last chapter in Section 4 provides a valuable perspective on comparative effectiveness research (CER) and personalized medicine. These are two of the latest initiatives (as this edition is published) that will be critical to any discussion of the future of health informatics and technology. Discussions and results of CER are already impacting health care decisions in many international health systems.

The final section of this edition is intended to inform readers about the status of nursing informatics on an international level. While all countries could not be highlighted in Section 5, key areas of the globe are addressed. The first chapter in this section primarily builds on the original chapter written about Canada in the 3rd edition and expands the discussion of how to move nursing's contributions from invisibility to visibility in health informatics systems globally. The second chapter in Section 5 provides a comprehensive view of health IT and nursing informatics (Health Telematics) in Europe. This section concludes with authors from Brazil and Asia who present a picture of the process and steps of moving the nursing and health informatics agenda forward within their respective countries.

The chapters for this book have been purposefully selected to paint a picture of both the efforts and outcomes of the TIGER initiative in phase II. In addition, the editors have attempted to offer a comprehensive perspective of nursing informatics as it is evolving in the United States and countries around the globe. There has also been a determined plan of selecting authors focusing on different dimensions within the nursing profession including educators, nursing leadership in a variety of settings, nurses in the policy arena, and non-nurses who have provided leadership historically in the field of nursing informatics. Additionally, we sought to include chapters from members of the interdisciplinary community, and by authors representing industry and health informatics organizations. Through this planned diversity, the editors believe and hope that the breadth of ideas and content will provide an appreciation of the complexities and different perspectives of nursing and health informatics in a time of major change in health care locally and globally.

Baltimore, MD   Marion J. Ball
Reisterstown, MD   Judith V. Douglas
Bethesda, MD   Patricia Hinton Walker

References

1. McKinsey Global Institute. Accounting for the cost of US health care: a new look at why Americans spend more. www.mckinsey.com/mgi; 2008.
2. Institute of Medicine. *Crossing the Quality Chasm: A New Health System for the 21st Century*. Washington, DC: National Academy Press; 2001.
3. McBride AB. Nursing and the informatics revolution. *Nurs Outlook*. 2005;53(4):183-191.
4. Porter ME, Teisberg EO. *Redefining Health Care*. Boston: Harvard Business School Press; 2006.
5. Herzlinger R. *Who Killed Health Care?* New York: McGraw Hill; 2007.
6. Baker ML. Duke Health uses IT to get beyond doctor's handwriting. CIO Insight. www.cioinsight.com; 2005.
7. Needleman J, Buerhaus PI, Stewart M, Zelevinsky K, Mattke S. Nurse staffing in hospitals: is there a business case for quality? *Health Aff (Millwood)*. 2006;25(1):204-211.

Acknowledgments

This book owes its soul to the work done by all of those who served the TIGER Initiative:

Patricia Abbott, Mervat Abdelhak, Stefanie Abernethy, Connie Adams, Fredrecker Adams, John Adcock, Ekta Agrawal, Joan Aiello, Deborah Aiton, Toni Akers, Ellen Albanese, Mirela Albertsen, Anna Alderuccio, Kelly Aldrich, Deborah Aldridge, Dana Alexander, Greg Alexander, Maryann Alexander, Samar Ali, Connie Allen, Peg Allen, Sue Allen, Sally Allred, Rose Almonte, Eileen Amruso, Hank Amundsen, Christel Anderson, Jackie Anderson, Jane Anderson, Mark Anderson, Thomas Andrews, Ida Androwich, Carlene Anteau, Deanna Anvoots, Margaret S. Argentine, Richard Aries, Diane Armon, Amber Arthur, Jeffrey Ashley, Cathy Aulgur, Robin Austin, Tami Austin, Carolyn Averill, Janis Aziz, Debra Backus, Lynn Bader, Sharlene Bagga, Donna Bailey, Mark A. Bailey, Dale Baker, Denise Baker, Janet Baker, Kathy Baker, L. Baker, Laurie Baker, Rema Balagangadharan, Marion Ball, Denise Banks, Janet Banks, Emily Barey, Michelle Bargren, Kim Barker, Nicole Barker, Janey Barnes, Karen Baron, Martha Barr, Patty Barrier, A. Barry, Melissa Foster Barthold, Robin Bartlett, Estelle Bartley, Ann Barton, Julia Barton, Beverly Barton-Pichardo, Nan Batten, Thomas Beach, Nancy Beale, Beth Beam, Donna Beaman, Margaret Beaubien, Patricia Becker, Dianne Bedecarre, Sharon Bee, Michele Behme, Anne Belcher, Beverly Bell, Magdalene Belury, Karla Benden, Marge Benham-Hutchins, Mary Benotti, Mari S. Berge, Amy Berk, Daria Berman, Susan Berry, Sue Berryhill, Debbie Betts, Carol Bickford, Sandi Bieganski, Sam Bierstock, Elizabeth Bigby-Artle, Mona Bingham, Nancy Blake, Kevin Blaney, Nora Blankenship, Elaine Blechman, Julie Bliss, Tamara Blow, Sandra Bodin, Susan Boedefeld, Barbara Boelter, Wendy Bohling, Charles Boicey, Linda Boles, Diane Bolton, Christine Boltz, Karen Boncha, Lisa Book, Roger Booth, Diane Bordas, Rose Bossman, Patricia Boston, Maria Botker, L. Bove, Marilyn Bowcutt, Ken Bowman, Marilyn Bowman-Hayes, Kelly Boyd, Deborah Braccia, Alicia Morton, Victoria Bradley, Ryan Bramhall, Susan Braverman, Judith E. Breitenbach, Patricia Brennan, Patti Brennan, Jo-Anne Brenner, Phyllis Brenner, Patricia Bresser, Olivia Breton, Karen Brewster, Jeneane Brian, Jessica Brier, Teresa Britt, Juliana J. Brixey, Jane Brokel, Kelly Brooks-Staub, Lisa Brophy, Eve Broughton, Jennifer A. Browne, Tammie Burroughs Browne, Christine Bruzek-Kohler, Susan Bullington, Patricia Burke, Jill Burrington-Brown, Melanie Burton, Kristin Butner, Christena Buttress, Terri Calderone, Pat Callard, Steve Calme, Rob Campbell, Barry Cannon, Kristi Canther, Jan Capps, Judy Carlson, Robyn Carr, Hyacinth Carreon, Diane Carroll, Karen Carroll, Winifred Carson-Smith, Christina Carter, Nancy Cartledge, Cate

Casey Lane, Margaret Cashen, Celeste Castle, Jim Cato, Kimberly Cavaliero, Jerry Chamberlain, Elissa Chandler, Suzanne Chandler, Polun Chang, Stella Charbakshi, Robin Chard, Pamela Charney, Kathleen Charters, Joseph Charuhas, Susan Chasson, Carol Chau, Barbara Cheh, Linda Chism, Patricia Cholewka, Lynn Choromanski, Marilyn Chow, Melissa Christensen, Sharon Christensen, Judith Church, Pam Cipriano, Maureen Clancy, Carla Clark, Hardy T. Clark, Placidia Clark, Rebecca Clark, Rita Clark, Tiffani Clark, Lori Clifton, Beth Clouse, Manuel C. Co Jr., Ed Coakley, Janet Fischer Cochran, Shannon Coghlan, Celia Cohen, Regina Cole, Adrienne Cole-Williams, Petrelia Ann Coleman, Elizabeth Colgan, Arne Collen, Marie Collins, Eli Collins-Brown, Karen Colorafi, Susan Conaty-Buck, Vickey Conley, Phyllis M. Connolly, Helen Connors, Colleen Conway-Welch, Deborah Cook-Altonji, Christine Cooper, Christina Coppola, Denny Cordy, Milton Corn, John Cornele, Fran Cornelius, Lucy Corral, Pamela Correll, Andrea Cotter, Joyce Cotton, Barbara G. Covington, Richard Cowan, Maggie Cox, Carole Crabtree, June Craig, Kathie Crane, Cindy Craven, Debora Cremin, Jessie S. Cristobal, Nicholas Croce, Phillip Crouch, Joan Culley, Chris Curran, Mary Ann Curtin, Lynn Czaplewski, Prudence Dalrymple, Robert Dalton, Nan Dame, Martha Dameron, Womack M.S. Dana, Nina Darisse, Theresa DaSilva, Zaldy David, Allison Davidoff, Janice Unruh Davidson, Denise Davis, Rhonda Davis, Kim Day, Jennie DeGagne, Carol DeBiase, Cathleen Deckers, Marguerite Degenhardt, Leslie Dela Cuz-Torio, Connie Delaney, Cheryl Dennison, Debra Derickson, Francis Desjardins, Nancy Dickenson Hazard, Linus Diedling, Linda Dietrich, Shelley DiGiacomo, Celeste DiMascolo, Sandra Dinwiddie, Emilie Dioneda, Joan DiOrio, Brian Dixon, Claire Dixon-Lee, Deborah Dodson, Penny Dodson, Rebecca Dodson, Peggy Doheny, Marsha Dolan, Mary Dominguez, Paul Donaldson, Donna M. Nickitas, Rebecca Donohue, Patricia Donohue-Porter, Douglas Dotan, Judy Douglas, Marina Douglas, Phyllis Doulaveris, Jack Dowie, Mary Doyle, Kim Draper, Kaeli Dressler, Jacqueline Drexler, Karen DuBois, Katherine DuBois, Debbie Duck, Melanie Duffy, Donna DuLong, Rebecca Duncan, Nancy Duphily, Stacie Durkin, Patricia Dykes, Patricia Ebright, Laurie Ecoff, Gail Edwards, Judith Effken, Margareta Ehnfors, Shirley Eichenwald Maki, Victoria Elfrink, Beth Elias, Stacey Eller, Jenny Elrod, Deborah Ely, Lisa Emrich, Elizabeth Enriquez, Sandra Eppers, Scott Erdley, Peggy Esch, Sharon Eshelman, Alberto Espinas, Rosario P. Estrada, Jo Evans, Danita L. Ewing, Nancy Fahey, Sharie L. Falan, Wang Fang, Ana Fano, Cathy Fant, Holly Farish-Hunt, Sarah Farrell, Gail Faso, Sally Fauchald, Veronica Feeg, Linda Feider, Kelly Feist, Eva Feldman, Iris Fernandez, Lisa Fetter, Trudy Finch, Julie Fine, Anita Finkelman, Melissa Finnegan, Angela Fiorentino, Cyndi Fischer, Sue Fischer, Regina Fish, Cheryl Fisher, Mark J. Fisher, Marion Fleck, Nancy Fleck, Sandy Fledderjohann, Lindsay Flowers, Patricia Fonder, Helen Fong, Valerie Fong, Mary Forman, Blanton Fortson, Susan Fossum, Joanne Foster, Melissa Foster Barthold, Bonnie Foulois, Bonnie Francis, Jean Francis, Deb Francisco, Joleen A. Frank, Beth Franklin, Terry Frederiksen, Sandra French, Colleen Frey, Barbara Friederichs, Phyllis Friend, Barbara B. Frink, Luis Fuertes, Patricia Fukuda, Susan Fulginiti, Theresa Fulginiti, Danniele J. Fullard, Sandy Fuller, Margaret Gadaire, Arceli Gagajena, Ann Gallagher, Mary Gallagher-Gordon, Colleen Gallogly, Michael Galloway, Christine Gamlen, Dianna Garcia-Smith, Julie Gardiner, Mary Garnica, Colette Garton, Carole A. Gassert, Travis Gates, Barbara Gawron, Michael Gay, Lynn Geren, Heather Gibson, Michelle Giles, Kandis Gillis, Bernadette Girello, Janet Given, Donna Gloe, Scarlet Glovasky, Cathleen

Glynn, Lisa B. Goben, Karen Goff, Barry Gogin, Francine Goitz, Laura Gokey, Denise Goldsmith, Diana Golzales, Laura Gonzalez, Valerie Gooder, Mary Goolsby, Janelle Goon, Candace Goulette, Randy Granata, Michelle Grate, Marilyn Graves, Pam Graves, Patty Graves, Catherine Gray, Jan Gray, Mary Gray, P. Allen Gray, Karen Graybeal, Laura Green, Karen Greenwood, Patricia Greim, Christine Greiner, Kathleen Gremel, Joyce Griffin-Sobel, Kathleen Griffis, Karen Grigsby, Charlyn Grosskopf, Anita Ground, Linda Grout, Margaret Groves, Kelly Grube, John Guare, Brian Gugerty, Lisa Gulker, Karl Gumpper, Brenda Hage, Cheryl Hager, Linda Hainlen, Karen Hajarian, Cynthia Hake, Marilyn Hall, Beth Halley, Sandy Halliburton, Cathy Halloran, Kelly Hammons, Angel Hampton, Ticia Handel, Jennifer Hanley, Sonya Hardin, Constance Hardy, Lee Harford, Lou Ann Hartley, Margaret Hassett, Susan Hassmiller, Janet Havey, Rtia Haxton, Sharon Healy, Linda Hebert, Michael Hedderman, Jane Hedrick, Laura Heermann, Diane K. Heine, Helen Heiskell, Linda Helfrick, Linda Hellie, Maria Hendrickson, Lori Hendrickx, Barbara Hennessy, Sherry Hendricks, T. Heather Herdman, Penni Hernandez, Elizabeth Herrman, Tonia Hewitt, Billie Hicks, Pamela Hietbrink, Helen Ann higgins, Jody Hignite, Sylvia Suszka Hildebrandt, Carole Hill, Martha N. Hill, Sharon Hill, Helena Hizon, Nancy Hoffart, Karen Hofmann, Tom Hogue, Victoria Holl, Cheryl Holly, Ivy Holt, Scott Holter, Katherine A. Holzmacher, Tracey Holzwarth, Laura Hood, Mary Hook, Elaine Hooper, Wanda Hooper, Malcolm Hopkins, Cariann Horstead, Valerie Howard, Melita Howell, Connie Huber, Christine A. Hudak, Margaret Hudock, Krysia Hudson, Cathy Huff, Janet Huff, Bonnie Hughes, Kathy Hughes, Janine Hulke, Susan Hull, Diane Humbrecht, Betsy Humphreys, Paula Humphreys, Reginald Humphries, Ellie Hunt, Karen Hunter, Kathleen M. Hunter, Claire Huntington, Carolyn Hutcherson, Anne Hutton, Brenda Illa, Susan Ilnicki, Dolly Ireland, Cathy Ivory, Eula Jackson, Ellen Jacobs, Susan K. Jacobs, Kim James, Lesley Janisse, Berit Jasion, Elvina Jeffers, Melinda Jenkins, Suzanne Jenkins, Helen Jepson, Bonnie Jerome D'Emilia, Sylvie Jette, Barbara Johns, Constance Johnson, Diane Johnson, Dionne Johnson, Ellen Johnson, Etta Johnson, Kellie Johnson, Kurt Johnson, Liz Johnson, Lynelle Johnson, Mark Johnson, Ruthann Johnson, Dorthy Jones, Josette F Jones, Kristenia Jones, Pat Jones, Sheri Jones, Lorene Jones-Rucker, Maryalice Jordan-Marsh, Jolly Jose, Lynda Joseph, Leland Jurgensmeier, Sheryl Juve, Linda Juzbasich, Lorraine Kaack, Mette Kjer Kaltoft, Marg Kampers, Pallavi Kantharia, Eva Karp, Sara Katsh, Gaye Kazmirski, Gail Keenan, Elise Kelcourse, Evelyn Kelleher, Valerie Kelley, Wanda Kelley, Myrtle Kelly, Loya Kelso, Mary Kennedy, Rosemary Kennedy, Julie Kenney, Chad Kent, Karlene Kerfoot, Nicole Kerkenbush, Sandra Kersten, Linda Ketchersid, Joan M. Kiel, Charles Killingsworth, Hongsoo Kim, Kathleen Kimmel, Mary Kimmel-Alexander, Christy Kindler, Stefanie Kingsley, Mary Kinneman, Dianna Kiraly, Jan Kirsch, Rebecca Kitzmiller, Cathy Kleiner, Barbara Klepfer, Julie Kliewer, Kay Kline, Margie Knappenberger, Karen Knoll, Linda Koharchik, Laura Kolkman, Irek Konefal, May Konfong, Susan Kossman, Allison Kozeliski, Margaret Kraft, Nancy Kranawetter, Jill Krcatovich, Mary Jane Krebs Turnbull, Dina A. Krenzischek, Kathie Krichbaum, Andrea Krzysko, Cindy Kugel, Mary Kujawa, Brenda Kulhanek, Sharon Kumm, Kyle Kurbis, Dina Kynard, Norma Lang, Caterina Lasome, Gail Latimer, Angela Lavanderos, Joann LaVenia, Marty LaVenture, Deb Lawrence, Karen Lawrence, Dawne Lazarek, Cyndi Leed, Chris Lehmann, Ann Leja, Kathy Lesh, Angela Lewis, Sharon Lewis, Carol Lightner, Beth Lindholm, Patricia Lindley, Karen Lipshires, Joan Lloyd-Collins, Tracy

Locke, Ann Lockhart, Sue Longacre, Maria Loomis, Margaret Louis, Gary Loving, June Lowe, Corrine Loyd, Lisa Lucas, Christine Lui, Cyndie Lundberg, Margaret Lunney, Dan Lutkenhouse, Craig Luzinski, Debra Lynch, Rebekah Lynch, Kay Lytle, Mary Mackenburg-Mohn, Linda Macomber, Lory J. Maddox, Rosalie Mainous, Sharon Majarowitz, Ellen Makar, Shirley Eichenwald Maki, Stacey Maloney, Myrna Mamaril, Diane Mancino, Peggy Mancuso, Andrea Mann, Pamela Manselle, Charlene Marietti, Abdel latif Marini, Susan Marino, Vickie Marise, Rex Markel, Anita Marshall, Susan Martens, Jasmine Martin, Jeanine Martin, Karen Martin, Lori Martin, Sherri Martin, Debi Martoccio, Nan Masterson, Darlene Mathis, Patricia Matthews, Heather May, Linda McCombe, Connie McAllister, Angela McBride, Kathy McCall, Kathleen McCarthy, Molly McCarthy, Patricia McCartney, Teresa McCasky, Harriet McClung, Margaret McClure, Marianne McConnell, Michael McCord, Kathleen A. McCormick, Cindy McCoy, Andy McDaniel, Teresa McDaniel, Jacqueline McDonald, Ann-Marie McDonough, Hawkeye McDougall, Sean McFarland, Regina McFerren, Jean McGill, Keri McGill, Michelle McGuire, Elizabeth McHugh, Shannon McIntire, Laura McIntosh, Debbie McKay, Nancy McKelvey, Erin McKenna, Shelli-Ann McKenzie, Jean McKoy, Sharon McLane, Wendy McLaughlin, Cheryl McLean, Barbara McLendon, Lois McMahon, Paula McNabb, Jane McNeive, Sandra McPherson, Hollie Shaner McRae, Jennifer McRaney, Ginny Meadows, Meg Meccariello, Deborah Medeiros, Eugenia Mena, Carol Mensch, John Meredith, Barbara Ann Messina, Peter Metcalfe, Terese Metzger, Brenda Meyer, Linda Meyer, Bonna Miller, Elaine Miller, Nancy Miller, Theresa A. Miller, Sharon Milligan, Mary Ann Millman, Andrew Mills, Mary Etta Mills, Cynthia Milo, Debbie Minor, Donna Mitchell, Shirley Mitchell, V.S. Mitchell, Nancy Moen, Judy Moffett, Nicole Mohiuddin, Patricia Montano, Carleen Moore, Oyweda Moorer, Margarita Morales, Rachelle Morales, Rob Morehouse, Kay Morgan, Lanette Morgan, Shirley Morgan, Vicki Morgan-Cramer, Liz Morris, Katherine Morrison, Beth Morrissette, Jacqueline Moss, Gretchen Moyer, Jan Moyers, Dale Mueller, Tina Mullard, Sharon Muller, Denise Mullins, Zona Mulvaney, Judy Murphy, Jane Mustain, Beth Ann Muthig, Roxane Myers, Eun-Shim Nahm, Ronald Napier, Walter Nasarek, Tina Nash, Steven E. Nasiatka, Diana Neal, Peggy Niedlinger, Betty Nelson, Pat Nelson, Ramona Nelson, Susan K Newbold, Ann Newman, Jacqueline Newton, Sergeant Nicholson, Donna M. Nickitas, Robert Nieves, Gunilla Nilsson, Kathleen Nokes, B.J. Noll, Anthony F. Norcio, Ruena Norman, Brian Norris, Dottie Norris, Michele Norton, Ogo Nwosu, Denise Bauer Nyberg, Liz Nye, Beth O'Connor, Nancy O'Connor, Tim O'Connor, Connie O'Daniel, David O'Dell, John O'Donnell, Ann O'Neill, Kate O'Toole, Sue Olenick, Nancy Olson, Randy Osteen, Judy Ozbolt, Jacqueline Pada, Carolyn Padovano, Tonya Pagel, M.D. Palladino, Karen K. Pancheri, Lynda Panerio, Hyeoun-Ae Park, Cheryl D. Parker, Joel Parker, Lynn Parsons, Rosemary Pascarella, Nancy Pasqualone, Rebecca Patton, Gary Paxson, Susan Payne, Karen Peddicord, Judith Pelletier, Darlene Perkins, Dave Perkins, Glenda Perry, Daniel Pesut, Judy Peters, Maureen Peters, Carol Petersen, Dorothy Phllips, Meihau Piao, Sandra M. Picard, Anne Marie Piehl, Carol Pierce, Louis Pilla, Nilsa Pineiro, Sayra Pingleton, Ronald Piscotty, Cheryl Pitman, Gail Pizarro, Joanne Pohl, Anna Poker, Lisa Polachek, Ellen Pollack, Gale Pollock, Lisa Porter, Keisha Potter, Jarethea Powell, Mollie Poynton, M. Christine Pratt, Diane Pravikoff, Melissa Precour, Ann Presley, Verline Price, Chuck Pritchard, Molly Procuniar, Mary Prosyniuk, Carla Provost, Maryann Prudhomme, Holly Pugh, Patricia Purfield,

Donita Qualey, Lisa Rabideau, Marcia Rachel, Robin S. Raiford, Daniel Ramos, Monifa Ramsay, Melissa Rank, Jan Rasmussen, Marcia Rau, Hollie Raycraft, Susan Raymond, Laurie Reagon, Matt Reavill, Linda Reeder, Susan Reese, Curtis Reeves, Kathleen Reeves, Roger Reeves, Stacey Reibsome, Patti Reid, Jim Reimer, Sally Remus, Rebecca Reynolds, Elizabeth Rhodes, Linda Ricca, Lygeia Ricciardi, Stephen Rice, Carolyn Richardson, Debora Richardson, Robin Richardson, Cathy Rick, Patrick J. Riley, Barbara Ripollone, Eileen Rissler, Sondra Rivera, Mary Anne Rizzolo, Debra Roach, Gail Robel, Nancy M. Robinson, Wanda Robinson, Wanda Rodriguez, Kathleen Rogers, Patti Rogers, Stephanie Rogers, Anne Rogerson, Stan Roller, Carol Romano, Claudia Ronayne, Luzviminda Ronquillo, Dona Rook, Beryl Rose, Susan Rosenberg, Doris Ross, Nancy L. Rothman, Jackie Rowland, Susan Runyan, Debbie Rupe, Gail Russell, Maureen Russell, Diana Ruzicka, Debra Ryan, Loretta Ryan, Virginia Saba, Kathleen Sabatier, Kay Sackett, Reonel 'Joon' Saddul, Karen Saewert, Johanna Salamandra, Kathleen Sanford, Jimmy Santiago, Kathleen Santos, Kathryn Sapnas, Teresa Sartain, Jeannette Sasmor, C. Anne Sass, Shirley Saunders, Denise Savell, Darla Saville, Terri Scharfe Pretino, Anne Scharnhorst, D. Schatzman, Shirley Schiavone, Ruth Schleyer, Vicky Schmidt, Mark Schneider, Joe Scholpp, Nancy Jean Schoo, Stephanie Schulte, Frances Shultz, Wendy Schultze, Cathy Schwartz, Pat Schwirian, Laura Seabury, Troy Seagondollar, Suzanne Sellards, Margaret Senn, Joyce Sensmeier, Tess Settergren, Jeanne Sewell, Paulette Seymour-Route, Patrick Shannon, Leighsa Sharoff, Patrick Sharpnack, Megan Shaw, Carol Sheldon, Thomas Shelton, Ann Shepard, Susan Sherman, Pamela Sherwill-Navarro, Nicole Shoemake, Barbara Showers, Florence Shrager, Sarah Shultz, Alice Shumate, Carol Siegler, Donna Silsbee, Sherri Simons, Beth Singleton, Harlow Sires, Nancy Sisson, Diane J. Skiba, Johanna Skuladottir, Andrea Smilski, Anne Smith, Deb Smith, Kathleen Smith, Linda J. Smith, Michael Smith, Pam Smith-Beatty, Ann Smith-Flango, Valerie Smothers, Paulette Snoby, Richad Snow, Susan Snyder, Lena Sorensen, Judie Spafford, Donna Speck, Fran Spivak, Cynthia Spradlin, Lance Spranger, Lee Stabler, Nancy Staggers, Julie Stanik-Hutt, Robert Stanley, Teresa Stanley, Janett Star, Carol Steiden, Amy Steinbinder, Stephanie Allard, Edward Stern, Gayle Stevens, Brian Stever, Stephanie Stewart, Linda J. Stierle, Sandy Stockey, Deborah Storlie, Melissa Stotts, Cindy Struk, Stanley Strzyzykowski, Tammy Stuart, Amy Stump, Mark Sugrue, Kevin Sullivan, I-Fong Sun, Sylvia Suszka, Darinda Sutton, Jill Sutton, Margaret Swanson, David Sweet, Linda Talley, Annelle Tanner, Sharron Tanner, Kathleen Tarleton, Laura Taylor, Olivia Taylor, Sheryl Taylor, Kathy Terman, Linda Thede, Lisa Thiemann, Annette Thies, Teri Thompson, Sue Thomson, Wendy Thomson, Jill Thurston, Mari Tietze, Jane Timm, Joann Tinio, Dante Tolentino, Beth A. Tomasek, Sergio Torres, Loree Towns, Portia Towns, Allison Tracey, Sandra Trakowski, Trish Trangenstein, Barbara Treusch, Michelle Troseth, Lois Tschetter, Sarah Tupper, Denise D. Tyler, Victoria Tyra, Judy Underwood, Leslie Underwood, Joy Upton, Avion Urbain, Nicholas Valadja, Mary Jinky Valdez, Barbara Van de Castle, Kimberly Van Duyse, Sharon Van Sell, Vickey Vance, Ruthann Vaughan, Teresa Vaughan, Susan Vaughn, Marcia Veenstra, Debby Velders, Cathie Velotta, Rujuta Vidal, Anne M. Vilhotti, Deb Vitins, Debra L. Waddell, Gina Wade, John Wade, Robert Wagner, Grafton Walker, John Walker, Mary Walker, Patricia Hinton Walker, Ruth Walker, Kathleen Walsh, Cathy Walter, Dru Anne Walz, Judith J. Warren, Janet Washo, Vashti Watson, Janis Watts, Barbara Weatherford, Angelique Weathersby, Charlotte Weaver, Lorene Wedeking, Kathleen

Welsh, George Welton, Ramona Wenger, Christine Werner, Bonnie Wesorick, Linda West, Bonnie Westra, Linda Weyenberg, Cynthia Wheelehan, Betty Wichman, Rita Wick, Karen Widneski, Pat Wierzbicki, Melinda Wiese, Dani Wiklund, Carol Wilhelm, Kirby Wilkerson, Kathleen Williams, Michelle Williams, Missi Willmarth, Danny M. Willoughby, Diana Willson, Bonnita Wilson, Kelly Wilson, Marisa L. Wilson, Shona Wilson, Angela Wiltse, Peggi Winter, Margo Winters, Mike Wisz, Juliana Withorn, Marty Witrak, Stan Woiczechowski, Julie Wolter, Shirley Woodhead, Sherri Woodward, Carrie Wright, Barbara Wroblewski, Dave Wyant, Christina Wyrwas, Susan Yamamoto, Amy Yates, Sharon Yearous, Johnny Yuen, M. Zalon, Mary Zasada, Deborah Zeller, Judith Zencka, Mary Zeringue, Rita Zielstorff, Kevin Zimmerman, Chris Zingo, Linda Ziolkowski.

Contents

Section I   Nursing Informatics: On the Move 1

1 Nursing Informatics: Transforming Nursing 5
Marion J. Ball, Judith V. Douglas, Patricia Hinton Walker,
and Donna DuLong

2 Strategies for Culture Change 13
Patricia Hinton Walker

3 TIGER Collaboratives and Diffusion 35
Diane J. Skiba and Donna DuLong

4 Networking Advancing Nursing Informatics 51
Susan K. Newbold

Section II   Workforce Imperatives 59

5 Education and Faculty Development 65
Diane J. Skiba and Mary Anne Rizzolo

6 Competencies: Nuts and Bolts 81
Connie Delaney and Brian Gugerty

7 Updated Academic Programs 93
Carole A. Gassert and Susan K. Newbold

8 Continuing Education and Staff Development 113
Joan M. Kiel and Elizabeth Johnson

9 Leadership Collaborative 133
Judy Murphy and Dana Alexander

10 Challenging Leadership Status Quo 155
Roy L. Simpson

11 Bridging Technology: Academe and Industry..................................... 167
Pamela R. Jeffries, Krysia Hudson, Laura A. Taylor,
and Steven A. Klapper

Section III   Infrastructure, Adoption, and Implementation 189

12 The Evolving National Informatics Landscape................................... 193
Carolyn Padovano and Alicia Morton

13 Standards and Interoperability 207
Joyce Sensmeier and Elizabeth Casey Halley

14 Usability and Clinical Application Design.. 219
Nancy Staggers and Michelle R. Troseth

15 Evidence-Based Clinical Decision Support.. 243
Diane Hanson

Section IV   Future Perspectives.. 259

16 Personal Health Record: Managing Personal Health 265
Charlotte Weaver and Rita Zielstorff

17 Disruptive Innovation: Point of Care... 291
John S. Silva, Nancy Seybold, and Marion J. Ball

18 Extending Care: Voice Technology.. 303
Debra M. Wolf, Amar Kapadia, and Pam Selker Rak

19 Nursing's Contribution: An External Viewpoint............................... 321
Mark Hagland

20 Transforming Care: Discovery Enabled by Health Information Technology........ 331
Barbara B. Frink and Asif Dhar

21 Local Global Access: Virtual Learning Environment 343
Beth L. Elias, Jacqueline A. Moss, Christel Anderson,
and Teresa McCasky

Section V   Global Initiatives.. 355

22 Invisibility to Visibility: Capturing Essential Nursing Information 359
Kathryn J. Hannah and Margaret Ann J. Kennedy

23 Health Telematics Europe 375
Ursula Hübner

24 Evolution: Nursing Informatics in Brazil 401
Heimar F. Marin, Denise T. Silveira, Grace Dal Sasso,
and Heloisa Helena C. Perez

25 Taiwan Model: Nursing Informatics Training 411
Polun Chang and Ming-Chuan Kuo

Appendix 429

Index 469

Contributors

Dana Alexander
GE Healthcare, Monument CO, USA

Christel Anderson
Clinical Informatics,
Healthcare Information and Management
Systems Society, Chicago IL, USA

Marion J. Ball
Healthcare and Life Sciences Institute,
IBM Research; Professor Emerita,
Johns Hopkins University School
of Nursing, Baltimore MD, USA

Polun Chang
Institute of BioMedical Informatics,
National Yang-Ming University,
Taipei, Taiwan, ROC

Connie White Delaney
University of Minnesota,
School of Nursing, Minneapolis MN,
USA

Arif Dhar
Deloitte Consulting and Deloitte
Center for Research Resources,
Bethesda MD, USA

Judith V. Douglas
Reisterstown Maryland 21136, USA

Donna DuLong
The Tiger Initiative, Denver CO, USA

Beth L. Elias
University of Alabama at Birmingham,
School of Nursing, Birmingham AL, USA

Barbara B. Frink
BB Frink and Associates LLC,
Bethesda MD, USA

Carole A. Gassert
College of Nursing,
University of Utah,
Salt Lake City UT, USA

John Glaser
Partners HealthCare, Boston MA, USA

Brian Gugerty
Gugerty Consulting LLC,
Arnold MD, USA

Mark Hagland
Chicago IL, USA

Elizabeth Casey Halley
MITRE Corporation,
McLean VA, USA

Kathryn J. Hannah
#11-2200 Varsity Estates Dr. N.W
Calgary Alberta, Canada T3B 4Z8

Diane Hanson
CPM Resource Center/Elsevier,
Hudsonville MI, USA

Patricia Hinton Walker
Uniformed Services University
of the Health Sciences,
Bethesda MD, USA

Ursula Hübner
Health Informatics and Quantitative
Methods, University of Applied Sciences,
Osnabrück, Germany

Krysia W. Hudson
Johns Hopkins University School
of Nursing, Baltimore MD, USA

Pamela R. Jeffries
Johns Hopkins University School
of Nursing, Baltimore MD, USA

Elizabeth O. Johnson
Applied Clinical Informatics,
Tenet Healthcare Corporation,
Dallas TX, USA

Amar Kapadia
Acute Care, Vocollect,
Pittsburgh PA, USA

Margaret Ann Kennedy
Standards, Canada Health Infoway,
Toronto ON, Canada

Joan M. Kiel
University HIPPA Compliance;
Health Management Systems,
Duquesne University,
Pittsburgh PA, USA

Steven A. Klapper
Johns Hopkins University School
of Nursing, Baltimore MD, USA

Ming-chuan Jessie Kuo
Cathay General Hospital,
Taipei, Taiwan, ROC

HeimardeFatima Marin
Federal University of São Paulo,
São Paulo SP, Brazil

Angela Barron McBride
Indiana University School of Nursing,
Lafayette IN, USA

Teresa McCasky
AORN - Association of peri-operative
Registered Nurses
2170 South Parker Road, Suite 300,
Denver CO USA

Alicia A. Morton
Department of Health and Human
Services, Bowie MD, USA

Jacqueline A. Moss
Clinical Simulation and Technology,
University of Alabama at Birmingham,
School of Nursing,
Birmingham AL, USA

Judy Murphy
Information Services, Aurora Health Care,
Milwaukee WI, USA

Susan K. Newbold
Vanderbilt University School of Nursing,
Franklin TN, USA

Carolyn Padovano
Health Information Technology,
Business & Technology Futures' Group
Research Computing Division,
Social, Statistical & Environmental Sciences,
Research Triangle Institute International,
701 13th Street N.W., Suite 750,
Washington DC, USA

Heloisa Helena Ciqueto Perez
Nursing School, University of São Paulo,
São Paulo, Brazil

Pam Selker Rak
CommuniTech, LLC,
Bridgeville PA, USA

Mary Anne Rizzolo
Professional Development, National
League for Nursing, New York NY, USA

Grace T.M. Dal Sasso
Federal University of Santa Catarina,
Florianópolis SC, Brazil

Joyce E. Sensmeier
Informatics, Healthcare Information
and Management Systems Society,
Chicago IL, USA

Nancy Seybold
Quartermark Consulting LLC,
Washington DC, USA

John S. Silva
Silva Consulting Services,
Eldersburg MD, USA

Denise Tolfo Silveira
Federal University of Rio Grande do Sul,
Porto Alegre RS, Brazil

Roy L. Simpson
Nursing, Cerner Corporation,
Kansas City MO, USA

Diane J. Skiba
University of Colorado Denver,
College of Nursing, Aurora CO, USA

Nancy Staggers
Informatics, College of Nursing,
University of Utah,
Salt Lake City UT, USA

Laura A. Taylor
Johns Hopkins University School
of Nursing, Baltimore MD, USA

Michelle R. Troseth
CPM Resource Center/Elsevier,
Grand Rapids MI, USA

Charlotte Weaver
Gentiva® Health Services,
Atlanta GA, USA

Debra M. Wolf
Department of Nursing,
Slippery Rock University,
Pittsburgh PA, USA

Rita D. Zielstorff
North Andover MA, USA

It is time to transform the nursing profession in the context of nursing informatics. The question is how? We cannot simply put a few computers on a few floors, or invite a few nurses to participate in decisions on information technology purchases. It is time to change the nursing profession and other health professions. Unfortunately, systems in place today all too often place onerous demands on the nurses and other clinicians who use them. In a sense, currently, the users serve the system because the technology is and has not been designed to serve the nurse or clinician. The burden of this servitude makes the caregiving process more time-consuming, and workloads increase for the nurse, the physician, and other point-of-care clinicians. At the end of the day, these systems do not improve the ability of the nurse to care for patients in a safer, faster, and more cost effective manner, as was the original intent of the "enabling" technologies. The decades-long reluctance of nurses and other clinicians to adopt health information technology (HIT) should come as no surprise. They want – and will embrace – HIT that provides them with information when, where, and how they need it (Ball et al. 2008).

In recent years, the California HealthCare Foundation (CHCF 2002) sponsored a report on the role of technology in addressing the nursing shortage, and the American Academy of Nursing (AAN 2003) published proceedings from its landmark conference on the use of technology to address staffing and safety concerns. In addition, the Robert Wood Johnson Foundation and the Institute of Health Care Improvement launched efforts to transform the practice environment for nurses and improve patient care (Ball et al. 2006).

We begin this fourth Edition of *Nursing Informatics*, newly subtitled *Where Technology and Caring Meet*, with four chapters that set the stage for the contributions the topics covered in following sections. At a time when informatics and technology are touted as much of the solution to the problems faced in health care today, these chapters provide the context and framework for the rest of the book.

Setting the Stage

In Chapter. 1, "Nursing Informatics: Transforming Nursing," Marion Ball, Judith Douglas, Patricia Hinton Walker, and Donna Dulong explain where and why the nursing profession must move forward in the area of technology and informatics, noting the Institute of Medicine's focus on patient safety. They examine the critical need for purposeful change in the nursing profession, identifying factors such as outcomes and cost that contribute to that need. With the nursing shortage expected to worsen significantly by 2020 (Robert Wood Johnson Foundation 2006), nursing informatics must take a leading role in energizing the profession of nursing and delivering high-quality care. The chapter explores the potential impact of health reform on nursing informatics, citing the American Recovery and Reinvestment Act of 2009 (ARRA) and the unprecedented $19 billion it provides for HIT (Blumenthal 2009). The goals of healthcare reform – improved quality, efficiency, and outcomes – all involve nurses, the nursing profession, and nursing informatics. And they all resonate with the vision set forth by the Technology Informatics Guiding Education Reform (TIGER) initiative and its nine collaboratives reported in detail elsewhere in this fourth edition of *Nursing Informatics*.

Charting the Course for Change

In order for the nursing profession and for other healthcare provider groups to embrace and meaningfully use the informatics and emerging technologies at the core of health reform, change in culture of health care and the U.S. health care delivery system is critical. In Chapter. 2, "Strategies for Culture Change," Patricia Hinton Walker provides a comprehensive view of the need for culture change and how it can be approached. Instead of recommending one approach, she describes five distinct perspectives. The first she discusses is the Technology Informatics Guiding Education Reform (TIGER) and its contributions related to the use of technology and informatics; this sets the stage for the description in Chapter. 3 of Roger's diffusion theory as demonstrated by the TIGER activities. The second perspective is education, both formal and continuing, with a special emphasis on education specific to nursing/health informatics. In setting forth the third perspective, Hinton Walker highlights organizational change models and the role of leadership, identifies the barriers to culture change, and presents three characteristics that support change via the socio-technical approach described as High Velocity Organizations (Spear 2009). The fourth perspective is that offered by research-based theoretical models, such as the Social Cognitive Theory (Bandera 1986), the Theory of Reasoned Action, the Theory of Planned Behavior, and the Technology Acceptance Model (TAM). Based on engineering science, TAM is particularly relevant to enhancing culture change related to the use of technology and is the basis for much of the literature on usability and clinical design cited in Chapter. 14. According to the literature, these models are good predictors of acceptance of technology (Ajzen 1991; Godin and Kok 1996). The fifth perspective involves innovation as social disruption (Hagel et al. 2008), and examines the impact of emerging technologies on health care and the nursing profession, citing examples (Brennan et al. 2007; Didnan 2008).

Chapter 2 also touches upon the potential of comparative-effectiveness research and personalized medicine – both receiving new attention under health reform – to totally 'disrupt' health care. Finally, it looks at the potential use of social media in health care, as suggested by the blog titled "Why Doctors and Nurses Should Use Social Media 21 September (2009). The chapter closes with a provocative perspective on the roles historic nursing leaders would play in culture change today.

Building and Using Social and Intellectual Capital

In Chapter. 3, "TIGER Collaboratives and Diffusion," Diane Skiba and Donna Dulong offer a brief history of the TIGER movement and the TIGER summit as background for their analysis of TIGER Phase II and its nine collaboratives. They describe how Phase II created and used intellectual capital, bringing together the collective knowledge of organizations to multiply the assets and outputs of the TIGER initiative (Nahapiet and Ghoshal 1998). In discussing the value of social capital, they describe how social networks and interaction can bring about cultural, economic, and political change (Cohen and Prusak 2001; Wenger 1999). To document the impact TIGER, a grassroots initiative, had on professional nursing organizations, Skiba and Dulong cite instances where informatics content was developed and/or integrated into their programs, presentations, and missions. They highlight the accomplishments of all nine TIGER collaboratives that are the topic of chapters elsewhere in this book, and conclude with a summary of lessons learned from the TIGER initiative and its success in enhancing both intellectual and social capital.

Networking for Advancement

In Chapter. 4, "Networking Advancing Informatics," Susan K. Newbold provides both a history and examples of how personal, organizational, electronic, and literature resources contribute to the evolution of nursing informatics (Newbold 2009). She lists helpful, up-to-date information, including the names and internet addresses of more than 20 professional organizations, electronic resources, and literature. In addition, she explains how the mentor program offered by the American Medical Informatics Association (AMIA) has enhanced personal resources in the informatics community over time. The chapter as a whole stands as guide to nursing informatics for students and faculty and for nursing informatics specialists, leaders, and practitioners.

References

American Academy of Nursing (2003) Conference proceedings: using innovative technology to decrease the nursing demand and enhance patient care delivery. Nurs Outlook 51(3):S1–S32

Ball MJ, Merryman T, Lehman CU (2006) Patient safety: a tale of two institutions. J Healthc Inf Manage 20(4):26–34

Ball MJ, Silva JS, Bierstock S et al (2008) Failure to provide clinicians useful IT systems: opportunities to leapfrog current technologies. Methods Inf Med 47(1):4–7

California HealthCare Foundation (2002). The nursing shortage: can technology help. www.chcf

Robert Wood Johnson Foundation (2006) Wisdom at Work: The Importance of the Older and Experienced Nurse in the Workplace. www.rwjf.org/files/pulications/other/wisdomatwork.pdf

Blumenthal D (2009) Stimulating the adoption of health information technology. N Engl J Med 10(1056) http://healthcarereform.nejm.org/?p=436 Accessed on 9 September 2009

Spear S (2009) Chasing the rabbit: official blog on electronic medical records, evidence-based medicine, and high velocity organizations... http://chasingtherabbittbook.mhprofessional.com/apps/ab/209/01/09/electronicmedicalrecords Accessed 29 May 2009

Bandura A (1986) Social Foundations of Thought and Action: A Social Cognitive Theory. Prentice-Hall, Englewood Cliffs, NJ

Ajzen I (1991), The theory of planned behavior. Organizational Behavior and Human Decision Processes 50:179–211

Godin G, Kok G (1996) The theory of planned behavior: a review of its applications to health-related behaviors. Amer J Health Promotion 11:87–98

Hagel J, Brown JS, Davison L (2008) Shaping strategy in a world of constant disruption. Harvard Business Review. Oct. Reprint R0801E. www.hbr.org. Accessed 23 May 2009

Brennan PF, Downs S, Casper G, et al. (2007) Project HealthDesign: stimulating the next generation of personal health records. AMIA Annual Symposium Proceedings. http://www.pubmed-central.nih.gov/articlerender.fcgi?artid=2655909. Accessed 28 May 2009

Didnan, L. (2008) Verichip goes Consumer with its implantable RFID chips; would you buy? Posted @ 6:06 a.m. Between the Lines. April 22, 2008. http://blogs.zdnet.com/BTL?p=8567 Accessed 28 May 2009

VoCollect (2009) Healthcare Systems http://www.vocollectcom/index.php/about/vocollect-health-care-systems. Accessed 29 May 2009

"Why doctors and nurses should engage in social media." 21 September 2009 blog. http://www.kevinmd.com/blog/2009/09doctors-nurses-engage-social-media.html Accessed 25 September 2009

The TIGER Initiative (2007) Evidence and Information Transforming Nursing: 3-Year Action Steps toward a 10-Year Vision. http://www.tigersummit.com. Accessed 28 September 2009

Nahapiet J, Ghoshal S (1998) Social capital, intellectual capital, and the organizational advantage. Acad Manage Rev 23(2):212–266

Cohen D, Prusak L (2001) In Good Company: How Social Capital Makes Organizations Work. Harvard Business School Press, Boston, MA

Technology Informatics Guiding Education Reform. (2009). Collaborating to Integrate Evidence and Informatics into Nursing Practice and Education: An Executive Summary. http://www.tigersummit.com/. Accessed 29 September 2009

Wenger E (1999) Communities of Practice: Learning, Meaning, and Identity. Cambridge University Press, New York, NY

Newbold SK, Westra BL (2009) American Medical Informatics Nursing Informatics History Committee Update. CIN: Computers, Informatics, Nursing 27(4):263–265

Nursing Informatics: Transforming Nursing

Marion J. Ball, Judith V. Douglas, Patricia Hinton Walker, and Donna DuLong

1

Informatics is no longer an option for nurses and other health care providers. It is a requirement. "The nation is at a tipping point in applying enabling technologies to health care … the time has come for health care to leave the manual tools of the past in the past."[1]

When nurses and the nursing profession are discussed, one of the first words to come to mind is the word "caring," which may seem the antithesis of technology. As nursing informaticists, we believe otherwise and look to the current drive for health care reform as an opportunity "to affect aspects of care that nurses have valued throughout history: coordinating care across the continuum, attention to prevention of disease and health promotion, attention to the role of the family and community, and empowering the voices of the patients (now clients/consumers/customers) in their own care."[2]

In this time of rapid change and investment in health information technology (HIT), nurses must rise to the challenge of leadership and harness their "caring" passion to the use of technology and informatics, improving the quality and safety of the care they provide to patients, families, and communities.

Health Reform and HIT

As this book goes to print, health care reform remains coutroversial in the United States and changes in the health care delivery system have yet to be folly implemented. Despite the uncertainy about the outcome, one aspect is very clear. The American Recovery and Reinvestment Act of 2009 (ARRA) provides for one of the largest investments ever made in HIT, an unprecedented $19 billion program to promote its adoption and use. To achieve the goal of transforming health care through the use of technology, the Office of the National Coordinator of Health Information Technology within the Department of Health and Human Services (DHHS) has been charged with developing a strategic plan for a nationwide interoperable health information system.[3]

M.J. Ball (⊠)
Healthcare and Life Sciences Institute, IBM Research, and Professor Emerita, Johns Hopkins University School of Nursings, Baltimore, MD, USA
e-mail: marionball@us.ibm.com

M.J. Ball et al. (eds.), *Nursing Informatics*,
DOI: 10.1007/978-1-84996-278-0_1, © Springer-Verlag London Limited 2011

What is the promise of health informatics and the HIT components of the stimulus package, labeled HITECH, in the law? The RAND Corporation estimates potential annual savings from HIT over the next 15 billion years at $80.9 billion, compared to annual costs of $7.6 million. According to the Business Roundtable Report,[4] the positive outcomes of this investment include:

- "More efficient transcription and documentation processes for doctors, nurses, and other clinical staff.
- Reduction in redundant laboratory testing and imaging services from multiple providers treating the same patient.
- Reduction in hospital length of stay due to faster record retrieval, scheduling, and coordination of care.
- Improved communication of patient history for better clinical treatment, especially in emergency departments.
- Reduced medical errors and adverse events in prescriptions and medication instructions.
- Reduced administration costs through electronic claims adjudication.
- More robust quality of reporting via electronic medical records.
- Enablement of remote decision making through electronic transmission of voice, data, and images.
- Portable, comprehensive personal health records.
- Security and privacy protocols not possible in a paper-based system."

Several important concepts and values imbedded in this list of promises from the HITECH investment are and have been important to nurses. Nurses have long cared about improving patient safety, quality, and access to care by informed health care providers and improving outcomes. Additionally, nurses and other health professionals have worked to make health care more efficient and cost-effective. This chapter highlights how HIT relates to these important issues, quality and patient safety, cost, and outcomes. Regardless of the final decisions regarding health insurance reform, the ARRA provides for significant changes in health informatics and technology.

The Institute of Medicine: Breaking the Ground

Groundbreaking reports by the Institute of Medicine (IOM) on patient safety, health care quality, and professional education made it clear that information technology and informatics skills are essential for all practicing nurses and nursing students. Beginning with the publication of *The Computer-based Patient Record: An Essential Technology for Health Care,*[5,6] the IOM mounted an initiative to change the nature of health care in the United States. The initiative gained momentum with the release of *To Err Is Human*[7] and *Crossing the Quality Chasm: A New Health System for the 21st Century,*[8] documenting the chilling problems of medical errors and the systemic obstacles to efficient and effective care for patients and presenting plans of action to address those problems, including detailed recommendations set forth in *Health Professions Education: A Bridge to Quality*[9] and *Keeping Patients Safe: Transforming the Work Environment of Nurses.*[10]

The IOM had a tremendous impact on the health care agenda for the United States, as evidenced by the 10-year drive toward the electronic patient record launched in 2004. But the IOM was alone. Its reports drew upon research conducted across health care for their findings and represented the input of experts from multiple disciplines and settings. What the IOM did was raise public awareness and voice a clear and coherent call for action at a time when action is sorely needed. As nursing leaders, we have, we admit, been singing this tune for a long time, as our contributions to earlier editions of this book show. But, increasingly, we are not singing alone. Frontline nurses have joined the chorus. Frontline nurses have joined in with the IOM. According to an online survey of registered nurses (RNs) conducted in 2005,[11] 72% believed that medication safety had improved in their hospitals since 2000 and 80% of those nurses cited information technology (IT) as a "major contributor" to those improvements.

In the eyes of many nurse advocates, the very life of the nursing profession is at stake. According to a 2006 white paper, the nursing shortage is expected to worsen, with one study predicting it to triple in the 13 years between 2007 and 2020, in part due to premature retirement.[12] Research studies on the impact of nurse staffing on the patient outcomes underscore the importance of such shortages and highlight the need for informatics for a number of reasons.

Outcomes

In 2003, an editorial in the *International Journal for Quality in Health Care* cited seven studies that found an association between hospital staff nursing and adverse patient outcomes and three that did not. Despite some "mixed conclusions" and varied methodologies, the studies "highlighted the vital contribution of nurses to the quality of patient care."[13] The reviewers' own study of discharge records for over six million patients concluded that "a higher proportion of hours or nursing care provided by RNs and a greater number of hours of care by RNs per day are associated with better care for hospitalized patients."[14] Another of the seven studies cited quantified the impact of staffing on postsurgical mortality, finding that "controlling for patient and hospital characteristics, the addition of one patient to a RN's workload was associated with a 7% increase in mortality."[15]

Other studies raised similar questions. Researchers who analyzed data from 232 acute care California hospitals and over 124,000 surgical patients found that an increase of one hour worked by RNs per patient day was associated with an 8.9% decrease in the odds of pneumonia and a 10% increase in the proportion of RNs was associated with a 9.5% decrease in the odds of pneumonia.[16] A study of nurse staffing and patient outcomes in Thailand that used a smaller sample of 2,531 medical and surgical patients and controlled for patient characteristics found the ratio of total nurse staffing to patients significantly related to in-hospital mortality.[17]

In 2007, a metaanalysis published by the Agency for Healthcare Research and Quality reported that nurse staffing had a direct effect on the quality of patient care: "Higher staffing levels were associated with less hospital-related mortality, failure to rescue, cardiac arrest, hospital acquired pneumonia, and other adverse events. The effect of increased RN staffing on patient safety was strong and consistent in intensive care units and on surgical floors. Greater RN hours spent on direct patient care were associated with decreased risk of hospital-related death and shorter lengths of stay."[18] Later that year, the same research team summarized their review of 27 studies of patient outcomes in relation to the nurse-to-patient ratio. An increase of one RN per patient day was associated with decreased odds ratios of hospital acquired pneumonia, unplanned extubation, respiratory failure, and cardiac arrest in intensive care units; and with a lower odds ratio for risk of failure to rescue in surgical patients. The increase of one RN per patient day shortened patients' length of stay by 34% in intensive care units and 31% in surgical patients. Extrapolating from their findings, they estimated that for every 1,000 hospital patients, the increase of one full-time RN per patient day would save five patient lives in intensive care units, five lives on medical floors, and six on surgical floors.[19]

Other studies strengthen the case and tease out some interesting highlights. According to a research review, safer care and fewer adverse events made hospital stays shorter and "higher knowledge and skill levels" of nurses reduced patient care cost through more effective care and reduced patient resource consumption (Thungjaroenkul et al. 2007). A study analyzing data to determine the relationship between peak hospital workloads and adverse events found that at one urban teaching hospital, where occupancy rates were over 100% for much of the year, admissions and patients per nurse were significantly related to the likelihood of an adverse event (P < 0.05) and an increase of 0.1% in the patient-to-nurse ratio led to 28% increase in the rate of adverse events.[20]

Costs

When viewed in strictly monetary terms, the business case for increased nurse staffing is not quite as clear. According to an article in *Health Affairs*, raising the proportion of nursing hours provided by RNs without an increase in total nursing hours reduced net costs, while increasing total nursing hours (with or without increasing the proportion of hours provided by RNs) reduced length of stay, adverse outcomes, and patient deaths, but increased hospital costs by up to 1.5%. The conclusion is compelling: "Whether or not staffing should be increased depends on the value patients and payers assign to avoided deaths and complications."[21]

Although this ethical and moral appeal is compelling, it may be unnecessary. As the nursing shortage looms, understaffing assumes critical significance.[22] And, job dissatisfaction and burnout among nurses carry very much real costs. According to a study of 10,319 nurses at 303 hospitals in the United States, Canada, Scotland, and England,[23] "Adequate nurse staffing and organization/managerial support for nursing are key to improving the quality of patient care, to diminishing nurse job dissatisfaction and burnout and, ultimately, to improving the nurse retention problem in hospital settings." A second study by Aiken and et al.[15] linked data from 10,184 staff nurses and 232,342 patients at 168 hospitals in Pennsylvania, adjusted for nurse and hospital characteristics, and found that "each additional patient per nurse was associated with a 23%…increase in the odds of burnout and a 15% increase…in the odds of job dissatisfaction…. In hospitals with high patient-to-nurse ratios, surgical patients experience higher risk-adjusted 30-day mortality and failure-to-rescue rates, and nurses are more likely to experience burnout and job dissatisfaction."

Although failing to find staffing a significant predictor of mortality or failure to rescue, a subsequent but smaller study (140 nurses, 2,709 patient) "reinforced" the importance of adequate staffing ratios and called for programs that support nurses in their practice environments.[24]

In 2008, to assess the impact of practice environments, Aiken et al. used the data from their earlier study and the practice environment scales of the Nursing Work Index to measure nurse job satisfaction, burnout, intent to leave, and reports of quality of care, as well as mortality and failure to rescue in patients. "Nurses reported more positive job experiences and fewer concerns with care quality, and patients had significantly lower risk of death and failure to rescue in hospitals with better care environments…. Care environment elements must be optimized alongside nurse staffing and education to achieve high quality of care."[25]

Understanding and managing nursing activities is critical to controlling costs, improving the environment in which nurses practice, and ensuring that patients receive safe, quality care.

Documentation is one such activity.[26] As the IOM reported in *Keeping Patients Safe: Transforming the Work Environment of Nurses* (2004), paperwork and documentation place a heavy burden on nurses. Although studies vary, this activity consumes from 13 to 28% of nurses' time.[27-30] Time spent on documentation cannot be spent on direct patient care.[31,32] Not surprisingly, nurses often find it frustrating and professionally unrewarding.

Based on observations, interviews, and focus group input, a study of 14 medical-surgical units identified more than one third of nurses' time as nonvalue-added (NVA), costing each unit an average of $757,000 in wages annually. More time went to support activities (coordinate care and manage clinical records) than patient care (assess, teach, treat, provide psychosocial support), and the least amount of time went to patient teaching and psychosocial support. These findings suggest that reducing NVA and support activities and increasing patient care time could improve clinical outcomes and control costs.[33]

Moreover, as recent literature reviews concluded, inadequate nurse staffing in the perioperative setting negatively affects patient safety and leads to nurse burnout, a concern in light of the growing nursing shortage.[34-36]

The evidence, we submit, is overwhelming. Nurses still have only limited experience using IT. As Weier[11] reported, only 32% had used online documentation at the point of care and still fewer had used electronic alerts or bar code medication administration (22 and 23%, respectively). And, this was despite the wave of studies advocating the use of IT to transform nursing. A systematic review of 23 studies[37] on the impact of electronic health records using a weighted average approach found that "The use of bedside terminals and central station desktops saved nurses, respectively, 24.5 and 23.5% of their overall time documenting during a shift." Yet another study found potential in the use of informatics tools to support evidence-based staffing.[38] The case could not be clearer: major changes have to be made in all aspects of the nursing profession in the context of a changing health care landscape.

HIT and the TIGER Initiative

One of the most significant responses to this critical need for change in the nursing profession has been the TIGER initiative. We and many of our colleagues believe this initiative, which began in early 2005, offers the best hope for the profession for the rapid and revolutionary change that the nursing profession has to make. The first step for TIGER was the organization of an invitational conference in 2006 at the Uniformed Services University of the Health Sciences in Bethesda maryland. More than 70 organizations participated in the TIGER Summit, and with masterful facilitators, this group of leaders developed a 10-year vision and a 3-year action steps and plan. Each of the participating organizations agreed to incorporate the TIGER vision and action steps into their organization's strategic plans; each fulfilled a critical role by distributing what is now called TIGER Phase I Summit Summary Report within their network to engage additional support for this agenda. Details of the 3-year plan and a list of participating organizations are available on the TIGER website at www.tigersummit.com/participants.

From the TIGER Summit in 2006 until now, these organizations, together with hundreds of additional volunteers and industry experts, have collaborated to complete the action steps necessary toward achieving the TIGER vision which addressed not only care in acute care settings, but also across the continuum of care. Although much of the discussion in this chapter is related to hospital-focused HIT investment, the TIGER initiative has embraced the practice of nursing in all health care settings, including primary care, long-term care, public health, and home health care. Health care reform is targeting both the electronic health record (EHR) and the personal health record (PHR). The emphasis is on improving preventive services, primary care, health promotion, and better management of individuals and families living with chronic illnesses. Nurses care passionately about these issues and are well qualified to address them as well as illness care. The HIT investment is relevant to nurse practitioners, nurse midwives, and home health nurses who will benefit from other ARRA investments made in the context of health reform. With enhanced interoperability previously mentioned in this chapter, additionally the capability to compare the effectiveness of different health care treatments and strategies will have significant implications for nurses in all types of settings. The $1.1 billion invested in comparative-effectiveness research and in improving individual health-related behaviors is sure to impact the role and practice of nurses in the future.

The TIGER Initiative remains focused on raising awareness of the need to engage nurses in all settings in the national effort to prepare the health care workforce toward effective adoption of electronic health records and to help shape the content within interoperable HIT systems through advocacy for the inclusion of nurse-relevant data elements. Presentations at regional, national, and international conferences have brought visibility of TIGER activities to nursing colleagues and continue to alert and educate nurses about the importance of the emerging and fast-moving HIT agenda. Also, leaders of the TIGER Phase II initiative enlisted an ever-growing cadre of nursing professionals in their efforts; they have focused their efforts in nine areas they call Collaboratives:

- Standard and Interoperability
- National Health Information Technology Agenda
- Informatics Competencies
- Education and Faculty Development
- Staff Development
- Usability and Clinical Application Design
- Virtual Demonstration Center
- Leadership Development
- Consumer Empowerment and Personal Health Record

Through their work, these nine Collaboratives have brought the nursing profession to the table at a time when health care itself is undergoing great changes. The subsequent chapters in this fourth edition of *Nursing Informatics: Where Technology and Caring Meet* provide a glimpse into the accomplishments of nursing leaders for each of these nine collaboratives. Additional chapters have been included to enhance the knowledge, expertise, and vision for the future, locally and globally. From across all the sectors of nursing – education, practice, industry, and government –, the sound we hear now is no longer a soprano chorus, but a powerful TIGER roar.

References

1. Ball MJ. Nursing Informatics of Tomorrow. Health Informatics. www.healthcare-informatics. com; 2005.
2. Hinton Walker P, Troseth M. Business coalitions: shaping health reform through technology and science. In: Slavik P, Moorhead S (eds), *Current Issues in Nursing*. 8th ed. St. Louis: Mosby; 2011.
3. Blumenthal D. Stimulating the Adoption of Health Information Technology. *N Engl J Med*. http://healthcarereform.nejm.org/?p=436; 2009. Accessed on 25.09.09.
4. Health Care Reform: The Perils of Inaction and the Promise of Effective Action. A Report to the Business Roundtable by Hewitt Associates LLC, September; 2009:19-20.
5. Institute of Medicine. *The Computer-Based Patient Record: An Essential Technology for Health Care*. Washington: National Academy; 1991.
6. Institute of Medicine. The Computer-Based Patient Record: An Essential Technology for Health Care. Revised ed. Washington: National Academy; 1997.
7. Institute of Medicine. *To Err Is Human*. Washington: National Academy; 2000.
8. Institute of Medicine. *Crossing the Quality Chasm: A New Health System for the 21st Century*. Washington: National Academy; 2001.
9. Institute of Medicine. *Health Professions Education: A Bridge to Quality*. Washington: National Academy; 2003.
10. Institute of Medicine. *Keeping Patients Safe: Transforming the Work Environment of Nurses*. Washington: National Academy; 2004.
11. Weier S. RNs Cite IT as 'Major Contributor' to Medication Safety Improvements. iHealth-Beat. www.ihealthbeat.org; 2005.
12. Robert Wood Johnson Foundation. Wisdom at Work: The Importance of the Older and Experienced Nurse in the Workplace. www.rwjf.org/files/publications/other/wisdomatwork. pdf; 2006.
13. Needleman J, Buerhaus P. Nurse staffing and patient safety: current knowledge and implications for action. *Int J Qual Health Care*. 2003;15(4):275-277.

14. Needleman J, Buerhaus P, Mattke S, et al. Nurse-staffing levels and the quality of care in hospitals. *N Engl J Med*. 2002;346(22):1715-1722.
15. Aiken LH, Clarke SP, Sloane DM, et al. Hospital nurse staffing and patient mortality, nurse burnout, and job dissatisfaction. *J Am Med Assoc*. 2002;288:1987-1993.
16. Cho SH, Ketefian S, Barkauskas VH, et al. The effects of nurse staffing on adverse events, morbidity, mortality, and medical costs. *Nurs Res*. 2003;52(2):71-79.
17. Sasichay-Akkadechanunt T, Scalzi CC, Jawad AF. The relationship between nurse staffing and patient outcomes. *J Nurs Adm*. 2003;33(9):478-485.
18. Kane RL, Shamilyan TA, Mueller C, et al. Nurse staffing and quality of patient care. *Evid Rep Technol Assess*. 2007;151:1-115.
19. Kane RL, Shamilyan TA, Mueller C, et al. The association of registered nurse staffing levels and patient outcomes: systematic review and meta-analysis. *Med Care*. 2007;45(12): 1126-1128.
20. Weissman JF, Rothschil JM, Bendavid E, et al. Hospital workload and adverse events. *Med Care*. 2007;45(5):448-455.
21. Needleman J, Buerhaus PI, Stewart M, et al. Nurse staffing in hospitals: is there a business case for quality? *Health Aff (Millwood)*. 2006;25(1):204-211.
22. Aiken LH, Clarke SP, Silber JH, et al. Hospital nurse staffing, education, and patient mortality. *LDI Issue Brief*. 2003;9(2):1-4.
23. Aiken LH, Clarke SP, Sloane DM. Hospital staffing, organization, and quality of care: cross-national findings. *Int J Qual Health Care*. 2002;14(1):5-13.
24. Halm M, Peterson M, Kandeis M, et al. Hospital nurse staffing and patient mortality, emotional exhaustion, and job dissatisfaction. *Clin Nurse Spec*. 2005; 19(5):241-251; quiz 252-254.
25. Aiken LH, Clarke SP, Sloane DM, et al. Effects of hospital care environment on patient mortality and nurse outcomes. *J Nurs Adm*. 2008;38(5):223-229.
26. Clancy TR, Delaney CW, Morrison B, et al. The benefits of standardized nursing languages in complex adaptive systems such as hospitals. *J Nurs Adm*. 2006;36(9):426-434.
27. Pabst M, Scherubel J, Minnick A. The impact of computerized documentation on nurses' use of time. *Comp Nurs*. 1996;14(1):25-30.
28. Smeltzer C, Hines P, Beebe H, et al. Streaming documentation: an opportunity to reduce costs and increase nurse clinicians' time with patients. *J Nurs Care Qual*. 1996;10(14):66-77.
29. Upenieks V. Work sampling: assessing nursing efficiency. *Nurs Manage*. 1998;29(4):27-29.
30. Urden L, Roode J. Work sampling: a decision making tool for determining resources and work redesign. *J Nurs Adm*. 1997;27(9):34-41.
31. Brooks J. An analysis of nursing documentation as a reflection of actual nurse work. *Medsurg Nurs*. 1998;7(4):189-198.
32. Brunt B, Gifford L, Hart D, et al. Designing interdisciplinary documentation for the continuum of care. *J Nurs Care Qual*. 1999;14(1):1-10.
33. Storfjell JL, Omoike O, Ohison S. The balancing act: patient care time versus cost. *J Nurs Adm*. 2008;38(5):244-249.
34. Aiken LH, Clarke SP, Sloane DM, et al. Nurses' reports on hospital care in five countries. *Health Aff (Millwood)*. 2001;20(3):43-53.
35. American Hospital Association. In Our Hands: How Hospital Leaders Can Build a Thriving Workforce. http://www.aha.org/aha/resource-center/Statistics-and-Studies/ioh.html; 2002.
36. Garrett C. The effect of nurse staffing patterns on medical errors and nurse burnout. *AORN J*. 2008;87(6):1191-1204.
37. Poissant L, Pereira J, Tamblyn R, et al. The impact of electronic health records on time efficiency of physicians and nurses: a systematic study. *J Am Med Inform Assoc*. 2005;12: 505-516.
38. Hyun S, Bakken S, Douglas K, et al. Evidence-based staffing: potential roles for informatics. *Nurs Econ*. 2008;26(3):151-158, 173.
39. Thungjaroenkul P, Commings GE, Embleton A. The impact of nurse staffing on hospital costs and patient length of stay: a systematic review. *Nurs Econ*. 2007;25(5):255-265.

Strategies for Culture Change

2

Introduction

The subtitle of this book, *Where Technology and Caring Meet,* reflects the next stage of challenges for nursing and other health professions in the midst of a rapidly growing need for health information technology (HIT) innovation and implementation. Significantly different cultural perspectives on the meaning of caring and technology for many health care professionals contribute to challenges related to implementation, acceptance, and meaningful use of technology and informatics in the provision of care to patients and consumers.

Why should we have a discussion about culture and cultural change as a major part of this 4th edition? In 2006, a group of nursing leaders organized an invitational meeting of nursing leaders across the profession to create a vision and shape strategies to implement technology and informatics within the nursing profession. This initiative was called Technology Informatics Guiding Education Reform (TIGER). In the preparation for the invitational symposium, TIGER leadership identified seven pillars which would frame the discussion of strategies for change: management and leadership, education, communication and collaboration, informatics design, information technology (IT), policy, and culture. Consensus was reached regarding themes and initial action steps for all the pillars except one, the pillar of Culture. As defined at the TIGER summit, culture is "a respectful open system that leverages technology and informatics across multiple disciplines in an environment where all stakeholders trust each other to work together towards the goal of high quality and safety."[1] The summit recommended the following actions as strategies to impact culture:

- Institute a national marketing campaign to promote the value of technology in a multi-disciplinary way that supports an accepting culture.
- Include HIT in every strategic plan, mission, and vision statement; use of HIT is embraced by executives, deans, all point-of-care clinicians, and students with goal of high quality care and safety.

P.H. Walker
Uniformed Services University of the Health Sciences, Bethesda, MD, USA
e-mail: phintonwalker@usuhs.mil

M.J. Ball et al. (eds.), *Nursing Informatics,*
DOI: 10.1007/978-1-84996-278-0_2, © Springer-Verlag London Limited 2011

- Establish multidisciplinary teams that embrace a shared vision and operate cohesively to push for broad technology integration within/across entire organizations.
- Develop mutual respect between/among clinicians who may bring different skills and knowledge, e.g., create/develop process in which experienced nurses can mentor new nurses, and also, the new nurses who are more technologically aware can mentor veteran nurses.

Summit participants agreed that these actions would derive their strength from the fact that a culture can support and promote the adoption of HIT and discourage "workarounds" by the users, if that culture is nonpunitive. In their view, when a user is striving to use HIT and avoid errors, the organization can learn from that experience.

As the TIGER summit came to an end, there was a clear consensus among the participants that "culture eats strategy for lunch every day." Success in facilitating transformational change, they agreed, was dependent upon not underestimating the significance of culture. Many key aspects of culture had yet to be discussed: the need for culture transformation, change theory and management, and the milestones to be reached as the nursing profession and other health care disciplines journey toward change.

There are many different perspectives on culture change, depending on which lens is used to view culture and which culture is being viewed. What is the health professional or nurse talking about? Is it the culture of the profession, or the education of new professionals, or the re-education of current practicing professionals? Is it the organizational settings where health care is provided or the home where innovative and disruptive technologies have shifted responsibility for care and decision making to the consumer? The literature offers insights into these many perspectives. Articles addressing the challenges related to changing health care and nursing culture in the context of technology and informatics cover a wide range of topics: professional initiatives, organizational culture and technology implementation, theoretical framework-designed approaches to addressing technology acceptance as a form of culture change, and technology innovation as disruption for social change applied to HIT issues. We need to view culture and culture change through the eyes of many different beholders, particularly when we discuss the use of informatics and technology where caring and technology actually do meet.

This chapter explores culture change from all of these perspectives, thereby essentially allowing the reader to "choose" the approach to culture change that is relevant to his or her particular lens, paradigm, practice, or perspective. Woven into the different approaches is the evidence of how professional initiatives like TIGER, individual nursing and medical professionals, health care organizations, researchers, and businesses are attempting to address the challenge of changing health care culture by maximizing the use of informatics and technology. New transformative technologies are emerging on the horizon, and nursing and the other "caring professions" traditionally dedicated to the value of caring must find ways to embrace informatics – or they will find themselves behind the power curve.

If the nursing profession rises to the occasion and gets in front of this tidal wave of emerging technology and embraces the cultural change required, nurses will be at the table reinventing the profession for a very different future. The result will be "meaningful use" of technology, a term that is still being debated in health professions, policy, and technology and business settings in the context of health reform. However, with proactive attempts to incorporate informatics and technology into practice, education, and research, the nursing profession can continue to improve the quality of care and the health status and care with the required cost-effectiveness that must be at the heart of any health reform initiative. Otherwise, nursing and other health professions will experience the difficulties all health professionals experienced with the "social disruption" called managed care where the business and financial minds responded more rapidly to the need for change in health care. This time, nurses and other health professionals must work *with* those shaping technological advances. Only then can "meaningful use" honor the charge to "do no harm" ethically, legally, and most of all, within the sacred context of the "caring" relationship.

Culture, Caring, and Technology

Culture

Culture is defined as "the cumulative deposit of knowledge, experience, beliefs, values, attitudes, meanings, hierarchies, roles…acquired by a group of people…. a way of life… the behaviors, beliefs, values, and symbols that they accept, generally without thinking about them…. Culture consists of patterns, explicit and implicit of and for behavior acquired and transmitted by symbols…."[2] Still another way of looking at culture is in reference to traditions, artifacts, rituals, and heroes. In the deep topic of culture, there are many differing views of what the term itself means. It is no wonder that nursing leaders at a 2-day TIGER summit could not come to a consensus regarding the concept of culture or cultural change(s). Initially, it depends on which body of knowledge, paradigm, or theoretical basis is used to talk about, explain, and/or try to write about cultural change.

When trying to focus this chapter on relevant roots of cultural change and after journeying through writings on culture that were based on sociology, anthropology, psychology, and other related sciences, this author landed on the term "socioculture" as a way to focus on the relevant roots of cultural change related to health care and more specifically the nursing profession. After sifting through the scientific and professional literature that used many different cultural change lenses, it seemed to this author that "socioculture" offered the best fit for the purposes of this chapter. Sociocultural evolution is an umbrella term used to describe how cultures and societies develop over time. Theories such as sociocultural evolution typically provide models to help understand the relationship between technologies, social structures, values of a society and of subcultures within a society, and how and why they change over time. Social structures within a sociocultural context involve groups or entities in relation to each other; social institutions and norms are embedded into social structures in ways that shape the behavior of actors in these systems. This theoretical explanation of sociocultural change further identifies the actors within these social systems as having roles: "The notion of social structure *as relationships between different entities or groups,* or as *enduring and relatively stable patterns of relationships* emphasizes the idea that society is grouped into structurally related groups or sets of roles, with different functions, meanings or purposes."[3]

Given nursing's history, roots, and evolution as a profession, the "notion of social structure" is relevant to discussions about cultural change in the context of caring and technology. Finally, within the context of sociocultural evolution, social scientists use sociotechnological theory to frame the cultural change and/or adjustment of a culture to the introduction and use of technology. We can apply their theories to our changing society in the context of social evolution impacted by technological change in an information-driven society. "Sociotechnical theory therefore is about *joint optimization*, with a shared emphasis on achievement of both excellence in technical performance and quality in people's work lives. Sociotechnical theory, as distinct from sociotechnical systems, proposes a number of different ways to achieve joint optimization. They are usually based on designing different kinds of organizations, ones in which the relationships between socio and technical elements lead to the emergence of productivity and wellbeing."[4]

Moving from the Industrial Age to the Information Age has not always been easy, particularly for groups, workers, professions, and institutions that adopted some form of the industrial age as a part of their culture. When the Industrial Age is mentioned, the first thought to come to mind is the automobile industry and similar industries that have become increasingly challenged in the Information Age. Although health care delivery is not necessarily seen as "industrialized," this begs a question of how managed care has "organized" the delivery of services. Patients in hospitals, surgical centers, and ambulatory care settings are moved along the "path" from pre-op to operative care to post-op. Systems in place in each of these settings are designed to have the patient come out of the care delivery area with "better parts" in some cases, and/or removal or repair of "nonfunctioning parts" in other cases. In like manner, primary and ambulatory care settings have "a time per station" for the health care providers, a frequent source of frustration for both providers and patients. In this industrial-type delivery system that many view as fragmented and lacking continuity of care, patient safety has become a major issue.

The question is whether or not health care delivery systems and providers can embrace the Information Age more completely. The evolution of the internet and the HIT industry and recent trends such as free personal health records (PHRs) available from both Google and Microsoft are rapidly moving health care into the Information Age. Health care reform, now being explored under the leadership of President Obama, portends to shift the focus to wellness care and prevention. Individuals and families are becoming increasingly more responsible for their own health care and having control of their own health records. All of these are surely challenging the "industrial-age" mental model. How can health care providers and systems embrace the information age more fully? Seven keys to success in the Information Age are suggested in the literature[5]:

1. Develop a positive attitude, acceptance of living in a new world, and learn to explore possibilities instead of resisting the changes.
2. Recognize that change is the dominant factor of the information age, that change becomes the culture, and by embracing change one can influence the future rather than always be adjusting to change.
3. Learn to be very flexible, and prepare yourself to deal effectively with the change that chooses you instead of trying to hang on to comfort zones and allow change to defeat you.
4. Become a communicator, recognizing that communication is the most powerful tool possessed in the information age, and focus on understanding, appreciating, and mastering all forms of communication.

5. Become a global networker and embrace the sources of new information, ideas, and options that broad networks can provide.
6. Focus on achieving goals, not just setting goals in order to become a better decision-maker by exploring new opportunities and using information provided through the use of technology.
7. Be a student for life and plan to stay ahead of the fast-paced information age game that means constantly acquiring new knowledge and skills and moving in new directions without focusing on the barriers, but the opportunities.

Given these seven keys for success in this technology-driven Information Age, nurses and other health care providers must find new ways of demonstrating "caring" and providing "care." This shift – not only in the way care is provided, but in how care is defined – will require a significant change in culture.

Caring and Technology

Nursing as a culture can be described as beliefs, values, norms, and laws related primarily to the practice of nursing.[6] Additionally, common group work, activities, processes, history, heroes, and rituals can further define the culture of a profession. The history of "caring" goes back to the seventeenth and eighteenth centuries and was fundamental to the beginning of the nursing and medical professions. The "caring relationship" was presented and is still recognized from the early "caring" of the Lady with the Lamp, Florence Nightingale.[7] Other heroes who play a significant part in nursing history include Lillian Wald, who expressed concern for the living conditions and health status of the poor and established the Henry Street Settlement and the first Visiting Nurse Service in 1893 (Biography.com 2007); Dorothea Dix, who championed for the needs of the mentally ill and those in prison settings with resulting changes in Canada and Europe and in over 15 states in the United States during the 1800s[8]; and Mary Breckenridge recognized the plight of rural America's mothers and babies and established the Frontier Nursing Service in the early 1900s.[9] These pioneering women not only brought about systems change, but also provided personal "caring" and compassionate touch to patients during their careers.

In a recent commentary on the science of care, Harris[10] highlighted the work of Francis Peabody and her call to physicians to provide personal care in the context of treating impersonal disease, reminding physicians that "the secret of the care for the patient is caring for the patient." This "caring" orientation is about personal and therapeutic relationships. Interaction is still at the core of nursing, medicine, and other health professions as well. For many health care providers, technological advances such as computers and informatics seem to take time away from the relationship with the patient and from what is described today as "patient care."

With this backdrop, the challenge of bringing together a culture of caring and technology becomes clearer. Further insight emerges from an examination of definitions. Terms that have been used when referring to a culture of caring include compassion, watchful oversight, commitment to the welfare of the whole person, attentive listening, comforting, touch, and relationship.[11,12] Technology, on the other hand, is generally defined as the use of tools and machines that may be used to help solve real-world problems.[13] It can also mean the use of technical methods, skills, and processes that can be both material and immaterial. Historically, technology has been used to change culture, sometimes positively, other times negatively.

Finally, there is the term IT which can be defined as a branch of engineering that deals with the use of computers and telecommunications to retrieve, store, and transmit data. It can also be described as the application of computer, communications, and software technology to the management, processing, and dissemination of information. Although most nurses and physicians have not focused on IT and data issues, they have historically been concerned with charting and recording their actions as providers and the reactions of their patients to the care and treatments delivered.

Recent discussions of the use of electronic medical records (EMRs), electronic health records (EHRs), and PHRs seem cold, distant, and impersonal compared to the more personal language of touch, comfort, and compassion. The differences between the language, definitions, and purposes of caring on the one hand and of technology on the other underscore the need to bridge the distance between them. This poses considerable challenges for nurses and other health professionals, educators, administrators, and policymakers. The TIGER Initiative, organized by nursing leaders and advocates, is one recent approach to bridge the divide between caring and technology.

For nurses and other health professionals, culture change to bridge the gap is critical to the adoption and meaningful use of technology. Unless key issues are addressed and specific strategies implemented, the results may have a negative impact on the delivery of quality care, continuity of care, cost-effectiveness of care, and the overriding issue of patient safety. In addition to the focus on the outcome of meaningful use (patient care), issues related to design, adoption, and successful implementation in social institutions connected to health care and education are also important, such as ensuring relevant input and participation in the development of these systems, attention to work flow and design, successful adoption, and meaningful use. According to Kilbridge and Classen,[14] "Effective use of informatics to enhance safety requires the establishment and use of standards for concept definitions and for data exchange, development of acceptable models for knowledge representation, incentive for adoption of EHRs, support for adverse event detection and reporting, and greater investment in research at the intersection of informatics and patient safety." Although much of this has been done, there is still the challenge of how to bring about cultural change within the health professions and specifically the nursing profession.

Approaches to Culture Change

Culture Change Through TIGER Initiative

The TIGER movement is a major effort that has already had a significant impact on culture change. When discussing technology, informatics, and culture, it is important to identify the contributions of the TIGER initiative in this context. TIGER is essentially a major grassroots initiative that was organized to significantly impact the culture of nursing and ultimately other health professions by creating a vision of and strategic approaches to "make informatics nursing's stethoscope of the twenty-first century".[15] Following the 2004 health IT summit convened by Dr. David Brailer, nursing informatics leaders shared their concerns that the nursing profession was not at the table when health IT was discussed and was behind in embracing technological advances and informatics in patient care. An informal group began to strategize about how to bring about a vision and define approaches to culture change related to informatics and technology to the nursing profession.

How was the initial plan for TIGER invitational summit related to cultural change? In the planning stages for TIGER, there were not many overt discussions of a specifically designed theory-based change process. However, the group actually applied several literature-based strategies for culture change in nursing, including diffusion of innovation theory.[16] They began with a strategy similar to what is known as "collective innovation–decision" and involves all individuals within a social system making a decision together. Acknowledging the impossibility of inviting everyone to the summit, its planners took great care to involve leadership and representation from all organizations and groups within the profession in order to have the decisions about the TIGER vision made collectively across the social system called nursing.

Further, using this theoretical approach, the first of the five stages of adoption in Roger's Diffusion of Innovation theory,[16] knowledge, persuasion, and decision, was carefully choreographed at the summit. Commitment to implementation came at the end of the meeting, with implementation beginning with TIGER Phase II through the use of collaboratives. These collaboratives were effectively assigned to groups according to the adoption categories together, such as innovators who are among the first to adopt an innovation; early adopters who have the highest degree of opinion leadership and are more socially forward than late adopters; early majority tends to be slower and adopt after contact with early adopters; late majority which will adopt after the average member of the society adopts with skepticism; and finally the laggards, who tend to stay focused on the "traditions" or more traditional rituals, mores, etc. of the nursing profession described earlier. Two other strategies used that were consistent with Roger's theory were the use of Opinion Leaders and communication channels by specifically focusing on presentations and publications throughout the profession to increase adoption. Implementation was also inherently part of the strategy of the TIGER invitational symposium and subsequent development of collaborative teams within TIGER Phase II was visibly similar to the use of diffusion of innovation by whether or not there was a specifically designed approach to culture change. Another approach that could be observed by students of culture change was the Culture Change Model described by Simon.[17] He describes a model with three strategies: the top-down approach, the grassroots approach, and the process champion approach. TIGER leaders wisely recognized that there was no "top-down" approach due to the diversity of individuals, groups, and practice within the profession of nursing and structured the symposium to rely on the grassroots and champions approach as a next step. To some extent, TIGER leaders did pay attention to the top-down approach by bringing the leaders of practice, education, and specialty and other national organizations together, anticipating that there would be some impact by the top-down approach over time. However, most of the change was focused on bringing grassroots individual players together to design recommendations and strategies for change, led by champions related to each new pillar or area of focus determined by a group survey.

The 2006 TIGER summit was held in Bethesda, Maryland, at the Uniformed Services University and consisted of approximately 100 leaders within the nursing profession. At that conference, the leaders identified a 10-year vision and created a 3-year map of strategies around the seven pillars mentioned in this chapter introduction with the exception of the pillar of culture. However, because of the implementation of the strategies addressed in TIGER's seven pillars, there is clearly an impact on culture and cultural change. The TIGER history, specifics of its initiative, and its subsequent recommendations are covered elsewhere in this book; however, as cultural change strategies are covered below, reference will be made to TIGER activities and recommendations, directing the reader to the relevant sections in this book for more detail.

Subsequently, TIGER Phase II was initiated with the development of nine collaboratives that were based on a grassroots vote of the priority issues that needed to be addressed to achieve the vision and strategic plan created at the 2006 summit. One of the most significant aspects of the beginning of this culture change was the process and participation of individuals and groups in each of these nine collaboratives. Over 1,000 grassroots nurses from many different health care settings and backgrounds participated in developing recommendations to achieve the 3-year strategic plan. Also during Phase II, many nursing organizations, including the National League for Nursing (NLN) and others, developed strategies for or approaches toward culture change.

This chapter focuses on TIGER's overall fit with approaches to culture change. Essentially, the TIGER II summary report and the recommendations of the various collaborative are consistent with strategies highlighted in this chapter. Consequently, reference is made to them that are relevant to the particular cultural change models and approaches to culture change under discussion.

Culture Change Through Education

Culture change has great possibilities through nursing education or health profession's continuing education settings. In addition to the nursing values, beliefs, and norms traditionally taught in nursing education settings, there is an opportunity to introduce and influence positive attitudes about the value of technology and informatics. During the educational process, nurses and health professionals not only learn theoretical aspects, but also experience the practical and clinical aspects of health care. Within the clinical learning experience, learners grow through real life experiences with patients, clients, and communities. Within the clinical setting, there is a great opportunity for nursing and other health profession students to be acculturated in the use of informatics and technology as a normal/expected part of the profession. Students are already exposed to a variety of tools and technologies that have been traditionally used in the delivery of patient care. If these tools and technologies can become ubiquitous and accepted, informatics-based point-of-care devices can also be introduced as integral to quality patient care.

The use of nursing education as a way to change culture is ideal for future generations of nurses and other health care professionals. It does not, however, change the settings in which many nurses will work. Currently, one of the major challenges between the educational experience/setting and the organization where practice occurs is that there is such a difference between "ideal nursing" and "reality nursing" which frequently confuses graduates and can have a negative impact on nursing retention. Using informatics and technology in both the educational setting and in the practice organization will transform the culture of nursing and potentially other health professionals. Consequently, it would not be that difficult to introduce the use of computers and health IT during the learning process so that it becomes part of the work process and patient care activities.

The TIGER initiative's focus on education was very successful. The National League for Nursing adopted a position related to advancing technology in educational programs. In addition, one of the TIGER collaboratives reviewed work already done on informatics competencies, clarifying and classifying them according to different levels of functioning. These leveled competencies motivate students and faculty to have competency-based learning activities integrated into the curriculum. With anticipated changes in health IT and emerging technologies that may change health care and nursing care, experience with health IT is a mandatory approach that should not be disconnected from the learning experience (see Chap. 6, "Competencies: Nuts and Bolts" by Connie Delaney and Brian Gugerty).

Other strategies that can have a significant impact on culture change are through changes in advanced nursing education, through continuing education, and certification. One major educational initiative that has emerged nationally is the focus on technology and informatics in Master's education programs. Currently, degree offerings in Medical Informatics, Health Informatics, and Nursing Informatics are (and have been) a significant part of the culture change. Nurse informatics specialists contribute in a significant way. According to Staggers and Thompson,[18] despite the fact that the field of nursing informatics is in its third decade, many definitions still exist to describe the field. Recent recruitment materials for the specialty[19] stated "Nurse programmers write and modify computer programs for use by nurses, nurse communicators work with other nurses to identify computer system needs or to assist in the training and implementation of those systems, informatics nurse managers manage or administer information systems, and nurse vendor representatives demonstrate systems to potential buyers." According to Bureau of Labor, salaries have risen in past few years and there in an increasing need for nursing informatics specialists. Certification for nurse informaticists is also evidence of progress in changing culture through education. Advanced education of nurses (and other health professionals) is necessary for clinicians such as nurses to become productive and critical members of the IT team.[20] In order to improve user interfaces and to address design according to clinical workflow, there is an important role for informaticists who can bridge clinical practice and systems engineering in health care.

Most of the changes that would be identified here are provided in the TIGER Phase II Collaborative on Competencies and Nursing Education/Faculty Development. Specifics that are particularly relevant to cultural change are addressed in the recommendations from the TIGER Phase I Report and more specifically in the TIGER Phase II Report, which are highlighted elsewhere in this book. In addition to programs that prepare specialists in Nursing Informatics (NI), what is required for culture change is that NI is "integrated into all four domains of nursing practice. The magnitude of change required on an individual, organization and professional levels points to the need for Nursing

Informatics education strategies on a national level."[21] A number of chapters in this book highlight TIGER Phase II accomplishments related to education, including Chap. 6 by Delaney and Gugerty mentioned previously. Three more other chapters in Sect. 2 address more specifically the role of educational initiatives in culture change: Chap. 5, "Education and Faculty Development" by Diane Skiba and Mary Anne Rizzolo; Chap. 8, "Continuing Education and Staff Development" by Joan Kiel and Elizabeth Johnson; and Chap. 7, "Updated Academic Programs," a two-part chapter including Carole Gassert's work that appeared in the 3rd edition of *Nursing Informatics* together with an update by Susan Newbold. Also in Sect. 2, Pamela Jeffries, Krysia Hudson, Laura A. Taylor, and Steven A. Klapper focus on strategies for the education of health care providers that enhance change of culture in the future in Chap. 11, "Bridging Technology: Academe and Industry." A more futuristic perspective on how education needs to change in order to integrate technology more effectively in both formal education and staff development appears in Chap. 21 in Sect. 4, "Local Global Access: Virtual Learning Environment" by Teresa McCasky, Beth Elias, Jacqueline Moss, and Christel Anderson.

Culture Change in the Context of Organizational Change

There is a great deal of literature discussing the relationship of organizational culture change with the use and adoption of informatics and technology. As in previous discussions regarding cultural change, there is very little consensus regarding the models and approaches for change within organizations. In fact, there is little agreement about what organizational culture actually is. Without agreement, it is easy to understand why there is little consensus about how to bring about organizational culture change. This section of the chapter identifies approaches to organizational culture change in the context of implementation of technology and informatics, specifically for the purpose of improving patient safety.

Schein[22] defines organizational culture in similar ways as culture has been defined earlier in this chapter with terms such as customs, rights, language, traditions, standards, and values. He further defines levels of culture including: artifacts described as those items seen, felt, and heard; espoused values described as shared values and social validation of the same; and basic assumptions that leaders and members pay attention to what things mean. According to Nellen,[23] organizational change for Schein[22] begins with "unfreezing" to find the motivation for change. Providing disconfirming data that can cause psychological discomfort is one way to increase awareness and motivation for change. Next is Cognitive Restructuring, which once "unfrozen" can result in such activities as trial and error actions, new learning, and retooling. The final stage is "refreezing" once the new behavior is fixed and will stay like it is until disconfirmation starts again when there is a need for the next organizational change.

According to Lorenzi et al.,[24] in the first stages of the technological revolution, most attention was focused on hardware/software development and business processes. The question of which came first, organizational development or technological change, is referred to "in a classic chicken-or-egg sense." Cutliffe and Lorenzi et al.[24,25] further ask whether technological advances are driving organizational change or "does the technology merely enable changes that are largely driven by nontechnical forces such as information systems designed to reduce costs?" Another model found in the literature described by Lorenzi et al.[24] is a four-stage model of organizational change that can be applied to the change related to informatics systems: (1) The steady state is affected by some reason for change which can be technical or nontechnical; (2) The organization identifies the desired outcomes and implements the change process; (3) The organization alters itself by the need for change; (4) Over time, the organization becomes the "new" initial state that is ready for the next change.

When considering the social-technical implications of change, particularly when computers and technology are involved, there are a number of considerations for cultural change. First is user involvement and participation in system development and adoption, which includes the following factors: cognitive including the knowledge of technology; motivational including interest, self-efficacy, or confidence; and situational including social norms toward technology, how the individual is treated relative to others, and the nature of user involvement. Another factor is user acceptance which is focused on perceived ease of use of the systems. The next set of factors measure the users' attitudes of satisfaction with their IT. Sometimes this is determined by the use of surveys. Finally, the usability factor refers to human factors and how the technology impacts the user's ability to work with the system. Effective change requires attention to these factors, particularly for technology change.

Scott et al.[26] when discussing organizational change related to the United Kingdom emphasizes group affiliation, teamwork, and coordination with attention to formal structures, regulations, and reporting relationships. Instead of focusing on a single dominant culture, the emphasis is also on subcultures related to departmental, occupational, specialty, wards, and clinical networks. The potential barriers to cultural change within organizations are described by these authors as lack of ownership, indicating that at some point the employees must buy into the culture change; complexity with consideration to realistic timeframes and attention to subcultures; external influence by paying attention to outside interests that may work against the cultural change needed by the organization; and lack of appropriate leadership highlighting transactional and transformational leadership as to main leadership styles. Two final potential barriers are cultural diversity and the need for careful consideration of the impact of change on specific groups and dysfunctional consequences which describe the sometimes unintended effects and consequences that can cause dysfunction within the organization.

Another sociotechnical approach that supports organizational change is known as High Velocity Organizations.[27] In the context of implementing EMRs, Spear describes three characteristics that make a difference: (1) when they design work, they make clear what they expect will lead to success and assess what may be differing from expectations; (2) work is improved in a disciplined, knowledge-building way; and (3) when leaders and members of high velocity organizations learn something locally, they share discoveries systematically.[28] The approach to organizational change based on Roger's Diffusion Theory was described earlier in the TIGER section of this chapter.

As mentioned previously, the purpose of bringing informatics and technology into organizations and changing the culture is to improve patient safety. Behind the patient safety agenda is the improvement of performance, effectiveness, and even communication.

When these aspects are improved within organizations, patient safety should benefit from these changes. Many of the specifics of organization change that could be identified here are provided in the TIGER Phase II collaborative related to leadership, management, and staff development. Specifics that are particularly relevant to cultural change are addressed in the recommendations from the TIGER Phase I report and more specifically in the TIGER Phase II report which are highlighted elsewhere in this book.

Of course, leadership at executive and middle management levels is a key to organizational culture change. Three chapters highlight the importance of leadership. The work of the TIGER Leadership Collaborative is presented by Judy Murphy and Dana Alexander in Sect. 2, Chap. 9, "Leadership Collaborative." Two more chapters provide perspectives on how critical leadership is to the advancement of technology and informatics. In Sect. 2, Chap. 10, Roy Simpson writes about "Challenging the Leadership Status Quo," and Mark Hagland provides a journalist's perspective in Sect. 4, Chap. 19, "Nursing's Contribution: An External Viewpoint."

Culture Change Framed by Theoretical Models

The use of theoretical models to explore how change related to technology implementation can be implemented is another approach to cultural change. Studies using a variety of theoretical models inform individuals, professional groups, and organizations about the design and, in some cases, the evaluation and testing of different implementation plans. Research conducted regarding adoption of technology also has cultural change implications.

Historically, much of the research framing patient safety is largely theoretical. Karsh[29] advocated for the use of theoretical models to guide and facilitate the adoption of health care systems and technologies, citing motivational theories such as Maslow's needs' classifications and decision-making theories such as Social Cognitive Theory.[30] Other theories involved in decision making include the Theory of Reasoned Action (TRA), the Transtheoretical Model of Change, and the Theory of Planned Behavior (TBI). Strong cases have been made that these models are very good predictors of actual behavior intention and acceptance of the use of technology. These models are used to explore attitudes and organizational support for the decision to participate in behavioral change related to the use of technology.[31,32]

A variety of theoretical models in the literature can guide the process of implementing and creating cultural change related to technological change and acceptance of technology and patient safety. However, the primary theoretical model that is highlighted in the literature is the Technology Acceptance Model (TAM). Models such as TAM are based on human factors engineering science. This includes the study of technology design and evaluation and has been used effectively to assess usability and acceptability of technology. According to Karsh,[29] it is important to understand the impact of new technologies on users, organizations, and work processes. According to TAM, ease of use and usefulness of technology are the key determinants of acceptance. Most of the research using TAM has examined technologies that could be used voluntarily, but in health care the issues of mandatory use have also been assessed. Karsh[29] identified technology characteristics that have a direct and indirect impact on acceptance as response time, flexibility, and breakdowns.

Wu[33] from Taiwan integrated staff training and two additional variables, trust and management support, into the TAM. Three nurses[34] expanded the use and an adaptation of this model called Information and Communication Technology Acceptance Model (ICTAM) to assess consumers' technology acceptance and usage behavior of online health information and related services. In the only article located on theoretical models in nursing, Killeen and King[35] advocated for a common nursing language that would unify nurses worldwide in the use of informatics taxonomies related to King's Goal Attainment Theory.

In addition to TAM, other models identified in the literature as making a difference include Innovation Diffusion Theory and Sociotechnical Systems Theory, both mentioned earlier. All of these theories share a number of patient safety-related factors that help ensure success of implementation based on the following considerations: "first, the system's usefulness; second, the system must be easy to use, intuitive and time-efficient; third, use must be seen as important enough to be adopted by others; and finally, aversive outcomes must be seen as eliminated."[36]

It is important to note two theoretical models that help researchers assess resistance to change or difficulties in implementation: (1) Equity Implementation Theory suggests users compare changes they must make in context of gain or loss in comparison to others within the organization; (2) Attribution Theory assesses external environmental influences and internal interpersonal influences combined with previous successes and failures to determine issues related to resistance and/or barriers to implementation.

Although Innovation Diffusion Theory and Sociotechnical Systems Theory are discussed earlier in this chapter, the concept of innovation is included in the final discussion related to cultural change. In this 4th edition, several chapters are relevant to the use of scholarly models and research findings as a key to culture change. Particularly relevant to this aspect of culture change is Chap. 14 by Nancy Staggers and Michelle Troseth, "Usability and Clinical Design." Another important design aspect of current and future health information systems is the availability of clinical decision support. Chapter 15, "Evidence-Based Clinical Decision Support," also in Sect. 3, by Diane Hansen addresses the value of scholarship and research in building evidence for practice. In the same section, Chap. 13 on "Standards and Interoperability," by Joyce Sensmeier and Elizabeth Haley, is based on scientific exploration of data elements, and as such, holds the key to future comparative effectiveness research. Chapter 20 in Sect. 4 offers a more detailed and futuristic view of comparative effectiveness research in "Transforming Care: Discovery Enabled by Health Information Technology" by Barbara Frink and Asif Dhar. This chapter also examines how personalized medicine can change culture through Innovation as social disruption.

Social (Cultural) Change Through Innovation and Disruption

The final approach to cultural change, the disruption-innovation model, was first mentioned in the *Harvard Business Review* in 1995 and has since been further described by Christensen et al.[37] In this model, disruptive changes are considered catalytic innovators that have five qualities: They (1) create systemic social change through scaling and replication; (2) address a need either overserved or not served at all; (3) offer products and services that are simpler and less costly than existing alternatives; (4) generate resources such as grants, investments, and intellectual capital; and (5) are often ignored or encouraged by existing players in the competitive marketing environment.[37]

In responding to disruptive changes, rather than take a reactive stance to technological change, many companies focus on proactive approaches called "shaping strategies".[38] In the past, technological innovations transformed industry and commerce, and businesses eventually learned to harness the innovation and create stabilizing infrastructures. According to Hagel et al[38], "conventional wisdom holds that in the absence of equilibrium, adaptation is the best strategy." Although acknowledging that rapid change may cause some organizational leaders to magnify risks and experience analysis paralysis, Hagel posits that successful leaders magnify hope and reduce fear, enabling them to take aggressive action in the form of shaping strategies. Two areas involving innovation as social disruption are covered by Frink and Dhar in Chap. 20, when they discussed the potential impact of comparative effectiveness research and personalized medicine on health care, specifically noting how clinical decision support will change as it moves beyond its current base on traditional evidence-based practice research.

A shaping strategy has three elements.[38] The first is shaping the view by altering mindsets. Notably, shapers start with a longer-term view that leaves room for refinement. The second element is the creation of a shaping platform. This involves developing defined standards and practices for activities that support the new direction. Shaping platforms provide leverage for both the shaper and participants. The third element is shaping acts and assets, which requires the shaper to demonstrate commitment in actions and in investment for the long term. The assets of the shaping company become a significant factor in persuading participants to invest time and other resources in the new direction.

The key is to continue to shape the turbulence around the organization or business in order to continue to move beyond the change process. Two examples of this focus on shaping strategies were presented recently at the National Library of Medicine (NLM) conference on the PHR. Despite the lack of consensus among the health professions on what the PHR should look like or accomplish, both Google and Microsoft are already engaged in shaping strategies with their Google Health and Microsoft Vault initiatives. They have been able to attract participants. Google has worked closely with the Cleveland Clinic,[28] and Microsoft Vault[39] has worked closely with the Mayo Clinic. Microsoft has also attracted investments and partners to shape the future in the context of health technology via the VeraChip.[40] This radio frequency identifier (RFID) Health Link microchip provides a PHR that gives emergency room doctors and nurses immediate access to vital medical and emergency contact information rapidly, accurately, and safely during an emergency.[41]

Another example in this category of innovation as social disruption is IndivoHealth, billed as the "world's first personally controlled record system, enabling a patient to own a complete, secure, copy of her medical record, integrating health information across sites of care and over time."[42] Funded by the National Library of Medicine, IndivoHealth is the medical record for Children's Hospital in Boston (Clinical and Public Health Informatics 2009). IndivoHealth is also partnering with vendors such as the Cerner Corporation to make their products compatible.

Sometimes the shaping of strategies in the context of innovation as social disruption is presented as altering mindsets. A prime example of this is the work of Dr. Patricia

Brennan.[43] Project Health Design is a national program designed to rethink the power and potential of PHRs with the intent of stimulating development of personal health management tools. Historically, PHRs were a collection of information from clinical encounters and self-collected observations. The Robert Wood Johnson Foundation provided grants to create a new vision of PHRs that would guide action for health and ultimately engage interdisciplinary providers in using HIT with the patient to improve health. This new record would complement information gathered at the point-of-care and be integrated around the patient, not the provider.

At the 2009 NLM conference on PHRs, Dr. Patricia Brennan[44] presented the new concept from her design team to the audience of experts in the field of PHRs. Challenging them to adopt a new mindset focused on *personal health*, rather than a *record* of encounters with the health care provider, Dr. Brennan focused on the personal health care needs of the person between encounters. The social disruption she proposed offers the nursing profession an opportunity to go back to its roots with a focus on health in the health-illness continuum. Dr. Brennan's concept is ahead of mainstream health informatics, other health care providers, and health care systems. Yet, given the focus from the Obama administration on "health" in health reform, there is potential for true social disruption through this innovative thinking. More on this important topic appears in Sect. 4 on Future Perspectives in Chap. 16, "Personal Health Record (PHR): Managing Personal Health."

Three more innovations promise to disrupt and reshape health care. One is a product by VoCollect[45] that uses voice-assisted technology to enter documentation directly (by voice deployment) into the centralized computer server. Used in long-term care settings and now being launched in acute care settings, this technology reduces the errors inherent in manual data entry and time-stamps interactions with patients. It also extends professional nursing level expertise through improved management, delegation, and follow-up. As an innovative disruption, this technology can change the industrial-like assembly-line care that has dominated nursing care delivery to date and transform nursing care delivery in the future. For a more complete description of this innovative technology, please refer to Chap. 18 in Sect. 4 by Debra Wolf, Amar Kapadia, and Pam Selker Rak, titled "Extending Care: Voice Technology."

Another disruptive innovation that reduces the need for manual interaction with the computer systems is the "neuro-chip." Now being deployed for patients, this has potential for application for the delivery and documentation of nursing care in the future. A technology that fuses brain cells with computer chips,[46] the neuro-chip is a bridge between living organisms and machines. Now being tested with amputees and wounded veterans returning from the Iraq and Afghanistan war zones, it has potential for the treatment of neurological disorders, including pharmaceutical trials testing the effect of drugs on neurons and possibly using a neuron's genetic instructions in treatment and care. Perhaps, like VoCollect, it has a future use with mind/machine connection for nurses and other health care providers to direct thoughts and further reduce the need for manual interaction with computer systems that have created such workflow problems for health care providers.

Another innovation that is already creating social disruption is the use of social media. This innovation is just emerging on the communications, health IT, and health care delivery scene. There are already studies on social media and the potential impact on population health with a focus on several groups. According to Health 2.0,[47] approximately 34% of

Americans turn to social media for health information using online forums, message boards, and other consumer-oriented social media sites. The social media also provide opportunity for social interaction, on twitter and on sites such as Facebook and MySpace.com, where teens, adults, and some cancer patients connect with peers and "patients like me."

According to the Pew Report, *The Social Life of Health Information,*[48] approximately 61% of American adults look online for health information. The Pew report calls these individuals "e-patients." Of these, about two-thirds are between the ages of 18 and 49 and are more likely than older e-patients to use mobile social media. Also, a growing number of social media sites are health-related or provide health information. One site on the internet[49] lists 25 health-related sites including two of the most popular sites, Healthranker, a health news site, and OrganizedWisdom, a health search term site. Other sites include PeoplesMD, a niche site where health and wellness research is shared; FitlLink which provides a workout journal; AmericanWell, the first online house call site; GroupLoop, for teens with cancer; and PatientsLikeMe where patients find others with similar health conditions. On diet-blog.com (2009) there are 35 sites for dieting and health concerns including Healthranker, MyFitBuddy, and support group forums such as 3FatChicks and SparkPeople. Instead of top-down provider-based news and information, for the most part sites like these provide information based on user-generated input. The latest news, research, support, and advice can also be found on many of these social networking sites.

The federal government and progressive provider groups have already identified several populations that can and are benefiting from the use of social media in health care. One such group is adolescents and another group includes those who are overweight and/or obese. It is important to note that women are more frequently research doctors and health professionals online. According to marketingcharts.com,[50] more than half of 25–34 years olds are influenced by social media and the majority of this group's hospital visits are maternity related. These young mothers are a particularly important group from a public health perspective that has been identified for prevention and health promotion social media content and interaction.

The Centers for Disease Control (CDC) and Department of Health and Human Services (HHS) began using social media to communicate and collaborate with providers and the public during the 2009 H1N1 influenza outbreak. At a symposium on "Driving Health IT Through Innovations in Social Media,"[51] speakers from CDC, FDA, Food and Drug Administration (FDA), and National Institutes of Health (NIH) provided information about the use of social media programs in the federal, state, and private health sectors. While some government groups still struggle with social interaction, many grassroots groups and visionaries "get it." These tools allow news and information to flow freely, collaboration to become second-nature, and support that is rapidly becoming as "pandemic as the diseases that threaten today's populations."[49]

In *The Innovator's Prescription,*[52] Christensen identifies three key lessons from the history of disruptive innovation related to health care. "First is that while the technological enablers almost always emerge from leading institutions in the industry, business model innovations do not. Almost always they are forged by new entrants to the industry. The second key lesson is that disruption rarely happens piecemeal, rather new value networks arise, disrupting the old." An example of the second key lesson is the emergence of miniclinics and retail clinics, at Walgreens, Wal-Mart, and elsewhere, that are now moving to be a part of the reimbursement system and seeking legitimatization. Third, there is a pervasive pattern that every industry is transformed through disruption. Finally, Christensen states that the technological enablers of disruption are always successfully employed against the industry's simplest problems first, and then they build commercial and techno-logical momentum. For a similar perspective in this text, read Chap. 17 in Sect. 4 by John Silva, Nancy Seybold, and Marion Ball in their chapter titled, "Disruptive Innovation: Point of Care".

Conclusion

The subtitle of the first three editions of this book was *Where Caring and Technology Meet*. However, this author believed that this 4th edition should be subtitled *Where Technology and Caring Meet*, and the current editors agreed it was time for a change. Since the indus-trial age is clearly in the rear-view mirror and the assembly-line mentality for many indus-tries fades into the distant past, we in health care and many other industries must make a difficult choice. Yes, health care has succumbed over the years to the assembly-line men-tality. We have 15 min office visits for nurse practitioners and physicians with people waiting in line for our care, for our procedures/protocols to "fix the parts," treat the symp-toms of the parts that are damaged or worn-out, clean dirty parts and apply dressings and other treatments to the parts that are broken, and even replace the parts. Even in the acute care setting, our time with this or that patient is "timed" and recorded (or supposed to be) and we move on to the next one. At the end of the "shift," we turn the "keys" over to the next shift of assembly workers. There are supervisors and workers who work in a team to get the patient out of the system according to a timetable on the clinical pathway or accord-ing to standards set through "peer review." This has caused nurses to try to run faster, work harder (not always smarter), and to try to cram more and more into 8–12 h of care.

With the global nursing shortage, even as the worldwide economy recovers, working in the same way into the future is not viable and the "caring" minds, hands, and relationships will be replaced (despite research that shows the higher educated RN is best for patient safety) by more faster, and cheaper hands to move the patient along on the assembly line of treatment in health care "factories." Brennan[44] had it right in her recently funded Robert Wood Johnson initiative on the PHR. Her vision, as mentioned previously, is not about *the record*, but about *personal health*. She envisions nurses caring for the patient during the episodes of care in primary care, acute, home, and long-term care settings, being involved in and facilitating *personal health* in the "in-between spaces." While focusing on the future, nurses need at the same time to look to past roots in home and community-based care.

Dr. Dale Smith, senior vice president of the Uniformed Services University and noted medical historian, would expand this vision to see the person's life as a background matrix and the health care provider (and/or scientific interventions emerging from health-related research) sprinkled throughout to comprise a "finite element matrix" – engaging with the patient's life and health actually one in the same from birth to death (Smith, (2009), Personal communication with Patricia Hinton Walker, 3 June, 2008). Instead of the health care worker being in charge, the person is in charge and needs the wisdom, knowledge, and experience of the health worker to improve quality of life and years of living in a healthy balance with nature and technology. What will it take for our "caring" professions to engage in this future, where we are not in control but truly do see the person who has allowed us to offer our presence to facilitate healing and use technology as our friend to make this happen in close or distant proximity?

Bioinformatic technology will continue development to provide more patient/computer interface. Implantation of neural chips, as mentioned previously, will provide computer support of biological functions and physical movement and possibly cognitive enhancements will be offered by caring professionals. Also, more sophisticated point-of-care devices will be networked and record instantaneously sensor readings and we will not need to "run down the hall" to document what was done on the assembly line today.

However, in the midst of the technological innovation as social disruption is already here and will become more and more dominant into the future, we must seriously engage. Nurses and other health care professionals must get in the front seat and help drive health care to ensure that the caring culture we value remains at its core. A major part of any culture is its history, values, and beliefs. In life, when we do not pay heed, learn, and take the lessons of the past into the future, we are doomed to repeat our past.

Nursing's history must continue to inform our future in the context of technology. First of all, when it came to assisting the nursing profession to make substantive change in its direction and embrace new ideas systematically, it took leadership, advocacy, and a vision for the future and championing actions within and outside nursing. Our founding Mother, Florence Nightingale, set the stage for others to follow. Florence would have been ecstatic if someone had provided a technological solution to monitoring the statistics in hospitals and also the decision support to remind professionals to wash hands between patients. Other key nursing pioneers such as Lillian Wald, Dorothea Dix, Clara Barton, and Mary Breckenridge would be right at the forefront as leaders to help create social disruption by re-envisioning how nursing can provide more health vs. illness care in the future. Lillian Wald would have been very excited about how technology could serve those in poverty and the homeless as in the days of the Henry Street Settlement. Today, she would be voicing concern about health literacy and access to computers for those underserved populations as she struggled to get funding to care for growing number of homeless, uninsured, and underinsured. Along with Lillian Wald, Dorothea Dix would be horrified by the numbers of homeless individuals who are on the streets and are mentally ill. Dorothea, Clara Barton, and Florence Nightingale, given their history of caring for those who serve their countries in times of war, would be particularly horrified with the plight of the number of homeless veterans. Mary Breckenridge would be very concerned about provider access to EMRs and patient/consumer access to PHRs in rural and remote communities and would be knocking on the doors of the policymakers to insist on access for these populations, not only to health care, but also health information and the continuity of care that technology has the potential to provide. Florence and Linda Richards, who earned their diploma as the first trained nurse in America in 1873, would be working diligently alongside the NLN and AACN to see that technology and changes in education would keep up with the changes in practice, so that nurses would be ready to practice effectively sooner when they transition from educational programming to the practice settings. Can you imagine these famous historical leaders taking on health care reform, working with the vendors to insist that nursing relevant data be included in the systems *and* lobbying for patients in all settings to benefit from PHRs?

Additionally, nursing's founding mothers in nursing theory have given us not only theory-based practice, but also theory-guided education and research (Hinton Walker and Redman 1999). These important figures include Neuman, Newman, Roy, Orem, Watson, Leininger, and King, among others.[53] The concepts they defined to organize nursing education, practice, and research are familiar to us all – the patient, client, and now consumer; the health and illness continuum; and the environment and the nurse.

In the context of social disruption, nurses have the opportunity to think ahead to old roles that would seem new. The recipient of our care would no longer be the patient, but the consumer or client. We would shift our focus on the health care continuum from the predominantly episodic and acute care to prevention, wellness, facilitating self care, and primary care with much less emphasis on tertiary care. We would use technology in new ways to assist families and communities in the management of chronic illness and conditions of aging populations. Much of this chapter focuses on the cultural change in the context of a rapidly changing environment, moving from the industrial model of the past to the technological and green ages of the future.

In this time of change, with increasing opportunities for the advanced practice role and caring for diverse populations within families and communities, it is critical that nursing stay connected to its caring roots. Nurses need to maintain the theoretical base that has helped the profession stay connected to the priority of providing holistic care and caring behaviors and relationships. It is important that we continue to bring together (as Betty Neumann would describe it) the physical, developmental, sociocultural, psycho-emotional, and spiritual dimensions of the patient/client, family, and the community. Other theorists have stayed true to holism using different language and paradigms; all have helped to keep nursing connected to its historical roots of caring in the midst of many changing environments and views of health-illness.

In conclusion, nurses must stay anchored in the roots of "caring" and "holism" with values of advocacy as we embrace technology, not trying to limit its boundaries and applications, but again to use the vehicle metaphor, get in the driver's seat, and continue to advocate for systems that record, value, and serve the personal health needs of the individuals, families, communities, and populations we serve locally and globally.

References

1. Technology Informatics Guiding Education Reform. TIGER Summary Report. http://tiger-summit.com/Action_Plan.html; 2007 Accessed 27.03.09.
2. Choudhury I. Culture definition. http://tamu.edu/classes/cosc/choudhury/culture.html; 2009 Accessed 6.10.09.
3. Wikipedia. Social Structure. http://www.answers.com/topic/socialcultural-evolution; 2009a Accessed 7.06.09.
4. Wikipedia. Socio-technical Systems Theory. http://www.answers.com/topic/sociotechnical-systems-theory; 2009b Accessed 6.10.09.

5. Love J. Seven keys to success in the information age. http://ezinearticles.com/?Seven-Keys-To-Success-In-The-Information-Age&id=51948; 2005 Accessed 7.06.09.
6. Suominen T, Kovasin M, Ketola O. Nursing culture – some viewpoints. *J Adv Nurs.* 1997;25(1):186-191.
7. Wikipedia. Timeline of nursing history. http://en.wikipedia.org/wiki/Timeline_of_nursing_history; 2009c Accessed 27.05.09.
8. Reddi V. Dorothea Lynde Dix 1802–1887. www.nursingadvocacy.org/press/pioneers/dix.html; 2005 Accessed 6.10.09.
9. Castlenovo G. Mary Breckenridge 1881–1965. www.nursingadvocacy.org/press/pioneers/dix.html; 2003 Accessed 6.10.09.
10. Harris JC. Toward a restorative medicine – the science of care. *JAMA.* 2009;301(16):1710-1712.
11. Vance T. Caring and the professional practice of nursing. RN Journal. http://rnjournal.com/journal_of_nursing/caring.htm; 2009 Accessed 29.05.09.
12. Watson J. Watson's theory of transpersonal caring. In: Walker PH, Neuman B, eds. *Blueprint for use of Nursing Models: Education, Research, Practice, and Administration.* New York: National League for Nursing Press; 1996:141-184.
13. Rocks S. Technology – definition and usage. http://hubpages.com/hub/technology-definition-and-usage; 2009 Accessed 6.05.09.
14. Kilbridge PM, Classen DC. Informatics opportunities: the intersection of patient safety and clinical informatics. *J Am Med Inform Assoc.* 2008;15(4):397-407.
15. McBride AB. Nursing and the informatics revolution. *Nurs Outlook.* 2005;53:183-191.
16. Wikipedia. Diffusion of innovations. Last modified 9 May 2008. http://en.wikipedia.org/wiki/diffusion_of_Innovations; 2008 Accessed 7.06.09.
17. Simon SI. Implementing culture change – three strategies http://www.culturechange.com/3strategies.pdf; 1990 Accessed 7.05.09.
18. Staggers N, Thompson CB. The evolution of definitions for nursing informatics. *J Am Med Inform Assoc.* 2002;9(3):255-261.
19. allnursingschools.com (2009) A nursing informatics career at a glance. Nursing informatics: learn about nurse informatics education & careers. http://www.allnursingschools.com. Accessed 6.06.09.
20. Ball M, Weiners W. Nurses: critical members of the IT team. Healthcare Inform. http://www.highbeam.com/doc/1P3-1108573941.html; 2006 Accessed 6.06.09.
21. Hebert M. A national education strategy to develop nursing informatics competencies. *Can J Nurs Leadersh.* 2000;13(2):11-14.
22. Schein EH. *Organizational Culture and Leadership.* 2nd ed. San Francisco, CA: Jossey-Bass; 1992.
23. Nellen T. Organizational culture and leadership by Edgar H. Schein. Notes compiled by Ted Nellen. http://www.tnellen.com/ted/tc/schein.html; 1997 Accessed 2.05.09.
24. Lorenzi NM, Riley RT, Blyth AJC, et al. *J Am Med Inform Assoc.* 1997;4(2):79-93.
25. Cutliffe SH. *New Worlds, New Technologies, New Issues.* Bethlehem, PA: Lehigh University Press; 1992.
26. Scott T, Mannion R, Davis H, et al. Implementing culture change in health care: theory and practice. *Int J Qual Health Care.* 2003;15:111-118.
27. Spear S. Chasing the rabbit: official blog on electronic medical records, evidence-based medicine, and high velocity organizations. http://chasingtherabbittbook.mhprofessional.com/apps/ab/209/01/09/electronicmedicalrecords; 2009 Accessed 29.05.09.
28. Lohr S. Google offers personal health records on the web. http://www.nytimes.com/2008/05/20/technology/20google.html; 2008 Accessed 28.05.09.
29. Karsh BT. Beyond usability: designing effective technology implementation systems to promote patient safety. *Qual Saf Health Care.* 2004;13:388-394.

30. Bandura A. *Social foundations of thought and action: a social cognitive theory*. Englewood Cliffs: Prentice-Hall; 1986.
31. Ajzen I. The theory of planned behavior. *Organ Behav Hum Decis Process*. 1991;50: 179-211.
32. Godin G, Kok G. The theory of planned behavior: a review of its applications to health-related behaviors. *Am J Health Promot*. 1996;11:87-98.
33. Wu JH, Shen WS, Lin LM, et al. Testing the technology acceptance model for evaluating healthcare professionals' intention to use an adverse event reporting systems. *Int J Qual Health Care*. 2008;20(2):123-129.
34. An JY, Hayman LL, Panniers T, et al. Theory development in nursing and healthcare informatics: a model explaining and predicting information and communication technology acceptance by healthcare consumers. *Adv Nurs Sci*. 2007;30:7-49.
35. Killeen MB, King IM. Viewpoint: use of King's conceptual system, nursing informatics and nursing classification systems for global communication. http://highbeam.com/doc/1P3-130482237.html; 2007 Accessed 6.06.09.
36. Holden RJ, Karsh B. A theoretical model of health information technology behavior. *Behavior and Information Technology*. 2009;28(1):21-38.
37. Christensen CM, Baumann H, Ruggles R, et al. (2006) Disruptive innovation for social change. Harvard Bus Rev. Reprint R0612E. www.hbr.org; 2006 Accessed 23.05.09.
38. Hagel J, Brown JS, Davison L. Shaping strategy in a world of constant disruption. Harvard Business Review, Oct. Reprint R0801E. www.hbr.org; 2008 Accessed 23.05.09.
39. Mintz J. Microsoft launches health records site. Posted 11:29 a.m. 10/4/2007. http://www.usatoday.com/tech/webguide/2007-10-04-microsoft-healthvault-n.htm; 2007 Accessed 2.05.09.
40. VeriChip Corporation (2008) selected by Microsoft to Offer Personal Health Record through Microsoft HealthVault. http://www.tradingmarkets.com/.site/news/Stock%20News/2028610/; 2008 Accessed 29.05.09.
41. Didnan L. Verichip goes Consumer with its implantable RFID chips; would you buy? Posted @ 6:06 a.m. Between the Lines. April 22, 2008. http://blogs.zdnet.com/BTL?p=8567; 2008 Accessed 28.05.09.
42. IndivoHealth. The Personally Controlled Health Record. http://indivohealth.org/; 2009 Accessed 29.05.09.
43. Brennan PF, Downs S, Casper G, et al. Project HealthDesign: stimulating the next generation of personal health records. AMIA Annual Symposium Proceedings. http://www.pubmedcentral.nih.gov/articlerender.fcgi?artid=2655909; 2007 Accessed 28.05.09.
44. Brennan P. Developing and testing personal health records. Slide presentation at Friends of the National Library of Medicine Conference on Personal Health Records, May 21, 2009. http://fnlm.org/Conference_Program_2009.html; 2009.
45. VoCollect Healthcare Systems. http://www.vocollectcom/index.php/about/vocollect-healthcare-systems; 2009 Accessed 29.05.09.
46. Than K. Brain cells fused with computer chip. Live Science. http://www.livescience.com/health/060327neurochipshtml; 2006 Accessed 29.05.09.
47. Health 2.0 Blog. http://www.health2blog.com/2008/01/people-who-need.html; 2008 Accessed 25.09.09.
48. Fox S. The social life of health information. http://www.pewinternet.org/Reports/2009/8-The-Social-Life-of-Health-Information.aspx; 2009 Accessed 15.07.09.
49. Medicine 3.0. 25 excellent social media sites for your health. http://nursingassistantguides.com/2009/25-excellent-social-media-sites-for-your-health/; 2009 Accessed 25.09.09.
50. Marketingcharts.com. One in four hospital, urgent care patients influenced by social media http://www.marketingcharts.com/television/one-in-four-hospital-urgent-care-patients-influenced-by-social-media;2009 Accessed 5.10.09.

51. Amplify Public Affairs (2009) Driving the adoption of health IT through innovations in social media. http://www.socialmediahit.com/agenda-july-16th-2009/h1n1-influenza Accessed 5.09.09.
52. Christensen C, Grossman JH, Hwang J. *The Innovator's Prescription: A Disruptive Solution for Health Care*. New York: McGraw-Hill; 2008.
53. Hinton Walker P, Neuman B. *Blueprint for nursing models*. New York: National League for Nursing Press; 1996.
54. Biography.com. Lillian D. Wald Biography. http://www.biography.com/articles/Lillian-D.-Wald-9521707; 2007 Accessed 27.05.09.
55. Clinical and Public Health Informatics. Intelligent Health Lab@ CHIP (children's Hospital Informatics program. http://chip.org/research/ig.htm; 2008 Accessed 29.05.09.
56. Foster J. 35+ social media sites for the health conscious. http://www.diet-blog.com/archives/2008/02/29/35_social_media_sites_for_the_health_conscious.php; 2008 Accessed 25.09.09.
57. Hinton Walker P, Redman R. Theory-guided evidence-based reflective practice. *Nurs Sci Q*. 1999;12(3):298-303.

TIGER Collaboratives and Diffusion

Diane J. Skiba and Donna DuLong

The Technology Informatics Guiding Education Reform (TIGER) Initiative started with a passionate dinner discussion among informatics colleagues after the announcement of the Office of the National Coordinator of Health Information Technology. These colleagues were determined to insure that nurses had the necessary knowledge and skills to practice in the "Decade of Health Information Technology" as it was being defined in July of 2004. From this conversation, a planning meeting was held in January of 2005 at Johns Hopkins University School of Nursing. The planning meeting brought together informatics colleagues from academia, health care institutions, the vendor community, and other federal entities. Many ideas were exchanged, but perhaps the most influential was from Dr. Angela McBride, who noted that the informatics community had many accomplishments but as a community we had not engaged our nursing colleagues. If we truly wanted to reach our goal of insuring that all nurses were prepared to practice, it was essential for us to engage the broader nursing community. Thus, the mission of TIGER was defined – to bring together leaders from various nursing specialty organizations to coalesce and create a vision plus an informatics agenda for the next 3 years and 10 years. This mission involved bringing together the intellectual and social capital of these specialty organizations with the informatics community to create an informatics agenda.

Intellectual and Social Capital

Throughout the literature on organizations, businesses, and communities, there are numerous articles explicating the various forms of capital associated with these entities. There can be physical, human, intellectual, and social capital. Each of these forms of capital contributes to the overall productivity and success of an organization or community. These forms of capital have become increasingly more important as society has progressed into the world of knowledge management. Specifically, the TIGER Initiative explored the use of intellectual and social capital to set and move forward an informatics agenda.

D.J. Skiba (✉)
University of Colorado Denver, College of Nursing, Aurora, CO, USA
e-mail: diane.skiba@ucdenver.edu

M.J. Ball et al. (eds.), *Nursing Informatics*,
DOI: 10.1007/978-1-84996-278-0_3, © Springer-Verlag London Limited 2011

According to the online business dictionary, intellectual capital is "the collective knowledge of individuals in an organization or society. This knowledge can be used to produce wealth, multiply output of physical assets, gain competitive advantage, and/or to enhance value of other types of capital. Intellectual capital includes customer capital, human capital, intellectual property, and structural capital." (http://www.businessdictionary.com/definition/intellectual-capital.html). Nahapiet and Ghoshal[1] also defined this term in a similar fashion by clearly relating it to the concept of human capital. Their definition is as follows, "Intellectual capital thus represents a valuable resource and a capability for action based in knowledge and knowing" (p. 245).[1]

More recently, Edvinsson and Malone[2] acknowledged that intellectual capital was composed of two major elements: *human capital* (the value of knowledge, skills, and experiences held by individuals) and *structural capital* (the underlying supportive infrastructure of human capital). Many, including McElroy[3] and Lesser,[4] noted that intellectual capital was necessary but not sufficient for increasing value and knowledge in an organization. There was an additional component, social capital that clearly added the value of relationships to the equation.

Social Capital is not a new idea. Its origin dates back to 1915. According to Cohen and Prusak,[5] the term was first introduced in a discussion on school community centers and was ultimately used by sociologists to describe neighborhoods and the growth of cities. In the 1970s, the term was used in relation to the development of social network and communities. Coleman,[6] in particular, argued that these networks along with their norms and values promulgated the idea that social capital contributes to the development of cultures and organizations. In the 1990s, it was Putnam's work that introduced the idea of the political and economic value of social capital that was later adopted by the World Bank. As more writings surfaced talking about knowledge management, the value of social capital began to increase. According to Cohen and Prusak[5] (p. 7), "we are beginning to discover the centrality of social interaction – of trust, personal networks and communities – to work of virtually all kinds." Wenger[7] also deemed social interactions among workers as an integral component in his work on communities of practice. Thus, social capital has evolved to include the missing ingredient of social relationships.

Here are some of the recent definitions.

> Social capital consists of the work of active connections among people: the trust, mutual understanding, and shared values and behaviors that bind the members of human networks and communities and make cooperative action possible (p. 4).[5]

> Social capital refers to connections among individuals – social networks and the norms of reciprocity and trustworthiness that arise from them. In other words, interaction enables people to build communities, to commit themselves to each other, and to knit the social fabric (p. 19).[8]

> Social capital is defined by its function. It is not a single entity, but a variety of entities with two elements in common: social structure and the actions of actors within the structure. Unlike other forms of capital, social capital inheres in the structure of relations between and among actors (persons).

Although there are other definitions,[9] these three have some common themes: trust, social norms, and social connections among people are key ingredients and that the interactions between people build the community that binds or knits the social fabric. Several authors[4,10] have noted that social capital has these three components: trust, norms, and networks. Trust is a key ingredient, and it is developed over time. Continuous interactions facilitate the development of trust and trust can be transferred within the network.[11] Norms, especially social norms, are defined "as shared understandings, informal rules and conventions that prescribe, proscribe or modulate certain behaviors in various circumstances" (p. 9).[12] According to Landry et al,[10] the norm that is most often mentioned in the literature on social capital is reputation of trustworthiness. In the case of social capital, the social norm is to contribute productively to sharing of knowledge and ideas for the greater good rather than retaining the knowledge for their individual opportunities.[4,10] Lastly, "a network is an interconnected group of people who usually have an attribute in common" (p. 9).[12] These networks or communities of practice help to facilitate the interactions among the actors so that trust can evolve and that norms can be spread across the network. As Huysman and Wulf[13] (p.6) stated, "investing in social capital means that long-term benefits such as social networks based on mutuality, trust, respect and appreciation will last much longer than engineered network such as organizational teams."

Lesser[4] noted that the recent focus on social capital is primarily being motivated by two drivers. The first is the growth of knowledge-based organizations. As knowledge becomes the "primary source of competitive advantage in the market, the ability to create new knowledge, share existing knowledge and apply organizational knowledge to new situations becomes critical"[4] (p. 9). The second driver is the rise in a networked economy.

Knowledge Management and Leadership

There is a fundamental shift in thinking about managing knowledge as a result of the combination of social capital and communities of practice.[14] According to Huysman and Wulf,[13] the first wave of knowledge management focused on human capital – gaining our individual knowledge, supporting individual capabilities to act on this knowledge, and learning. The goal centered on supporting the exchange of human capital to avoid knowledge redundancy and to fill in knowledge gaps.[15] What was missing from this form of knowledge management was the acknowledgment that people wanted to share their knowledge and learn from each other. Thus, the second wave of knowledge management focused on the addition of social capital where a group uses mechanisms such as social networks, trust, reciprocity, and shared norms and values to facilitate collaboration and cooperation.[13]

In the late 1980s and early 1990s, informatics as a discipline was clearly in the first wave of knowledge management. The focus was on the development of a discipline and that being recognized as a clinical specialty. The work focused on defining nursing informatics and distinguishing itself from medical informatics. It was the time when the roles and responsibilities of nursing informatics specialists were articulated in the Scope and Standards of Practice published by the American Nurses Association (ANA). The development required the conduct of research and the generation of knowledge. In this phase, the informatics community was very insular and not well connected to the larger nursing community. The informatics community had its own network for knowledge development and sharing, but it did not cross the boundaries to the larger nursing community. The larger nursing community was unaware of the accomplishments in informatics and did not understand the discipline. In many instances, the discipline was equated solely with computer technology. Many in the nursing community viewed computer technology as a means to replace nurses.

As we examine the TIGER initiative, it is apparent that the informatics community has embraced the second wave of knowledge management where communities advance social capital as a means to share knowledge and develop a network of trust to further collaboration of a shared agenda. What follows is a description of the various components of the TIGER Initiative and how intellectual and social capital combined to create an informatics agenda for the nursing community.

The TIGER Initiative

An outcome of our first planning meeting in 2005 was the creation of TIGER's mission. Dr. Angela McBride shaped our mission by acknowledging that although nursing informatics had a lot of accomplishments, the discipline was invisible to the nursing community. There was a need to engage the nursing community as a whole, if the goal was to insure that all nurses were prepared to practice in a consumer-centric, informatics-intensive environment. Thus, the mission of TIGER was to bring together leaders from various nursing specialty organizations to coalesce and create a vision plus an informatics agenda. This mission required bringing together the intellectual and social capital of the nursing community with the informatics community to not only create an informatics agenda, but to carry forward this agenda in all aspects of nursing.

To accomplish this mission, an invitational conference was considered the most effective strategy to bring the two communities together. Since there is no one organization to represent nursing's voice, it was important to determine the most efficacious method to get nursing representation. To this end, the Nursing Organization Alliance (NOA) served as a basis for the initial invitations. To insure there was broad nursing representation, invitations were sent to elected leaders (Chair, President or their designees) or Executive Directors of the numerous specialty organizations represented in NOA. Additionally, other specialty organizations were solicited from the TIGER executive committee and its corresponding committees. If we were to reach the majority of practicing nurses in the country, we needed representation that reached beyond the nursing informatics community and represented the majority of nursing stakeholders. Therefore, the summit invitations were focused on creating a representative list of nursing leaders who had the social capital within their respective organizations to reach most nursing professionals. To that end, invitations were also sent to representatives from key federal agencies (Veteran's Administration, Military, and Division of Nursing, Health Services Resources Administration) and industry. There was one rule enforced during the invitation process. There should be more nurse representatives in attendance than informatics representatives.

The TIGER Summit

Over 100 participants attended the TIGER Summit in October 2006. The participants represented 39 different specialty organizations, leaders from the informatics organizations, vendor representatives, and leaders from various federal agencies, the military, and other nonprofit organizations. There were also representatives from the National Library of Medicine, American Dietetics Association, and the American Health Information Management Association (AHIMA). A decision was reached early in the selection of the invitees that this summit would focus on nursing rather than inviting a variety of disciplines. The rationale for this was to build upon our shared norms such as the commitment to provide safe and quality care to all patients throughout the continuum of care. Each of the participants had an equal vote during the summit, and each organization represented had the social capital and infrastructure to disseminate TIGER's activities afterwards. The goal was to use the organization's social capital to share knowledge.

External consultants used open-space facilitation to guide the community to reach consensus about a vision and an action plan. Diverse members from various health care sectors, specialty, and informatics organizations were divided into small work groups. The small group work fostered interactions and allow for building trust across the diverse community members. To start the summit, a structured experience called a gallery walk allowed all the attendees to experience state-of-the-art demonstrations of the latest health information technologies. This inquiry-based gallery walk provided an opportunity for all participants to create a shared knowledge base. It also provided an opportunity for small groups to begin to share their knowledge and experiences. To help the large group come to consensus, interactive audience response systems were used for voting. The use of these anonymous voting systems allowed the community to acknowledge all ideas and build their trust with the community.

At the conclusion of the Summit, the attendees developed a vision statement and action plan to be completed within the next 3 years. The TIGER vision has two pillars:

Allow informatics tools, principles, theories and practices to be used by nurses to make health care safer, effective, efficient, patient-centered, timely, and equitable.
Interweave enabling technologies transparently into nursing practice and education, making information technology the stethoscope for the twenty-first century.

To achieve this vision, summit attendees defined specific activities that should be completed within 3 years for each of the pillars and ranked the priorities of these activities using a wireless audience response system.

Management and Leadership

The TIGER attendees envisioned *revolutionary leadership that drives, empowers, and executes the transformation of health care* as the highest priority of the TIGER Summit. In order to achieve this outcome, the attendees recommended that the industry identifies

strategies for increasing the power, influence, and presence of nursing on health information technology (HIT)-related activities. Building upon the social capital in their professional organization, nurses can influence colleagues as well as governmental and legal
bodies. As national attention remains focused on health care reform enabled through the
use of HIT, there are numerous activities for nurses to lead and participate in public discussions, forums, and policy committees. To initiate this action, the attendees recommended
publication and widespread dissemination of the TIGER Summit report to nursing leaders,
especially through professional networking organizations. Another recommended strategy
was to highlight educational programs for nursing leaders that emphasize informatics and
information management competencies.

Education

Education reform, targeted at all levels of nursing preparation, remains the primary purpose of the TIGER Initiative. The participants described their vision for education as *collaborative learning communities that maximize the possibilities of technology toward
knowledge development and dissemination, driving rapid deployment and implementation
of best practices.* To accomplish these goals, the participants suggested numerous strategies starting with acquiring funding to develop and implement learning innovations, fostering faculty development, and ensuring necessary infrastructure. Faculty acceptance of
technology, a critical success factor, will require education and training, incentives, and
necessary support. Integrating computer competencies, information literacy, information
management, and informatics will require nursing curriculum reform and the infusion of
technologies for learning. New collaborative partnerships among public and private academic, service, and industry enterprises will be required to provide ongoing access to new
technologies. In addition, the participants recommended that a national group be convened
to develop strategies for the recruitment, retention, and training of current and future work-
forces in informatics education, practice, and research.

Communication and Collaboration

As nurses are central to communication and collaboration with other members of the health
care team, the participants envisioned *standardized, person-centered, technology-enabled
processes to facilitate teamwork and relationships across the continuum of care.* Nursing
needs to work with all other stakeholders to establish, disseminate, and support a shared
vision, core values, and goals related to the use of HIT. One of the best ways to achieve this
objective is through the use of demonstration projects that model collaborative relationships across the continuum of care. Other examples are local TIGER teams or regional
sharing among practice, education, and research teams. The industry would benefit from
the publication and dissemination of the successes and failures of these demonstration
programs and establish replicable models for others to follow.

Informatics Design

The TIGER Summit attendees acknowledged that HIT does not fully support state-of-the-art and the science of nursing practice. However, they were able to describe their future HIT vision as *evidence-based, interoperable intelligence systems that support education and practice to foster quality care and safety.* Nurses, by involving themselves in future informatics design, will have a crucial role in helping to realize this vision. In addition, it is necessary to include multidisciplinary end-users in the design and integration/incorporation of informatics that is intuitive, affordable, usable, responsive, and evidence-based across the continuum of care. Future HIT systems must be designed that promote the mining and use of data for analysis, clinical decision making, and measurement to improve the quality of care. This will require the creation and implementation of multidisciplinary, multilingual standards. Best practices can be shared with others by developing guidelines for integrating informatics infrastructure, including but not limited to intelligence systems, IT hardware architecture, data documentation and warehousing, universal database, and portals of knowledge.

Information Technology

A clear vision for health IT emerged as *smart, people-centered, affordable technologies that are universal, useable, useful, and standards-based.* This demands the integration of interoperability IT standards to clinical standards in both practice and education. A strong need exists to educate practice and education communities on IT standards and establish hard deadlines for adoption. The need for security, privacy, and interoperable systems must drive the ongoing development and implementation of standards across all health care settings, and nurses must be at the table to prioritize, develop, and evaluate all standards development efforts.

Policy

The attendees envisioned policy needs related to HIT as *consistent, incentives-based initiatives (organizational and governmental) that support advocacy and coalition-building, achieving, and resourcing an ethical culture of safety.* Above all, this will require nurses' involvement in a National Health IT agenda, congressional testimony, and participation in policy decisions at all levels toward technology that supports ethical, safe patient care. Nursing must have a strong, unified voice to endorse consistent, agreed-upon IT standards. Other priorities include obtaining funding for curriculum expansion, research, and practice in nursing informatics and HIT, as well as identifying incentives that support the adoption of innovative technologies. Finally, the attendees support the use of a personal health record (PHR) for every person in the United States.

At the end of the summit, each leader was asked to identify action plan goals that could be accomplished by their particular organization. Each leader signed the Commitment Wall (see Fig. 3.1) acknowledging their pledge to share the work of this Summit and to promote that the TIGER action plans be incorporated into their organization's strategic goals.

The postsummit activities were designed to build upon the intellectual capital of the various organizations. The participants developed a common vision and action plan to share with their respective organizations through the use of their established social networks. The voice of nursing was strengthened by having all organizations deliver the same, clear message to their constituents that nurses need to be prepared for the decade of health information technology. Thus, the social capital of the professional organizations was harnessed to advance the TIGER agenda. This dramatically changed the industry dynamic, as it was no longer just an agenda being espoused by informatics professionals, but one that was supported by the profession of nursing.

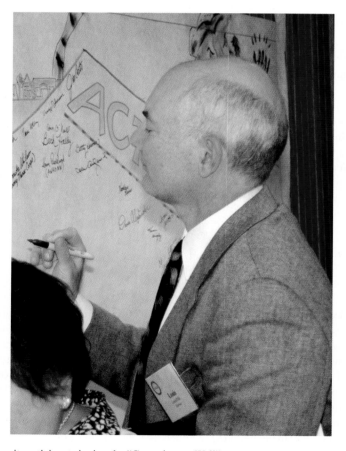

Fig. 3.1 Summit participant signing the "Commitment Wall"

The TIGER Summit Report

The work of the summit was widely disseminated in the summary report, "Evidence and Informatics Transforming Nursing: 3-Year Action Steps toward a 10-Year Vision,"[16] available online at http://www.tigersummit.com. The report published the action plan with a series of recommendations targeted to various audiences: professional nursing organizations, nursing education, information technology vendors, government and policy makers, health care delivery organization, health information management professionals, and health sciences librarians.

The most critical aspect of moving the TIGER agenda forward was put into motion. In order to reach the entire nursing community and achieve the TIGER vision, the agenda and action plan had to engage the broader nursing community through the social networks already established. Each of the participants committed to taking the TIGER vision to their members and implementing an action plan. As Putnam[8] acknowledged, the real value of social capital is the degree to which the message is circulated among the professional nursing organizations.

TIGER Phase II

As the 70 organizations that participated in the TIGER Summit started to integrate the action steps into their organization's strategy and disseminate the TIGER Summit Summary Report within their network, it became clear that TIGER needed to organize and leverage the groundswell of industry support. Phase II of TIGER was initiated 6 months after the TIGER Summit. Phase II was designed to harness the efforts of hundreds of additional volunteers and industry experts that joined TIGER, as well as better support the activities of the participating organizations. A proliferation of TIGER-related articles and presentations at regional, national, and international conferences raised the awareness of the need to engage nurses in the national effort to prepare the health care workforce toward *effective adoption of electronic health records*. The TIGER action plan was reorganized into nine key areas, and nine TIGER collaborative teams were formed. They include:

1. Standards and Interoperability
2. National Health Information Technology (IT) Agenda
3. Informatics Competencies
4. Education and Faculty Development
5. Staff Development
6. Usability and Clinical Application Design
7. Virtual Demonstration Center
8. Leadership Development
9. Consumer Empowerment and Personal Health Record

Each collaborative team was assigned coleaders with particular expertise in their area of focus. Members of the collaborative teams were recruited from the participating organizations, bringing a diverse set of interests and backgrounds to each team and helping to accelerate the progress within the organizations.

The goals set forth by each collaborative team were addressed from the overall perspective of "What does every practicing nurse need to know about this topic?" The teams identified resources, references, gaps, and areas that need further development and provided recommendations for the industry to accelerate the adoption of health IT for nursing. All teams started by building upon and recognizing the work of organizations, programs, research, and related initiatives in the academic, practice, and government sector within their topic area.

Each of the nine collaborative teams developed their own wikis, similar to a website, to share information. The wikis were used as a project workspace and resource to communicate among the team, to other collaborative teams, and with the public. Most of the communication with the teams was done via webinars, or web meetings, teleconferences, electronic surveys, and email lists. The idea of shared space and public dissemination were indicators of the trust and reciprocity developed within each of the collaborative teams. A TIGER Advisory Council, comprised of the collaborative leaders and the program director, met monthly to coordinate activities and review progress. By early 2009, over 1,500 individuals had joined the TIGER effort and are helping to achieve the TIGER vision throughout the health care community. The diverse communities that make up the TIGER Initiative accomplished most of this outreach.

Collaborative Team Results

After 15 months of virtual work, the nine collaborative teams developed recommendations focused on raising awareness with nursing stakeholders in three areas:

1. Workforce development
2. Improve technology used by nurses
3. Engage nurses in HIT policy discussions

A comprehensive summary of these recommendations, as well as the detailed report for each collaborative team, can be found on the TIGER website at http://www.tigersummit. com. In addition, each collaborative team has described their efforts in respective chapters of this book. In this chapter, we describe the impact of the collaborative teams and how they used social and intellectual capital to move the TIGER agenda forward.

The collaborative work was critical in bringing more focus and momentum to the TIGER activities. It is impossible to develop widespread nursing support for an agenda defined at one meeting; continual contact with the participants is necessary to support their respective efforts and refine the action plan to keep up with changes in the health care landscape. As Lesser[4] (p.8) states, "social capital requires maintenance to remain productive." It was also necessary to build trusting relationships among the professional organizations. It was also important to recognize the changing landscapes of health care, technology, and the economy. Since 2004, health care reform and the national push for adopting electronic health record have accelerated with a new administration putting financial incentives and penalties in place to ensure compliance. New studies that correlate a higher rate of mortality and morbidity in hospitalized patients with a lower skill mix of nursing continues to challenge nursing leaders facing an impending workforce shortage. In the midst of a severe economic downturn, the emphasis on providing safe, high quality, effective patient care will continue to be at the forefront of the political agenda and the media's attention. It is even more important today to ensure that the nursing workforce has the necessary technology and informatics skills to use HIT effectively and efficiently to enhance nursing practice.

TIGER Impact

The social capital within different communities impacted the dissemination strategies and mechanisms used to gain support within their members. Organizations had a unique opportunity to participate in a variety of activities and methodologies. Some of the examples are listed below, although as momentum builds it is possible to anticipate that new techniques will develop.

Nursing Informatics Community

Nursing informatics organizations embraced the opportunity to support the TIGER agenda within the industry. The American Medical Informatics Association (AMIA) and Healthcare Information and Management Systems Society (HIMSS) organized TIGER presentations at several national, regional, and international conferences. The Alliance for Nursing Informatics (ANI), an umbrella organization for the nursing informatics community, provided financial and strategic support to TIGER for the collaborative teams. Nursing informatics organizations such as CARING, American Nursing Informatics Association (ANIA), MInnesota Nursing INformatics Group (MINING), and New England Nursing Informatics Consortium (NENIC) not only welcomed TIGER presentations at their meetings, but also were essential for distributing TIGER surveys and requests for information, and they were active participants on the collaborative workgroups.

Practice Specialty Community

Specialty organizations also presented on TIGER at their regional and national conferences. For example, the Association of periOperative Registered Nurses (AORN), the National Association of Clinical Nurse Specialists (NACNS), and the Oncology Nursing Society (ONS) accepted TIGER presentations at their national conferences. Many participating organizations also presented on TIGER at specialized conferences within their organizations, such as state chapter meetings or conferences focused on technology. Numerous articles were published in journals distributed to nurses, including Nursing

Outlook, CIN (computers, informatics, nursing), Nursing Management, and Journal of Health Information Management. Several organizations published articles in their member newsletters or journals, including the American Society of Peri-Anesthesia Nurses (ASPAN), Association of Women's Health, Obstetric and Neonatal Nurses (AWHONN), and the ONS. Ongoing work within the specialty organizations is planned. For instance, the National Nursing Staff Development Organization (NNSDO) has plans to further develop the informatics competencies recommendations. The AHIMA is planning a similar conference to engage allied health professionals in adopting informatics competencies.

Nursing Leadership Community

Nursing leadership organizations provided critical support for TIGER, enhancing visibility and access to nursing executives. The ANA supported TIGER on several committees and provided strategic support through the ANI. The American Nurses Credentialing Center, a division of ANA, scheduled a TIGER workshop at their National Magnet™ Conference, as did Sigma Theta Tau International (STTI). AONE provided access to nurse executives for the TIGER Leadership survey and also facilitated TIGER presentations at both state and national conferences. Long-term care nurse executives contributed numerous articles and presentations related to technology and the TIGER effort through their alliance with the National Association Directors of Nursing Administration in Long Term Care (NADONA/LTC). The American Academy of Nursing (AAN) publishes a monthly column on technology and devoted an entire issue of Nursing Outlook to nursing informatics.

Educational Community

Nearly a fourth of the leaders and participants on the TIGER collaborative teams came from the academic community. As described in the TIGER Education and Faculty Development Collaborative Case Study, all major stakeholders were active participants in the TIGER action plan. Numerous presentations to this community were done at national, state, and local levels. The two major nursing education organizations, National League for Nursing and the American Association for Colleges of Nursing, were responsive to insuring that informatics competencies were incorporated into nursing educational programs. Academic partnerships with industry are proliferating, and the National League for Nursing is helping to foster faculty development in informatics through the development of a faculty toolkit. The Health Resources and Services Administration (HRSA) Division of Nursing has also funded seven faculty development collaboratives through their Integrating Technology into Nursing Education and Practice Initiative. There were also many statewide initiatives to bring together academia with nursing practice to address informatics challenges. Minnesota developed a statewide approach to TIGER – bringing together stakeholders in an annual Minnesota TIGER conference. Other states have also brought together the key organizations to discuss issues related to the preparation of nurses with informatics knowledge and skills, including Massachusetts (Massachusetts Organization of Nurse Executives), North California, and California.

Vendor Community

Health care IT vendors that develop technology were active with TIGER in numerous ways. Many of the leaders of the TIGER collaborative teams were supported by the vendor community. The vendor sponsors of the TIGER Summit developed an interactive "Gallery Walk" to demonstrate technology capabilities to the attendees and supplied demonstrations and presentations to the TIGER Virtual Demonstration Center. Several vendors, such as GE Healthcare, McKesson, Cerner, CPM Resource Center, and others, presented TIGER at their user group conferences or via webinars focused on their nursing community.

The above examples demonstrate how the TIGER grassroots effort was able to capitalize on the intellectual capital from numerous organizations to leverage their social capital to promote an informatics agenda. "The success of the TIGER Initiative will depend largely upon the extent to which the social capital of the broader nursing community is leveraged. The shared values and rules for social conduct expressed in personal relationships, trust, and a common sense of "civic" responsibility within the nursing community creates the "common voice" and makes nursing more than just a collection of individuals",[15] (p.16). It was apparent at the end of this phase that the informatics agenda was a joint effort between the nursing and informatics communities.

Lessons Learned

Several strategies promoted the success of the TIGER initiative. These learnings can serve as a guide for others who want to harness the power of intellectual and social capital to influence policy decisions and move an agenda forward.

1. *It is essential to clearly identify the beneficiary (or target) of the agenda.* In the case of the TIGER Initiative, the entire nursing workforce served to benefit if successful. Historically, nursing informatics specialists were both the driving force and the perceived target for education of technology and informatics. Widespread adoption of EHRs demands that all nurses need health IT knowledge and skills, thus widening the target to all practicing nurses.
2. *All stakeholders, especially the beneficiaries, need to be represented and included in the creation of the agenda.* Their buy-in will be critical to the success of the program. For the TIGER Initiative, it was difficult to find one nursing organization that was truly representative of the needs of all nursing professionals. Historically, nurses participate in professional organizations that are linked to their specialty practice (e.g., critical care, peri-operative, nurse executives, clinical nurse specialists, oncology, obstetric, nurse practitioners, educators, etc.). Each of these different nursing specialties represented different intellectual and social capital. In organizing the TIGER

summit, it was critical to have representation from each of the nursing specialty organizations. The impact of the TIGER agenda could be much broader as each participating organization had the potential to reach thousands of additional nurses within their respective membership. In addition, their members were more likely to adopt recommendations coming from one of their peers. As the TIGER Initiative asked for a commitment from each organization to integrate the shared vision and action plan into their strategic goals, it was important to invite the person within the organization that had the authority (e.g., president or officer) to develop their strategy.

3. *To accelerate the development of an agenda, involve subject matter experts.* Use the best advice available in developing a plan, as eventually experts will be called upon to evaluate the quality and comprehensiveness of the program. Therefore, it pays to know and include their opinion up front. In the TIGER Collaborative teams, it was critical to pair up nursing specialty experts with nursing informatics experts to develop a message and action plan that resonated with the specialty organization members.

4. *Establish the common mission/goal and values up front.* This is the reason why the stakeholders will get engaged and remain engaged. Focus should be on an issue that strikes at people's emotions. In the case of the TIGER Initiative, common values that helped to cement broad nursing support was the desire to create a patient-centered, quality, and safe health care delivery system that better supported nursing activities. Federal mandates called for health IT to facilitate health care reform. The threat of this reform occurring without nursing at the table is the reason that the issue became so urgent for nursing leaders to become involved.

5. *Define the issue in a way that the participants easily understand it.* The expected outcome of the TIGER Initiative was to raise awareness within the entire nursing community of the need for all nurses and nursing students to obtain a minimum set of competencies related to computer literacy, information literacy, and information management skills. The TIGER Initiative used the analogy of the computerization being as essential to nursing practice as the stethoscope was in the twenty-first century. Early introduction of the stethoscope met with some skepticism, but over time it became so commonplace that you rarely see any health care provider practicing at the bedside without this enabling tool.

6. *Create a sense of urgency.* It is impossible to quickly mobilize people to support your agenda if you do not have a burning need to act. The President established the timeline for the TIGER Initiative when demanding that health care will be delivered with Electronic Health Records (EHRs) by the year 2014. This action became the catalyst for organizing nursing leaders to develop a strategy.

7. *Time your activities to coincide with natural opportunities to influence the outcomes.* Be aware of budget cycles and grant opportunities in pursuing funding. Often there is a defined timeline for "public comments" to new policies, and you will want to be prepared to provide input during these critical review cycles. For example, the TIGER Initiative had to pursue other funding strategies when we could not meet the budget cycle defined by the Institute of Medicine. In another example, the TIGER Initiative provided input during the review cycle for public comments on several use cases being developed by the Office of the National Coordinator's agencies. The TIGER

Education Collaborative also provided input while AACN was revising their "Essentials for Baccalaureate Education" to include informatics requirements.

8. *Align your recommended policy with the larger, strategic picture.* For example, the TIGER Initiative was aligned with the IOM recommendations and the Federal Office of the National Coordinator's strategic plan from its inception. The passage of the American Reinvestment and Recovery Act in 2009 passed by the Obama Administration added even more momentum to the need to build a national health IT infrastructure and prepare the workforce to use new technologies. Policy makers look favorably upon opportunities to build upon previous work, and the context of the policy fitting into larger strategic initiatives gives you the opportunity to link onto their efforts. It will also allow you to gain the support of the related initiatives. Several people have leveraged the TIGER Summary reports when building their strategy to secure ARRA funds for health IT projects.

9. *Develop a dissemination plan for your agenda in order to gain larger industry support.* In the case of the TIGER Initiative, the plan was for each participating organization to commit to bringing the work back to their respective organization and develop their own action plan to be completed within 3 years. This short timeframe resulted in more than hundred TIGER-related presentations at conferences and meetings nationally, regionally, and even internationally within 2 years.

10. *Provide continuous opportunities to share materials, lessons learned, and best practices with the participants.* As the participants continue to develop their plan, sharing these materials within the TIGER community via the website and publications allows all organizations to benefit from the collective leverage of the program. Each subsequent presentation, article, and contact identifies new potential participants and new opportunities. The new participants might have questions or want materials to share with their colleagues. As in viral marketing, it is necessary for them to access a reliable source of materials and share their success stories.

Conclusion

The TIGER summit established a common understanding of the problem and developed the action plan necessary to achieve the vision that was shared across the nursing and informatics community. The inclusion of numerous professional organizations and motivated nurses from academia and other sectors of health care was a key to advancing the informatics agenda. The intellectual capital of these organizations was able to provide the context and value of the informatics agenda to their memberships. The social capital of these professional organizations was harnessed to disseminate the agenda and corresponding action plan. This wide dissemination and the work of the Phase II collaboratives engaged the nursing community, fostered new networks where social connections among nurses were based on trust and reciprocity, and increased the interactions between people to build a community that binds them all to the informatics agenda. The need to prepare all nurses with the necessary knowledge and skills in practice in an ever-increasing technology-rich environment is now a nursing agenda.

References

1. Nahapiet J, Ghoshal S. Social capital, intellectual capital, and the organizational advantage. *Acad Manage Rev.* 1998;23(2):212-266.
2. Edvinsson L, Malone M. *Intellectual Capital.* New York: Harper Business; 1997.
3. McElroy M. Social Innovation Capital: Part 1. Redefining Intellectual Capital (Draft). http://www.macroinnovation.com/images/SIC3.07.01.pdf; 2001 Accessed 7.09.09.
4. Lesser E. Leveraging social capital in organizations. In: Lesser E, ed. *Knowledge and Social Capital: Foundations and Applications.* Woburn: Butterworth Heineman; 2000.
5. Cohen D, Prusak L. *In Good Company: How Social Capital Makes Organizations Work.* Boston: Harvard Business School Press; 2001.
6. Coleman J. Social capital in the creation of human capital. *Am J Sociol.* 1988;94(1):95-123.
7. Wenger E. *Communities of Practice: Learning, Meaning, and Identity.* New York: Cambridge University Press; 1999.
8. Putnam R. *Bowling Alone: The Collapse and Revival of American Community.* New York: Simon & Schuster; 2000.
9. Adler P, Kwon S. Social capital: the good, the bad, and the ugly. In: Lesser E, ed. *Knowledge and Social Capital: Foundations and Applications.* Woburn: Butterworth Heineman; 2000.
10. Landry R, Amara N, Lamari M. Does social capital determine innovation? To what extent? Fourth International Conference on Technology Policy and Innovation. http://kuuc.chair.ula-val.ca/francais/pdf/apropos/publication5.pdf; 2000 Accessed 7.09.09.
11. Fountain JE. Social capital: a key enabler of innovation. In: Branscomb L, ed. *Investing in Innovation: Towards a Consensus Strategy for Federal Technology Policy.* Cambridge: MIT Press; 1997.
12. Commission P. *Social Capital: Reviewing the Concept and its Policy Implications. Research Paper.* Canberra, Australia: AusInfo; 2003.
13. Huysman M, Wulf V. *Social Capital and Information Technology.* Cambridge: MIT Press; 2004.
14. Ackerman M, Pipek V, Wulf V, eds. *Sharing Expertise: Beyond Knowledge Management.* Cambridge, MA: MIT Press; 2003.
15. Skiba D, Dulong D. Using TIGER vision to move your agenda forward. *Nurs Manage.* 2008;39(3):14-16.
16. The TIGER Initiative. Evidence and Information Transforming Nursing: 3-Year Action Steps toward a 10-Year Vision. http://www.tigersummit.com; 2007 Accessed 7.09.09.
17. Technology Informatics Guiding Education Reform. Collaborating to Integrate Evidence and Informatics into Nursing Practice and Education: An Executive Summary [Online]. http://www.tigersummit.com/; 2009 Accessed 7.09.09.

Networking Advancing Nursing Informatics

4

Susan K. Newbold

The number and type of resources have grown over the years to help the informatics nurse and any nurse, for that matter, learn about integrating informatics into their practice. The resources are in the categories of people resources, organizational resources, electronic resources, and the literature. This chapter highlights those resources for the nurse and the informatics nurse.

People Resources

There are official and unofficial resources for learning about and mentoring for nursing and health care informatics. The American Medical Informatics Association (AMIA) offers a mentoring program the benefits of which are shown in Table 4.1.

In addition to formal programs, you can develop informal programs of networking with colleagues. Consider a habit of periodically keeping in touch with informatics professionals. This might include meeting a colleague for lunch or simply telephoning an informatics colleague. Make certain you have a supply of business cards available at all times. If you do not have one through your work place, you can easily create your own using a template and card stock purchased from an office supply store.

Your colleagues may be the best source of information about a job opportunity or information about a problem you are having at your worksite. Seek out opportunities to attend events where these colleagues gather.

Organizational Resources

Over the last 30 years, many organizations have developed which will help with education and networking in health care informatics. Table 4.2 lists many of the groups related to health care and nursing informatics.

S.K. Newbold
Hospital Corporation of America®, Nashville, TN., USA
e-mail: sknewbold@comcast.net

M.J. Ball et al. (eds.), *Nursing Informatics*,
DOI: 10.1007/978-1-84996-278-0_4, © Springer-Verlag London Limited 2011

Table 4.1 Benefits of the AMIA Mentorship Program for mentees and mentors

By participating, mentees have the opportunity to
  Improve their networking skills and build their network
  Learn more about AMIA
  Build communication and leadership skills
  Learn about informatics in general
  Learn more about their informatics areas of interest
  Obtain a position
  Pitch a project
  Obtain a specific referral
  Obtain a professional recommendation
  Engage in a project collaboration

By participating, mentors have the opportunity to
  Get to know great newer trainees
  Help newer trainees with some/all of the above in highly manageable way
  Mold newer trainees and provide guidance they wish they had had
  Stay in touch with the Mentee base
  Brush up their own networking skills and build their network
  Look for potential project collaborators and candidates for hire
  Encourage bright minds to stick with informatics, thereby strengthening the field
  Serve and strengthen AMIA, their professional home

There are other groups, which may not have a direct nursing informatics component, but can still be of value to the nurse. They include AHIMA (American Health Information Management Association)(www.ahima.org), and the American Nurses Credentialing Center (ANCC) for information on Informatics Nurse certification(www.nursingworld.org/ancc). Several of the regional groups host local meetings on informatics topics.

To highlight one of the oldest and most geographically disperse organizations, see CARING at www.caringonline.org. CARING is a national nursing informatics organization with international membership from 34 countries which began over 26 years ago in the Washington, DC area, but now has a far-reaching impact. The mission of CARING is to advance the delivery of quality health care through the integration of informatics in practice, education, administration, and research. CARING and ANIA plan to merge by 2010 offering benefits to a larger number of nurses. Benefits of membership include:

- Access to a network of over 3,300 informatics professionals in 50 states and 34 countries
- An active e-mail list with the option to have messages in digest format
- An online, searchable membership directory
- Quarterly newsletter indexed in CINAHL, Thomson, and EBSCO
- A toll free number to contact the CARING Board
- Job bank with employer-paid postings
- Reduced rate for the Computers, Informatics and Nursing (CIN) Journal
- Annual CARING luncheon during AMIA and annual dinner during SINI
- Membership in the Alliance for Nursing Informatics (www.allianceni.org)
- An annual joint conference with ANIA and networking events around the nation and the world

Table 4.2 Healthcare and nursing informatics groups

Alliance for Nursing Informatics (ANI), www.allianceni.org
American Medical Informatics Association (AMIA), www.amia.org
ANIA-CARING, www.ania-caring.org
Association of periOperative Registered Nurses (AORN), www.aorn.org
Association of Women's Health, Obstetric and Neonatal Nurses (AWHONN), www.awhonn.org
Brazilian Nursing Association Nursing Informatics Group
British Computer Society Nursing Informatics Nursing Specialist Group, www.bcs.org
Canadian Nursing Informatics Association (CNIA), http://www.cnia.ca/
Center for Nursing Classification and Clinical Effectiveness (CNC), http://www.nursing.uiowa.edu/excellence/nursing_knowledge/clinical_effectiveness/index.htm
Central Savannah River Area Clinical Informatics Network (CSRA – CIN), www.csra-cin.org
Cerner Nursing Advisory Board, www.cerner.com
Connecticut Healthcare Informatics Network (CHIN)
Croatia Nursing Informatics Association (CroNIA)
Delaware Valley Nursing Computer Network (DVNCN), www.dvncn.com
Health Informatics of New Jersey (HINJ), www.hinj.net
Health Informatics New Zealand Nursing Informatics Working Group, www.hinz.org.nz
Healthcare Information and Management Systems Society (HIMSS), www.himss.org/ni
Informatics Nurses From Ohio (INFO), http://informaticsnursesohio.info/
International Medical Informatics Association (IMIA) Special Interest Group Nursing Informatics, http://www.imiani.org
MEDITECH Nurse Informatics program, www.meditech.com
Midwest Nursing Research Society (MNRS) Nursing Informatics Research Section, www.mnrs.org
Minnesota Nursing Informatics Group (MINING), www.miningonline.org
NANDA International, www.nanda.org
New England Nursing Informatics Consortium (NENIC), www.nenic.org
North Carolina State Nurses Association Council on NI (NCNA CONI), http://www.ncnurses.org/Practice_CoNI/practice_CoNI_home.asp
Nursing Informatics Europe, www.nicecomputing.ch/nieurope/index.html
Perinatal Information Systems User Group (PISUG)
Puget Sound Nursing Informatics (PSNI), www.psniwa.org
SNOMED CT Nursing Working Group, www.ihtsdo.org
South Carolina Informatics Nursing Network (SCINN), www.scinn.org
Utah Nursing Informatics Network (UNIN), www.utahnursinginformatics.org

Conferences

Several of the Informatics organizations listed offer national and international conferences, workshops, and symposia. Here follows a bit about some of the major events.

American Medical Informatics Association (AMIA), (www.amia.org)

AMIA holds an interdisciplinary Annual Symposium. Many of the events are held in Washington, DC with other locations included. The AMIA 2010, 2011, 2013, and 2014 Annual Symposiums will be held in Washington, DC, with the 2012 event in Chicago, IL. In addition to tutorials, workshop, multiple tracks, and exhibitors, working group events are held. The Nursing Informatics Working group makes sure that nursing-focused content is available.

American Nursing Informatics Association (ANIA)(www.ania.org) and CARING (www.caringoline.org)

These two organizations, due to their merger in 2010, jointly host an annual conference in the spring. Generally, every other year (i.e., 2011) it is held in Las Vegas, NV. The 2012 Conference will be held in Orlando, FL., USA. This conference offers multiple tracks, general sessions with top-notch speakers and exhibitors, and poster sessions. Several pre-conference events are offered. The focus is on clinical informatics.

Healthcare Information Management and Systems Society (HIMSS) (http://www.himss.org/asp/topics_nursingInformatics.asp)

HIMSS offers a huge Annual Conference and Exhibition in the spring attracting over 27,000 attendees. Other smaller events are held around the world. The location for these conferences rotate and have been held in Atlanta, GA, Chicago, IL, Dallas, TX, Orlando, FL, and San Diego, CA. The event offers multiple tracks, multiple preconferences, and a Nursing Informatics Symposium. In addition, HIMSS hosts Webinars and Audio Conferences on a variety of topics. Recently, there has been a Virtual Conference with Online Presentations.

International Medical Informatics Association (IMIA) Special Interest Group Nursing Informatics (NI) (http://www.imiani.org)

IMIA NI hosts a major international conference every 3 years. The 2012 event will be in Montreal Canada, 23–27 June 2012, hosted by the AMIA (www.ni2012.org). The conference in 2015 will be hosted in Taipei, Taiwan. In addition, IMIA holds a conference every 3 years, soon changing to a 2-year cycle. The next MedInfo conference will be held in Copenhagen (www.imia.org)

Summer Institute in Nursing Informatics (SINI), (http://nursing.umaryland.edu/sini/)

This annual conference is hosted by the University of Maryland School of Nursing and held yearly in July in Baltimore, Maryland. In 2010 the conference celebrated its 20th year. The event offers preconference sessions, webcasts for those who cannot attend in person, multiple tracks, and poster sessions. Also included are a walking tour of Baltimore, tours of the simulation laboratory, vendor exhibitions, and other networking events.

In addition to the major conferences, also look for User group conferences hosted by vendors, the Weekend Immersion in Nursing Informatics, and TEPR.

Electronic Resources

Nursing-related electronic mailing lists are a way to communicate with nurses from around the world. The most active e-mail list is hosted by CARING (www.caringonline.org), with over 2,000 subscribers and an average of 8 messages posted daily. Other groups with nursing informatics-focused lists are AMIA and HIMSS. Nursing-L (http://mailman.amia.org/listinfo/nrsing-l) is a free list hosted by AMIA.

Nursing Informatics History Project

The American Medical Informatics Association Nursing Informatics Working Group (AMIA NI-WG) has undertaken a large project to document and preserve the history of nursing informatics. See www.amia.org/niwg-history-page. This is occurring through three activities:

1. Nursing informatics pioneers and nursing informatics organizations have been solicited to preserve their materials in an archive at the National Library of Medicine started by Dr. Virginia Saba in 1997.
2. Stories of the pioneers in nursing informatics are being videotaped and made available through AMIA's web site.
3. Historical research is planned to document the evolution of informatics as a specialty in nursing.

TIGER

Technology Informatics Guiding Educational Reform (TIGER) (www.tigersummit.com) is a major resource for nursing informatics competencies and is discussed elsewhere in this edition. The purpose of TIGER is to integrate informatics to the practice of every nurse.

Daily e-news Bulletins

Several informatics journals and organizations offer bulletins to help keep professionals apprised of happenings in the health care informatics industries. The California Health Foundation – iHealthBeat (www.chcf.org), Modern Healthcare Magazine (www.modern-healthcare.com), Health Data Management (www.healthdatamanagement.com), AMIA (www.amia.org), and HIMSS (www.himss.org) are among the organizations that send out daily, weekly, or monthly bulletins. Some are benefits of membership, but others are free.

Nursing Informatics Web Sites

See the various organizations for access to resources online. For example, AMIA hosts a list of job descriptions for informatics nurses at http://www.amia.org/working-group-nursing-informatics/working-group-nursing-informatics-roles. HIMSS has a collection of documents including those for project management, a salary survey, and an introduction to nursing informatics at www.himss.org/ni

Resources have started to appear on social networking sites such as Facebook, Twitter, and LinkedIN. Time will tell whether these become valuable resources for the informatics nurse.

Informatics Literature

Although books may not be as up-to-date as electronic resources, there is still much value in the printed word for educating nurses about informatics. Also, look at proceedings of the conferences mentioned in this chapter available in either print or electronic form. These are some of the books and journals used in this author's practice and teaching.

In addition to informatics books, look for content-specific books like those on project management and systems analysis.

Suggested Reading

American Nurses Association. *Nursing Informatics: Scope & Standards of Practice*. Silver Spring: American Nurses Association; 2008.
Ball MJ, Hannah KJ, Edwards MJA. *Introduction to Nursing Informatics*. 3rd ed. New York: Springer; 2006.
Ball MJ, Hannah KJ, Newbold SK, Douglas JV, eds. *Nursing Informatics: Where Caring and Technology Meet*. 3rd ed. New York: Springer; 2000.
Computers, Informatics, Nursing (CIN). Philadelphia: Lippincott Williams & Wilkins.
Englebardt SP, Nelson R, eds. *Health Care Informatics: An Interdisciplinary Approach*. St. Louis: Mosby; 2002.
Hebda T, Czar P. *Handbook of Informatics for Nurses & Healthcare Professionals*. 4th ed. Upper Saddle River: Pearson Prentice Hall; 2009.
Hunt EC, Sproat SB, Kitzmiller RR. *The Nursing Informatics Implementation Guide*. New York: Springer; 2004.
Newbold SK, Westra BL. American Medical Informatics Nursing Informatics History Committee Update. *Comput Inform Nurs*. 2009;27(4):263-265.
O'Neil CA, Fisher CA, Newbold SK. *Developing Online Learning Environments in Nursing Education*. 2nd ed. New York: Springer; 2009.
Saba VK, McCormick KA. *Essentials of Nursing Informatics*. 4th ed. New York: McGraw-Hill; 2006.
Thede LQ, Sewell J. *Informatics and Nursing: Opportunities & Challenges*. 3rd ed. Philadelphia: Lippincott Williams & Wilkins; 2009.

Weaver CA, Delaney CW, Weber P, Carr R. *Nursing and Informatics for the 21st Century: An International Look at Practice, Trends and the Future*. Chicago: Healthcare Information and Management Systems Society; 2006.

Westra BL, Newbold SK. American Medical Information Association Nursing Informatics History Committee. *Comput Inform Nurs*. 2006;24(2):113-115.

Section

Workforce Imperatives

From its inception, Technology Informatics Guiding Education Reform (TIGER) recognized the role that workforce development would have to play in transforming the nursing profession. As Hart (2008) explained, "technology advancements have increased at a dramatic rate, while attempts at incorporating a basic set of technology and information science competencies for nurses at various levels of education and practice have been dragging."

Competencies were thus critical to the transformation of health care in the 21st century. When TIGER launched Phase II, the Competencies Collaborative was the first to move forward, identifying the base that was subsequently adopted by three other TIGER collaboratives focused on workforce issues. This base was the European Computer Driver's License (ECDL), now known in the United States as the International Computer Driver's License (ICDL), where testing sites are being established. The Ohio Learning Network had 17 active centers as of 2009, and ICDL had been delivered to universities in California, Michigan, Colorado, and Massachusetts. At this writing, ICDL Testing and Courseware can be accessed through their website @ www.ICDLUS.org (Keating 2009). The three collaboratives to build upon the work of the Competency Collaborative are Education and Faculty Development, Continuing Education and Staff Development, and Leadership Collaborative; chapters reporting on their efforts are also in this section.

Earlier, Rick and colleagues (2003) reported success in using online learning to deliver informatics-related training, coaching, and mentoring to nurses at the largest integrated healthcare system in the nation, the Veterans Administration (VA). Still, obstacles remained, including workforce shortages, high patient acuity, increasing ancillary duties, and layers of administrative work in addition to clinical practice responsibilities (Rick et al. 2003). When Pravikoff et al. (2005) evaluated the readiness of the clinical nursing workforce for evidence-based practice, their findings were grim: many lacked essential informatics skills. According to Skiba (2004), most nurses lacked information literacy skills, and data-driven models of care would be ineffective if nurses and nursing leadership did not understand the need for such skills in healthcare delivery settings. As a solution, Simpson (2001) advocated collaboration between and among educational institutions, healthcare organizations, and health information systems vendors as a way to foster the growth of technology-enabled practice. Connors et al. (2007) reported on one such collaboration and its use of a clinical information system to create "IT [information technology] savvy healthcare providers who will cross the quality chasm." Two other examples of partnerships between industry and academic systems developed to impact student learning, nursing practice, and nursing research are: the collaboration between Eclypsis and the University of Pennsylvania School of Nursing (Reuters 2009); and earlier between Cerner, the Aurora Health System and the University of Wisconsin, Madison (AScribe 2004).

The need for leadership development in the area of nursing informatics and technology is obvious and critical, according to Hart (2008). Stein and Deese (2004) argued that nurse leaders can play a key role in exploring how technology can support nursing practice and development and address work environment issues key to the recruitment and retention of nurses. This section of *Nursing Informatics: Where Technology and Caring Meet* builds upon these findings from the literature and adds significantly to them. This is true not only of the four chapters that report the work of the TIGER collaboratives, but of the other three chapters as well. All contribute to the growing understanding of how nurse leaders and educators can address informatics workforce development issues in education and practice settings.

Education and Faculty Development

In Chapter 5, the anchor chapter for this section, Diane Skiba and Mary Anne Rizzolo describe educational initiatives that will impact nursing workforce development in the future. Based on work of the Education Collaborative, "Education and Faculty Development" highlights the need for, and process of, faculty development and identifies the changes needed in nursing education. As evidence of some of these changes, the authors cite the national leadership roles played by two nursing accreditation organizations in advancing the TIGER agenda. The National League for Nursing (NLN) has approved a position statement outlining 23 informatics-related recommendations for nursing school administrators, faculty, and the organization itself, while the American Association of Colleges of Nursing (AACN) has incorporated informatics as "essential" elements in both baccalaureate (BSN) and doctor of nursing practice (DNP) programs. Drawing from a survey of State Boards of Nursing, Skiba and Rizzolo conclude the chapter with a rich discussion of state initiatives that advance the informatics educational agenda and the development of the future nursing workforce.

Competencies

Chapter 6, "Competencies: Nuts and Bolts" by Connie Delaney and Brian Gugerty, is based on the work of the TIGER Informatics Competencies Collaborative (TICC). This work served as a lynchpin for that of the three other collaboratives presented in this section. In a complicated process, TICC sorted through all the competencies in the literature to identify an easily usable strategy for organizing those competencies. The model they developed consists of three parts: Basic Computer Competencies, Information Literacy Competencies, and Information Management Competencies. After developing the framework, collaborative members set about finding and sorting through existing resources to meet the competencies it contained. In one of the most important contributions, they iden-tified the European Computer Driving License Foundation (ECDL) as a way of addressing basic computer competencies. The authors specify other resources in this chapter and pro-vide a lengthy list of competencies for the more advanced levels in the TICC model.

Academic Programs

Chapter 7, the third chapter in this section and the accompanying update, "Update Academic Programs," are included to provide perspective on the progress in nursing infor-matics. In the chapter, brought over from the 3rd Edition of *Nursing Informatics*, Carole Gassert relates the history of nursing informatics and reviews the development of aca-demic and continuing education programs in the field. In the new addendum, Susan Newbold includes an updated definition of nursing informatics (ANA 2008) and updated lists of programs that offer courses and/or specialty education in nursing informatics. Newbold also discusses the essentials related to nursing informatics for the new Doctor in Nursing Practice (DNP) programs (80 as of this writing) and offers updated information on continuing education opportunities. Gassert's chapter and Newbold's addendum touch upon issues addressed elsewhere in this section, including the first two chapters on educa-tion and competencies, and the fourth chapter on staff development.

Staff Development and Continuing Education

Chapter 8, the fourth chapter in this section, "Continuing Education and Staff Development" by Joan Kiel and Elizabeth Johnson, represents the work of the TIGER Staff Development Collaborative. The authors open with a compelling case for staff development and continu-ing education, citing data from the American Academy of Nurses Workforce Commission study related to the use of technology. They highlight "viewpoints from the field," the results from 210 responses to an online TIGER survey. Designed to obtain feedback on computer literacy, computer training, and computer skills for nurses employed in a variety of healthcare settings, the survey yielded results that are a must read for anyone interested in staff development and continuing education. Four rich case studies from four healthcare delivery systems and specific recommendations for successful approaches to clinical sys-tems training conclude the chapter.

Leadership

Chapters 9 and 10, the next two chapters in this section, address leadership as a key factor in the advancement of the nursing informatics agenda. In chapter 9, "Leadership Colla-borative" by Judy Murphy and Dana Alexander, these authors report on the TIGER

Leadership Collaborative, which began its work by identifying the health information technology related issues that nursing leaders face. Building on the findings of the Competency Collaborative described in the chapter by Delaney and Gugerty, Murphy and Alexander take a leadership perspective on the TIGER Nursing Informatics Competencies model, focusing on how nursing leaders can use this model to address workforce development issues. The chapter also describes leadership development programs for nurses who are now in leadership positions or who aspire to lead in the future, and discusses the results and recommendations from the TIGER leadership survey of chief nurse executives.

Chapter 10 in this section is also on leadership, and it offers a different and provocative perspective. Author Roy Simpson in his chapter "Challenging Leadership Status Quo," challenges nurse leaders to go beyond general knowledge related to nursing informatics to being able to debate the nursing-specific benefits of one clinical system over another. He further makes the case that nurse leaders need additional competencies to evaluate vendors and vendor relationships, such as detailed knowledge of patient-care workflow, the predictable technology adoption lifecycle, the power of relational databases, and the power of relational databases. These competencies are essential if leaders are to make the best decisions for their delivery systems. In closing, Simpson urges nursing leaders to adopt an entrepreneurial *and* a public policy-oriented mindset—and to address the implications of both.

Collaboration

The final chapter, Chapter 11, in this section brings together the differing aspects of workforce development mentioned throughout this section. In "Bridging Technology: Academe and Industry," Pamela Jeffries, Krysia Hudson, Laura Taylor, and Steven Klapper describe a collaboration involving an educational institution, a vendor, and a simulated healthcare delivery system. The chapter opens by identifying the benefits of simulation and a framework for simulation in nursing education. It then describes the challenge of implementing clinical interventions in a simulated environment using scenario-based clinical information systems, and discusses using Second Life and Micro Sim for evaluation purposes. The case study presents details of the relationship between the Johns Hopkins University School of Nursing and the Eclipsys Corporation in the use of the Sunrise Clinical Manager, an electronic health record product donated for educational purposes. The authors provide specific examples of how the donated hardware, software, and consultant time, and training were integrated into a curriculum so that nursing students could experience real-world, nursing informatics incorporated into their clinical practice experience.

The chapters in this section echo the themes introduced in the first four chapters of this book—transformation, culture change, social and intellectual capital, and networking. These themes will resound throughout the rest of the book, with chapters that drill deeper and pursue new perspectives on the future nursing informaticians and TIGER participants who envision for health care and the nursing profession.

References

AScribe Newswire (2004 Apr 13) Technology to deliver nursing best practices at point of care. AScribe Business and Economics News Service. http://www.accessmylibrary.com/coms2/summary_0286-6217494_ITM. Accessed 26 September 2009

Connors H, Warren J, Weaver C (2007) HIT plants SEEDS in healthcare education. Nurs Adm Q 31(2):129–133

Hart MD (2008) Informatics competency and development within the US nursing populations workforce: a systematic literature review. CIN: Computers, Informatics, Nursing 26(6): 320–329

Keating J (2009) Personal communication of Patricia Hinton Walker with John Keating, Regional Development Executive EMEA, ECDL Foundation, Dublin, Ireland, September 2009

Pravikoff D, Tanner A, Pierce S (2005) Readiness of U.S. nurses for evidence-based practice: many don't understand or value research and have had little or no training to help them find evidence on which to base their practice. Amer J Nurs 105(9):40–51

Rick C, Kearns MA, Thompson NA (2003) The reality of virtual learning for nurses in the largest integrated health care system in the nation. Nurs Adm Q 27(1):41–57

Reuters (2009 Jan 14) University of Pennsylvania School of Nursing and Eclipsys form academic partnership to bring HIT to nursing education curriculum. http://www.reuters.com/article/pressRelease/idUS144526+14-Jan-2009+BW20090114. Accessed 26 September 2009

Simpson RL (2001) Technology enabling the service/education partnership. Nurs Adm Q 26(1):87–91

Skiba DJ (2004) Informatics competencies. Nurs Educ Perspectives 25(6):312

Stein M, Deese D (2004) Addressing the next decade of nursing challenges. Nurs Econ 22(5):273–279

Education and Faculty Development

5

Diane J. Skiba and Mary Anne Rizzolo

Introduction

The topic of ensuring that all nurses had computer knowledge and skills dates back to the work of Anderson, Gremy, and Pages[1] and Ronald.[2] These articles not only called upon the profession to address the necessary knowledge and skills, but also provided information about the first nursing course that offered computer literacy in the profession. In the early 1987s, the call to action was for nurses to have computer literacy skills.[3,4] To address this, Ronald and Skiba[5] wrote a monograph that provided an educational framework to teach three different levels of learners (informed user, proficient user, and developers) about computer education. The monograph provided content outlines and resources for teaching.

Since that time, the discipline of informatics was introduced in the health arena and the focus was more than just computers and automation. The concentration in the early years was on the creation of the discipline of nursing informatics and preparing specialists in the field. It was important to begin to prepare graduate level specialist, as most in the field were educated through on-the-job training. In the 1980s, two graduate programs were started at the University of Utah and University of Maryland. An important event was the first scope and standards document developed by the American Nurses Association (ANA 1994) outlining the clinical specialty in nursing informatics. Since then, numerous graduate programs have come into existence, and the scope and standards have been revised three times with the newest version in 2008 distinguishing between an informatics nurse and an informatics nurse specialist (ANA 2008).

Throughout the last 30 years, numerous articles appeared in the literature on the importance of informatics for nursing and the need to include this content in the nursing curriculum. In 1997, the National Advisory Council on Nurse Education and Practice[6] issued a report to the Secretary of the Department of Health and Human Services calling for a national informatics agenda for nursing education and practice. Numerous studies

D.J. Skiba (✉)
University of Colorado Denver, College of Nursing, Campus Box C-288-03, Education 2 North, 3120 E. 19th Avenue, Aurora, CO 80045, USA
mail: diane.skiba@ucdenver.edu

J. Ball et al. (eds.), *Nursing Informatics*,
DOI: 10.1007/978-1-84996-278-0_5, © Springer-Verlag London Limited 2011

examined the extent to which informatics has been incorporated into the nursing curriculum.[7-13]

These studies continued to document over time that there was relatively little in the nursing curriculum focused on informatics. If there were courses, required or elective, it was because an individual with knowledge of informatics pushed to have the content covered in the curriculum. In addition, although accreditation bodies talked about computers, it was framed as communication or usage in research rather than an informatics emphasis. There were also a series of articles highlighting the necessary competencies for nurses,[14-19] nurse managers,[20] and nurse practitioners.[21] "Now, despite 20 plus years of accomplishments, nursing informatics in nursing education remains an elusive concept" (p. 301).[22]

But the right forces began to converge in the early years of the new millennium. One of the driving forces was a series of reports by the Institute of Medicine (IOM). As Warren and Connors (p. 58)[23] reported, the first of these, *To Err is Human*, served as a catalyst to call for a transformation of health care practices. This report[24] as well as subsequent reports[25-27] set the stage for the demand to use information technology (IT) to mitigate error, improve safety, and insure quality care. Each report highlighted the increasing value of health IT and the need for health care professionals to properly use them as clinical decision tools in the provision of safe and quality care. One particular report outlined the five core competencies all health care professionals need to practice in the twenty-first century, stressing the need for patient-centered care, interdisciplinary teams, and evidence-based practice together with quality improvement and informatics tools.[26] These reports, coupled with the creation of the Office of the National Coordinator of Health Information Technology in 2004 by the federal government, served as catalysts to bring informatics into the forefront. It was no longer hidden in the background.

As a result of these driving forces, the Technology Informatics Guiding Education Reform (TIGER) initiative was formed in 2004 to "bring together nursing stakeholders to develop a shared vision, strategies, and specific actions for improving nursing practice, education, and the delivery of patient care through the use of health information technology."[28] One of the primary goals was insuring that all nurses were prepared to deliver care in a consumer-centric informatics intensive health care environment. In 2006, the TIGER steering committee gathered over 100 leaders who represented nursing organizations, administration, practice, education, technology, government agencies, and other key stakeholders to "create a vision for the future of nursing that bridges the quality chasm with IT, enabling nurses to use informatics in practice and education to provide safer, higher-quality patient care."[29] Using small group work, report-outs, and a wireless audience response system, the group came to consensus on seven components that form the Seven Pillars of the TIGER Vision:

1. Management and Leadership
2. Education
3. Communication and Collaboration
4. Informatics Design
5. Information Technology
6. Policy
7. Culture

Recommendations were developed for all of the constituencies represented at the Summit and representatives of nursing organizations pledged to incorporate the TIGER vision into their respective organizations' strategic plans. Following the Summit, in an attempt to involve as many leaders as possible in implementing the vision, volunteers were solicited and hundreds of individuals offered their time to participate on nine collaborative teams:

1. Standards and Interoperability
2. National Health Information Technology Agenda
3. Informatics Competencies
4. Education and Faculty Development
5. Staff Development
6. Usability and Clinical Application Design
7. Virtual Demonstration Center
8. Leadership Development
9. Consumer Empowerment and Personal Health Records

This chapter provides an overview of the activities of the Education and Faculty Development Collaborative.

TIGER's Education and Faculty Development Collaborative

Based on the TIGER Summit Final Report, the objectives listed below were established for the Education and Faculty Development collaborative. The emphasis chosen by the collaborative was to focus on faculty development and prelicensure education of nurses. In addition, whenever possible, the need for more nursing informatics specialists was also emphasized in a variety of venues, particularly at meetings and conferences held by the Health Services Resource Administration.

Faculty Development and Education Collaborative Objectives

1. Use the informatics competencies, theories, research, and practice examples throughout nursing curriculums.
2. Create programs and resources to develop faculty with informatics knowledge, skill, and ability and measure the baseline and changes in informatics knowledge among nurse educators and nursing students.
3. Develop a task force to examine the integration of informatics throughout the curriculum.
4. Develop strategies to recruit, retain, and train current and future nurses in the areas of informatics education, practice, and research.
5. Improve and expand existing nursing/clinical/health Informatics education programs.

6. Encourage existing Health Services Resources Administration (HRSA) Division of Nursing to continue and expand their support for informatics specialty programs and faculty development.
7. Encourage foundations to start programs that provide funding for curriculum development, research, and practice in nursing informatics and IT adoption.
8. Collaborate with industry and service partners to support faculty creativity in the adoption of informatics technology and offer informatics tools within the curriculum.

To address these objectives, several working groups were established. At the conclusion of their work, the Collaborative held two webinars to provide interested educators with information about how schools of nursing were incorporating informatics into their curriculums and about different approaches to forming partnerships to teach students about electronic health records and clinical documentation.

National League for Nursing

The National League for Nursing (NLN), through its Educational Technology and Information Management Advisory Council (ETIMAC) and ETIMAC's task groups, is one organization that is providing the leadership to forward TIGER's agenda and prepare nurses to practice in a digital environment. The NLN has a long history of promoting informatics with its first council being organized in 1984.

In 2006, ETIMAC's Task Group on Informatics Competencies, chaired by Roy Simpson, completed a comprehensive review of the literature on informatics competencies for various levels of nursing education, then developed a survey to determine the extent to which informatics was included in the curriculums of all types of nursing education programs. The survey that was sent to administrators and faculty achieved a response rate of 25% for administrators and 12% for faculty during the 1-month period it was open, and those responding represented the mix of programs offering nursing education programs, from practical nursing through graduate level.

Survey results[13] revealed that only 15% of programs required students to own a computer, and even fewer (6%) required personal digital assistants (PDAs). Sixty-one percent of the programs had a computer literacy requirement; 42% had an information literacy requirement. Responses to questions related to the integration of informatics in the curriculum, however, yielded some disturbing data. Fifty-eight percent of faculty and 56% of administrators said that informatics was integrated throughout several courses, and 51% of faculty and 65% of administrators said students were exposed to informatics in their clinical experiences. However, comments made by faculty and administrators indicated that many were unclear on the definition of informatics. Those comments (e.g., "all courses are web-enhanced") indicated that members of both groups confused informatics with educational technology. Questions about faculty knowledge of informatics revealed that 81% were self-taught; again, comments like "took online course in WebCT" further document confusion about the definition of informatics.

Based on these results, the Task Group began work on a position statement, and in May 2008, the NLN Board of Governors approved *Preparing the Next Generation of Nurses to Practice in a Technology-Rich Environment: An Informatics Agenda*. It outlined 23 recommendations for nursing school administrators, faculty, and for the organization itself.

For Nurse Faculty

- Participate in faculty development programs to achieve competency in informatics.
- Designate an informatics champion in every school of nursing to: (a) help faculty distinguish between using instructional technologies to teach vs. using informatics to guide, document, analyze, and inform nursing practice, and (b) translate state-of-the-art practices in technology and informatics that need to be integrated into the curriculum.
- Incorporate informatics into the curriculum.
- Incorporate ANA-recognized standard nursing language and terminology into content.
- Identify clinical informatics exemplars, those drawn from clinical agencies and the community or from other nursing education programs, to serve as examples for the integration of informatics into the curriculum.
- Achieve competency through participation in faculty development programs.
- Partner with clinicians and informatics people at clinical agencies to help faculty and students develop competence in informatics.
- Collaborate with clinical agencies to ensure that students have hands-on experience with informatics tools.
- Collaborate with clinical agencies to demonstrate transformations in clinical practice produced by informatics.
- Establish criteria to evaluate informatics goals for faculty.

For Deans/Directors/Chairs

- Provide leadership in planning for necessary IT infrastructure that will ensure education that prepares graduates for twenty-first century practice roles and responsibilities.
- Allocate sufficient resources to support IT initiatives.
- Ensure that all faculty members have competence in computer literacy, information literacy, and informatics.
- Provide opportunities for faculty development in informatics.
- Urge clinical agencies to provide hands-on informatics experiences for students.
- Encourage nurse-managed clinics to incorporate clinical informatics exemplars that have transformed nursing practice to provide safe quality care.
- Advocate that all students graduate with up-to-date knowledge and skills in each of the three critical areas: computer literacy, information literacy, and informatics.
- Establish criteria to evaluate outcomes related to achieving informatics goals.

For the National League for Nursing

- Disseminate this position statement widely.
- Seek external funding and allocate internal resources to convene a think tank to reach consensus on definitions of informatics, competencies for faculty and students, and program outcomes that include informatics.
- Participate actively in organizations that focus on education in nursing informatics to ensure that recommendations from those organizations are congruent with the NLN's positions on curriculum.
- Use ETIMAC and its task groups to: (a) develop programs for faculty, showcasing exemplar programs, and (b) disseminate outcomes from the think tank.
- Encourage and facilitate accrediting bodies, regulatory agencies, and certifying bodies to reach consensus on definitions related to informatics and minimal informatics competencies for practice in the twenty-first century.

The Position Statement was widely disseminated to the nursing education community. A press release received significant media coverage (http://www.nln.org/newsreleases/informatics_release_052908.htm), and an interview with NLN CEO Beverly Malone on the topic was televised by iHealthBeat. A webinar was offered to faculty in the fall 2008. During the 2008 American Academy of Nursing Meeting that took place from November 6 to 8 in Scottsdale, AZ, the Expert Panel on Nursing Informatics unanimously endorsed the NLN's Position Statement, *Preparing the Next Generation of Nurses to Practice in a Technology-rich Environment: An Informatics Agenda.* The full text of the Position Statement is available at http://www.nln.org/aboutnln/PositionStatements/index.htm. To learn more about the work of this Council, link to https://www.nln.org/getinvolved/AdvisoryCouncils_TaskGroups/etimac.htm

ETIMAC also established the Task Group on Faculty Development related to Informatics Competencies.[30] Their purpose is to formulate a comprehensive plan for faculty development related to the integration of informatics into the nursing curriculum. Specific tasks to be completed by the end of 2009 included the following:

1. Identify exemplars and examine how innovative schools of nursing have integrated informatics into the curriculum and prepared their graduates to practice in the current practice environment.
2. Develop curriculum guidelines related to incorporating informatics as a core competency in the nursing curriculum across all educational levels.
3. Develop a web resource site that provides information and links to teaching strategies, assignments, exercises, active learning experiences, case studies, and software that is available and targeted to specific informatics learning outcomes.
4. Draft a comprehensive plan for a faculty development series that would prepare faculty to incorporate best practices for integration of informatics competencies into the curriculum.
5. Establish and monitor an electronic "eCommunity" on strategies and best practices to integrate informatics competencies into the nursing curriculum.

For more information and updates on this task force's work, link to http://www.nln.org/getinvolved/AdvisoryCouncils_TaskGroups/informatics.htm

American Association of Colleges of Nursing

The American Association of Colleges of Nursing is also advancing the TIGER vision by incorporating informatics as an "Essential" element of baccalaureate and the doctor of nursing practice education.

In 2008, a consensus-building technique was used to reach agreement about the essential elements of baccalaureate education for professional nursing practice. This document, *Essentials of Baccalaureate Education for Professional Practice*, can be accessed on their web site at http://www.aacn.nche.edu/Education/bacessn.htm. One of the nine *Essentials* focuses on Information Management and Application of Patient Care Technology. For each essential element, a rationale is provided along with expected competencies and sample content. It is the expectation that all baccalaureate education programs will incorporate the new "Essentials" into their curriculum.

Baccalaureate Essential IV: Information Management and Application of Patient Care Technology

The baccalaureate program prepares the graduate to:

1. Demonstrate skills in using patient care technologies, information systems, and communication devices that support safe nursing practice.
2. Use telecommunication technologies to assist in effective communication in a variety of healthcare settings.
3. Apply safeguards and decision-making support tools embedded in patient care technologies and information systems to support a safe practice environment for both patients and health care workers.
4. Understand the use of CIS systems to document interventions related to achieving nurse sensitive outcomes.
5. Use standardized terminology in a care environment that reflects nursing's unique contribution to patient outcomes.
6. Evaluate data from all relevant sources, including technology, to inform the delivery of care.
7. Recognize the role of IT in improving patient care outcomes and creating a safe care environment.
8. Uphold ethical standards related to data security, regulatory requirements, confidentiality, and clients' right to privacy.
9. Apply patient care technologies as appropriate to address the needs of a diverse patient population.
10. Advocate for the use of new patient care technologies for safe, quality care.

11. Recognize that redesign of workflow and care processes should precede implementation of care technology to facilitate nursing practice.
12. Participate in the evaluation of information systems in practice settings through policy and procedure development.

In addition, the AACN previously incorporated informatics into their *Essentials of Doctoral Education for Advanced Nursing Practice*. One of the eight essentials is focused on Information Systems/Technology and Patient Care Technology for the Improvement and Transformation of Health Care. Again, the rationale, expected outcomes, and sample content are provided. To learn more, go to http://www.aacn.nche.edu/Education/essentials. htm.

Essential IV: Information Systems/Technology and Patient Care Technology for the Improvement and Transformation of Health Care

The DNP program prepares the graduate to:
1. Design, select, use, and evaluate programs that evaluate and monitor outcomes of care, care systems, and quality improvement including consumer use of health care information systems.
2. Analyze and communicate critical elements necessary for the selection, use, and evaluation of health care information systems and patient care technology.
3. Demonstrate the conceptual ability and technical skills to develop and execute an evaluation plan involving data extraction from practice information systems and databases.
4. Provide leadership in the evaluation and resolution of ethical and legal issues within health care systems relating to the use of information, IT, communication networks, and patient care technology.
5. Evaluate consumer health information sources for accuracy, timeliness, and appropriateness.

Accreditation Bodies

It is notable that both accrediting agencies for schools of nursing have updated their standards for accreditation of program to include technology. The Commission on Collegiate Nursing Education (CCNE) does so by requiring schools to incorporate the "Essentials" into their curriculums. Links to all of the CCNE standards for accreditation of programs documents can be found on the CCNE website at http://www.aacn. nche.edu/accreditation. The National League for Nursing Accrediting Commission (NLNAC) revised their standards and criteria for accreditation of programs in 2008; new language specifies that the curriculum reflects technological advances. A link to the 2008 NLNAC standards and criteria can be found at http://www.nlnac.org/manuals/ SC2008.htm.

Associate Degree Nursing Committee

Three members of the Education and Faculty Development Collaborative explored the issues and challenges of incorporating informatics into associate degree curricula via two avenues: they gathered data by posting the following message on the National Organization for Associate Degree Nursing (N-OADN) electronic mailing list and also discussed the topic informally with members during the N-OADN annual convention in November of 2007. The message read,

> Do you have an ADN initiative that addresses the education of students and/or faculty in preparing them with the necessary computer skills, information literacy skills and informatics skills to work in a technology-rich health care environment? I am interested in initiatives, resources, learning activities and examples you may have. What learning outcomes do you expect of the ADN grad regarding informatics?

The following themes and challenges emerged and represent the opinions of approximately 75 associate degree faculty who responded via the electronic mailing list or during informal discussions at the N-OADN conference.

Many associate degree nursing faculty said that they recognize the need to incorporate informatics into the curriculum because they know that this content has been added to the NCLEX test plan, but one program director questioned what competencies were appropriate for AD graduates. Most reported that informatics is integrated throughout the curriculum, but a few reported having a stand-alone course, and one program collaborates with the business and technology division to provide an informatics course. Faculty also reported that while electronic medical records (EMRs) are used in many of the hospitals and agencies where students have their clinical practice, most small rural hospitals have limited computerization so their knowledge and use of informatics are limited, but evolving.

Several faculty remarked about student computer literacy skills. Most participants said their schools did not have a required computer literacy course, but they are observing that each new group of students enters their program with increased levels of competency. One faculty member asserted that computer literacy skills are as essential as cardiopulmonary resuscitation (CPR) skills; another reported that her college is investigating the addition of a computer literacy test for all students prior to admission. Some faculty reported that they are administering more tests on the computer and are requiring students to use technology when doing presentations in class.

Several participants mentioned that both students and faculty are using PDAs. They are purchasing digital copies of reference books for these devices and using them in the clinical area. Some schools obtained funding to purchase the PDAs.

Those faculty members who are aware of the need to incorporate informatics concepts into the curriculum reported that it is difficult to get older faculty to embrace informatics and incorporate the use of EMRs into clinical practice. They report that resistant faculty questions the value of having students spend time learning the hospital's EMR system since it reduces time spent in patient care, but they wonder if their reluctance is more related to feelings of incompetence. Several faculty reported that health care agencies restrict the use of EMR documentation to faculty only, placing an unreasonable load on the faculty and reducing the time available for clinical teaching. Very few schools have EMR software in their computer labs, and most felt that the cost of such products was prohibitive.

State Boards of Nursing

Another subgroup of the TIGER Education and Faculty Development Collaborative was charged with investigating existing or pending requirements from state boards of nursing regarding integration of informatics into educational programs. In November 2007, the work group developed an online survey and sent an email to the educator coordinator or administrator of each board of nursing, requesting their participation. Those who did not respond to the online survey were contacted by phone for their responses. Thirty-eight states provided data.

In response to the question "Does your state board of nursing have any curriculum and/or practice requirements related to the use of technology in the clinical practice setting?," 12 boards indicated that they had a requirement. When asked what technology was specified, 52.6% identified informatics, 21.1% specified simulation, and 15.8% selected basic computer skills. Nearly two-thirds indicated "other" technology requirements, but did not provide any further information.

Another question asked the state boards if they had curriculum and/or practice requirements related to some specific technologies. The majority had no requirements or recommendations. Only two have a requirement that prelicensure program graduates have proficiency in basic computer software use, and another state board recommends it. Two boards have recommendations that prelicensure programs include computerized nursing documentation. One state board recommends that prelicensure programs provide computer access to patient data.

Other survey questions were related to information literacy and specific informatics content. Again the majority had no requirements or recommendations. Regarding the use of evidence-based knowledge databases, four state boards had a prelicensure requirement; one had a recommendation. Four boards had a requirement for online access to find and use information; two had recommendations. Four state boards also had a requirement related to knowledge of privacy and security standards, and three had recommendations. Requirements of understanding the link between IT and safety exist in four states; three additional states have recommendations. Using IT to support clinical workflow is a prelicensure requirement in three states. Defining the role of informatics in nursing and health care is a requirement of prelicensure programs in two states; it is a recommendation in two others.

It is important to recognize that all state boards of nursing have language in their regulations stating that prelicensure educational programs provide content that reflects current nursing practice. Since current practice involves the use of technology and knowledge of informatics to provide safe, quality patient care, these regulations do not need to include specifics of curriculum content. Indeed, if specific content is mandated, regulations need to be reviewed and modified more frequently to keep up with a rapidly changing health care environment. It is certainly the responsibility of faculty to be aware of current practice and emerging trends and develop curriculums that go beyond current practice and prepare students for the future. The National Council of State Boards of Nursing can take a leadership role by informing the state boards of changes in health care environments and keeping them aware of best practices and emerging trends. Armed with this knowledge, members of the state boards can evaluate the curriculums of schools and hold them accountable for providing content that reflects the most current nursing practice.

State Initiatives

Another important stakeholder in education is statewide initiatives that occur across educational institutions, such as the Oregon Statewide Initiative.

From the TIGER perspective, there were four states that had either initiatives focused on informatics or had the infrastructure in place to begin informatics initiatives. One state formed the Minnesota TIGER. In addition, a State Initiatives committee, chaired by Dr. Paulette Seymour-Route (University of Massachusetts), brought together two additional states (North Carolina and California) to examine current and potential work in the area of informatics. Both Massachusetts and California had statewide initiatives for faculty related to teaching with technology, in particular using simulations in nursing education. Both states have a readily available statewide infrastructure in place to begin a campaign to incorporate informatics into nursing education.

Minnesota TIGER

The Minnesota TIGER is one such state initiative. Under the leadership of Drs. Connie Delaney and Bonnie Westra, the Minnesota TIGER was created to translate the vision of the national TIGER initiative into action in the upper-Midwest. The flowing organizations, University of Minnesota, the MINING (Minnesota Nursing Informatics Group), MOLN (Minnesota Organization of Leaders in Nursing), MACN (Minnesota Association of College of Nursing), Minnesota Nurses Association, and the Informatics Group, sponsor the yearly summit. More information is available at http://www.nursing.umn.edu/MNTiger/.

North Carolina

The State Board of Nursing in North Carolina is leading the charge by requiring that all schools of nursing begin to incorporate the five IOM core competencies, including informatics, into their nursing curriculum. Their State Board of Nursing web site (http:// ncbon. com), under their Education Rules, Administrative Code, Chapter 36 Board of Nursing, Rule 21NCAC 36.0321(b)(1) CURRICULUM, states that didactic content and supervised clinical experience appropriate to program type shall include: Using informatics to communicate, manage knowledge, mitigate error, and support decision making, as well as the four other IOM Competencies. Their early efforts and the work of the Quality and Safety Education for Nurses (QSEN)[31] position North Carolina as a pioneering leader in promoting informatics at all levels of nursing education.

Massachusetts

The Board of Higher Education and the Massachusetts Organization of Nurse Executives convened a conference, *Creativity and Connections: Building the Framework for the Future of Nursing Education and Practice*. The focus was to address two questions: How can higher education institutions graduate more nurses and what competencies will be required of the nurse of the future? An outcome of this conference was the creation of a formal coalition to create a seamless progression through all levels of nursing that is based on consensus competencies that include transitioning nurses into their practice settings. Another result was the creation of core competencies for the *Nurse of the Future*. Their work builds upon the IOM's five core competencies and "competencies collected from other states, current practice standards; education accrediting standards; national initiatives and projected patient demographic and healthcare profiles for Massachusetts" (Massachusetts Department of Higher Education Nursing Initiative 2007, p. 2). To learn more, visit http://www.mass.edu/currentinit/currentinitNursingNurseFuture.asp.

California

Like Massachusetts, the *California Institute for Nursing & Healthcare* had a statewide initiative focused on the transformation of nursing education. In 2008, they released their *Nursing Education Redesign for California: White Paper and Strategic Action Plan Recommendations*. In their recommendations, they call for the inclusion of informatics in the nursing curriculum and their support for minimal competencies in the area. This statewide infrastructure is positioned to leverage its network and resources to move the TIGER informatics agenda. To read more about their work, go to http://www.cinhc.org/index.html.

Health Services Resources Administration (HRSA)

The TIGER Initiative has worked closely with the Division of Nursing within HRSA. During the planning phase of the TIGER Summit, we approached Dr. Denise Geolot, then Deputy Director of the Division of Nursing, for their involvement. A representative from Division of Nursing attended the TIGER Summit. There are three major accomplishments associated with HRSA's Division of Nursing.

The first is the creation of the Division of Nursing Faculty Develoment: Integrating Technology into Nursing Education and Practice Initiative (ITNEP). This initiative made funds available for projects to provide education in new technologies, under Title VIII,

Section 831 of the Public Health Service Act, as amended by the Nurse Reinvestment Act of 2002. According to the grant announcement, the use of information and other technologies in nursing education and practice includes informatics, telehealth, mannequin-based and patient simulators, computer-based instructions, virtual simulation, interactive simulated case studies, advanced 3D graphics, and e-learning technologies. The monies were to support what HRSA called nursing collaboratives for faculty development. The purpose is to use information and other technologies to expand the capacity of schools of nursing to educate students for twenty-first century health care practice. To date, six collaboratives have been funded, as shown in Table 5.1.

Given the high demand, especially the number of applicants to the HITS program, HRSA received additional funding for two more collaboratives. These collaboratives are one solution to provide faculty with the necessary knowledge and skills to teach about technology and with technology.[32]

The National Advisory Council on Nurse Education and Practice (NACNEP) advises the Secretary of the U.S. Department of Health and Human Services and the U.S. Congress on policy issues related to the Title VIII programs administered by the HRSA Bureau of Health Professions Division of Nursing, including nurse workforce supply, education, and practice improvement. The focus of their 2007 spring meeting was on "Challenges facing the Nursing Workforce in a Changing Environment." In particular, this meeting focused on Information Technology in Nursing Education and Practice. A product of that meeting is the Seventh Report to the Secretary of Health and Human Services and the Congress. This soon-to-be-released report focuses on teaching about and teaching with technology. The first component targets the preparation of a workforce capable of practicing in a technology-rich health care environment. The second component discusses the use of technology to facilitate the educational preparation of nurses. For more information, go to http://bhpr.hrsa.gov/nursing/nacnep.htm

Table 5.1 ITNEP Collaboratives

University of Wisconsin at Madison PI: Dr. Patricia Brennan
Duke University PI: Dr. Barbara Turner http://www.tip-nep.org/
The HITS Program (University of Kansas, University of Colorado Denver, Indiana University & NLN) PI: Dr. Helen Connors http://www.hits-colab.org/
University of Pittsburgh PI: Dr. Helen Burns http://www.nursing.pitt.edu/elite/index.jsp
Drexel University PI: Dr. Linda Wilson
University of Washington PI: Brenda Zierler

In addition, HRSA along with the Office of the National Coordinator have made the preparation of an informatics workforce an important facet of their agenda. At two national grantee meetings, there was an emphasis on the preparation of health care professionals in health IT and the preparation of a health IT workforce that included informatics specialists in nursing. The first conference, held in November 2007, was targeted to grantees funded by the Office of Health Information Technology and Health Resources Services Administration Grantee Meeting, focused on *Promoting HIT Adoption in the HRSA Community: Success Through Collaboration.* To view slides, go to http://www.blsmeetings.net/OHIT/presentation.cfm (Select Day 2).

The second conference, held in February of 2008, was a HRSA All Grantee meeting in which there was a session on the *Emerging role of HIT in the delivery & quality of Health Care & Health Care Training.*

Innovators in Nursing Education

Another group of important stakeholders were innovative educators who were moving the informatics agenda by adding informatics content to their nursing curriculum or by providing their students with hands-on experiences with electronic health record systems. These innovative faculty presented two webinars as part of the Education and Faculty Development Collaborative. The first webinar highlighted three different approaches to incorporating informatics into the nursing curriculum. The webinar, *Getting Started: Adding Informatics to the Nursing Curriculum,* featured three speakers: Dr. Jane M. Brokel, Assistant Professor, University of Iowa; Dr. Josette Jones, Assistant Professor, Indiana University; and Dr. Trish Trangenstein, Professor, Vanderbilt University. The first presentation by Brokel described an individual course that was developed for the undergraduate program at the University of Iowa. Dr. Josette Jones presented how informatics competencies were integrated throughout the BS curriculum. The last speaker, Dr. Trish Trangenstein, explained how their Bridge Students were users and integrators of NI tools and explained the toolkit they developed for their program. Their slides are available at http://tigereducation.pbwiki.com/.

The second webinar focused on three unique partnerships to help faculty prepare students to use electronic documentation and electronic health records. The first partnership was between a department of nursing and a department of computer sciences at a community college. Karin Sherrill, RN, MSN, CNE and Diana Breed, RN, MSN of Maricopa Community Colleges District Nursing Program-Mesa Campus explained the development and pilot testing of their Health Assessment Nursing Documentation System. This unique partnership demonstrated what can be done with limited time (less than 1 year) and virtually no real budget. The second was a 10-year partnership between a School of Nursing and one of their clinical agencies, Cardinal Health. Dr. Kay Hodson of Ball State University and Dlynn Melo of Cardinal Health System described a decade-long collaboration that has provided a WIN-WIN situation for both partners. The School of Nursing has gained access to Cardinal Health's electronic documentation system for all their students. The presentation cited the cost savings for Cardinal Health and the satisfaction of the students learning in this environment. The last presentation was an example of a partnership between academia and business. Drs. Helen Connor and Judith Warren of the School of Nursing at the University of Kansas presented their Simulated E-hEalth Delivery Systems (SEEDS), a collaboration between the School of Nursing and Cerner Corporation that began in 2001. The goal was to redesign the Cerner's current clinical information systems to fit the educational workflow of baccalaureate nursing students. The success of this partnership has expanded and now includes a consortium of over 12 schools of nursing. A video of SEEDS is available for viewing at http://www2.kumc.edu/healthinformatics/video.html and presentation slides can be found at http://tigereducation.pbwiki.com/.

Summary

The TIGER Education and Faculty Development Collaborative accomplished many of the goals set forward by the initial TIGER Summit. These goals were accomplished through the work of many volunteers in nursing education and health IT that represented the various stakeholder groups. There is no doubt that informatics has moved from the background to the foreground in nursing education. After a long rich history, its time has come. The necessary knowledge and skills in informatics are clearly delineated for all nurses. The nursing education community will now need to incorporate the necessary content and informatics experiences to insure that all new graduates are prepared to practice in a consumer-centric technology-rich health care environment.

References

1. Anderson J, Gremy F, Pages J. *Education in Informatics of Health Professionals*. New York, NY: Elsevier Publishing; 1974.
2. Ronald JS. Computers in undergraduate nursing education: a report of an experimental introductory course. *J Nurs Educ*. 1979;18(9):4-9.
3. Ronald JS. Guidelines for computer literacy curriculum in a school of nursing. *J N Y State Nurses Assoc*. 1983;14(1):12-18.
4. Skiba D. Computer literacy: the challenge of the 80s. *J N Y State Nurses Assoc*. 1983;14(1):6-11.
5. Ronald J, Skiba D. *Guidelines for Basic Computer Education in Nursing*. New York, NY: National League for Nursing; 1987.
6. National Advisory Council on Nurse Education and Practice. *Report to the Secretary of the Department of Health and Human Services: A National Informatics Agenda for Nursing Education and Practice*. Washington, DC: Author; 1997.
7. Carty B, Rosenfield P. From computer technology to information technology. Findings from a national study of nursing education. *Comput Nurs*. 1998;11:122-126.
8. McNeil BJ, Odom SK. Nursing informatics education in the United States: proposed undergraduate curriculum. *Health Informatics J*. 2000;6(1):32-38.
9. Hobbs S. Measuring nurses' computer competency: an analysis of published instruments. *Comput Inform Nurs*. 2002;20(2):63-73.
10. Russell A, Alpay L. Practice nurses' training in information technology: report on an empirical investigation. *Health Informatics J*. 2000;6:142-146.

11. McCannon M, O'Neal P. Results of a national survey indicating information technology skills needed by nurses at time of entry into the work force. *J Nurs Educ.* 2003;42(8):337-340.

12. McNeil BJ, Elfrink VL, Bickford CJ, et al. Nursing information technology knowledge, skills, and preparation of student nurses, nursing faculty, and clinicians: a U.S. survey. *J Nurs Educ.* 2003;42(8):341-349.

13. Thompson B, Skiba D. Informatics in the nursing curriculum: a national survey. *Nurs Educ Perspect.* 2008;29(5):312-316.

14. Staggers N, Gassert CA, Curran C. A Delphi study to determine informatics competencies for nurses at four levels of practice. *Nurs Res.* 2002;51(6):383-390.

15. Staggers N, Gassert CA, Curran C. Informatics competencies for nurses at four levels of practice. *J Nurs Educ.* 2001;40(7):303-316.

16. Hebert M. A national education strategy to develop nursing informatics competencies. *Can J Nurs Leadersh.* 2004;13(2):11-14.

17. Jiang WW, Chen W, Chen YC. Important computer competencies for the nursing profession. *J Nurs Res.* 2004;12(3):213-226.

18. Smedley A. The importance of informatics competencies in nursing: an Australian perspective. *Comput Inform Nurs.* 2005;23(2):106-110.

19. Barton AJ. Cultivating informatics competencies in a community of practice. *Nurs Adm Q.* 2005;29(4):323-328.

20. Bickford C. Informatics competencies for nurse managers and their staff. *Semin Nurse Manag.* 2002;10(2):110-113.

21. Curran C. Informatics competencies for nurse practitioners. *AACN Clin Issues.* 2003;14:320-330.

22. Skiba D. Moving forward: the informatics agenda. *Nurs Educ Perspect.* 2008;29(5):300-301.

23. Warren J, Connors H. Health information technology can and will transform nursing education. *Nurs Outlook.* 2007;55(1):58-60.

24. Kohn LT, Corrigan JM, Donaldson MS. *To Err is Human: Building a Safer Health System.* Washington, DC: National Academies Press; 2000.

25. Committee on Quality Health Care in America, Institute of Medicine. *Crossing the Quality Chasm: A New Health System for the 21st Century.* Washington, DC: National Academy Press; 2001.

26. Greiner A, Knebel E. *Health Professions Education: A Bridge to Quality.* Washington, DC: National Academies Press; 2003.

27. Aspden P, Corrigan J, Wolcott J, et al. *Patient Safety: Achieving a New Standard of Care. Report of the Committee on Data Standards for Patient Safety, Institute of Medicine.* Washington, DC: National Academies Press; 2004.

28. Technology Informatics Guiding Education Reform. The TIGER initiative: collaborating to integrate evidence and informatics into nursing practice and education: an executive summary. www.tigersummit.com/; 2009. Accessed 28.09.09.

29. Technology Informatics Guiding Education Reform. The TIGER initiative: evidence and informatics transforming nursing: 3-year action steps toward a 10-year vision. www.tigersummit.com/; 2007. Accessed 28.09.09.

30. Skiba D, Rizzolo M. National League for Nursing's informatics agenda. *Comput Inform Nurs.* 2008;27(1):66-68.

31. Cronenwett L, Sherwood G, Barnsteiner J, et al. Quality and safety education for nurses. *Nurs Outlook.* 2007;55(3):122-131.

32. Skiba D, Connors H, Jeffries P. Information technologies and transformation of nursing education. *Nurs Outlook.* 2008;56(5):225-230.

Competencies: Nuts and Bolts

6

Connie Delaney and Brian Gugerty

Nurses are expected to provide safe, competent, and compassionate care in an increasingly technical and digital environment. Since the landmark 1999 Institute of Medicine (IOM) report *To Error is Human*,[1] health care professionals and consumers have been inundated with follow-up IOM reports,[2-5] popular press, and clear visibility of broken health care systems fraught with errors and need for transformation. Information and communication technologies have been identified as core prescriptions for addressing safety and quality. Nurses are directly engaged with information systems and technologies as the foundation for evidence-based practice, clinical decision support tools, and the electronic health record (EHR).

To help practicing nurses be responsive to the changes in their practice environments, a specialty called Nursing Informatics has emerged over the past 20 years. This specialty has had an impact on all roles, functions, clinical care, education, and research/scholarship throughout nursing and in all nursing specialties. The most recent 2008 American Nurses Association (ANA) Nursing Informatics Scope and Standards defines nursing informatics as the integration of nursing science, computer and information science, and cognitive science to manage communication and expand the data, information, knowledge, and wisdom of nursing practice. In sum, nurses certified in Nursing Informatics[6] (ANA 2008).

- Are skilled in the analysis, design, and implementation of information systems that support nursing in a variety of health care settings
- Function as translators between nurse clinicians and information technology personnel
- Insure that information systems capture critical nursing information

These specialized nurses add value to an organization by[6] (ANA 2008)

- Increasing the accuracy and completeness of nursing documentation
- Improving the nurse's workflow

C. Delaney (✉)
University of Minnesota, School of Nursing, Minneapolis, MN, USA
e-mail: delaney@umn.edu

M.J. Ball et al. (eds.), *Nursing Informatics*,
DOI: 10.1007/978-1-84996-278-0_6, © Springer-Verlag London Limited 2011

- Eliminating redundant documentation
- Automating the collection and reuse of nursing data
- Facilitating the analysis of clinical data, including indicators established by the Joint Commission for Accreditation of Healthcare Organizations, core measures, federal or state mandated data, and facility-specific data

While Nursing Informatics is a highly specialized field, there are foundational informatics competencies that all practicing nurses and graduating nursing students should possess to meet the standards of providing safe, quality, and competent care.

Formed as part of the Technology Informatics Guiding Education Reform (TIGER) initiative, the TIGER Informatics Competency Collaborative (TICC) developed informatics recommendations for all practicing nurses and graduating nursing students. This chapter describes those recommendations and the process that yielded them.

Approach and Strategy

An extensive review of the literature and of nursing informatics education, research, and practice groups provided the base for the TIGER Nursing Informatics Competencies Model. This review, which defined informatics competencies for practicing nurses and nursing students, was supplemented by surveying over 50 health care delivery organizations for competencies. The efforts, described on the TICC Wiki (http://tigercompetencies.pbwiki.com), yielded over 1,000 individual competency statements. These were boiled down to form the three parts of our TIGER Nursing Informatics Competencies Model: Basic Computer Competencies, Information Literacy, and Information Management.

Once the model was developed, TICC aligned each component with an existing set of competencies maintained by standard development organizations or de facto standards. This process identified very good fits with four existing sets of standards maintained by three standard-setting bodies that developed them. Those bodies and the standards they continue to evolve are:

- The European Computer Driving Licence (ECDL) Foundation: Basic competencies
- Health Level 7 (HL7): The electronic health record functional model clinical care components
- The American Library Association (ALA): Information literacy standards

Building on these three sets of competencies, TICC focused on developing recommendations for standards that would be, first, relevant to nurses and, second, sustainable over time. The three standard-setting bodies TICC identified have all put tremendous thought, energy, and expertise into their recommended competencies. When those competencies aligned with the informatics competency needs for nurses, TICC adopted theirs, thus adding strength, rigor, and validity to the TICC recommendations (Table 6.1).

Table 6.1 TIGER competencies, standards, and standard-setting bodies

Component of the TIGER nursing informatics competencies model	Standard	Standard-setting body
Basic Computer Competencies	European Computer Driving Licence	European Computer Driving Licence Foundation
Information Literacy	Information Literacy Competency Standards	American Library Association
Information Management	Electronic Health Record Functional Model – Clinical Care Components	Health Level Seven (HL7)
	European Computer Driving Licence – Health	European Computer Driving Licence Foundation

Standards Set 1: Basic Computer Competencies

A "digital native" has grown up with digital technology such as computers, the Internet, mobile phones, and MP3. A "digital immigrant" grew up without digital technology and adopted it later. There are a substantial number of digital immigrants in the nursing workforce who have not mastered basic computer competencies. Also, many digital natives have gaps in their basic computer competency skill set.

Europeans realized this shortcoming in the workforce across many industries and acted on it. The ECDL Foundation set basic computer competencies in the late 1990s and again in this decade. About nine million Europeans have now taken the ECDL exam and become certified in basic computer competencies. Effectively a global standard in basic computer competencies, the ECDL syllabus addresses basic computer competencies in seven modules.[7] They are:

Module 1: Concepts of Information and Communication Technology (ICT)

These competencies establish understanding of general knowledge of information and communication technology, including basic hardware and software concepts.

An example knowledge item for module 1 is *"Know the main parts of a computer like: central processing unit (CPU), types of memory, hard disk, common input and output devices."*

Module 1 has 61 knowledge items.

Module 2: Using the Computer and Managing Files

These competencies establish that a candidate's knowledge of concepts needs to operate and manage a personal computer.

An example knowledge item for module 2 is *"Understand how an operating system organizes drives, folders, files in a hierarchical structure."*

Module 2 has 54 knowledge items.

Module 3: Word Processing

These competencies demonstrate a candidate's ability to use a word processing application to create and manage documents.

An example knowledge item for module 3 is *"Open, close a word processing application. Open, close documents."*

Module 3 has 66 knowledge items.

Module 4: Spreadsheets

These competencies establish understanding of a candidate's ability to use a spreadsheet to enter data, calculate basic mathematical functions on data, and produce outputs.

An example knowledge item for module 4 is *"Create formulas using cell references and arithmetic operators (addition, subtraction, multiplication, division)."*

Module 4 has 66 knowledge items.

Module 5: Using Databases

These competencies demonstrate a candidate's knowledge of key database concepts and ability to use a database application.

An example knowledge item for module 5 is *"Understand how a database is organized in terms of tables, records and fields."*

Module 5 has 66 knowledge items.

Module 6: Presentation

These competencies demonstrate that a candidate's competence is using a presentation software application.

An example knowledge item for module 6 is *"Understand Create a new presentation based on a default template."*

Module 6 has 72 knowledge items.

Module 7: Web Browsing and Communication

These competencies involve web browsing skills, internet concepts, e-mail, and other information technology-mediated communication options.

An example knowledge item for module 7 is *"Enter a URL in the address bar and go to the URL."*

Module 7 has 92 knowledge items.

At the end of its year-long collaboration, TICC arrived at a consensus-based decision to recommend adoption of the ECDL competencies for all practicing nurses and graduating nursing students. Recognizing that ECDL certification requires 30+ hours of study and costs more than some institutions may be able to afford, TICC ranked the relative importance of ECDL syllabus items and identified the following modules as first steps to basic computer proficiency that are feasible and affordable. They also will provide the basic competencies that will allow nurses to go on to obtain other TICC competencies:

* Module 1: Concepts of Information and Communication Technology (ICT)
* Module 2: Using the Computer and Managing Files
* Module 3: Section 3.1. Word Processing: "Using the application"
* Module 7: Web Browsing and Communication (Table 6.2)

Table 6.2 Recommendations for ECDL certification with timelines for adoption

Recommendation	Timeline for adoption
All practicing nurses and graduating nursing students gain or demonstrate proficiency in ECDL modules 1, 2, and 7, as well as ECDL Category 3.1	By January 2011
All practicing nurses and graduating nursing students become ECDL certified or hold a substantially equivalent certification	By January 2013

Resources are available to help nurses as they work to attain basic competencies. The non-profit ECDL Foundation (http://ecdl.com) maintains and periodically updates the ECDL syllabus and makes arrangements with entities in various countries to localize the ECDL syllabus. Outside of Europe, ECDL is known as International Computer Driving Licence (ICDL).

In the United States, it is available through CSPlacement (www.csplacement.com). CSPlacement offers CSP Basic, an e-learning course and a certification exam that is sub-stantially equivalent to the TICC recommendation of a first and significant step toward basic computer competency, and CSP, an e-learning course and a certification exam that is substantially equivalent to the entire ECDL syllabus.

Also in the United States, the Healthcare Information and Management System Society (HIMSS, www.himss.org) has a certificate called Health Informatics Training System (HITS). The HITS program of e-learning, testing, and certification contains content that is substantially equivalent to the TICC recommendation of a first and significant step toward basic computer competency, as well as other content.

Standards Set 2: Information Literacy

Information literacy builds on computer literacy. Information literacy is the ability to

- Identify information needed for a specific purpose
- Locate pertinent information
- Evaluate the information
- Apply it correctly

Information literacy is critical to incorporating evidence-based practice into nursing prac-tice. The nurse/provider must be able to determine what information is needed. This involves critical thinking and assessment skills. Finding the information is based on the resources available, which can include colleagues, policies, and literature in various for-mats. Evaluating or appraising the information also involves critical thinking and the abil-ity to determine the validity of the source. The actual implementation of the information results in putting the information into practice or applying the information. The evaluation process is necessary to determine whether the information and its application resulted in improvements. Thus, information literacy competencies are fundamental to nursing and evidence-based practice (Table 6.3).

Some institutions may find these competencies difficult to implement in their entirety immediately. Therefore, as a first and significant step toward information literacy in nurses, the TICC recommends focusing on the first three competencies for the first year. Once these are achieved by nurses in a particular organization, the other two can be added. TICC has set a timeline for adoption of January 2011; by that date, all nurses will all five compe-tencies and incoming nurses will demonstrate or will be helped to obtain all five.

Resources available to help nurses attain this goal include the ALA. Its report, *Information Literacy Competency Standards for Higher Education*, identifies

Table 6.3 Recommendation for information literacy competencies with timelines for adoption

Recommendation	Timeline for adoption
All practicing nurses and graduating nursing students will have the ability to	By January 2011
Determine the nature and extent of the information needed	
Access needed information effectively and efficiently	
Evaluate information and its sources critically and incorporates selected information into his or her knowledge base and value system	
Individually or as a member of a group, use information effectively to accomplish a specific purpose	
Evaluate outcomes of the use of information	

the competencies recommended above as standards. The report also lists performance indicators and outcomes for each standard. A faculty member or instructor can effectively use this report to create a more detailed syllabus and/or lesson plan(s) to implement the TICC information literacy competencies. The ALA makes these available on its website at www.ala.org/ala/mgrps/divs/acrl/standards/informationliteracycompency.cfm.

In addition, the Information Literacy in Technology website at http://www.ilitassessment.com offers a tool to assess a student's ability to access, evaluate, incorporate, and use information. Commercially available, this iLIT test may be of use in demonstrating proficiency in information literacy.

Standards Set 3: Information Management

Information management is the principle upon which TICC Clinical Information Management Competencies are built. Information management is a process consisting of (1) collecting data, (2) processing the data, and (3) presenting and communicating the processed data as information or knowledge.

An underlying concept for information management is the data-information-knowledge continuum. *Data* are discrete, atomic-level symbols, for example, the number 120. *Information* are data that are grouped or organized or processed in such a way that the data have meaning, for example, a blood pressure of 120/80. *Knowledge* is information transformed or combined to be truly useful. An example of knowledge is that a blood pressure of 120/80 is dangerously hypertensive in a neonate.

Nurses manage information in a variety of ways, but more and more the preferred or required method is through information systems. We define an information system as being composed of human and computer elements that work interdependently to process data into information. The most relevant, important, and fundamental information management competencies for nurses are those that relate to the electronic health record system (EHRS).

Using an EHRS will be the way nurses manage clinical information for the foreseeable future. That said, however, nursing responsibilities are not changing in the shift to increased use of EHRSs. For example, nurses are still required to exercise due care in protecting patient privacy. But the manner in which these responsibilities to patients and communities are upheld may be different. Therefore, all practicing nurses and graduating nursing students are strongly encouraged to learn, demonstrate, and use information management competencies to carry out their fundamental clinical responsibilities in an increasingly safe, effective, and efficient manner.

The most rigorous as well as practical work on enumerating the relevant parts of the EHRS for clinicians was done by HL7 Electronic Health Record (EHR) Technical Committee and was published in February 2007 as an approved American National Standard (ANSI) publication titled *The HL7 EHR System Functional Model, Release 1*, sometimes referred to as ANSI/HL7 EHR, R1-2007.

The direct care component of the HL7 EHR System Functional Model serves as a basis of the clinical information management competencies for practicing nurses and graduating nursing students listed at the end of this chapter (see Appendix). Although the list of competencies for proficient use of EHRs is long, it merely makes explicit the clinical nursing responsibilities required of practicing nurses and graduating nursing students today in a paper information management environment or a mixed paper and electronic environment.

The direct care component of the HL7 EHR System Functional Model is not quite sufficient by itself to cover the information management responsibilities of nurses in the digital era. What is needed, in addition, is a set of competencies that address the importance of electronic health record and like systems to nurses and the "due care" that nurses need to take in managing information via these systems. Again, to address these concerns, the ECDL Foundation has come up with a set of items they call the ECDL-Health syllabus.

A high-level outline of ECDL Health includes four areas including Concepts, Due Care, User Skills, and Policy and Procedures. Transformed into TICC competencies, these are as follow:

- Concepts
  - Verbalize the importance of health information systems (HIS) to clinical practice
  - Have knowledge of various types of HIS and their clinical and administrative use
- Due Care
  - Assure confidentiality of protected patient health information when using HIS under his or her control
  - Assure access control in the use of HIS under his or her control
  - Assure the security of HIS under his or her control

- User Skills
  - Have the user skills outlined in the HL7 EHRS model, which includes all of the ECDL/ICDL-Health User Skills of navigation, decision support, output reports, and more

- Policy and Procedure
  - Understand the principles upon which organizational and professional HIS use by health care professionals and consumers are based

Despite some overlap, items in User Skills ECDL l ICDL-Health syllabus are complementary to the HL7 EHRS model items. Importantly, the ECDL-Health syllabus items add an important "awareness" component through a range of topics. For example, Why is the EHRS important; What it is; What its parts are; How does the EHR relate to other health information technology; why it is important to protect data, confidentiality, and privacy while using an EHRS; as well as how to do that, and more. Together, the ECDL-Health syllabus items and the HL7 EHRS model clinical care items create a robust set of information management items for all practicing and graduating nursing students (Table 6.4).

The primary resources for this third set of standards include HL7 and ECDL. The HL7 EHR System Functional Model is available at www.hl7.org/EHR. This ANSI standard can be used by nursing instructors in schools of nursing and health care delivery organizations to develop curriculum to impart the recommended information management competencies to all practicing nurses and graduating nursing students.

The ECDL-Health Syllabus is available at www.ecdl.com by clicking on products, then on ECDL Health. A significant portion of the HL7 EHR System Functional Model is covered by the ECDL-Health Syllabus. The ECDL-Health Syllabus was developed by the ECDL Foundation to extend the foundation of basic computer competency skills that are not industry-specific to the health care industry.

The ECDL/ICDL-Health syllabus is localized by countries for use in that country. The American Medical Informatics Association (AMIA) endorsed Digital Patient Record Certification (DPRC), available at http://dprcertification.com, which covers many of the same general ECDL/ICDL-Health syllabus items, is specific to the US health system. For example, it includes HIPAA content. DPRC covers the "awareness" as well as other TICC information management competencies.

The HIMSS offers users a more international version of the ICDL-Health syllabus for its eLearning Academy, i.e., the HITS. It is accessible through its website at www.himss.org.

Both the DPRC and HITS certifications are a substantial first step toward achieving clinical information management competencies for U.S. nurses and graduating nursing students.

Table 6.4 Recommendation for clinical information management competencies with timeline for adoption

Recommendation	Timeline for adoption
Schools of nursing and health care delivery organizations will implement the clinical information management competencies listed at the end of this chapter	By January 2012
Schools of nursing and health care delivery organizations will implement the transformed ECDL-Health syllabus items listed above	By January 2012

The Way Forward

Nurses are the "ground troops" in efforts to transform our health care system into a safer, higher quality one characterized by evidenced-based practice and patient-centered care. In order to meet their potential to be key contributors in these efforts, nurses need to be fully empowered to effectively and efficiently use health information technology which is now permeating all areas of nurses' practice.

A set of informatics competencies that establishes a ground floor of proficiency by nurses was needed. The TICC established such a set of informatics competencies for all practicing nurses and graduating nursing students that is composed of three elements: basic computer, information literacy, and information management competencies. Adoption of these competencies will enable nurses to have a minimum set of competencies to more fully engage in the informatics revolution that is transforming health care.

Acknowledgments   The members of the TIGER Informatics Competency Collaborative (TICC) are too numerous to mention here. They can be viewed on the TIGER web site. All TICC members had some part in the research and deliberations from which this report was drawn.

The authors also acknowledge TICC members Anne Coleman, Donna DuLong, Wanda Kelly, Sarah Tupper, and Denise Tyler for their contributions to this chapter and thank Marie McCarren, not a TICC member, for her editing.

Appendix

Clinical Information Management Competencies

TICC has transformed the Direct Care components of the HL7 EHR System Functional Model into recommended Clinical Information Management Competencies for nurses as shown below.

Using an EHRS, the nurse can:

Identify and Maintain a Patient Record
Manage Patient Demographics
Capture Data and Documentation from External Clinical Sources
Capture Patient-Originated Data
Capture Patient Health Data Derived from Administrative Data
Interact with Financial Data and Documentation
Produce a Summary Record of Care
Present Ad Hoc Views of the Health Record
Manage Patient History
Manage Patient and Family Preferences
Manage Patient Advance Directives

Manage Consents and Authorizations

Manage Allergy, Intolerance, and Adverse Reaction Lists

Manage Medication Lists

Manage Problem Lists

Manage Immunization Lists

Interact with Guidelines and Protocols for Planning Care

Manage Patient-Specific Care and Treatment Plans

Manage Medication Orders as Appropriate for His/Her Scope of Practice

Manage Nonmedication Patient Care Orders

Manage Orders for Diagnostic Tests

Manage Orders for Blood Products and Other Biologics

Manage Referrals

Manage Order Sets

Manage Medication Administration

Manage Immunization Administration

Manage Results

Manage Patient Clinical Measurements

Manage Clinical Documents and Notes

Manage Documentation of Clinician Response to Decision Support Prompts

Generate and Record Patient-Specific Instructions

Manage Health Information to Provide Decision Support for Standard Assessments

Manage Health Information to Provide Decision Support for Patient Context-Driven assessments

Manage Health Information to Provide Decision Support for Identification of Potential Problems and Trends

Manage Health Information to Provide Decision Support for Patient and Family Preferences

Interact with Decision Support for Standard Care Plans, Guidelines, and Protocols

Interact with Decision Support for Context-Sensitive Care Plans, Guidelines, and Protocols

Manage Health Information to Provide Decision Support Consistent Healthcare Management of Patient Groups or Populations

Manage Health Information to Provide Decision Support for Research Protocols Relative to Individual Patient Care

Manage Health Information to Provide Decision Support for Self-Care

Interact with Decision Support for Medication and Immunization Ordering as Appropriate for His/Her Scope of Practice

Interact with Decision Support for Drug Interaction Checking

Interact with Decision Support for Patient-Specific Dosing and Warnings

Interact with Decision Support for Medication Recommendations

Interact with Decision Support for Medication and Immunization Administration

Interact with Decision Support for Nonmedication Ordering

Interact with Decision Support for Result Interpretation

Interact with Decision Support for Referral Process

Interact with Decision Support for Referral Recommendations

Interact with Decision Support for Safe Blood Administration

Interact with Decision Support for Accurate Specimen Collection

Interact with Decision Support that Presents Alerts for Preventive Services and Wellness

Interact with Decision Support for Notifications and Reminders for Preventive Services and Wellness

Manage Health Information to Provide Decision Support for Epidemiological Investigations of Clinical Health Within a Population.

Manage Health Information to Provide Decision Support for Notification and Response regarding Population Health Issues

Manage Health Information to Provide Decision Support for Monitoring Response Notifications Regarding a Specific Patient's Health

Access Healthcare Guidance

Interact with Clinical Workflow Tasking

Interact with Clinical Task Assignment and Routing

Interact with Clinical Task Linking

Interact with Clinical Task Tracking

Facilitate Interprovider Communication

Facilitate Provider-Pharmacy Communication

Facilitate Communications between Provider and Patient and/or the Patient Representative

Facilitate Patient, Family, and Care Giver Education

Facilitate Communication with Medical Devices

The above list comes from the Direct Care components of the HL7 EHR System Functional Model. In some cases functional statements were not changed as they can also serve as competencies. For example, the HL7 EHR System Functional Model statement of "Access Healthcare Guidance" was unchanged, except for the preamble that applies to all Clinical Information Management Competencies as "Using an EHRS, the nurse can: Access Healthcare Guidance." The HL7 EHR System Functional Model statement of Communication with Medical Devices was changed from "Communication with Medical Devices" to "Facilitate Communication with Medical Devices" to make it a Clinical Information Management Competency.

References

1. Institute of Medicine. *To Error Is Human*. Washington: National Academy; 1999.
2. Institute of Medicine. *Crossing the Quality Chasm*. Washington: National Academy; 2000.
3. Institute of Medicine. *Improving the Quality of Long Term Care*. Washington: National Academy; 2001.
4. Institute of Medicine. *Keeping Patients Safe*. Washington: National Academy; 2003.
5. Institute of Medicine. *Knowing What Works in Health Care*. Washington: National Academy; 2008.

6. American Nurses Association. Nursing Informatics: Scope and standards of practice. Silver Spring, Maryland: ANA; 2008.
7. The European Computer Driving Licence Foundation. European Computer Driving Licence/ International Computer Driving Licence Syllabus Version 5.0. http://www.ecdl.org/; 2009.

Updated Academic Programs

Carole A. Gassert and Susan K. Newbold

Academic Preparation in Nursing Informatics

Nursing informatics (NI) has become well-established as a specialty within nursing and health informatics, the broader category of informatics practice. (This part of Chap. 7 is reprinted as it appeared in the 3rd edition of *Nursing Informatics* (2000) with the following disclaimer, "The views expressed in this chapter are solely those of the author and not necessarily those of the Health Resources and Services Administration (HRSA), Department of Health and Human Services." Dr. Gassert was at that time Informatics Nurse Consultant in the Division of Nursing, HRSA.) NI practice focuses on the representation of nursing information and its management and processing within the health informatics community. It is one example of a domain-specific informatics practice. Medical, dental, and consumer informatics are other examples.

Informatics experts, including nurses, are being sought to help employees manage information more competitively. Increased recognition of the need for collecting and aggregating healthcare information has created exciting opportunities for nurses. They are crucial contributors to the development and implementation of the information structures and technology needed in today's healthcare environment.

Since the words "nursing informatics" first appeared in the literature in 1984, the field of practice has been named, defined, and recognized as a specialty by the nursing profession. Academic programs to prepare nurses within the field have also been developed. In addition, standards for the practice of NI have been written. Finally, a certification examination has been developed to certify those individuals who demonstrate beginning levels of competency in NI as informatics nurses (IN).

The purpose of this chapter is to discuss the educational preparation of nurses in NI. Although the focus is on describing academic opportunities in NI, it is necessary to examine NI as a specialty, discussing its definition, specialty attributes, scope of practice, and standards as they influence academic program development.

C.A. Gassert (✉)
University of Utah, College of Nursing, Salt Lake City, UT, USA
e-mail: carole.gassert@earthlink.net

M.J. Ball et al. (eds.), *Nursing Informatics*,
DOI: 10.1007/978-1-84996-278-0_7, © Springer-Verlag London Limited 2011

Evolving Definition of Nursing Informatics

Since the 1970s, nurses have been contributing to the design of information systems, consulting with healthcare agencies about selecting and using information technology and helping install and use information systems in hospitals. In 1992, their roles were professionally acknowledged when the American Nurses Association (ANA) recognized NI as an area of specialty practice in nursing.[1] Although many nurses practice in the specialty, others are still asking, "what is NI?"

The delineation of NI has been dynamic, changing to reflect growth within the field. As initially identified in the literature by Ball and Hannah,[2] NI was defined as the discipline of applying computer science to nursing processes. A year later, NI was described as a focus that uses information technology to perform functions within nursing.[3] This later definition was easily understood and therefore widely dispersed in nursing to explain the new practice area. Although useful, the definition failed to acknowledge NI activities beyond the use of computer applications.

Subsequent definitions represented a more widely delineated practice, including reference to a theoretical basis for practice. In 1988, Grobe described NI as the "application of the principles of information science and theory to the study, scientific analysis, and management of nursing information for purposes of establishing a body of nursing knowledge" (p. 29).[4] A more widely disseminated and accepted definition appeared in a classic article that describes the study of NI. In their article, the authors define NI as "the combination of nursing science, information science, and computer science to manage and process nursing data, information, and knowledge to facilitate the delivery of health care" (p. 227).[5] Computers are acknowledged as *tools* used in the NI field.

Both the Grobe definition and the Graves and Corcoran definition are important for three reasons. First, they more accurately describe the field, allowing such issues as information processing, language development, application of the systems life cycle, and usability to be identified as part of NI. Second, these definitions have implications for the content to be included in curricula used to prepare INs. Finally, these definitions serve as a foundation for the ANA's definition. The ANA scope of practice document states that NI "is the specialty that integrates nursing science, computer science, and information science in identifying, collecting, processing, and managing data and information to support nursing practice, administration, education, research, and the expansion of nursing knowledge (p. 3)."[6]

Specialty Attributes of Nursing Informatics

Designation of an interest area of nursing as a specialty is a multifaceted process.[7] The following attributes must be demonstrated:

- A differentiated practice
- A research program
- Representation of the specialty by at least one organized body
- A mechanism for credentialing nurses in the specialty
- Educational programs for preparing nurses to practice in the specialty

Different focal points separate NI practice from other nursing specialties. NI focuses on the structure and algorithms of information used by nurses in their practice, while other nursing specialties focus on the content of information management and the technology needed to effectively implement those processes.

Nurses have worked in informatics roles for more than two decades. Although the purchase and implementation of information technology in healthcare settings continue to demand considerable attention from INs, such activities do not define the entire domain of NI practice. Nursing language development, implementing NI educational programs, establishing telehealth systems, and solving systems usability issues are other examples of NI practice. These examples reflect the diverse and differentiated nature of NI practice.

By establishing a specific research program, NI has fulfilled a second attribute required for recognition as a specialty. When Schwirian[8] proposed a research framework for NI, there was little reported scientific inquiry in the field. Since that time, however, an increasing number of NI researchers have reported their work at national and international conferences and in the literature. Recently, several authors have reported on the development of nursing language.[9-14] Others have studied the impact of systems on patient care,[15] examined the design of information systems[16], or developed and evaluated NI models.[17-22] NI researchers have also investigated the decision-making processes of nurses[23,24]. All of these examples support topics identified as research priorities for NI by the National Institute for Nursing Research at the National Institutes of Health.[25]

A third attribute needed for qualification as a specialty is to be represented by at least one professional body. Three major nursing organizations, the ANA, the National League for Nursing (NLN), and the American Organization of Nurse Executives, have established special interest groups that target NI. An interdisciplinary organization, the American Medical Informatics Association (AMIA), also has a nursing informatics working group (NIWG). At the international level, the International Medical Informatics Association (IMIA) has an NI special interest group with representation from member countries. There are also many regional NI organizations that promote information sharing among NI members. The formation and maintenance of NI special interest groups are extremely important in providing information exchange, mentoring, and educational experiences for nurses who are new to the field. With the support of so many organizations, NI has more than met the attribute of representation by a professional body.

The fourth attribute needed for recognition of representation as a specialty is a mechanism for credentialing members of an interest area. This certification process for NI has been developed through the ANA and its affiliate, the American Nurses Credentialing Center (ANCC). Two separate task forces of nurses representing NI practice, education, and administration were appointed by the ANA to develop the scope of practice document and standards for NI practice. The ANA Council for Nursing Systems and Administration (formerly the Council of Computer Applications in Nursing) coordinated the task forces, and a certification examination for credentialing nurses as generalists in NI was developed under the direction of the ANCC. Although an NI specialist certification examination was originally planned, to date it has not been developed.

As a final attribute, a specialty must have educational programs to prepare nurses to practice within that field. NI education will be discussed later in this chapter.

Nursing Informatics Practice

The scope of practice document outlines in detail what is and is not NI practice. In terms of educational preparation, it is important to note that although INs are expected to be competent in the use of information technology, NI practice should not be defined solely by the use of technology. The scope of practice document further describes the boundaries, core, intersections, and dimensions of NI. In essence, the document states that while the field focuses on the nursing perspective of data, information, and knowledge, NI also recognizes that collaboration within the larger umbrella of health informatics is requisite to developing integrated information tools that will benefit both providers and recipients of healthcare.[6] Hence NI education should be interdisciplinary.

Authorizing legislation passed in 1992 prohibited further funding of nursing administration educational programs by the Division of Nursing, the federal agency charged with nursing work force preparation. This led to discussion of whether NI practice is clinical or administrative in nature.[26] Some have defined clinical NI and administrative NI as distinct entities, a distinction that seems artificial. Because NI activities have as a foundation the handling of clinical data and information, it seems best to describe all NI as a practice in which the informatics practitioner moves back and forth between a direct or indirect practice focus depending on patient and client needs. Handling individual patient data in the clinical setting would be considered direct informatics practice, whereas handling aggregate-level data for allocating resources would be indirect informatics practice. Educational programs in NI should provide students with knowledge and experience from both direct and indirect practice.

NI is generally practiced in one of five arenas: healthcare agencies, consulting firms, vendor corporations, academic settings, and private businesses practices. As healthcare shifts its focus to nontraditional environments (such as outpatient and home care) and to the use of telehealth systems to deliver care, NI practice needs to move into these areas. Specific practice activities may vary from one setting to another, but the following list of activities generally describes NI practice:

- Developing applications, tools, processes, and structures that help nurses manage data
- Evaluating applications, tools, processes, and structures to determine their effectiveness for nursing
- Adapting existing information technologies to meet nurses' and clients' needs
- Managing systems selection, implementation, and evaluation
- Collaborating with other healthcare informatics professionals in developing solutions to previously identified information needs for nurses and clients
- Using informatics theories and principles to develop and test computerized educational systems, such as those delivered through the World Wide Web
- Developing and testing informatics models and theories pertaining to handling, communicating, or transforming nursing information
- Developing a taxonomy or naming system to describe and order nursing phenomena
- Conducting research to advance the knowledge base of NI
- Consulting with patients and clients of NI
- Teaching the theory and practice of NI

As the field of NI practice expands, different activities may be added to the list. With such a large scope of practice, it is not uncommon for INs to try to focus their practice in a way that allows for the development of one or two areas of expertise. Some INs have developed expertise in building taxonomies, while others have refined the processes associated with systems implementation. Increasingly, INs will need to share their expertise within interdisciplinary teams. Limited resources and the need to develop information technology solutions that are common to all clients are fostering interdisciplinary practice.

Informatics Nurse Specialist Role

According to the scope of practice document, nurses who practice in the field of NI are designated as either INs or informatics nurse specialists (INS), depending on whether they are prepared at the baccalaureate or graduate levels in nursing.[6] This specification is consistent with ANA requirements that specialists have graduate education in nursing. Many INs have graduate preparation in fields that are outside of but support NI, such as business or computer science.[27,28] Regardless of their academic degree, almost all INs and INSs bring clinical practice experience to their roles.

Nurse specialists have traditionally described their roles by identifying different components or facets of their jobs. It seems appropriate, therefore, to describe INS roles in terms of the components of practice, consultation, research, marketing, education, and management. The practice component covers such activities as design, development, selection, testing, implementation, enhancement, and use of information technology. The consultation component includes advising and helping others reach solutions related to information technology. The research component covers investigation of such problems as research methodology, symbolic representation of data, clinical decision-making, ergonomics, usability issues, and information system impact. Marketing activities include selling both products and ideas related to information and information technology.

The educational role component includes training, presentation of both informal and formal programs in informatics, and development of learning technologies. Management, the final component, involves overseeing issues of change, quality, redesign, adoption and innovation, project planning, and cost. Just as the activities depend on the practice setting, the INS' primary role component may change with the setting or priorities of the employer. A discussion of competencies needed to practice in the field of NI follows.

Nursing Informatics Competencies

A competency is defined as "having sufficient knowledge, judgment, skill, or strength (p. 4)."[29] Identifying competencies for a specialty and certifying nurses who meet those competencies promotes higher quality in specialty practice.[30] IMIA's Work Group on NI initially identified levels of informatics competencies.[31] The statements of competency were intended to describe preparation of the general population of nurses relative to informatics as they accomplished their roles of clinician, nurse administrator, nurse educator, and nurse researcher.[32] The Work Group's designation of levels of preparation, however, has been used as the basis for organizing specialty programs in NI at the University of Maryland at Baltimore (UMB).[33]

Nurses prepared with level 1 competencies are considered to be information technology users. These individuals know, understand, use, and interact with computer applications and healthcare information systems. These nurses must also be prepared to collect relevant data for patient care, access information needed for providing nursing services, and implement policies to ensure privacy, confidentiality, and security of data. Such preparation should take place in baccalaureate (basic) nursing programs. The scope of practice for NI states that these competencies are required for all nurses.[6] Historically, nursing education programs have been slow to incorporate informatics competencies into the curriculum, and many practicing nurses still lack "user level" competencies.

Nurses with level 2 competencies are recognized as information technology modifiers, who analyze, manage, critique, develop, modify, and evaluate information technology for nursing. In addition to information technology skills, modifiers apply theoretical knowledge of nursing science, information science, computer science, and business to their practice. Modifiers' practices are focused in NI, and they are expected to conduct research to contribute to the body of knowledge. Modifiers are the INSs prepared at the master's level in graduate specialty programs in NI.

Nurses with level 3 competencies are identified as information technology innovators. These nurses design and develop research-based information technology for nursing, analyze and define the structure of nursing language, and explain the processing of information by nurses as they make both clinical and administrative decisions. Innovators are prepared at the doctoral level in nursing. With highly sophisticated preparation in research, nursing science, and information and computer science, innovators should contribute significantly to the body of NI knowledge and design information technology that truly supports nurses in delivering patient care.

Nursing Informatics Standards of Practice[34] defines the responsibilities for practice and professional performance for which generalist-level (initially competent) INs are held accountable. There are six standards that address the practice activities of INs. Eight standards speak to the professional performance of INs, and six additional standards delineate expectations for performance relative to the domain or field of NI. INs are expected to meet each of the 20 standards but not every measurement criterion within each of the standards. The scope of practice document, competency lists, and standards should serve as the basis for developing educational programs in NI.

Nurse educators interested in NI programs should consider using lists of expected competencies requisite to developing the curriculum. Such lists are available in Peterson and Gerdin-Jelger's publication[31] and in the ANA scope of practice document.[6] The standards are also distributed through the ANA.[34]

Nursing Informatics Education

Nurses frequently ask how they can learn more about informatics education. The NIWG of AMIA maintains a Web page that lists educational opportunities.[35] Generally, educational opportunities can be divided into six categories, as shown in Table 7.1.

Table 7.1 Models of nursing informatics education

Type	Programs
Continuing education and professional development	AMIA congresses NLN conferences HIMSS annual conference IMIA international NI meeting New York University NI conference Rutgers University international conference University of Maryland summer institute
Graduate programs with a specialty in NI	New York University Saint Louis University University of Maryland University of Utah
Post-master's certificate in NI	Duke University New York University Saint Louis University University of Arizona University of Iowa University of Maryland
Graduate programs with NI concentrations and minors	Northeastern University University of Arizona University of Iowa
Post-master's fellowships in NI	Partners HealthCare System Harvard Medical School and Deaconess Medical Center
Informatics courses	Graduate and undergraduate courses

Continuing Education in Nursing Informatics

Many professional development (continuing education) opportunities are available in NI through workshops and conferences sponsored by professional nursing organizations and universities. The ANA has included NI educational sessions at its biennial convention. The NLN Council for Nursing Informatics (CNI), an active special interest group, has sponsored an annual conference focusing on NI. In 1998, the CNI implemented an exciting conference and membership meeting through a webcast.[36]

An interdisciplinary organization, Healthcare Information and Management Systems Society (HIMSS), has conducted an annual informatics conference that includes informatics issues pertinent to nursing. The organization also invites nurses to learn about clinical information systems issues by joining an interdisciplinary special interest group.

AMIA, another interdisciplinary organization, has a very active NIWG that offers workshops, seminars, and other educational sessions in conjunction with spring and fall meetings. The NI Special Interest Group of IMIA sponsors an excellent international NI conference every 3 years. The 2000 meeting will be held in New Zealand, and Brazil will host the 2003 meeting. IMIA also sponsors MedInfo, an interdisciplinary international informatics conference, every 3 years.

Several universities have offered continuing education in NI. For more than 10 years, New York University (NYU) Medical Center conducted an NI conference each spring. NYU now offers a fall meeting through the nursing department. Rutgers University also has hosted a spring NI conference for 17 years.

While directing NI at the UMB School of Nursing, this author collaborated with the director of the campus Information Resources Division to develop a summer institute in 1991.[28] The institute continues to focus on information technology and its effects on administrative and clinical nursing practice, information systems selection and evaluation, strategies for systems implementation, and informatics trends and issues from the nursing perspective.

Increased informatics educational opportunities are evidenced by the number of workshop and conference announcements distributed through traditional and electronic mail. Most conferences provide an excellent opportunity to learn about state-of-the-art technology and informatics issues, but some nurses, particularly those who enter informatics without academic preparation in the field, are looking for programs to help them learn how to perform their role. In addition, few conferences focus on the theories and concepts nurses need to practice NI as delineated by the standards.

Courses in Nursing Informatics

To prepare nurses in informatics, nursing schools are adding informatics to undergraduate and graduate curricula. For example, Travis and Brennan[37] describe a series of courses that prepare undergraduate students to be sophisticated "users" of information and information technology. Earlier literature describes informatics courses that prepare practicing nurses and graduate students to be "users" of information technology.[38,39] The web lists NI courses offered by Lewis University, Loyola University, Georgia State University, Wichita State, and Hunter College.[35] Given the importance of appropriate information management in healthcare and the prevalence of using information technology to process information, one would expect all nursing schools to include informatics in the curriculum. Surprisingly, Carty and Rosenfeld[40] found that less than one third of nursing schools in a stratified random sample of NLN-accredited schools included informatics in the curriculum.

Master's Specialization in Nursing Informatics

Not only is there a need for basic informatics preparation for nurses, but with the growing sophistication of information technology in nursing, there is also a need for specialized NI education. The purpose of graduate specialization in NI to prepare INSs and individuals who can modify information management processes, data structures, and the technology needed to support information processing.

Master's specialty education in NI is built on several assumptions. First, one major area of coursework must be nursing science. Students must have baccalaureate preparation in nursing to allow them to increase their nursing knowledge at the graduate level. Increased theoretical understanding of nursing and nursing research facilitates the INS' ability to represent nursing's view of informatics issues and solutions accurately. Another assumption is that coursework must have an interdisciplinary focus on either information systems management or biomedical computing. This concentration of coursework builds students' knowledge base of technical and management issues related to information and information systems. Learning with another discipline also prepares the INS to work with other disciplines to identify problems and offer solutions from an interdisciplinary perspective. The result should be more representative and integrated information management solutions for all clinicians.

A third assumption is that state-of-the-art technology must be available to support students' technological growth. Not only must students have access to the latest technologies, they must also be able to use technologies from different technical environments. The INS must be flexible and able to move with advances in technology. Implied in the third assumption is that NI programs will have personnel available to support students (and faculty) technologically. The NI faculty can help with technological support, but additional personnel are needed.

The fourth assumption is that adequate numbers and a variety of practicum sites must be available to students. Sites in traditional and nontraditional healthcare agencies, vendor corporations, and consulting firms should be available. Having additional sites in organizations that set informatics policy, academic settings, and entrepreneurial NI practices would allow students to match career interests with available NI activities as they apply newly acquired knowledge during guided experiences.

The final assumption is that students must be prepared in basic computer competencies before starting NI specialty and interdisciplinary courses. The NI scope of practice document indicates that graduates of basic nursing programs should be able to use informatics applications that have been designed for the clinical practice of nursing.[6] To expand on this thinking, if students decide to *specialize* in NI, which uses the computer as a tool, they should have basic microcomputer skills in word processing, spreadsheet applications, database manipulation, e-mail, World Wide Web, and presentation graphics. Furthermore, rather than being intimidated by computers, they should be inquisitive and self-directed in learning to use new applications and technologies.

This author developed the curriculum and implemented the first graduate specialization program in NI at UMB in 1988.[41,42] This program was funded as a prototype for NI education within nursing administration. In 1990, the University of Utah was funded as a second model of NI education because of its focus on clinical nursing.[43] These two programs received their start-up funding from the Division of Nursing, HRSA. For several years, only UMB and Utah awarded master's degrees in NI,[27] but additional NI specialty programs are now open. In 1998, NYU opened an NI specialty program at the graduate level. Saint Louis University also offers a specialty program in NI.

All the four programs build on a master's core that emphasizes scientific inquiry, theoretical bases for advanced nursing practice, and healthcare delivery systems. Consistent with the philosophy of the informatics community, all of the programs emphasize the need for their students to understand interdisciplinary approaches to informatics courses in departments outside of nursing. Utah utilizes an interdisciplinary approach within the NI courses and encourages students to take elective courses outside of nursing.

The total number of credit hours of specialty courses varies among the four NI programs, but the content is similar. The UMB program requires 30 semester credit hours of coursework in informatics (Table 7.2). There are 15 credits allocated to the NI major and 15 credits of information science support. The total NI program requires 40 credits.

The master's specialization program at the University of Utah requires 25–26 semester credit hours of coursework in informatics (Table 7.3). Students take six credits of systems core courses and 19–20 credits of specialty area courses. Utah students also take six credits of a thesis or master's project focused in informatics. The NI program requires a total of 38–39 credits.

The NI program at NYU requires students to complete 21 semester credit hours in the specialty. Courses are listed in Table 7.4.

The final NI specialty program to be covered is at Saint Louis University. It requires a total of 41 semester credits. Students in the program take 29 credit hours of informatics courses from the schools of nursing, business and administration, and public health (Table 7.5).

Some nurses who are masters prepared in other specialties have asked the academic community to allow them to attend informatics courses along with the NI specialty students. This has resulted in the development of post-master's certificate options in NI. Such options are available at schools of nursing at Duke University, Saint Louis University, NYU, University of Arizona, University of Iowa, and UMB.

Table 7.2 University of Maryland at Baltimore nursing informatics courses

Major courses
Organizational Theories
Managerial Health Finance
Computer Applications in Nursing and Health Care
Concepts in Nursing Informatics
Practicum in Nursing Informatics
Support courses[a]
Structured Systems Analysis and Design
Project Management
Database Program Development
Data Communications and Networks
Decision Support Systems

[a]Support courses could also focus on expert systems, neural networks, telehealth, or interface design

Table 7.3 University of Utah nursing informatics courses

Systems core courses
Program Planning and Development
Program Management and Evaluation
Required specialty area courses
Introduction to Nursing Informatics
Clinical Systems Analysis and Design
Clinical Decision Support
Clinical Database Design
Clinical Systems Implementation
Practicum in Nursing Informatics
Master's Project or Thesis

Table 7.4 New York University nursing informatics courses

Nursing Informatics: An Introduction
Assessment and Analysis of Clinical and Nursing Information Systems
Database Design and Decision Support in Clinical and Nursing Systems
Implementation, Management and Evaluation of Clinical and Nursing Systems
Nursing Informatics Internship

Table 7.5 Saint Louis University nursing informatics courses

Health Information Systems
Practicum in Nursing Informatics
Administration of Care Systems I and II
Database Management Systems
Information Systems in Public Health
Nursing Informatics Concepts
Systems Analysis and Design
Programming
Introduction to Object-Oriented
Program Development Techniques

Master's Programs with Nursing Informatics Concentrations and Minors

Three programs indicate that their graduate curricula include courses in NI along with other requirements for other specialties in nursing.[35] Northeastern University requires their nursing administration majors to take three NI courses. The University of Arizona offers an MS degree with Role Development Option for Systems Management. Within this major, informatics is one of the emphasis areas. Finally, the University of Iowa offers a 20-semester credit hour certificate in informatics within the administration focus.

Doctoral Specialization in Nursing Informatics

The purpose of a doctoral program in NI is to prepare innovators or NI scientists. The NI scientist will be prepared to

- Conceptualize nursing information requirements for the future
- Design effective nursing information systems
- Create innovative information technology
- Conduct research regarding integration of technology with nursing practice, administration, education, and research

- Develop theoretical, practice, and evaluation models for NI
- Augment work to develop taxonomies and lexicons for atomic-level nursing data

Given the expected activities, the NI scientist focuses on the role components of researcher and designer/developer. Employment opportunities could be available as appointments in academic institutions, directors of research and/or information systems in healthcare facilities, research and development for software companies, appointments to government agencies, and consultants in research for information systems.

Doctoral programs should be built on several assumptions. Because of the informatics activities expected from these innovators, the doctoral program should build on a master's degree in NI. Included in this assumption is a belief that students must have sophisticated information management and technology competencies before entering the doctoral program. Because the number of master's specialization programs is limited, students may need to be admitted without such a background, but they should take additional courses to build their knowledge base in NI.

A second assumption for a doctoral program is that an interdisciplinary approach must be maintained. Students should take doctoral-level courses required for information systems students with an emphasis on improving their capabilities in designing and developing information technology. A third assumption is that adequate state-of-the-art technology and technological support must be available to students, as discussed previously. In addition, the physical environment should allow doctoral students to be assigned to their own computer and working space to facilitate design and development efforts. The final assumption of doctoral study is that adequate informatics researchers must be available in the academic community to support student research activities.

As of this writing, only UMB offers a doctoral program with a prescribed curriculum in NI.[33] Many universities, however, provide an opportunity for doctoral students to develop a program of study in informatics. Examples are the University of Utah, University of Texas at Austin, University of California-San Francisco, University of Wisconsin-Madison, and University of Iowa.

Postgraduate Fellowships

Since 1993, a 1-year fellowship in NI has been offered by the Massachusetts General Hospital (MGH) and, since the merger of MGH and Brigham and Women's Hospital, by Partners Health Care System. The fellowship, directed by Rita Zielstorff, is designed to promote the development of NI practitioners by allowing them to gain additional informatics experience of their choosing. Fellows are selected from qualified applicants. Admission preference is given to graduates of master's or doctoral programs in NI.[35] Fellows have included Mimi Hassett, RN, MS, from UMB, 1993–1994; Emily Welebob, RN, MS, from UMB, 1995–1996; Andrew Awoniyi, RN, ND, from University of Colorado Health Sciences Center, 1996–1997; Beth Tomasek, RN, MS, from UMB, 1998; and Cheryl Reilly, RN, PhD, from University of California-San Francisco, 1999.

A second fellowship, the Douglas Porter Fellowship in Clinical Computing, is available to nurses through the Harvard Medical School and the Divisions of Medicine and Nursing at Beth Israel Deaconess Medical Center. This fellowship is 3 years in length and multidisciplinary in focus. Nurses who apply must have at least a master's degree, should have a strong clinical background, and should be interested in advancing the practice of nursing using technology and information science. Fellows have included Denise Goldsmith, RN, MS, and Heimar Marin, RN, PhD.

Nursing Informatics Education in the Future

This chapter has described NI education in the United States. In the past few years, more educational opportunities have become available in academic centers, and nurses now have choices about the type and location of NI programs they wish to enter. Federal legislation passed in 1998 allows the Division of Nursing to fund administration; we anticipate that more schools will apply for NI funding in the future. The National Advisory Council on Nurse Education and Practice[44] has also recommended a national informatics agenda to the Secretary, Health and Human Services. These activities and the ubiquitous nature of technology are of increasing interest in NI.

With all these changes, it is interesting to ponder what the NI program of the future will look like. Will NI programs exist, or will all informatics professionals be educated through interdisciplinary programs? Will existing programs require students to take courses in the broad range of informatics topics available, or will specialization within the field be encouraged? Finally, will individual schools continue to spend precious resources on isolated programs, or will they collaboratively pool informatics resources from across the nation or across the world to develop new NI education models? The evolution of NI education over the next 5–10 years will be fascinating to follow.

Summary

NI has become well-established as a specialty within nursing and health informatics. Development of scope of practice and standards documents and NI educational models has facilitated further curriculum development within the field. A mechanism for certification has added legitimacy to the specialty. Finally, NI educational opportunities include specialty programs, post-master's certificate programs, programs with a minor in NI, fellowships, continuing education, and individual courses.

Update on Academic Programs

INs have many opportunities for advancing their education in nursing and healthcare informatics. There are more NI degree programs available. Many of the degree programs are available partially or totally online. Informatics education is more integrated into the educational preparation of every nurse. The focus of education is moving from training INs to training all nurses. Schools of nursing offer courses at the undergraduate, master's, and doctorate levels in NI, although not always mandatory.

Updated Definition of Nursing Informatics

In 2008, the ANA[45] NI Work Group Members updated the definition of NI:

NI is a specialty that integrates nursing science, computer science, and information science to manage and communicate data, information, knowledge, and wisdom in nursing practice. NI supports consumers, patients, nurses, and other providers in their decision-making in all roles and settings. This support is accomplished through the use of information structures, information processes, and information technology.[45]

The new definition differs from the previous 2001 version in that it adds the concept of "wisdom" to the continuum of data-information-knowledge-wisdom. Decision-making is a newly identified component in the process. The last sentence of the definition is a new addition referring to how information technology supports the use of vocabulary and terminologies, information management, and information technology.

An international definition of NI was put forth by the International Medical Informatics Association Nursing Informatics Special Interest Group (IMIA NI SIG) in 1998: "Nursing informatics is the integration of nursing, its information, and information management with information processing and communication technology, to support the health of people worldwide."[46] The definition is now being revised by the IMIA NI SIG.

Nursing Informatics as a Specialty

NI continues to grow as a nursing specialty. More INs are prepared at the PhD level to conduct research and at the master's level to guide practice. All NI specialty groups in the United States have aligned to form the Alliance for Nursing Informatics (ANI; www.allianceni.org) promoting one voice for issues of national interest regarding information technology and patient care. Credentialing of INs continues at the generalist level by the ANCC but has not progressed to the specialist level. For those not licensed as a registered nurse in the United States, international certification is available through IMIA NI SIG. For this certification, a portfolio is reviewed by the IMIA NI Education Working Group.

Nursing Informatics Practice

The scope and standards of practice for INs were combined into one document and greatly expanded.[45] The document has a bigger emphasis on informatics competencies.

There is no one standard job description for the informatics nurse. An informatics nurse can wear many hats including that of project manager, researcher, educator, implementer, consultant, or project developer. At this time, there is no consensus on titles for these professionals. In 2008, there was an attempt by the AMIA NIWG (http://www.amia.org/working-group/nursing-informatics) to classify NI under a government standard occupational classification (SOC) system. Despite documentation and interviews with INs, the code was not approved. CARING is an NI organization advancing the delivery of quality healthcare through the integration of informatics in practice, education, administration, and research (www.caringonline.org). In the CARING membership database in July 2009, there were 1979 members holding 1,110 unique titles! No wonder there is confusion about the role of the informatics nurse.

Nursing Informatics Competencies

The TIGER Initiative (Technology Informatics Guiding Education Reform) had pulled together extensive work on defining the computer literacy and information literacy competencies needed by all nurses (http://www.tigersummit.com/). The informatics competencies are described elsewhere in this book.

Nursing Informatics Education

Nurses who are seeking to expand their traditional education regarding informatics have many opportunities for learning. AMIA NIWG maintains a web page listing educational opportunities (see http://www.amia.org/mbrcenter/wg/ni/resources/academic.asp). Originally the list was divided into six categories, but now an increasing number of schools are offering programs, and the divisions are somewhat blurred. An updated model of NI education is presented in Table 7.6.

Continuing Education in Nursing Informatics

Professional nursing organizations, informatics organizations, and universities continue to hold NI workshops and conferences. The American Academy of Nursing has a Nursing Informatics Expert Panel dedicated to improving the health and safety of patients. The National League for Nursing Technology and Information Management Advisory Council has hosted clinical and educational informatics conferences. The Healthcare Information Management and Systems Society (HIMSS) hosts an annual NI conference attached to the main annual conference and exhibition held each spring. AMIA is an interdisciplinary organization that threads nursing content through the Spring Conference and Congress and Annual Symposium. AMIA is the United States representative to the IMIA. The NI special interest group of IMIA holds an international informatics conference every 3 years. The next conference, hosted by AMIA, will be held in Montreal Canada. In 2015, it is expected that the conference will be in Asia. IMIA continues to sponsor MedInfo, the next one scheduled for 2010 in Cape Town, South Africa. Due to the need to emphasize healthcare informatics in the changing healthcare environment, there is a movement to host MedInfo every 2 years instead of every 3 years.

The University of Maryland School of Nursing hosts an excellent 3 day conference in Baltimore. The twentieth event will be held in 2010. The American Nursing Informatics Association and CARING have formed a partnership to host an annual NI conference. This one is held each spring and in Las Vegas, NV in alternate years.

Table 7.6 Models of nursing informatics education

Type	Programs
Continuing education and professional development	American Medical Informatics Association (AMIA) Congress and Annual Symposium ANIA-CARING Annual Conference and Webcasts National League for Nursing (NLN) Conferences Healthcare Information and Management Systems Society (HIMSS) Annual Conference and Exhibition International Medical Informatics Association (IMIA) International NI Conferences University of Maryland School of Nursing Summer Institute in Nursing Informatics (SINI) Weekend Immersion in Nursing Informatics (WINI)
Graduate programs with a specialty in nursing informatics	Columbia University Duke University Excelsior College Loyola University, Chicago Pace University University of Alabama, Birmingham University of Arizona College of Nursing University of Colorado Health Sciences Program, School of Nursing University of Delaware Nursing The University of Iowa Center for Nursing Classification & Clinical Effectiveness University of Kansas School of Nursing University of Maryland School of Nursing University of Medicine and Dentistry, New Jersey University of Utah College of Nursing University of Washington School of Nursing Vanderbilt University School of Nursing Walden University

Courses in Nursing Informatics

In addition to a greater number of schools offering courses, the courses are moving toward the online environment. Some schools, like Vanderbilt University School of Nursing, have the programs almost entirely online. At Vanderbilt, the students with a bachelor's degree gather in the physical campus only two–three times during the three semester intensive program. Courses are conducted through a learning management system with some synchronous components.

The doctor of nursing practice (DNP) degree has gained popularity with over 80 programs in 2009 and more planned. The American Association of Colleges of Nursing (AACN) has outlined competencies for the DNP in the areas of technology and information literacy. According to the AACN,[47] the DNP graduate must:

- Demonstrate information literacy in complex decision-making
- Translate technical and scientific health information appropriate for user need and
- Participate in the development of clinical information systems

There is no standard for how the programs must carry out these goals. There is a wide variety of ways in which the schools interpret these requirements. For example, courses range from 1 to 4 semester credits.

Nursing Informatics Education in the Future

The American Recovery and Reinvestment Act of 2009, signed by President Obama on 17 February 2009, includes $19.2 billion in provisions for healthcare information technology. This will necessitate the education and training of nurses for informatics positions. All nurses need to have some level of knowledge about informatics and the impact on quality patient care and improved safety. Different teaching/learning environments will need to be developed to prepare nurses in informatics.[48]

Summary

NI is an established specialty within nursing and healthcare informatics. The scope and standards of practice documents have been updated. Certification continues for INs. educational opportunities have expanded and include online delivery mechanisms.

References

1. Milholland DK. Congress says informatics is nursing specialty. *Am Nurs.* 1992;July/August:1
2. Ball MJ, Hannah KJ. *Using Computers in Nursing*. Reston: Reston; 1984.
3. Ball KJ. Current trends in nursing informatics: implications for curriculum planning. In: Hannah KJ, Guillemin EJ, Conklin DN, eds. *Nursing Uses of Computer and Information Science*. Amsterdam: Elsevier Science; 1985:181-187.
4. Grobe SJ. Nursing informatics competencies for nurse educators and researchers. In: Peterson HE, Gerdin-Jelger U, eds. *Preparing Nurses for Using Information Systems: Recommended Informatics Competencies*. New York: National League for Nursing; 1988:25-33.
5. Graves JR, Corcoran S. The study of nursing informatics Image. *J Nurs Scholarsh.* 1989;21(4):227-231.
6. American Nurses Association. *Scope of Practice for Nursing Informatics*. Washington: American Nurses Publishing; 1994.
7. Panniers TL, Gassert CA. Standards of practice and preparation for certification. In: Mills ME, Romano CA, Heller BR, eds. *Information Management in Nursing and Health Care*. Springhouse: Springhouse; 1996:280-287.
8. Schwirian PM. The NI pyramid – a model for research in nursing informatics. *Comput Nurs.* 1986;4(3):134-136.

9. Grobe SJ. The nursing intervention lexicon and taxonomy: implications for representing nursing care data in automated patient records. *Holist Nurs Pract*. 1996;11(1):48-63.

10. Henry SB, Warren JJ, Lange L, et al. Review of major nursing vocabularies and the extent to which they have the characteristics required for implementation in computer-based systems. *J Am Med Inform Assoc*. 1998;5(4):321-328.

11. Martin KS, Norris J. The Omaha system: a model for describing practice. *Holis Nurs Pract*. 1996;11(1):75-83.

12. McCloskey JC, Bulechek GM, Donahue W. Nursing interventions core to specialty practice. *Nurs Outlook*. 1998;46(2):67-76.

13. Ozbolt JG. From minimum data to maximum impact: using clinical data to strengthen patient care. *Adv Pract Nurs Q*. 1996;1(4):62-69.

14. Saba VK. Why the home health care classification system is a recognized nursing nomenclature. *Comput Nurs*. 1997;15(suppl 2):S69-S76.

15. Brennan PF. Improving health care by understanding patient preferences: the role of computer technology. *J Am Med Inform Assoc*. 1998;5(3):257-262.

16. Zielstorff RD. Online practice guidelines: issues, obstacles, and future prospects. *J Am Med Inform Assoc*. 1998;5(3):227-236.

17. Gassert CA. Structured analysis: a methodology for developing a model for defining nursing information system requirements. *Adv Nurs Sci*. 1990;13(2):53-62.

18. Gassert CA. Defining information requirements using holistic models: introduction to a case study. *Holist Nurs Pract*. 1996;11(1):64-74.

19. Gassert CA. A model for defining information requirements. In: Mills ME, Romano CA, Heller BR, eds. *Information Management Nursing and Health Care*. Springhouse: Springhouse; 1996:7-15.

20. Gassert CA. Using a revised model to identify information requirements for cardiac surgery patients operating mobile computing technology. In: Gerdin U, Tallberg M, Wainwright P, eds. *Nursing Informatics: The Impact of Knowledge on Health Care Informatics*. Amsterdam: IOS; 1997:172-175.

21. Staggers N, Parks P. Description and initial applications of the Staggers & Parks nurse-computer interaction framework. *Comput Nurs*. 1993;11(6):282-290.

22. Turley JP. Toward a model for nursing informatics. *Image J Nurs Sch*. 1996;28(4):309-313.

23. Fonteyn ME, Grobe SJ. Expert system development in nursing: implications for critical care nursing practices. *Heart Lung*. 1994;23(7):80-87.

24. Thompson CB. Use of Iliad to improve diagnostic performance of nurse practitioner students. *J Nurs Educ*. 1997;36(1):36-45.

25. National Council on Nursing Research (NCNR) Priority Expert Panel for Nursing Informatics. *Nursing Informatics: Enhancing Patient Care*. Bethesda: National Institutes of Health; 1993.

26. Simpson RL. Shifting perceptions: defining nursing informatics as clinical specialty. *Nurs Manage*. 1993;24(12):20-21.

27. Carty B. The protean nature of the nurse informaticist. *Nurs Health Care*. 1994;15(4):174-177.

28. Gassert CA. Summer institute: providing continued learning in nursing informatics. In: Grobe SJ, Pluyter-Wenting ESP, eds. *Nursing Informatics '94: an International Overview for Nursing in a Technological Era*. Amsterdam: Elsevier Science; 1994:536-539.

29. Grobe SJ. Introduction. In: Peterson HE, Gerdin-Jelger U, eds. *Preparing Nurses for Using Information Systems: Recommended Informatics Competencies*. New York: National League for Nursing; 1988:4.

30. Parker J. Development of the American Board of Nursing Specialties (1991–1993). *Nurs Manage*. 1994;25(1):33-35.

31. Peterson HE, Gerdin-Jelger U. *Preparing Nursing for Using Information Systems: Recommended Informatics Competencies*. New York: National League for Nursing; 1988.

32. Grobe SJ. Nursing informatics competencies. *Methods Inf Med*. 1989;28(4):267-269.
33. Gassert CA, Mills ME, Heller BR. Doctoral specialization in nursing informatics. In: Clayton PD, ed. *Proceedings of Fifteenth Annual Symposium on Computer Applications in Medical Care*. New York: McGraw-Hill; 1992:263-267.
34. American Nurses Association. *Nursing Informatics Standards of Practice*. Washington: American Nurses Publishing; 1995.
35. Nursing Informatics Working Group, American Medical Informatics Association. Education in nursing informatics. http://amia-niwg.org; 1999.
36. Nelson R, Curran CE, McAfooes J, et al. The NLN webcast: developing and implementing an online conference and business meeting. *Nurs Health Care Perspect*. 1999;20(3):122-127.
37. Travis L, Brennan PF. Information science for the future: an innovative nursing informatics curriculum. *J Nurs Educ*. 1998;37(4):162-168.
38. Magnus MM, Co MC, Derkach C. A first-level graduate studies experience in nursing informatics. *Comput Nurs*. 1994;12(4):189-192.
39. McGonigle D, Eggers R. Establishing a nursing informatics program. *Comput Nurs*. 1991;9(5):184-189.
40. Carty B, Rosenfield P. From computer technology to information technology: findings from a national study of nursing education. *Comput Nurs*. 1998;16(5):259-265.
41. Gassert CA. Opportunities to study nursing informatics. *Input Output*. 1989;5(2):1-2.
42. Heller BR, Romano CA, Moray LR, et al. Special follow-up report: the implementation of the first graduate program in nursing informatics. *Comput Nurs*. 1989;7(5):209-213.
43. Graves JR, Amos LK, Huether S, et al. Description of a graduate program in clinical nursing informatics. *Comput Nurs*. 1995;13(2):60-70.
44. National Advisory Council on Nurse Education and Practice. *A National Informatics Agenda for Nursing Education and Practice: A Report to the Secretary of the Department of Health and Human Services*. Rockville: Department of Health and Human Services; 1997.
45. American Nurses Association. *Nursing Informatics: Scope and Standards of Practice*. Silver Spring: American Nurses Publishing; 2008.
46. International Medical Informatics Association Nursing Informatics Special Interest Group. http://www.imiani.org/; 1998.
47. American Association of Colleges of Nursing. The essentials of doctoral education for advanced nursing practice. www.aacn.nche.edu; 2006.
48. O'Neil CA, Fisher CA, Newbold SK. *Developing Online Learning Environments in Nursing Education*. 2nd ed. New York: Springer; 2009.

Continuing Education and Staff Development

8

Joan M. Kiel and Elizabeth Johnson

Introduction

Paul Starr, in his Pulitzer Prize winning book, *The Social Transformation of American Medicine*, wrote, "…medicine is also, unmistakably, a world of power where some are more likely to receive the rewards of reason than are others." Starr noted that this power is rooted in both knowledge and competence (Starr 1982). Thus, it is imperative that nursing professionals gain the required knowledge in order to secure organizational power. In medicine, it is the nurse who spends direct time with patients and their families and interacts with all members of the health care team including physicians, therapists, pharmacists, dietitians, and allied health providers. Nurses need to have the most current health care system knowledge and information which can be accomplished through innovative and effective staff development and continuing education programs.

This chapter focuses on staff development and continuing education programs in information technology and informatics for nurses. Cases studies are presented illustrating successful programs and also the "learning pains" that were involved. Survey results (both qualitative and quantitative data) are presented. Lastly, the effects of information technology on patient safety, quality, and efficiency are all reviewed as key reasons to engage in nursing staff development and continuing education.

The American Recovery and Reinvestment Act (ARRA) of 2009 economic stimulus bill recently passed by the U.S. Congress allocates some $19 billion dollars to incentivize medical practices to adopt and implement electronic health records (EHR). Starting in 2011, physicians deemed to be "meaningful users" (an eligibility criteria still being defined) can potentially receive 75% of that year's Medicare and Medicaid charges up to a maximum of $15,000 ($18,000 if the first year of implementation is 2011 or 2012). The ARRA is predicted to be one of the most significant drivers of caregiver adoption of HER in history and will increase demands for staff training in health technology skills in the near and intermediate future.

J.M. Kiel (✉)
Duquesne University, 600 Forbes Avenue, Pittsburgh, PA 15282, USA
e-mail: kiel@duq.edu

M.J. Ball et al. (eds.), *Nursing Informatics*,
DOI: 10.1007/978-1-84996-278-0_8, © Springer-Verlag London Limited 2011

The Need

National Nursing Organization Viewpoints

Computers, information technology, and informatics are inherent parts of the current and future health care delivery system. Key national nursing organizations such as the National League of Nursing (NLN), American Academy of Nurses (AAN), American Association of Colleges of Nursing (AACN), and the American Organization of Nurse Executives (AONE) have expressed their need for present and future nurses to possess information technology knowledge, skills, and ability. As interdisciplinary health care team members and patient advocates, nurses need to obtain and utilize these skills and contribute to the advancement of the health care delivery system.

The NLN elaborated on ten trends that are and will continue to affect professional nurses. The second trend was the "technological explosion." Explosion is an accurate description as the NLN views technology as all-encompassing in the nursing profession. From the personal computer to digital technology used in telehealth and telemedicine to nanotechnology, nurses will play an active role and lead at the cutting edge of the art due to their direct patient contact. Supporting nursing is the electronically accessible clinical data, the electronic medical record, and electronic commerce. The NLN cites some schools are using distance learning; thus nurses are learning and utilizing computers and electronic data to enhance their knowledge and support their profession. If nursing is to continue being an integral player in delivering quality patient care and interacting with the health care team, gaining technology skills and knowledge is not an option.[1]

The AAN Workforce Commission completed a time study on the effect of technology products that nurses utilize in patient care. The study includes observations of nursing practice at 25 hospitals and health systems. The conclusion presented a picture of an inefficient work process allowing nurses to spend only 30% of their time on direct patient care. As a result, the study identified that by the use of technology, care delivery and coordination, communication, documentation, and other critical nursing daily tasks could be enhanced.[2]

The white paper published by the AACN on the Education and Role of the Clinical Nurse Leader demonstrated a broad range of information and health care technology needs for nurses. From the more traditional use of information technology to retrieve information to the need of technology for evidence-based medicine, nurses have a great need to be fully engaged in the learning and use of technology. The report stated in part that "…health literacy is the foundation of independence, health promotion, and disease prevention, all of which are hallmarks of excellence in nursing practice." As clinical leaders, technology is a vital part of their daily jobs and the advancement of the profession of nursing.[3]

The AONE random survey of its membership concurred with the other organizations. They found new nurses needed to know how to utilize e-mail, Microsoft Windows, database searches, and clinical software for documentation and medication administration.[4] Here again, the need for technology use spans from the daily tasks to information literacy.

The Institute of Medicine, although not a nurse-specific organization, has been a champion for quality health care delivery. At the Health Professions Education Summit, leaders from a variety of health professions, including nursing, came together to discuss the educational needs of the health care practitioner. The group found that in order to deliver high quality and safe health care, workers need to be adequately prepared. Specifically, five core areas were identified[5]:

1. Delivering patient-centered care
2. Working as part of an interdisciplinary team
3. Practicing evidenced-based medicine
4. Focusing on quality improvement
5. Using information technology

It is evident from these organizations and industry experts that information technology and informatics are vital to the delivery of health care. In addition, it is critical that the nursing profession be at the table among their interdisciplinary health care team members. This can only happen if nurses embrace the utilization of technology by developing a comprehensive skill set in health care technology through well-designed continuing education and staff development programs.

The TIGER Survey

In order to collect viewpoints from the field, the TIGER Staff Development and Continuing Education group conducted an online survey. The purpose of the survey was to obtain feedback on computer literacy, computer training, and computer skills for nurses employed in a variety of health care settings. Two hundred and ten surveys were returned with the majority of respondents (45.2%) having an administrative/management role within the organization. Out of that, 18.6% were staff development/professional development personnel and 7.1% staff nurses (Table 8.1).

The majority of respondents worked in a hospital setting (47.6%) followed by a long-term care facility (34.3%) (Table 8.2).

The settings were evenly divided, classified as a teaching facility with 49.8% answering "yes" and 50.2% answering "no" (five respondents did not answer). Although most settings were urban (48%), the remaining were divided between suburban (28.7%) and rural (23.3%) (eight respondents did not answer).

What did differ greatly was the facility size as seen in Table 8.3.

Table 8.1 Role within the organization

Administration/management	45.2%
Staff development/professional development	18.6%
Information technology services	9.5%
Staff nurse	7.1%
Other	19.5%

$n=210$

Table 8.2 Practice environment

Hospital	47.6%
Long-term care facility	34.3%
Ambulatory care	1.4%
Home care	1.0%
Other	15.7%

$n=210$

Table 8.3 Facility size by bed count

1–100	14.5%
101–299	40.1%
300–499	14.0%
500+	19.3%
Not applicable	12.1%

$n=207$

The survey objective was to obtain responses from a wide variety of institutions based on size, type, and location in order to provide a full representation of professional nursing's contribution to the results on computer education.

Organizations were asked to self report the general level of computer literacy for their staff nurses (Table 8.4).

The majority of nurses have midlevel computer literacy with very few nurses reporting minimal basic computer knowledge. What was surprising, given that nurses did have some computer proficiency, was that just over half (57.7%) of the facilities offered basic computer training for the nurses. Therefore, nurses are acquiring computer skills outside of their place of employment. For those who do receive in-house training, it was the responsibility

Table 8.4 General level of computer literacy for staff nurses

1	1.0%
2	1.9%
3	9.0%
4	11.4%
5	20.5%
6	19.5%
7	18.6%
8	10.5%
9	5.2%
10	2.4%

Scale: 1–10 with 10 being the highest
$n=210$

of the staff development office predominantly (41.3%), followed by the information technology department, (30.2%), nursing colleagues, (18.0%), and vendors (4.8%).

The results were similar for organizations offering training to nurses on how to access online clinical information resources such as literature, practice protocols, procedures, references, or evidence. Of the facilities, 62.7% offered training, with the staff development office performing 37.6% of the training sessions. In this area, however, nursing colleagues did 15.2% of the training, followed by the medical librarians 10.2%, information technology department 8.1%, and the vendors 0.5%.

In regard to computer clinical applications, 85.3% of facilities offered in-house training for nurses. This included training on order entry, documentation, laboratory results review, and medication management. Again, the staff development office provided the most training (45.3%) followed by the information technology department (22.1%), nursing colleagues (17.1%), and vendors (3.3%).

The TIGER Survey results demonstrate that nurses are receiving training in information technology and it is predominantly being performed by the staff development personnel. As technology, whether it be basic computer applications, information literacy, or clinical applications, continues to change, more resources will be required for nursing staff development.

Other National Surveys

Another national survey conducted by the Healthcare Informatics Research Series group identifies low adoption rates for electronic documentation among U.S. nurses. Nursing professionals arguably document the majority of patient care delivered in both inpatient and outpatient facilities. However, this survey indicates that less than half of all nurses use some form of electronic documentation in their daily clinical practice. Such a finding represents a significant challenge – and also a training opportunity – for continuing education and staff development efforts nationally. Unless nursing professionals help lead (rather than follow) the development of EHRs, they will not earn the level of organizational credibility and power to which they would otherwise be entitled (Fig. 8.1).

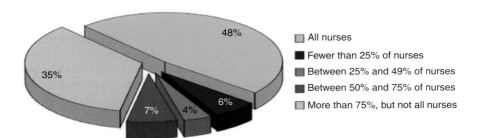

Fig. 8.1 Percentage of nursing staff using e-documentation. *Source*: Healthcare Informatics Research Series found at: http://links.mkt1408.com/servlet/MailView?ms=MzM0MTkxNDgS1& r=NzYwMTMxMjE0S0&j=NTE0ODA0NjMS1&mt=1&rt=0t

Case Studies: Who Is Doing What, Where, and How

Staff development and continuing education programs are delivered via a variety of instructional strategies. It is important to assess the learning gap at all levels and identify best learning methods relative to the needs of the audience involved. Assessment also includes physical resources such as trainers, equipment, online access, and fully equipped training rooms required for successful training. In addition, it includes the question as to whether the organization will provide the training on-site (classroom), offsite (classroom or online), or commit to a totally external approach such as college classes or conferences. This section of the chapter presents a myriad of examples of successful staff development and continuing education opportunities.

Weekend Immersion in Nursing Informatics

The Weekend Immersion in Nursing Informatics (WINI) Conference is a Friday to Sunday, 3-day intensive computer training experience. Developed in 1995, the conference is presented in different cities across the country. Its objectives are as follows[6]:

1. Examine theories, models, and frameworks that could be used in health care and nursing informatics practice, education, administration, and research domains
2. Distinguish among the terms human factors, ergonomics, and human–computer interaction and usability
3. Discuss system planning concepts
4. Describe available hardware, software, and communication components for a health care information management solution
5. Identify strategies to establish a solution
6. Develop an implementation plan and project management plan for an information systems plan
7. Evaluate the implementation of a health care Information System solution
8. Identify opportunities to contribute to local, state, national, and international informatics initiatives
9. Assess readiness to complete the American Nurses Credentialing Center (ANCC) certification examination for nursing informatics

The objectives focus both on the theory and practice of computer literacy, information technology, and information systems to give the learner a wide range of learning. The conference assists an applicant preparing to take the Nurse Informaticist (NI) Certification Examination offered by the ANCC. This credential can prove to be vitally important in establishing the professional nurse's credibility as knowledgeable in health care technology.

An Academic Health Center

From a weekend format to a 6-week pilot study at a large urban academic health science center, a need was recognized to train nurses in information literacy. Five competencies were the objectives for this training[7]:

1. Recognizing when information is needed and effectively communicating the need
2. Understanding original research, the distinct research methodologies for one's discipline, and the process involved in publishing scholarly information
3. Recognizing that information stored in collections must be organized in order to be useful and that libraries use systematic methods to accomplish this
4. Recognizing that information sources come in a variety of forms, exhibit different characteristics, and appear in various physical formats
5. Effectively using a variety of search tools, understanding and applying essential information seeking concepts and practices, and acknowledging that the research process is nonlinear and iterative and requires flexibility

This training consisted of staff development and library personnel participating in weekly sessions with five or six participants per session over 6 weeks. The main topics were accessing health information from databases such as CINAHL and MEDLINE and from credible Internet sites. In addition, a dedicated computer with internet access and a printer was installed on each unit.[7] Although this pilot study used a small sample ($n=32$) and suffered the data loss due to a server crashing, the results obtained can still be extrapolated over other populations. The pilot study showed that nurses can make modest enhancements in their information literacy capabilities. But what must be considered when doing in-house training are the interruptions that nurses commonly experience in their daily work experiences. For example, a nurse logged log into the database to perform a literature search was called away for patient care.[7] The process workflow of a typical nurse's day specific to the specialty unit and the time constraints needs to be considered when designing training programs.

Cleveland Clinic

Moving from training nurses on computer skills and information literacy to a full scale implementation of computerized nursing applications, the plethora of technology will be demonstrated. From its inception in 1988, the Cleveland Clinic Department of Nursing Informatics has had an interdisciplinary approach to technology.[8] The department is comprised of not only nurses, but also educators, systems analysts, and system administrators. The focus of the information technology is on positive patient outcomes and nurse workflow.

The training consists of a variety of methods. Nurses provide training to other nurses on the use of clinical applications on each nursing unit. Classes are held in a computer laboratory with self study manuals and instructor-led sessions. Computer-based training modules are also available (provided both on-site or from any external computer such as the home or library). With all of these methods, the nursing staff can be adequately prepared to use the information technology in their daily jobs. The Cleveland Clinic nurses utilize information technology for electronic medical records, order entry, documentation, medication dispensing and administration, and results reporting.

The Cleveland Clinic has taken the training and utilization of information technology one step further with their Nursing Unit of the Future. Here, nurses use "trial and error" information technology that they have the possibility of using in the future – as a result they have a vested interest in providing feedback. The technologies are evaluated based on the following criteria:

- How devices withstand normal wear and tear
- How easily information is gathered and recorded
- User friendliness
- Clinician satisfaction
- Time efficiency vs. existing methods
- Impact on patient safety
- Impact on patient satisfaction
- Impact on caregiver satisfaction

Nurses at the Cleveland Clinic are immersed in information technology. They extend their passion for technology to the patients and families by lending laptops, assisting patients to access their e-mail while an inpatient, log on to chat groups related to their condition, or look up general medical information.

Lancaster General Hospital

Lancaster General Hospital (LGH) is a 638-bed, nonprofit, community-based institution. In training personnel on a new documentation system, many lessons were learned. The intended users of the system are nurses who use the documentation system for daily charting, unit clerks who chart on the discharge instructions, and other health care providers who may have a "View Only" access to the system. LGH used a blended learning approach utilizing both instructor-led classes and online instructional modules.

The classes were organized into three phases. The first phase was for discharge instructions training and consisted of mandatory classes. The second phase focused on admission assessments and offered an educational choice of either a computer-based learning module or a 2-h instructor-led class. The final phase focused on shift assessments and required mandatory classroom attendance due to the more complex components of the system. The classes included a review of the basic tenets of the system and offered practice time in the "test" system, so that participants could practice the newly acquired learning outside of a "live" production environment. During go-live for each unit, on-site nursing support was available which promoted staff buy-in and point-of-care assistance. During the go-live phase of discharge instructions, support personnel were present from 7 a.m. to 9 p.m. For admission and shift assessments, on-site support was available 24/7 for 1 full week.

With any training and staff development initiative, some phases receive good evaluations; still "negative" feedback can be extremely valuable in analyzing how the training efforts could be improved. What worked well was a phased-in approach which allowed users to become familiar with the basic system and then move to more advanced aspects of documentation. Another positive outcome was the finding that as one unit completed a successful implementation, subsequent initiatives benefited from the initial efforts which hoped to clarify support questions and issues. Lastly, blended education options of both online and live classes allowed users to choose what instructional strategy worked best for them.

Potential improvements in the implementation process would have been identified earlier had more information services staff dedicated to the project. Second, the education of the physicians related to discharge instructions could be helped by having a physician champion on the team developing the views of instructions that their peers will see. Lastly, the physicians resisted moving vital signs to an online format, so they are still on paper. A physician change agent or champion may have been helpful to handle their resistance to the change.

Summa Health System

Summa Health System is a multifacility acute care hospital. The two main facilities are Akron City Hospital and St. Thomas Hospital, both located in Akron, OH. They are teaching facilities and serve as tertiary care centers for the area with approximately 1,500 credentialed physicians and 1,800 nurses at the two facilities.

In July 2005, Summa Health System began implementing a Computerized Physician Order Entry System (CPOE) with limited nursing documentation. The system was first implemented at the Akron City Hospital campus. Akron City Hospital, the larger of the two facilities, initiated the project with a single pilot unit, continuing through March 2006 rolling out application to the other 19 units at the City campus. In January 2007, the application was implemented at the St. Thomas campus, bringing up four to six nursing units at a time. They generally were in related areas (i.e., all the obstetric or critical care units).

During this activation schedule, the Clinical Information Systems Education team was charged with training all of the users for the application. The training included physicians, residents, medical students, nurses, nursing students, and all allied health departments such as respiratory, radiology, and dialysis. Because Summa was going from paper and pencil order entry to CPOE, this was a very significant undertaking.

Project leaders worked with the Chief Medical Information Officer (CMIO), a physician, to design the initial training for the physicians. Classes were scheduled for 1.5 h for groups of physicians with the CMIO providing training for many of the large classes. All physicians are required to attend this initial training session to get their log-in and password. They are also finger-printed at that time because Ohio required reliable authentication procedures for electronic order entry submission. All other users were scheduled for classes based on the amount of interaction each user type would have with the system. Nurses receive a total of 8.5 h of classes, whereas nursing assistants received 1.5 h of class. All classes were conducted in the computer labs at the two large facilities. Each classroom was equipped with 12–14 computers and classroom needs specific to computer training.

The project assembled a team of two full-time Clinical Information Systems staff who were the Education Team and a full-time education consultant who had experience in training for CPOE. One paid full-time trainer supported the training process for 18 months. In addition, there were four to six staff nurses who had expressed an interest in teaching the classes or were designated by the pilot unit manager as trainers. The staff nurses were used on a per diem basis. Generally, the nurses' time was scheduled first and the Education Team picked up the classes the nurses were unable to teach.

The physician classes were scheduled 2–4 weeks prior to the activation date. The class schedules were determined by the number of physicians who needed to be trained and required access to the system. The classes were basically a very generic introduction to the system.

Nursing and Allied Health classes were scheduled anywhere from 4 to 6 weeks prior to the activation date based on the number of staff for the designated areas. The Allied Health classes were gradually phased out as more and more of the units were activated. So for the last several activations, we only offered classes for new staff as needed. Nursing Unit Managers also designated specific nurses to serve as Super Users for their unit. These Super Users were given an additional 8 h of training and then served as experienced resources for their peers.

All of the classes include handouts with specific instructions for the various functions based on their role. The physicians receive a pocket guide with instructions on basic functionality. It clearly displays the physician support phone number on the cover for easy reference.

As group of units were activated, Clinical Information Systems staff and Consultants provided support on each unit 24 h a day for the first 2 weeks. The Support team was able to address specific issues with individual physicians and staff members as needed. After the 2 weeks of activation support, the units reverted to the standard support provided by Clinical Information Systems. That involves a team of eight nurse analysts taking calls from the Computer Support Desk and calling the person back and working with them individually. The nurse analysts rotate call (on-call for a week at a time and answer calls 24/7). They have the ability to remotely access the end user's computer, allowing visualization of the end user's computing environment that promotes effective assistance with specific issues and questions.

In addition to the traditional means of accessing the nurse analyst on-call, there is a specific cell phone set up for physician only calls. The physicians are provided with a specific number while at the hospital and the call is forwarded directly to the nurse analyst via a cell phone (this phone support is available 24/7). The point-of-contact assistance through activation support and the physician phone has been the most successful strategies for physician adoption of the system. There is also a group of nurse analysts who serve as physician liaisons and handle the phone calls to the support line during business hours. These nurses are able to develop a relationship with the physicians and helps better meet physician needs. The Physician Liaisons also meet with the various physician departments on a regular basis to share new information and updates as well as handle their concerns from that formats.

With these strategies, Summa has been able to achieve:

- Ninety-five percent physician adoption within 4 months of implementation
- Four percent reduction in overall length of stay, with an estimated $3 million savings
- Thirty-eight percent reduction in pulmonary embolus after implementation of VTE protocols
- Improved compliance for AMI core measures achieving over 90% compliance for all measures
- Improved antimicrobial selection for pneumonia patient through utilization of Clinical Decision Support

For nursing, there are regular meetings for "Super Users" for them to hear about new uses of the system, learn the new aspects of the application as appropriate, and share concerns/questions that have come up on the units. This strategy has been used successfully for implementation of the upgrade of the CPOE application, a diagnostic hand-off report between nursing and the ancillary areas. Super Users were also provided with detailed handouts and the handouts were made available on a reference site on the proprietary intranet.

There are dedicated analysts for lab, radiology, and other ancillary areas. These analysts meet with their departments regularly and/or make rounds to the various areas to address individual user concerns/issues.

There are regular newsletters published for both nursing and physicians. These are distributed to various departments and users via e-mail, on the intranet site, in the departments, and at Super User meetings.

Very early in the project, physicians were offered a computer-based training module. The requirement for attendance at an initial class was maintained, but the module was to function as a quick review. It has had only limited use, but is still available.

The Education Team trains students in every discipline in addition to regular hospital staff. Annually, this involves approximately 1,500 nursing students, 300 medical students, and 48 students from other disciplines. A computer-based module was developed for the nursing students. Each group is scheduled for computer lab time and given a short introduction to the system, log-in instructions, and a review of security issues. They then complete the CBT in a proctored environment. Other students are trained in traditional computer class sessions as needed.

Scheduling for the large number of nurses who needed training was a challenge initially, with numerous e-mails, voice mails, and paper schedules floating around. To ease scheduling, a system was purchased that allowed unit managers to schedule their own staff in advance and produced clear, legible class rosters for sign-in sheets. Unfortunately, the system did not interface with the Human Resources application that was the central storage for all training records. As a result, a fair amount of manual data entry was still required. Fortunately, Nursing Education and Staff Development authorized their receptionists to enter the data into that system. The fact remains that the ease of interface should have been considered when the system was purchased.

Now in a "maintenance" mode for training, Summa is down to a limited number of staff and rarely uses the staff nurse trainers who assisted during activation. One of the most significant challenges now is training temporary staff, particularly nurses, who still need 8.5 h of training. Training is scheduled monthly, but when temporary nursing staff training is needed, it is often on a short-notice basis and usually for a very limited number of nurses. This has required using a significant amount of resources to train a very limited number of people.

Summa still wants to create a computer-based training program for these temporary staff that allows the Education team to be available as a resource rather than as the trainer for one person. The time factor is a big drawback here: it takes a significant amount of time to create a single hour of computer-based training.

St. Vincent Mercy Medical Center

St. Vincent Mercy Medical Center has implemented an electronic medication system, EHR, and online training systems. In McKesson's Admin Rx, hand-held scanners replace paper Medication Administration Records (MARs), potentially decreasing medication errors and assisting nurses with the medication process. Orders are placed in the system, verified by the nurse by checking the original order in the EHR, and compared to the physician order form. The process is completed with the nurse noting the orders as in the paper world. Bar-code technology printed on the patient armbands is used with these scanners providing positive patient identification and direct viewing of the patient medication profile.

Every new hire or agency nurse must go through proper training by Nursing Staff Development for use of the system. Policy requires every nurse to attend this class before being allowed to practice. Classes are scheduled with nursing orientation, with additional classes offered for agency nurses and clinical affiliates from nursing schools. Nursing students may administer medications only with the instructor.

Most significant positive outcomes observed were:

- All staff members were educated and system rolled out in groups of nursing units, not all at once.
- Support staff was available 24/7 during implementation time. With unit Super Users in place and a person rounding on the units identifying issues, training support was very effective.

Most significant improvements needed were identified as the following:

- Refresher for staff who have been identified as missing processes
- Replacement of equipment timeframe for turnaround or changes
- Adjustments to programs that did not interface or talk to each other, causing issues with information systems

St. Vincent also implemented an electronic health record (HER) for patients, rolling it out for all staff and physicians. Nurses were educated in two separate sessions, one for patient history and the other for CPOE and accessing information.

All nurses and new hires were educated in both applications in two separate classes taught by staff who helped build the system. All new hire staff are educated in the system and its proper usage. The most significant positive outcome was that education was mandatory for all nurses. Also, support by "Red Coats" (Super Users) was always available (via pager) to assist in navigating the system and answer practice questions 24/7 for both physicians and nurses. In spite of this, major improvements were still needed. Some staff members struggling due to a lack of computer skills needed to be offered training. Physicians needed to place all orders in the system, not just selective orders, in order to decrease verbal orders and decrease errors, while increasing consistency for staff. Last, too many updates and changes are coming out with other nursing practice changes, overwhelming the staff.

Last, St. Vincent education system was revamped. They have had computer-based training since 2004 and struggled with nurses and computer skills. The addition of Admin Rx and EHR really improved their skills as they used these systems every day. Some do still struggle. Transition from the former learning management system to a new system occurred in 2006. "Go-Live" was delayed many times due to system issues. Midyear 2006, the system was ready to transition, but not all nursing staff members had completed the online competency assessment. A 4-day delay was required for all content to be revised and packaged for the new system.

Educating staff was difficult due to the variety of work schedules and no mandatory training was identified. Educators distributed handouts to the units and worked with staff by teaching them more on a 1:1 basis rather than in the classroom. In 2007, the team developed a research study for nursing satisfaction and web-based competencies. All content and testing relating to competency are placed in the learning management system. They no longer offer paper–pencil testing for adult competency. There were neither enough resources available to educate the large group of staff, nor would we have gotten compliance with attendance, as it was not mandatory.

What went well was the short transition to repackage the content and upload. But improvements were needed as there are still struggles with learners and navigation (system issue vs. learner understanding). Second, personnel resources to assist have so many other responsibilities that they are not accessible when needed to solve issues. Lastly, the system overall has issues and requires more intervention by administrators.

Tenet Healthcare: Creating a Training Team

Tenet Healthcare (THC) is a national integrated health care system with more than 50 acute care facilities in its network. Recognizing the need for a standardized training program involving a variety of clinical systems applications, Tenet set a corporate-level goal to create a national Training Team using customized portions of a corporate training plan that would have sufficient flexibility to address unique facility needs of individual hospitals in the network.

The controlling objective for the training plan was that all pertinent staff and providers would receive training and demonstrate competency in using all applications appropriate for each to perform their job duties in a confident, comfortable, and accepting manner.

The Training Team was comprised of Implementation Training Specialists working in coordination with various application Project Managers and Implementation Specialists who developed a core Training Plan for implementation of all applications for Tenet Healthcare IMPACT Project. Each facility under the direction of the Site Project Manager customized portions of the Training Plan to address unique facility needs and subsequently execute the plan.

The team faced many challenges in this project. Training can be the most expensive part of any implementation. There are direct costs of removing individuals from their regular duties to develop training materials related to the project, and direct costs related to removing individuals from the workplace for training and replacing them during their training. In addition, there are also the indirect costs of staff not being properly trained and wasting time trying to figure out how to do something or being frustrated by not understanding the system. There is also the cost of rework when errors occur and the cost of lost revenue if charges are lost or cannot be billed because of inaccurate entry.

The purpose of the Training Plan is to recommend an approach to support the IMPACT Project, vendor-specific implementation requirements, and the hospital-specific needs. Recommendations are based on the best method of delivering knowledge to the diverse audience of physicians and staff, while aligning the approach with project and organizational goals, conversion schedules, best learning practices, and learning resources. The Learning Plan benefits are that it does the following:

- Provides an organized approach (step-by-step process) and improves credibility for the Project Team
- Allows adequate time for trainer development
- Gives the hospital staff confidence in the project leadership's ability to provide quality materials and learning opportunities
- Allows for the identification of risk factors allowing for timely modifications
- Makes the job of the training easier and more efficient with the development of the comprehensive plan
- Makes for less resistance to change within the organization through the use of effective marketing and change management techniques
- Provides a more accurate estimate of resources (computers, learning) available to conduct the training
- Provides the best foundation available to plan for training
- Addresses specific needs of the learners within Sierra Providence Eastside Hospital
- Gives target dates for training that will mesh with the implementation timeline and assist with keeping the project on track
- Identifies the need for decision making
- Increases end-user willingness to participate in training
- Allows for successful implementation with minimal end-user frustrations
- Increases cost-effectiveness of training due to efficient use of existing and contracted resources

Training Team

End users must be prepared for the changes they face during and after conversion. A comprehensive training plan that includes talented staff and top-notch learning materials will lead to the success of the implementation. To that end, a Training Team was formed using an interdisciplinary team, including nursing, respiratory, dietary, lab, radiology, scheduling, pharmacy, surgery, and ancillary units.

Learning Gap Analysis; Computer Skills Assessment

A basic computer and Windows self-assessment tool was provided to each hospital at the commencement of the project for all associates to be using the new system. The self-assessment tool aided in the identification of associates requiring a Basic Computer/Basic Windows Class prior to the new system training. Very few associates required this training in 2008 and none was identified for 2009.

Training Delivery Methods

The primary and preferred delivery method for end-user training is a well-blended approach of web/computer-based training (WBT) with trainer and instructor-led training (ILT), supported by continuing access and self-exploration exercises in the train domain for reinforcement and expansion. Super Users are present to help assist End Users during instruction and CBT. Super Users facilitate learning in the department or unit-specific processes and skills within each application. This occurred preconversion and postconversion in the train domain. Super Users also assist Staff Development Specialists with any ILT. Application training for physicians is conducted using a one-to-one basis at the nursing station and/or independent learning lab times and physician lounge computers as requested by the physicians.

Training Schedules

Criteria used to set training schedules include:

- The number of users to be trained, and the ability to complete training in the 6 weeks prior to conversion
- The audience identified, with consideration given to job title, location, work hours, prerequisite skills, and complexity of the application
- Competency requirements for each application
- Number of available computer classrooms and trainers
- Availability of a training domain within the new applications, including ongoing support and updates
- Support of hospital leadership for user training attendance

Super User Training

To increase motivation for the Super Users, the Training Team recommended the several methods of recognition, which are in compliance with the overall plan and specific "Super Users" and Trainer responsibilities. The first involved sending each Super User a *Welcome Letter* welcoming them to the team. The letter defines their responsibilities and invites them to ask about their teaching concerns (get these out in the open where they can be dealt with). Second, each Super User was to receive recognition both prior to kickoff and after *training* has occurred. And third, Super Users were to attend a *special tools* class for coaching and mentoring skills. In considering the special needs of Super Users, the following are included in the curriculum:

- Job Aids for End Users
- Job Aids with special Super User issues
- Think about when it is just better to coach – not instruct
- Acknowledge gaps, concerns, and fears
- Ways to have student "go through" tasks for hands-on experience – performance

- Team work for facilitating and then for success on the floor
- Point out documentation for future reference (such as books, learning aids, and quick reference cards)

Success Criteria

- All pertinent personnel received the right training at the right time (trained according to timeline and target dates)
- All pertinent personnel demonstrated competency
- An effective class attendance and scheduling process in effect
- A process was in place to accurately document, monitor, and report attendance tracking
- An effective ongoing, postconversion training process was defined
- Training materials were customized and site-specific
- Training was congruent with corporate guidelines
- Class evaluations demonstrate learning occurred
- Ninety percent of users report satisfaction with training
- End users demonstrate acquisition of the cognitive skills and any other objectives of the training program on the day of the class or at the end of the training program
- End Users demonstrated the ability to perform the skills and any other objectives of the training program in the work setting (measured at 4–6 weeks)
- An Improvement in business results was demonstrated as defined by metrics indicating overall project success (measured at 6–9 months out from conversion). Measure the impact of the training program in relationship to business needs and goals

Outcomes: Quality of Care, Patient Safety, and Operational Issues

Since the release of two landmark publications by the Institute of Medicine, *To Err Is Human: Building a Safer Health System* and *Crossing the Quality Chasm,* both the health care industry and consumers have become very much interested and engaged in the national dialog regarding patient safety and quality of care.

Subsequently, the Institute of Medicine's Committee on Data Standards for Patient Safety released recommendations on the utilization of information technology in addressing patient safety and quality of care. These data standards have further intensified national interest in the implementation of new clinical technologies as a means to resolve these health care safety and quality concerns. The report[9] included the following recommendations:

- *Recommendation* 1: *Americans expect and deserve safe care.* Improved information and data systems are needed to support efforts to make patient safety a standard of care in hospitals, doctors' offices, nursing homes, and in every other health care setting. All health care organizations should establish comprehensive patient safety systems that:

- Provide immediate access to complete patient information and decision support tools for clinicians and their patients.
- Capture information on patient safety – including both adverse events and near misses – as a by-product of care and use this information to design even safer care delivery systems.
- *Recommendation* 2: A national health information infrastructure – a foundation of systems, technology, applications, standards, and policies – is required to make patient safety a standard of care.
  - The federal government should facilitate deployment of the national health information infrastructure through the provision of targeted financial support and the ongoing promulgation and maintenance of standards for data that support patient safety.
  - Health care providers should invest in EHR systems that possess the key capabilities necessary to provide safe and effective care and to enable the continuous redesign of care processes to improve patient safety.

These recommendations are rooted in the expectation that nurses will have adequate information technology knowledge and skills. Therefore, the education and staff development programs are critical to the success of these implementations. A study conducted in a Davenport, IA, health system found that information technology enhancements allowed nurses more time with the patients at the bedside.[10] While at the bedside, nurses are able to practice evidenced-based medicine which promotes the quality of care and cost-effective utilization of health care services.

Innovations in information technology are transforming the nursing profession and can significantly influence the delivery and efficacy of medical services. Both patients and nursing professionals can potentially find greater satisfaction in this new technical environment.

Recommendations for Successful Clinical Systems Training Approaches

A 2009 national survey of EHR adoption rates in U.S. acute care hospitals indicated that only 17% of all facilities had adopted an EHR system. Barriers to adoption most often cited by respondents included high capital investment requirements, high system maintenance costs, and staff training costs.[11] The ultimate clinical and financial success of any new clinical technology system will depend in large part upon rigorous preimplementation analysis and planning along with appropriate staff training prior to the "go-live" event as a means to reduce the influence of these barriers.

The following effective clinical provider training programs for nurses, physicians, and allied health and unit-based clerical staff tend to share common staff preparation and training strategies as part of a successful project:

- *Utilize a structured analysis of the care environment's workflows*: Many health care organizations have found value in using the Six Sigma process methodology which provides a structured method of defining current vs. future clinical workflows. It is imperative that implementation planners first assure that the current paper-based work-flows and characteristics are appropriately analyzed and documented. This will typi-cally include development of baseline "metrics" and "mapping" of provider workflows, user needs, and system resources. The Six Sigma methodology is a frequently utilized method of conducting this analysis.

- *Secure participation and enthusiasm of clinical users*: Use of "Super Users" and "Super Trainers" (physicians and nurses who are respected by peers, enthusiastic about the new technology/system, skilled in its use, and are noted to be good communicators) can be vital to a successful staff training program that results in producing not only technical system use skills, but also excellent attitudes regarding the value to patient care designed into the new system. Identification of these key training team members should begin in the first phases of planning for an implementation.
- *Identify training strategies*: A combination of traditional classroom instruction and computer-based training is probably the most effective approach. Creation of a central-ized training "War Room" staffed 12 h a day by "Super Trainers" with scheduling and content flexibility for end users appropriate to their individual availability and current computer skills can greatly enhance the staff training effort. A "nurses train nurses" and "physicians train physicians" approach helps to promote user confidence in both the training staff and also the clinical system.
- *Implement only one clinical area at a time*: Using a clinical area with the most favorable characteristics (e.g., existing level of computer knowledge excellence, prior enthusiasm in adopting new technology or procedures, managers in area have confidence of subor-dinates, etc.) as an initial pilot is highly preferable over a facility-wide approach. This "test bed" area will provide an excellent "laboratory" for identifying unanticipated implementation problems/needs that will be of invaluable assistance in future efforts.
- *Make every effort to see that the first implementation site is a success for all classes of end users*: Training support and planning associated with the first site should be espe-cially intense. A positive result for all involved will yield rich results in successfully engaging subsequent users in later efforts.

Conclusion

Despite currently discouraging rates of adoption of clinical systems in health care environ-ments, well-designed staff development and continuing education training programs can greatly increase the successful implementation of new clinical technology. A review of the past implementation experience of other facilities as reported in the literature combined with the development of a comprehensive end user training plan is the foundation for assuring a positive effect on the quality of patient care and patient safety provided by new information technologies.

The training and continuing education functions are of particular value in this effort. If end users are not sufficiently skilled in systems use or are not enthusiastic about its value in clinical care, the implementation effort is more than likely to fail despite any inherent technical advantages it may possess.

Acknowledgments   The authors wish to acknowledge Rhoda H. Denlinger, BSN, RN, Staff Educator for Computers, Lancaster General Hospital, Lancaster, Pennsylvania; Megan Shaw, BSN, MEd, RN-BC, Coordinator, Clinical Information Systems Education, Summa Health System, Akron, Ohio; and Kathleen McCarthy, St. Vincent Mercy Medical Center, Toledo, Ohio. Each contributed invaluable insights on programs on their individual institutions.

References

1. Heller BR, Oros MU, Durney-Crowley J. The future of nursing: ten trends to watch. http://www.nln.org/nlnjournal/infotrends.htm#2; n.d. Accessed 03.04.08.
2. ihealthbeat. IT could help nurses boost efficiency, safety study finds. http://www.ihealthbeat.org/articles/2007/11/8/IT-Could-Help-Nurses-Boost-Efficiency-Safety-Study-Finds.aspx?topicID=53; 2007. Accessed 03.04.08.
3. American Association of Colleges of Nursing. *White Paper on the Education and Role of the Clinical Nurse Leader*. Washington, DC: AACN; 2007.
4. Barton A. Cultivating informatics competencies in a community of practice. *Nurs Adm Q*. 2005;29(4):323-328.
5. Institute of Medicine. *Health Professions Education: A Bridge to Quality*. Washington, DC: National Academy Press; 2003.
6. Wini Conference. http://www.winiconference.net/id11.html; 2008. Accessed 08.04.08.
7. Rosenfeld P, Salazar-Riera N, Vieira D. Piloting an information literacy program for staff nurses – lessons learned. *Comput Inform Nurs*. 2002;20(6):236-241.
8. Cleveland Clinic Nursing Informatics. http://cms.clevelandclinic.org/nursing/body.cfm?id=8; 2008. Accessed 09.04.08.
9. Aspden P, Corrigan J, Wolcott J, et al. *Patient Safety – Achieving a New Standard of Care*. Washington, DC: Institute of Medicine; 2004.
10. Healthcare IT News. http://www.healthcareitnews.com/story.cms.id=8265; 2008. Accessed 15.04.08.
11. Ashish J, DesRoches C, Campbell E, et al. Use of electronic health records in U.S. hospitals. *NEJM*. 2009;16(360):1628-1638.
12. Starr P. *The Social Transformation of American Medicine*. New York, NY: Basic Books; 1982:4.

Leadership Collaborative

9

Judy Murphy and Dana Alexander

Overview

Health information technology (HIT) is a key enabler for health care reform. Effective use of HIT will enable nurse executives to ensure nursing care that is safe, of high quality, efficient, and patient-centric, as well as help them deal with a looming workforce shortage. Today's leaders are often expected to transform their organization's values, beliefs, and behaviors. Technology is an underpinning for the needed changes, but adoption of technology does not happen without leadership that is educated and prepared to lead care transformation initiatives that are based on technology implementation. This requires vision, influence, risk taking, clinical knowledge, and a strong expertise of professional nursing practice.

In 2006, the TIGER Initiative held an interactive summit to gather leaders from the nation's nursing administration, practice, education, informatics, technology organizations, government agencies, and other key stakeholders to create a vision for the future of nursing that bridges the quality chasm with information technology, enabling nurses to use informatics in practice and education to provide safer, higher-quality patient care. One of the highest priorities identified at the TIGER Summit was to develop *revolutionary leadership that drives, empowers, and executes the transformation of healthcare.*

The TIGER Leadership Development Collaborative team engaged stakeholders from various levels of nursing leadership in both practice and educational settings to identify effective leadership development strategies related to the use of HIT. Building on the TIGER Informatics Competencies Collaborative recommendations, the Leadership Development Collaborative completed an inventory of existing leadership development programs to determine how informatics competencies were integrated into their curriculums. They surveyed nursing leaders to gain perspective on knowledge gaps related to HIT in their management teams and identify their most urgent development needs.

As technology introduces opportunities for change that impact many aspects of the role of the nurse and since nursing leadership is responsible for developing a culture that is innovative and ready to embrace the change, the TIGER Leadership Development

J. Murphy (✉)
Aurora Health Care, 3031 West Montana Street, Milwaukee, WI, 53215, USA
e-mail: judy.murphy@aurora.org

M.J. Ball et al. (eds.), *Nursing Informatics*,
DOI: 10.1007/978-1-84996-278-0_9, © Springer-Verlag London Limited 2011

Collaborative aligned with the Magnet® Recognition Program and collected dozens of examples of how organizations are using HIT to demonstrate aspects of their Magnet Journey. The Leadership Development Collaborative team used the exemplars, together with the input on knowledge gaps in informatics competencies, to formulate a core set of recommendations for ongoing program development.

During the last decade, information technology (IT) has transformed every aspect of life, affecting businesses in every industry and empowering consumers to change the way they work, bank, shop, and travel. However, this profound change has been slow to penetrate the health care system infrastructure. As a result, major reform is needed in how health care is delivered in the future – changes that affect organizational values, beliefs, and behaviors.

Industry and National Imperatives

The urgency for health IT is well established. Several major studies and organizations have demonstrated the link between technology and safety and quality. In 1999, a group of large employers came together to form a group, The Leapfrog Group, to assess health care by certain quality indicators. Officially launched in November 2000, this group is supported by the Business Roundtable and the Robert Wood Johnson Foundation and many other industry and corporate groups. One of the four "leaps" in hospital quality, safety, and affordability includes the presence of computerized order entry (CPOE) as a measure shown to reduce serious medication prescribing errors by more than 50%.

The federal government is supporting the use of technology as a critical tool to reform health care delivery. The U.S. Department of Health and Human Services (DHHS) states that the broad use of health IT will:

- Improve health care quality
- Prevent medical errors
- Reduce health care costs
- Increase administrative efficiencies
- Decrease paperwork
- Expand access to affordable care

As a direct result of the American Recovery and Reinvestment Act of 2009, national attention has turned to HIT and incentives to encourage the implementation, adoption, and use of Electronic Health Records (EHRs) to achieve these defined benefits by Health and Human Services and to stimulate health care reform. Major advocacy issues include Certification, Meaningful Use, and Quality Reporting. Defining "Meaningful Use" and "Meaningful Users" of EHRs is in process and critical to achieving goals for patient outcomes and population health. It is expected that more requirements for quality outcomes and population health and quality reporting will be defined over time. "Meaningful Use" and the government-driven stimulus package initiative include both reimbursement incentives and penalties that will impact nursing.

There is no doubt that new technologies have the potential to create a safer and more efficient work environment for nurses. Health IT will also play a key role in our ability to deal with a looming workforce shortage. While HIT is expected to help realize process improvements that contribute to better patient care outcomes, it must be used in conjunction with other tools and techniques to have an effect on care. As health IT is central to health care reform and nurses comprise the largest group of clinical users of an HIT system, nurse executives must play a critical role and remain engaged throughout the lifecycle of system selection, implementation, and optimization. Additionally, the health care team will look to the nurse executive to drive adoption and articulate the goals and anticipated benefits of the technology implementation to guide health care reform.

Involvement of Nurse Leaders

From a policy and legislative perspective, nursing has the opportunity to be at the table to influence policy and standards for health IT. Examples of nursing leaders influencing HIT at the national level include:

- *Connie Delaney, PhD, RN, FAAN, FACMI* was appointed to the HIT Policy Committee and *Judy Murphy, RN, FACMI, FHIMSS* was appointed to the HIT Standards Committee by the Director of the U.S. Department of Health and Human Services (HHS). Both are helping to guide the incentives for implementation of EHRs for all Americans by the year 2014, as part of the HITECH (HIT for Economic and Clinical Health) component of the American Recovery and Reinvestment Act of 2009.
- *Mary Wakefield, PhD, RN, FAAN* was appointed as Administrator of the Health Resources and Services Administration (HRSA) by President Obama in 2009.
- *Linda J. Stierle, MSN, RN, NEA-BC,* Chief Executive Officer of the American Nurse Association, continues to work toward achieving meaningful health care reform through her participation with the Health Reform Dialogue group.
- *Deborah Parham Hopson, PhD, RN, FAAN,* was appointed as a member of the new Federal Coordinating Council for Comparative Effectiveness Research, to help guide spending on health care research that was allocated in the American Recovery and Reinvestment Act of 2009.

Additionally, there are state level initiatives to foster nursing knowledge at the policy/legislative level as well educating the practicing nurse. For example, the State of Iowa, in response to legislation for the Iowa Health Information Technology System, included a practicing nurse (nurse practitioner) and a nurse informaticist to the electronic health information advisory council and the executive committee as the representatives of entities involved in EHRs.

Background: The Tiger Leadership Collaborative Vision

The TIGER vision for leadership was defined at the 2006 summit as the state of "Revolutionary Leadership that drives, empowers, and executes the transformation of health care through the use of IT." Two action steps were identified to help achieve the leadership vision:

- Create leadership, management, education, and development strategies to support nursing leaders in transforming care through technology initiatives.
- Identify strategies to increase the power, influence, and presence of nursing leadership in IT initiatives, both locally and nationally, at their own organizations through their professional organizations, as well as governmental and legal bodies.

A call for participation in the Leadership Development Collaborative identified a broad range of individuals with expertise in nursing leadership and interested in working with virtual tools such as wikis and webinars to develop strategies for leadership development.

One of the team's first strategies was to identify common issues that nursing leaders face within their scope of practice related to health IT. These activities often are the responsibility of the nurse executive, and examples are listed in Table. 9.1. In order to prepare nursing leaders to address these issues, the team established three strategic objectives as a framework for their recommendations:

1. Increase nursing leadership's awareness regarding the transformation enabled by HIT.
2. Empower nursing leadership to use HIT knowledgeably.
3. Facilitate nursing leadership to understand, promote, own, and measure the success of technology projects.

Four key action steps were identified by the Leadership Collaborative:

1. Develop an inventory of existing resources for HIT in current nursing leadership development programs.
2. Define informatics competencies for nurse leaders.

Table 9.1 Common issues that nursing leaders face related to health IT

Nursing leader activities related to health IT
Development of a convincing ROI for IT around patient safety
The need to overcome financial and cultural barriers related to IT
Identification of funding sources, i.e., grants, to support IT projects
Create a strategy and rationalization for implementation of IT
Supporting and providing leadership development on IT topics
Articulating the importance of IT and its link to safety
Support clinical IT staff to develop a product that enables workflow and clinical decision support, and to train clinicians
Improving patient safety through point-of-care decision support
Assure that safety features, evidence-based practice standards, and outcomes are incorporated. All are key elements of a successful clinical information system
Exercising research opportunities that substantiate the business case for nursing
Insist on technological advances that fully integrate and automate nursing information into clinical decision support

3. Identify and describe synergies and linkages between the Magnet Program and Health IT.
4. Determine and prioritize leadership development needs.

Nursing Leadership Development Programs

In order to develop a U.S. nursing workforce capable of using EHRs to improve the delivery of health care, an investment must be made in people to build an informatics-aware health care workforce. As reported in *Building the Workforce for Health Information Transformation*, "A work force capable of innovating, implementing, and using health communications and information technology (HIT) will be critical to healthcare's success." Even more critical will be equipping the health care executives to effectively lead this transformation.

The leadership collaborative team developed an inventory of leadership development resources from a variety of sources, including a comprehensive literature review, ongoing research programs, expert resources, and review of known leadership development programs. The comprehensive literature review was completed using the MeSH and CINAHL headings (nursing management, leadership, informatics, and expert resources) as search terms. This research uncovered several different types of leadership development programs that provide background education and training for nurses in health care informatics. The programs and options for nursing administration and health services management provide nursing leaders opportunities to prepare nurses to engage in team roles to meet the demands and expectations of the evolving health care industry and the technologies and knowledge that will support this industry.

The collaborative identified five categories of leadership development programs for nurses:

1. Academic Graduate Programs for Nursing Administration with Informatics Education
2. Organizational Fellowship Programs for Nurse Executive Education and Mentorship
3. Health Industry Network Programs for Nursing Management Education
4. Technology Vendor-Sponsored Programs for Nursing Leadership
5. Self-education Opportunities for Nurse Executives and Managers.

Once identified, each program type was evaluated for the inclusion of informatics competencies within the program. The findings from this analysis are described within each program type.

Academic Graduate Programs for Nursing Administration with Informatics Education

The U.S. News and World 2008 Report ranked the top eight graduate level nursing programs that focus on nursing service administration. From this list, seven of the eight programs required graduate level informatics course for their master's degree in nursing administration (University of Iowa, University of Pennsylvania, University of North

Carolina-Chapel Hill, University of Illinois-Chicago, University of Michigan, University of Maryland, and University of California-San Francisco).

The informatics courses have a focus on standards and information systems' life cycle and management; along with clinical and administrative decision making. Additionally, online distance education programs are now meeting the leadership and clinical informatics' objectives listed above on a broader scale.[1]

Across the nation there are approximately 179 Masters programs, 46 PhD programs, and 64 certificate programs focusing on nursing service administration. Whether or not any or all of these programs have informatics-related courses in their curriculum is not known at this time, but this is an opportunity for future analysis. It is our hope that potential students will review curriculums and select those programs that include this very important body of knowledge.

Organizational Fellowship Programs for Nurse Executive Education and Mentorship

In a second type of program, the American Organization of Nursing Executives (AONE), Sigma Theta Tau, and the American Medical Informatics Association (AMIA) have provided leadership development programs and conferences for nursing leaders. In 2006, nursing executives identified organizational process workflow redesign and technology applications such as EHR, computerized provider order entry (CPOE), clinical documentation, organization-wide information technology solutions, bar coding for medication administration, and picture archiving and communication system as major priorities which drove the early leadership development needs.[2]

Health Industry Network Programs for Nursing Management Education

Some large health systems and hospitals offer nurse manager leadership development programs, internships, and fellowships for students and graduates, such as Massachusetts General Hospital and the Institute for John Hopkins Nursing Academy, who provide programs with emphasis on managing people. Kaiser Permanente Nursing Leadership Institute partners with the Advisory Board to offer a program. The Advisory Board Leadership Academy offers a broad scope of training topics for its members that includes measurement of performance, improvement of processes, and addresses strategic and operational challenges. Overall, the inclusion of technology, information management skills, and knowledge are not uniformly integrated into the current nursing management education. An opportunity exists to define and establish a common foundation across all program types.

Technology Vendor-Sponsored Programs for Nursing Leadership

There are national and international educational programs sponsored by technology vendors for nursing leadership development through conferences, workshops, and user groups. Nurse leaders reported in 2006 that current systems did not adequately address workflow complexities and standardization.[3] Mechanisms exist where HIT vendors sponsor programs associated with training leaders through networking with health systems for learning through collaborative sharing at conferences and web-based user groups. Vendor-sponsored programs have been a valuable contribution to the education of nurse leaders for information technology.

Self-Education Opportunities for Nurse Executives and Managers

Ball[4] and Brokel[5] reported that consistent self-education is necessary to endure the lifecycle of technology and informatics changes today. After formal education, the need to keep pace with HIT advancements is possible through journals such as Nursing Management, Nursing Outlook, the *Journal of the American Medical Informatics Association, Computers Informatics Nursing, Health Informatics Journal*, and *Journal of Healthcare Information Management* who provide current topics for the field.

Informatics Competencies

The explosion of HIT and new technology at the point-of-care has created dramatic change in health care delivery. IV pumps and patient beds are "smart" with built-in rules to automatically adjust to patient changes; robots roam hospital halls to do rounds and deliver medications and supplies; and hospital resources such as health care personnel, medications, supplies, and even patients are identified with barcodes or radio-frequency identification tags. This trend is not unique to health care; in fact, there is a national shift toward a "knowledge-based workforce." Critical to the success of this transition is ensuring that the workforce is adequately trained with the skills necessary to perform their duties with the new technologies.

Nurses need to be equipped to integrate technology seamlessly within their workflow and need better tools to work safely, more efficiently, and communicate more effectively with the patient and other health care providers. Nurses are directly engaged with information systems and technologies as the foundation for evidence-based practice, clinical decision support tools, and the EHR. As nurses are at the center of health care delivery, they are constantly responding to requests for information, assistance from patients, family members, physicians, and other health care staff. As communication mechanisms make the digital shift, the nurse has to quickly master these tools to function in their role. All health care providers today need the knowledge and skills to work with electronic records, including basic computer skills, information literacy, and an understanding of informatics and information management capabilities.

Education Is Essential

A comprehensive approach to education reform is necessary to reach the current workforce of nearly three million practicing nurses. The average age of a practicing nurse in the U.S. is 47 years. These individuals are "digital immigrants" as they grew up without digital technology, had to adopt it later, and some may not have had the opportunity to be educated on its use or be comfortable with technology. This is opposed to "digital natives," younger individuals who grew up in the digital age, with technology such as computers, the internet, mobile phones, and MP3. There are a number of digital immigrants in the nursing workforce who have not mastered basic computer competencies, let alone information literacy and how to use HIT effectively and efficiently to enhance nursing practice. In addition to the rising age of the health care workforce, the past 2 years have shown the greatest increase in the number of nurses returning to the workforce in the past several decades. The nurse executive must be aware of the unique educational requirements of staff who may not be as comfortable or familiar with computer technology prior to introducing a significant HIT project such as an EHR, as the success will depend upon adequate support and educational resources.

Nursing leaders need to assess the capabilities of their workforce and support efforts to address any gaps that limit the ability of their staff to use HIT capabilities necessary for the delivery of safe and effective patient care. The TIGER Initiative has identified and published a minimum set of informatics competencies that all practicing nurses need to have to succeed in today's digital environment. In support of this initiative, the Leadership Development Collaborative team directed a work group to further identify the minimum informatics competencies that all nurses need to include informatics knowledge and skills that are essential for today's nursing leader. The following outlines the work group's recommendations and educational resources to help achieve these objectives.

Nursing Informatics Competencies Models

Following an extensive review of the literature and survey of nursing informatics education, research, and practice groups, the TIGER Informatics Competencies Collaborative identified three primary categories of informatics competencies that all nurses need: basic computer skills, information literacy, and information management or the ability to effectively use an EHR. They described the categories as components and developed the TIGER Nursing Informatics Competencies (TNIC) model as illustrated in Table 9.2 to describe the alignment of each component with an existing set of competencies maintained by standard development organizations or de facto standards. More details on the research and

Table 9.2 TIGER nursing informatics competencies model

Component of the model	Standard	Source (standard-setting body)
Basic computer competencies	European Computer Driving License (ECDL)	European Computer Driving License Foundation www.ecdl.org
Information literacy	Information Literacy Competency Standards	American Library Association www.ala.org
Information management	Electronic Health Record Functional Model – Clinical Care Components	Health Level Seven (HL7) www.hl7.org
	International Computer Driving License – Health	European Computer Driving License Foundation www.ecdl.org

recommendations of the TIGER Informatics Competencies Collaborative team can be found on the TIGER website at www.tigersummit.com.

The TIGER Leadership Development workgroup for Informatics Competencies further evaluated each component to determine if there was a need to expand the competencies' requirements specifically for nursing leaders. Below is a review of each component of the TNIC model and the recommendations that are most relevant to different leadership roles within nursing practice.

Basic Computer Skills

There are a substantial number of nurses practicing today who either have not mastered basic computer competencies or have gaps in their basic computer competency skill set. Other industries have realized this shortcoming in the workforce and developed comprehensive training programs to address it. One such organization with extensive experience in this area is the European Computer Driving License (ECDL) Foundation. The ECDL identified basic computer competencies and developed an educational course and certification exam nearly two decades ago. To date, about seven million Europeans have now taken the ECDL exam and become certified in basic computer competencies.

The ECDL is known as the International Computer Driving License (ICDL) in the United States and elsewhere outside Europe. The ECDL/ICDL is composed of seven training modules that are outlined in Table 9.3. The concepts include basic computer use (e.g., turning the computer on/off), file management, word processing, spreadsheets, databases, presentation tools, and communication technologies. The knowledge and skills recommended by the ECDL training guide will set a baseline of computer competencies that individuals can use in almost any setting. *The TIGER Informatics Competencies Collaborative recommends that all practicing nurses and graduating nursing students become ECDL/ICDL certified or hold a substantially equivalent certification by 2013.*

They further recommended a phased-approach to completing this education by prioritizing some of the modules to be completed by all nurses by 2011.

The TIGER Leadership Development workgroup felt that all nurses in a leadership position should be competent in all seven components of these computer skills as soon as they assume a management role. The responsibilities of nurses in leadership roles necessitate general familiarity with spreadsheets (budgeting, evaluating metrics), advanced

Table 9.3 European/International Computer Driving License modules

ECDL/ICDL syllabus
Module 1: Concepts of information and communication technology (ICT)
Module 2: Using the computer and managing files
Module 3: Word processing
Module 4: Spreadsheets
Module 5: Using databases
Module 6: Presentation
Module 7: Web browsing and communications

communication skills (through technology as well as presentations and written documentation), and a basic understanding of information management practices such as databases. While it is common to conduct a skills-and-needs assessment for clinical nurses entering a new position in a health care facility or system, it is uncommon for nurse leaders to provide a self-assessment of their informatics competencies. The workgroup recommends that new manager/leader orientation includes all seven modules of the basic computer competencies. In addition to demonstrating these competencies, the work group recommends that the competencies be incorporated into job descriptions and performance evaluations.

Virtual Communication Tools

One area of basic computer competencies that the work group identified as needing further development for nursing leaders is related to advanced information communication tools or "virtual tools." Sigma Theta Tau International describes this as "virtuality," or the various technologies that support managing and leading people in a virtual space that transcends a physical location and time. The workgroup recommended that nurse leaders master the competencies needed to support, maintain, and sustain leadership in virtual communities that use the mass collaboration tools, social networking, and wireless communication networks.

Information Literacy

The American Nurses Association recognizes that nurses are "knowledge workers," and as a result, need to access information and apply knowledge appropriately to deliver high-quality nursing care. The ability to find, evaluate, and apply evidence at the point-of-care is a necessary skill for any practicing nurse. Clinical reasoning and evidence-based decision making prepares nurses at the frontlines, whether at the service level as a direct care provider or as an indirect care provider in management, academic, or research role. Information literacy assists the professional nurse to interpret data and synthesize a plan of action based on the nursing process. Data must be interpreted within its framework and context in order to be meaningful. Data-driven decision making is one of the most essential skills for the nurse leader.

As illustrated in Fig. 9.1, there are five levels of information literacy. The TIGER Informatics Competencies Collaborative recommends that all practicing nurses and graduating nursing students have the ability to:

1. Determine the nature and extent of the information needed
2. Access needed information effectively and efficiently
3. Evaluate information and its sources critically and incorporate selected information into his or her knowledge base and value system
4. Individually or in a group, use information effectively to accomplish a specific purpose
5. Evaluate outcomes of the use of information

Framework for Application of Information Literacy and Evidence-Based Practice to Nursing Process					
Curriculum Pattern	**Level 1**	**Level 2**	**Level 3**	**Level 4**	**Level 5**
Information Literacy	Identify information needed	Find needed Information	Appraise Information	Implement information into practice	Evaluate outcomes of info use
	◄ – ►				
Nursing Process	Assessment	Planning	Intervention	Implementation	Evaluation
	◄ – ►				
Evidence-Based Practice	Develop researchable Question	Search for Evidence	Appraise Evidence	Implement findings into practice	Evaluate outcomes & process

Fig. 9.1 Framework for application of information literacy to nursing process. Courtesy of Susan Pierce

The TIGER Leadership Development Collaborative fully supports the adoption of these five levels of information literacy competencies by 2011. The nurse leader will need to demonstrate the ability to maximize clinical reasoning tools and optimize access to data for the delivery of patient care and adopting best practice models of care. It is further recommended that the competencies be incorporated into job descriptions and performance evaluations.

Information Management

Information management describes how a nurse interacts with an electronic or personal health record and requires a mastery of computer skills and ability to find and apply knowledge to practice. Information management is a process consisting of (1) collecting data, (2) processing the data, and (3) presenting and communicating the processed data as information or knowledge. These are fundamental skills for nurses as knowledge workers, and using EHRs will be the way nurses manage clinical information in the foreseeable future.

Although the navigation and arrangement of data in the patient record may be different in a digital world, this is not a significant shift in nursing responsibilities. For example, nurses are required to exercise due care in protecting patient privacy. But the manner in which these responsibilities to patients and communities are upheld may be different across environments or organizations. Therefore, all practicing nurses and graduating nursing students are strongly encouraged to learn, demonstrate, and use information management competencies and EHRs to carry out their fundamental clinical responsibilities in an increasingly safe, effective, and efficient manner.

The TIGER Informatics Competencies Collaborative team found the most rigorous and practical work when enumerating the relevant components of EHRs upon which to base competencies. For clinicians, this was done by the Health Level 7 (HL7) EHR Technical Committee and was published in February 2007 as an approved American National Standard (ANSI) publication, titled "The HL7 EHR System Functional Model, Release 1," and known as ANSI/HL7 EHR, R1-2007.

The direct care component of the HL7 EHR System Functional Model serves as a basis of information management competencies for practicing nurses and graduating nursing students. The detailed competencies are available in the TIGER Informatics Competencies Collaborative report on the website at www.tigersummit.com/competencies.

Although the information management competencies are numerous, they make explicit competencies for proficient use of EHR's clinical nursing responsibilities that practicing nurses and graduating nursing students are responsible for today in a paper information management environment or a mixed/hybrid paper and electronic environment. The direct care component of the HL7 EHR System Functional Model is not quite sufficient by itself to cover the information management responsibilities of nurses in the digital era. What is additionally needed is a set of competencies that address the importance of EHR and like systems for nurses and the "due care" that nurses need to take in managing information via these systems. Again, the ECDL Foundation has come up with a preliminary set of items that address these concerns, with ECDL-Health – also available on the TIGER website at www.tigersummit.com.

Expanded Competencies for Nurse Leaders

The TIGER Leadership Collaborative team found considerable dissonance in external expectations placed upon nurse leaders regarding their use, knowledge, and access to patient-level EHRs. Most of the controversy stemmed from the difference in roles and responsibilities at varying defined levels of nursing management. For example, staff nurses and charge nurses are intimately involved in entering and retrieving data in the EHR for patient care documentation and chart- or peer-review purposes. On the other hand, unit-level managers and/or supervisors or directors are less likely to be involved in entering data for patient care purposes than they are in periodic and ongoing chart review to assess staff practice and documentation compliance, monitoring and analyzing quality trends, and helping to resolve performance issues. In contrast, nurse executives are more likely to be involved in synthesizing aggregate data gathered from the EHR in report format vs. reviewing patient-level documentation. These expanded competencies are summarized in Table 9.4.

The Leadership Development Collaborative recommends that *all levels of nursing management* must have fundamental knowledge and basic navigation skills related to the EHR and understand how EHR interactions impact nursing workflow, even if not directly involved in the delivery of patient care.

Table 9.4 TIGER expanded nurse management informatics competencies

Competency	Management level	Examples
Develop "dashboards" to manage outcomes	Charge Nurse Unit-Manager or Director Nurse Executive	Use data from the electronic health record (EHR) and national standards to develop "dashboards" or clinical summary reports to demonstrate critical nursing measures, patient safety metrics, and identify patient outcomes Identify discrete data needs, obtain from available data, link interventions to outcomes, and demonstrate progress on meeting outcomes as well as outliers
Proficient in the use of electronic support systems	Charge Nurse	Proficient in the use of electronic support systems including staffing, scheduling, acuity, other clinical IS such as patient location and tracking systems
	Unit-Manager or Director	Identify the educational requirements, time commitment, and resources necessary to use electronic support systems and manages plan to implement with development, testing, education, support, and sustainability processes addressed
	Nurse Executive	Proficient in aggregate budgeting, financial planning, unit metrics/monitoring, quality measurement, clinical decision support tools, and others Understands the skills and resources necessary to optimize the use of electronic support systems
Support research that advances nursing and the delivery of patient care	Unit-Manager or Director Nurse Executive	Review, plan, and evaluate care delivery compared to outcomes and identify process improvements Develop organizational vision for care delivery that incorporates advancing new evidence and research into delivery of care
Develop goals, benefits, and anticipated outcomes for adoption of new technologies	Unit-Manager or Director Nurse Executive	Use knowledge of best practices and standards of care to articulate care processes impacted and desired patient and organizational outcomes Ongoing monitoring of adoption of technology toward achieving defined goals and benefits
Sustain the focus on the patient care delivery model through EHR transformation	Unit-Manager or Director Nurse Executive	Define nursing care delivery and clinical documentation model impact with EHR Apply continuous quality improvement to care delivery model and interdisciplinary plan of care

(*continued*)

Table 9.4 (continued)

Competency	Management level	Examples
Develop and support adequate educational and support resources for new technology implementation	Unit-Manager or Director	Provide operational management of scheduling and resource allocation for provision of care *and* incorporation of new technologies
	Nurse Executive	Advocate enterprise-wide resource planning for implementation based on strategic goals/activities
Share knowledge with collegues to improve best practice evidence	Unit-Manager or Director	Collaborate within the organization and industry to share knowledge of best practices and patient care models that fully realize the benefits of technology to deliver safer, higher-quality patient care
	Nurse Executive	Collaborate with industry, policy-making, and regulatory organizations to share knowledge of best practices and patient care models that fully realize the benefits of technology to deliver safer, higher-quality patient care

As nurses are usually the largest group of clinical users of an HIT system, the nurse executive is expected to fully understand and articulate the goals and anticipated benefits of the technology implementation. Additionally, the nurse executive must remain engaged throughout the lifecycle of system selection, implementation, and optimization. Nurse leaders are often required to make tactical and purchasing decisions about EHRs. These decisions can have widespread impact, both positive and negative, depending upon the nurse executive's understanding of the system requirements, ability to integrate with existing HIT, degree of training, support, and practice changes necessary to accommodate the system, and impact upon the bedside nurse's workflow.

The American Nurses Association further clarifies the nurse executive's role in data collection, assessing the effectiveness and understanding the impact on care delivery and workflow. Recent studies have emphasized the importance of evaluating workflow, usability, and human factor principles prior to implementing any new technology in order to measure and mitigate any untoward effects secondary to the technological solution. The TIGER Usability Collaborative team has published recommendations and provided helpful resource in their summary report, available on the TIGER website at www.tigersummit.com/usability.

The TIGER Leadership Collaborative identified additional informatics competencies that are recommended for nursing management at the level of unit-manager, director, or nurse executive. First, the ability to obtain and evaluate outcome-related data is a necessary requirement with expanding regulatory and quality reporting criteria. The volume and extent of the reporting metrics, especially related to nurse-sensitive indicators and "present on admission," demand access to this information in an electronic media. It is anticipated that the requirements for regulatory and quality metrics will increase as more emphasis is placed on "Meaningful Use," EHR adoption, and comparative effectiveness research.

The nurse executive will require an expanded knowledge of the budgetary, regulatory, safety, security, and privacy policies related to the use of EHRs. New policies will be developed as "meaningful use of certified EHRs" is defined, as incentives and reimbursement rates will be determined by the 2009 American Reinvestment and Recovery Act. The Joint Commission, Center for Medicaid Services, and individual state regulatory bodies will require new reporting requirements and may expand their inspection requests or visits. It is anticipated that the nurse executive will have direct responsibility for demonstrating compliance, as the chief executive for patient care services, and need proficiency in accessing this reportable data.

Magnet Program Collaboration

Technology introduces change to many aspects of the role of the nurse, and nursing leadership is responsible for developing a culture that is innovative and ready to embrace change. Fortunately, a well-recognized professional model that engages nurses at all levels to incorporate change into their culture already exists. The TIGER Leadership Development Collaborative found significant alignment with the Magnet® Recognition Program, developed by the American Nurses Credentialing Center (ANCC). The Magnet Program exemplifies a model for change (see Fig. 9.2), recognizes health care organizations that provide nursing excellence in the delivery of quality patient care, and demonstrates innovation in professional nursing practice.

As many HIT-savvy nurse leaders recommended correlating the Magnet Forces® to HIT implementation and adoption success, the TIGER Leadership Development Collaborative collected dozens of examples of how organizations used HIT to demonstrate aspects of their Magnet Journey. These examples help to illustrate how technology can achieve each

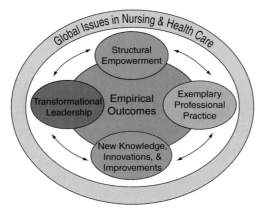

Fig. 9.2 The magnet model

of the 14 forces of magnetism as well as transform the nursing organization to use technology for their benefit. The exemplars were meant to demonstrate the creativity and flexibility to transform the practice of health care delivery by rethinking current tools through gaining access to collective organizational experiences improved through fully automated integrated health care processes.

One goal of the TIGER Leadership Development Collaborative team was to leverage innovative programs involving hospitals from around the United States to act as a gateway for other hospitals as they carry forward with implementing technology to benefit patients and nursing practice.

Nursing Leadership Survey

At the initial TIGER Summit, one of the important activities identified to move the nursing discipline forward was to empower nurse leaders to effectively practice in this electronic era. Data from the Nursing Leadership Survey conducted by the TIGER Leadership Collaborative team provided background data for developing programs aimed toward enhancing a leader's ability to promote technology in their respective areas of practice.

Methodology

A survey for distribution to Chief Nurse Executives was determined as a strategy to review the current status of executives' knowledge and skills about technology. The goal identified was to have a tool which would identify areas of opportunity for program development to meet the needs of nurse leaders as opposed to point deficiencies. Background for survey development included AONE's statement on "Guiding Principles for the Nurse Executive in the Acquisition and Implementation of Information Systems" (2006) and AONE's 2006 Technology Committee Survey. These documents provided guiding information for the formulation of indicators of knowledge and skills. Sections focused on Basic Computer and Technology, Communication Strategies, Project Management, and Change Management and included indicators for each section. The survey was distributed electronically.

Results

Participants in this survey scored Chief Nurse Executives as having proficiency in utilizing technologies and the basic mechanics of developing technologies. Participants identified the following areas for development: locating/interpreting information in chart and information on the advances in technology as it affects nursing practice, implications of a technology implementation, technology's impact on workflow, and policies and procedures.

Participants in the survey scored the Director level as having proficiency in utilizing technologies in their work for the areas under their purview. Areas identified for development for the director/associate dean role include: utilizing data for improving patient care, updating policies and procedures for clinical systems, information on advances in technology as it affects nursing practice and workflow, implication of technology implementation, and providing resources for staff for innovation/adoption of technology.

Participants scored the Nurse Manager role as having adequate knowledge utilizing technologies and basic mechanics. Areas needing improvement include utilizing data to improve patient care, updating policies and procedures for clinical systems, information on advances in technology as it affects nursing practice and workflow, utilizing data from information systems for decision making, and providing resources for staff for innovation/adoption of technology.

The role participants identified as requiring the biggest potential for development is the charge nurse role. Most indicators did not score with proficiency and were identified as areas for development. This reported area represents significant opportunity area for improving care/efficiencies since the charge nurse locus of control often represents the daily/shift care of a patient population and the flow of work on the unit often rests on the skills and knowledge of this nurse.

The nurse informaticist's role was also scored by participants and the role scored as performing with adequate knowledge or above.

Survey Recommendations

The survey provides a glimpse into potential areas in each leadership role which may benefit for further knowledge/skills. Beyond the narrative below, Table 9.5 summarizes the HIT competencies for these three levels of nursing leaders.

Charge Nurse Role

Develop leadership competencies focusing on computer skills. Programs which focus on the daily workflow and skills of running a unit for a shift in which the work is touched or influenced by a computerized process would be targeted. These skills might include interpreting clinical data in its electronic form, policies and procedures, and allocation of staff for pre and postimplementations.

Director/Manager Role

The director/manager level role identified opportunities in viewing/accessing information and data interpretation. If leaders in the director/manager roles are afforded the opportunities to improve and incorporate these knowledge and skills locating and analyzing data, the nurses and workflows under their prevue would improve.

Chief Nurse Executive and Dean Roles

Even though participants identified chief nurse executives as having proficiency technologies and skills in the arena of locating/interpreting data and technology, there are opportunities for increasing knowledge as it affects developing nursing practices, workflow, policies and procedures, and implementation knowledge. These areas directly impact an institution's work toward utilizing technology to provide for information/patient safety practices; the chief nurse executive creates the vision that permeates the care delivered. It is often the executive's role that assumes the direction/priorities of an institution and it is the nurse executive who can provide the resources and direction to have the staff achieve and excel at these skills as their institutions move toward electronic records (Table 9.5).

Table 9.5 HIT competencies for nursing leadership levels

	Charge Nurse	Manager or Director or Associate Dean	Chief Nurse Executive or Dean
Navigation of electronic patient record	✓	✓	✓
Basic computer competencies (see subcategories)	✓	✓	✓
Demonstrate information literacy competency: maximize clinical reasoning tools and optimize access to data for the delivery of patient care and adopting best practice models of care	✓	✓	✓
Electronic Support System staffing, scheduling, acuity, other clinical IS such as pharmacy, lab, radiology, location and tracking systems, budgeting, financial planning, unit metrics/monitoring, quality measurement, clinical decision support tools, and others	✓	✓	✓
Major care delivery processes supported by technology initiatives and determine the goals, benefits and anticipated outcomes of the adoption and use of technology implementations		✓	✓
Sustain focus of patient care delivery model		✓	✓
Support educational process new technology implementation: back-filling patient care providers when mandating participation of all nurses attending training sessions on the new technology processes		✓	

Table 9.5 (continued)

	Charge Nurse	Manager or Director or Associate Dean	Chief Nurse Executive or Dean
Social networking and mass collaboration tools both within the organization and within the nursing profession to facilitate the sharing of knowledge around best practices and patient care models that fully realize the benefits of technology to deliver safer, higher-quality patient care	✓	✓	✓
Solid understanding of security and privacy issues: comprehensive policies related to medical record access	✓		✓
Capable to lead nursing team to informatics	✓	✓	✓
Lead role in Steering Committee for electronic records These activities include involvement with planning the budget and developing financial and clinical impact measures	✓	✓	✓
Subcategories for basic computer competencies			
Concepts of communication and IT *(Hardware, Software, Networks, Electronic/ Digital Environment, Privacy and Security, Ethics, Copyrights)*	✓	✓	✓
Computer use and file management *(Operating System, File Management, Utilities, Printing)*	✓	✓	✓
Word processing software *(Application Use, Creating Documents, Formatting, Tables, Graphics , Printing)*	✓	✓	✓
Spreadsheet software *(Application Use, Cells, Formulas/Functions Formatting, Charts, Printing)*	✓	✓	✓
Database software *(Common Database Use, Retrieving Information, Reports)*	✓	✓	✓
Presentation software *(Application use, Developing a Presentation, Text, Charts, Tables, Graphics, Views, Print Management)*	✓	✓	✓
Web browsing and communication *(Internet, Browsers, World Wide Web (Forms, Information retrieval), E-Mail Management, Print Management)*	✓	✓	✓

Leadership Development Needs

In summary, although we are well on our way in many areas, there is still much work to do to realize the vision of the TIGER summit in 2006. If we are to develop *revolutionary leadership that drives, empowers, and executes the transformation of health care*, the nursing profession will need to consume the recommendations and strategies in this chapter to prepare our leaders of tomorrow and ensure that they have the informatics competency education and development that are needed. Below are the four key recommendations to achieve that vision:

- Develop programs for nurse executives and faculty that stress the value of information technology and empower them to use HIT knowledgably.
- Expand and integrate informatics competencies into Nursing Leadership Development Programs.
- Promote sharing of best practices using HIT effectively to improve the delivery of nursing care and the overall care delivery team
- Promote alignment with the Magnet Recognition Program as a mechanism to demonstrate nursing excellence in using technology to improve nursing practice and the delivery of safer, more effective patient care.

AONE's Technology Task Force

One of the most promising efforts to equip nursing leaders with the necessary resources to promote health IT adoption is the Technology Toolkit that AONE's Technology Task Force is creating. This dynamic toolkit will focus on topics related to standards, IT contingency planning for disasters, wireless technology, return on investment, competencies for managers and executives, job descriptions, and share key learnings. More information can be found at www.aone.org.

Acknowledgments   The authors would like to acknowledge and extend their thanks to the volunteers and nursing professional organizations who lent their leadership, expertise, and support to the *TIGER Leadership Development Collaborative*. They would also like to thank the workgroup chairs and participants, whose names appear elsewhere in this book, who brought their expertise, experiences, review, and hands-on support to the effort.

References

1. Kenner C, Androwich IM, Edwards PA. Innovative educational strategies to prepare nurse executives for new leadership roles. *Nurs Adm Q*. 2003;27(2):172-179.
2. Androwich IM, Haas S. American organization of nurse executives' 2006 survey on nursing and information technology. *Nurse Lead*. 2007;5(2):17-23.

3. Weaver CA, Skiba D. ANI connection. TIGER initiative: addressing information technology competencies in curriculum and workforce. *Comput Nurs*. 2006;24(3):175-176.
4. Ball MJ. Nursing informatics of tomorrow: one of nurses' new roles will be agents of change in the healthcare revolution. *Healthc Inform*. 2005;22(2):74.
5. Brokel J. Technology: creating sustainability of clinical information systems: the chief nurse officer and nurse informatics specialist roles. *JONA*. 2007;37(1):10-13.
6. American Nurses Association. *Scope and Standards of Practice for Nurse Administrators*. Washington, DC: American Nurses Publishing; 2004.
7. American Nurses Association. *Scope and Standards of Practice for Nursing Informatics*. Washington, DC: American Nurses Publishing; 2008.
8. American Nurses Credentialing Center Magnet Recognition Program®. http://www.nursecredentialing.org/Magnet/NewMagnetModel.aspx; 2008. Accessed 27.10.08.
9. American Organization for Nurse Executives. Guiding principles for acquisition and implementation of information technology. http://www.aone.org/aone/pdf/GuidingPrinciplesforAcquisitionandImplementationofInformationTechnology.pdf; 2006. Accessed 14.01.08.
10. American National Standards Institute. ANSI/HL7 electronic health record-system (EHR-S) functional model. www.ansi.org; Accessed 12.08.08.
11. Bohinc M, Gradisar M. International perspectives: decision-making model for nursing. *JONA*. 2003;33(12):627-629.
12. CMS Information Related to the Economic Recovery Act of 2009. http://www.cms.hhs.gov/Recovery/11_HealthIT.asp; 2009. Accessed 11.07.09.
13. Curran CR. The informatics nurse: helping to build the knowledge infrastructure for nursing. *Nurse Lead*. 2004;2(3):26-29.
14. Department of Health and Human Services website about HIT – Health Information Technology for the Future of Health and Care. http://healthit.hhs.gov/portal/server.pt; Accessed 11.07.09.
15. Effken JA. An organizing framework for nursing informatics research. *Comput Nurs*. 2003;21(6):316-325.
16. European Computer Driving License (ECDL). http://www.ecdl.org/publisher/index.jsp; Accessed 08.08.08.
17. European Computer Driving License Health model. http://www.ecdl.nhs.uk/resources/ecdl-health-unit/healthunitsyllabus.pdf; Accessed 12.08.08.
18. Farmer LA. Situational leadership: a model for leading telecommuters. *J Nurs Manag*. 2005;13(6):483-489.
19. Harris K, Huber D, Jones R, et al. Future nursing administration graduate curricula, Part 1. *JONA*. 2006;36(10):435-440.
20. Hawley SR, Molgaard CA, Ablah E, et al. Academic-practice partnerships for community health workforce development. *J Community Health Nurs*. 2007;24(3):155-165.
21. Heller BR, Drenkard K, Herr MB, et al. Educating nurses for leadership roles. *J Contin Educ Nurs*. 2004;35(5):203.
22. Herrin D, Jones K, Krepper R, et al. Future nursing administration graduate curricula, Part 2: foundation and strategies. *JONA*. 2006;36(11):498-505.
23. Hertzler B. Informatics leadership: what chief nurse executives need to know. In: Weaver C et al., eds. *Nursing and Informatics for the 21st Century: An International Look at Practice, Trends and the Future*. Chicago, IL: Health Information and Management Systems Society; 2006.
24. The Leapfrog Group. http://www.leapfroggroup.org/; 2009. Accessed 11.07.09.
25. McCartney PR. Leadership in nursing informatics. *J Obstet Gynecol Neonatal Nurs*. 2004;33(3):371-380.
26. Phillips J. Knowledge is power: using nursing information management and leadership interventions to improve services to patients, clients and users. *J Nurs Manag*. 2005;13(6):524-536.

27. Pierce ST. Framework for application of IL and EBP to nursing process, slide 32. In: Pierce ST, Moore D, Shelton D, et al., eds. *Curriculum Enhancement: Integrating Information Literacy for Evidence-Based Practice*; 2001. http://www.nsula.edu/watson_library/shreve/curri_enhanct.ppt#270,32Slide. Accessed 12.08.08.
28. Prensky M. Digital natives, digital immigrants. In: *On the Horizon*. www.marcprensky.com/writing/; 2001. Accessed 27.09.09.
29. Romano CA, Heller BR. Nursing informatics: a model curriculum for an emerging role. *Nurse Educ*. 1990;15(2):16-19.
30. Sensmeier J. Survey demonstrates importance of nurse informaticist role in health information technology design and implementation. *Comput Nurs*. 2007;25(3):180-182.
31. Sigma Theta Tau International Nursing Honor Society. Resource Paper and Position Statement on Leadership and Leadership Development Priorities. http://www.nursingsociety.org/aboutus/Documents/position_leadership.doc; n.d. Accessed 31.07.08.
32. Snyder-Halpern R, Corcoran-Perry S, Narayan S. Developing clinical practice environments supporting the knowledge work of nurses. *Comput Nurs*. 2001;19(1):17-26.
33. Wilkinson A. New age informatics & the management of perioperative nursing documentation. *Dissector*. 2007;35(1):20-23.

Challenging Leadership Status Quo

10

Roy L. Simpson

Organizational structures in corporate business differ fundamentally from those found in a hospital or health care facility. Nurse executives would be wise to understand the organizational structures that come into play and even wiser to remember that titles do not always accurately reflect authority within an organization. For example, holding a line position in a corporation entitles that individual to decide how to deploy resources to achieve the corporation's business goals. Employees in staff positions provide information and advice to those in line positions. In matrix-based organizations, project managers select from a pool of employees to work on specific assignments, which often results in a single employee working for several managers.

Outside these structures, most corporations have individuals whose titles belie their influence. For example, while a person who serves as the chief executive's "right hand" might not have line or staff responsibility; that individual likely wields more authority than other executive-titled professionals. In that context, one perspective is that today's Chief Nursing Officers (CNOs) and nursing executives have "tunnel vision" when it comes to technology and the nursing profession. For reasons unknown, forward thinking clinical executives fail to understand the role of the nurse informatician and the unique perspective that only this dual professional can apply to the practice of nursing.

One good question is how many CNOs are familiar with the scope of practice for nurse informaticians as laid out by the American Nursing Association (ANA)? This author challenges the traditional nursing executives to embrace a broader perspective of leadership and executive roles within the profession. Thought leaders in our profession believe there is no downside to delegating technology management to a staff member. Note that the reference here is to "technology management."

Why is this important? The following questions are relevant to ask nurse executives in reference to technology management. Does delegating a nursing-critical function to a staff member without understanding the scope, impact, and relevance of that function make sense? Without a thorough understanding of the function, how will the nurse executive gain the organization's backing for that function? How effective can a technology-crippled

R.L. Simpson
Vice President, Nursing Informatics at Cerner Corporation, 2800 Rockcreek Parkway, Kansas City, MO 64117, USA
e-mail: rsimpson@cerner.com

M.J. Ball et al. (eds.), *Nursing Informatics*,
DOI: 10.1007/978-1-84996-278-0_10, © Springer-Verlag London Limited 2011

nurse executive be when it comes to advocating for funding, staff, and other investments in that function? Is there a single nurse executive who *can create* a budget or read a spreadsheet?

Probably not. But the question is how many nurse executives can debate the nursing-specific benefits of one clinical system over another? Perhaps a handful at best. Technology investments continue to be one of the largest line items in any health care organization's budget, yet the level of most nurse executives' related knowledge is low – dismally low. That lack of knowledge, coupled with political pressure, often prompts nursing to acquiesce to physicians during the selection process. As a result, nursing has to use systems that are less than ideal for nursing functions.

This situation not only needs to be remedied in short order, but the nursing profession as a whole also needs to embrace technology and the accountability that comes with it. Until and unless nursing can define the unique contribution it makes to patient care, our profession will be marginalized, making us generic health care workers. To avoid the generic health care worker scenario, CNOs and nursing's other executive leaders need to champion a fundamental shift in the profession. Starting now, the future of nursing depends on redefining its role and contribution in ten areas specific to information technology (IT). Each of these areas represents a fundamental capability or understanding that is currently lacking in the nursing profession. Gaining competency in each of the areas will push nursing forward, enabling professional nurses to harness the power of IT.

CNOs and Other Nursing Leaders Must Become Acutely Knowledgeable About IT Systems' Ability to Support Patient Care

Consider nursing leadership's role in IT evaluation and selection. Unfortunately, many CNOs and other nursing leaders shy away from meeting with vendors, listening to their presentations, and actively discussing the merits of each. Nursing executives need more than a working knowledge of the systems under review; they must be able to know the systems at such a deep level that they can compare like releases of the products from each of the considered vendors. Being able to determine functional parity, or the lack of parity, in the systems being considered is critical when it comes to identifying value for the IT dollar spent.

Nurse executives do not operate the nursing department based on what the organization's annual report says, yet a one-page executive "order" from the chief information officer is what defines nursing's technical support. A major concern is that the governing of nursing's key functions is frequently abdicated to an executive outside nursing – an executive who has little, if any, understanding of nursing operations. If the profession's leaders do not make known the technology assistance they need, who will?

However, functionality discussions represent only the beginning of a true vendor evaluation effort. CNOs need to exert the same level of due diligence over a system selection as they would for an acquisition of another health care operation or facility. For example, the CNO needs to be able to answer the following questions, which are certain to be posed by the facility's executive team when a system or vendor is providing information regarding the use of a particular system in his/her agency:

- Which vendor has demonstrated the most accurate and thorough understanding of the hospital's business and financial goals?
- What is each vendor's ability to help the facility overcome market and competitive pressures?
- Each vendor has an "ideal customer." Which profile most clearly maps to our health care organization?
- How do the vendors "stack up" in two critical areas: delivering on time and on budget? (Note: This question needs to be answered in terms of customer references with particular attention paid to remarks from "like" facilities.)
- How do vendors' pricing models compare? For instance, vendors offering "fixed costs" give nurse executives a better handle on expenses that contracts built around a "time and materials" model.
- Which vendor's technology roadmap best supports the hospital's 5- and 10-year business plans?
- Which vendors operate from a strong financial footing? (Note: CNOs would be wise to recruit the hospital's chief financial officer to weigh in on this determination. Because most IT vendors are public companies, reports from trusted financial analysts can provide detailed insights into each company's financial health.)
- How will the merger and acquisition climate in IT influence each vendor's technology roadmap, financial position, and customer base?

One specific way to gain this depth of knowledge involves engaging with the nurse executive from each of the vendor companies. An absence of a nurse executive on the vendor side should make nursing leadership think long and hard about eliminating the vendor from the "short list." However, the absence of a nurse executive on the vendor side does not eliminate vendors from consideration "in the real world." It is during vendor presentations that nurse executives can ask probing questions, not only about system functionality and the direction of future development, but also about the degree of influence that each vendor's nurse executive brings to bear on the priorities that drive system development timelines. In addition, vendor presentations are an ideal time to inquire about how concerns voiced by the nurse executive will be escalated within the health care organization itself and to the vendors under consideration.

Many nurse executives' lack of a core competency in IT prevents them from appropriately evaluating the systems under consideration, leaving them to struggle for years with systems that meet the requirements of other special interests within the health care organization, but not their own. One example in nursing departments is that nursing executives lacking process knowledge of cross-state licensure issues will be hardpressed to determine an IT system's telehealth capabilities. As telehealth becomes ubiquitous, the very issues that need to be planned for could be undermined by an IT decision made years ago. Another example is that nurse executives generally possess a thorough working knowledge of the regulations and licensure issues that come into play during accreditation. However, IT executives/leaders generally do not. Nurse executives need to work with IT to share this knowledge early in the system selection process.

Nursing Must Embrace a Universal Approach to Nomenclature and Taxonomy

Taking a standard approach to how decisions are documented is crucial if the unique contribution nursing makes to patient care is quantified. Nurse executives should evangelize, champion, and advocate for a standardized approach to nomenclature and taxonomy – one for which all nurses are trained and tested. Using a standard set of descriptions adds structure to the process of documenting care and allows each chart entry to codify that care. Workflows and data dictionaries represent two additional areas where standards are imperative.

From an enterprise view, the myriad of hospital IT and clinical systems perfectly illustrate why nursing's leadership must demand standards. Given the high number of connection points and interdependencies that emerge as data flows through a typical hospital information system, standards provide the most effective and efficient way to assure the integrity of the all-important clinical data repository. Standards for documenting nursing care and data exchange help improve patient care as data points accumulated in the repository become information and trends emerge as knowledge.

Nurse Executives Should Recast Their Strategic Vision to View Information Technology as a Tool to Help Nursing Do its Job Better

This recognition of IT as an enabler will prompt nurse executives to spend more "up front" time planning how systems and technologies will work and interact with each other. Standardizing the processes and their documentation, supported by strategic thinking, will help ensure the quality of care. This uniformity not only shapes patients' expectations for care, but also minimizes the need to create manual "work arounds" that actually break processes.

Only Nursing Can Architect How the Comprehensive Process of Patient Care Should Flow

Nurse executives who oversee how care is delivered are uniquely qualified to analyze workflow and recommend efficiencies that streamline care. It is essential that this analysis examines care across the continuum of care – from its beginning in the patient's home to its end with self-care in the home. Only this beginning-to-end analysis can give the proper context and perspective to planning and managing care-related workflow.

For example, once the CNO delegates documentation of the process, it is likely that the nursing staff will describe the process based on their perspective of "today's" practice, not in alignment with the organization's strategic plan for the flow process for care across the continuum. These "silos" of nursing expertise mean that a staff nurse in Med/Surg is not likely to know the best process for homecare. However, discharging a patient from a Med/Surg area to home is a transition of care and handoff which is key to a successful outcome.

Nurse Executives' Understanding of IT Should Span from System Development Through to Maintenance and Migration, Ending at Obsolescence, Disposition, and Replacement

While IT vendors support and maintain systems for a usually undisclosed period of time, the health care organization is obligated to continue paying maintenance fees and keeping current on supported versions of applications, databases, and system administration tools to receive that support. Failure to stay current on supported system components (including but not limited to application software, operating system, database, and hardware) launches the health care organization into a "no man's land" where the facility is literally on its own for maintaining its systems. To avoid this scenario, most health care organizations implement upgrades in system components to "keep current."

Every IT system evolves along a predictable lifecycle – one that nursing leaders should understand and anticipate. When nursing understands how the lifecycle works, nurse executives can leverage that knowledge in the budgeting process and system upgrade and replacement plans, as well as in nursing practice. At some point, every piece of technology in use today will be obsolete. Being able to plan for that obsolescence puts nursing leadership in a position to drive change, not respond to it.

As Fig. 10.1 shows, the lifecycle of any technology begins with planning and ends with disposition. Because obsolete technologies are replaced, the lifecycle never ends when you consider the "replacement" phase. In addition to its lifecycle, each technology also falls

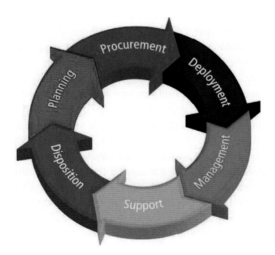

Fig. 10.1 Technology lifecycle

into a predictable "Adoption Lifecycle." It is critical that CNOs understand where their hospital and nursing organization fit in this cycle because the organization's adoption profile, consciously or unconsciously, influences technology evaluations.

Geoffrey Moore's legendary technology tome, *Crossing the Chasm,*[1] forever changed the way technology inventors, manufacturers, and distributors view their markets. Moore's seminal work, and his identification of five technology adopter groups, now guides many of the leading technology vendors in the world as they design, build, and bring to market different versions of their products, many of which are "tuned" to the needs of each group: Innovators, Early Adopters, Late Adopters, Late Majority, and Laggards.

As Moore suspected, each of the five types has its own profile, priorities, and perceptions that influence technology adoption and use. The first group, the smallest of the five, is the Innovators, who view being on the "leading edge" of technology as equivalent with power and status. These individuals pride themselves on being "the first on the block" to try new technologies and have a high tolerance for system glitches. Innovators were the first to rely on in-dash navigation in their cars and, when it failed to guide them to their chosen destination, could be found on the side of the road, laughing but happy to have been "assisted."

Early Adopters, the second and larger group, value new technologies as well, but they are more comfortable being a bit later in the adoption cycle – benefitting from the work Innovators did to remedy early system vulnerabilities. While they avoid 1.0 releases of products, they embrace later versions which they expect to be functional and reliable. Those in the Late Majority wait until all the kinks have been worked out. They want more than just functionality and reliability; they expect these proven technologies to be easy to use. These adopters, who prize for value for dollar spent, delight in paying half what the Early Adopters did for the same product.

Laggards, as Moore defined them, are just that. They want "tried and true," trusted technology products that operate reliably. They have no tolerance for downtime and are the group most likely to become vocal when the manufacturer stops supporting the release they own. They are upgrade-adverse. In addition to the individual adoption profiles Moore delineated, each health care organization has an "institutional adoption profile." Using the characteristics of the institutional profile, savvy nurse executives can identify the likely period of time within which senior management is comfortable – technically, operationally, and competitively – with its systems. In planning for IT obsolescence, nurse executives must take into account senior management's appetite for change.

As one can see, technology obsolescence is not as easy to define as it once was. For example, if a particular health care facility prides itself on being the first entity in town to have the latest gear in the surgical suite, that hospital probably sees "obsolescence" sooner than the hospital across town that rarely mentions it technology-enabled capabilities. Being able to anticipate senior management's arrival near the end of its comfort zone will enable nurse executives to research vendors and capabilities before that knowledge is needed. This proactive approach makes it more likely that nurse executives will be able to influence the all-important "short list" of vendors for consideration, rather than having to deal with vendors who were selected without nursing's input.

Technology systems' selection represents a key opportunity to up level nursing's productivity, efficiency, and job satisfaction – not a time to settle for being able "to live with" either system. CNOs need to know which system supports nursing practice best and why. System selection requires solid analytical assessment on the part of nursing leadership because this decision will affect the practice of nursing for many years to come.

Nurse Executives Need to Know How to Exploit the Power Inherent in Relational Databases

Advanced information systems revolve around an industry standard – a relational database. The power of relational databases comes from being able to precisely locate and report specific data. For example, when a user requests certain set of data, the relational database searches entire files, extracting only the requested data. That data can be sorted and displayed in virtually unlimited combinations of reports, greatly increasing the speed and efficiency of comparative analysis.

A special language called structured query language (SQL) allows relationship databases to operate in conjunction with each other. A standard relational database houses information in thousands of tables. Each table includes column-displayed data and the database's "relational" power allows it to create new tables based on user queries.

Nurse executives who want to avoid some of the cost of custom tailoring the reporting capabilities of their clinical systems would be wise to consult with their nurse informatician. That dual expert easily bridges the worlds of nursing and technology perfectly positioning her to be the resident "reporting" guru when it comes to tapping into the power of relational databases.

Nurse Executives Must Fully Understand and Appreciate the Differences Between Research Analysis and Operational Analysis

It is critical that nursing's leadership distinguishes between the purest forms of academic analysis that researchers perform to prove a theory. This analysis can be extrapolated to larger population. Operational analysis, on the other hand, examines the current and historical performance of an operational (or steady-state) investment, measuring that performance against an established set of cost, schedule, and performance parameters. By its very nature, operational analysis is less structured than performance reporting methods applied to developmental projects (such as Earned Value Analysis) and more creative. It prompts considerations of how the objectives could be better met, how costs could be saved, and whether, in fact, the organization should even be performing a particular function. An operational analysis should demonstrate that you have actually done a thorough examination of the need for the investment, the performance being achieved by the investment, the advisability of continuing the investment, and alternative methods of achieving the same investment results.

Extending beyond the baseline developmental performance measures of "Are we on schedule?" and "Are we within budget?," operational analysis answers more subjective questions in the specific areas of strategic and business results, financial performance, and innovation.

Engage in the Technology Acquisition and Utilization Process Early and Often to Balance the Organization's Business Drivers with Nursing's Priorities

Executive leadership's vision for the organization, along with the capabilities needed to drive the operation forward competitively, guides the technology acquisition and utilization process. Engaged nurse executives push to have nursing's vision incorporated into the organization's priority set – not just during technology acquisition periods, but throughout the use of that technology. Nursing's strategy should be to engage early and often in the technology acquisition process to ensure that nursing priorities are communicated to vendor providers of IT. Nurse executives need to tell vendors what they need and engage with executives of the IT vendors' user groups to learn more about the customer experience. Nursing needs a clear strategy for influencing the future development of the selected vendor's clinical systems.

Know How Organizational Changes, Yours and Theirs, Can Impact IT Systems

While some long-term IT changes can be expected based on the health care organization's institutional adoption profile, new organizational directions may be short-term shifts as well. For example, replacing a single corporate-level executive can bring a new perspective to IT scrutiny. Acquisitions of or mergers with another facility may or may not mean an IT change is coming. It usually depends on the organization's status in the transaction.

Finally, realize there can be organizational changes on the vendor's side that warrant an IT move by your health care organization. Consider the impact of a new chief executive officer or chief technology officer at your vendor of choice. That is one organizational change that can trigger an entirely new technology roadmap, which may not dovetail with the facility's vision and direction. If the IT vendor is acquired, one can expect to see support timeframes for legacy and "noncompliant systems" shorten – sometimes drastically. (Note: "Noncompliant systems" is vendor-speak for an acquired company's systems that do not support the acquiring company's technology roadmap.)

Fully Understand Total Cost of Ownership (TCO) to Project with Accuracy

When calculating the cost of technology acquisition for clinical deployment, nurse executives need to account for all the pricing elements that contribute to the total cost of ownership (TCO) of the IT being considered. While most nurse executives list annual license fees, consulting expenses to tailor the system, and initial training and annual maintenance costs, it is easy to overlook additional expenses which occur over time. These expenses include, but are not limited to, acquisition of additional hardware, deployment of upgrades, upgrade-specific training and retraining, and consulting time to migrate custom code. Other related expenses include the cost of attending annual user conferences and regional user group meetings. Attendance at those gatherings is crucial if you intend to influence the direction of future development of the system.

Once the total is calculated, the debate about which budget or, in some cases, budgets will be tapped for initial acquisition costs and subsequent, ongoing expenses. It is just as true in health care organizations as it is in the "real world" – she who has the gold rules. By contributing a greater proportion of the financing, nursing can claim and exert more influence over the IT system's use, future development, and even disposition.

Understand the Entrepreneurial Mindset

Nurse executives who understand the business of health care beyond the four walls of their facilities tend to better understand the impact of organizational changes on IT than those who have a nursing-specific view of the health care industry. For example, knowing the business drivers that influence how IT providers work will help savvy nurse executives prepare for the surprises that can come up during systems use.

The constant innovation needed to keep pace with changing regulatory mandates shortens system lifecycles, attracting entrepreneurial thinkers to the field of health care informatics and technologies. Constant changes in the regulatory requirements mean that application software must be updated on what seems to nursing like a continual basis. Frequent compliant-related changes, along with automating processes that are ill-defined and involve a multitude of user groups, also make the industry appealing to entrepreneurs.

Clearly, entrepreneurs' rewards come from commercializing their ideas for a profit. Indeed, without profitable commercialization, entrepreneurs would be out of business – literally. That understanding acknowledges the commercialization and profit that drive the entrepreneur's business model. CNOs must remember that entrepreneurs simply thrive on change; they welcome and embrace it – even when that change impacts *your* particular health care systems team. They do not see turnover on the vendor side as significant, but account team turnover almost always means nursing has to restart the knowledge ramp-up for the new team.

In addition to that challenge, health care systems vendors crave business process pre-dictability. The simpler and less complex the task, the easier it is to automate it. For that reason alone, nurse executives need to be alert to the fact that engineers by design want to quantify nursing into a rote role with workflow they think is efficient because that scenario is easier for the engineer to program. Nursing's critical thinking expands decision-tree options, making programming difficult and interconnectivity with other hospital systems complex. Only nursing can provide the critical thinking that forms the basis for quality patient care, and it is up to nurse executives to advocate for more enabling technologies to support critical thinking, not fewer technologies.

Nursing's role as a cocreator of clinical systems routinely generates valuable intellectual property (IP) in the form of workflows, nomenclature, taxonomies, and data dictionaries. Not being entrepreneurs themselves, most nurse executives do not realize the market value of system capabilities they codevelop, and more importantly, they do not negotiate for rights and royalties to that IP. If the contract between the health care organization and the technology vendor does not state that the health care organization retains control over nursing-created IP, the technology vendor is entitled to assume worldwide rights for that IP. Nursing would be wise to consult with the health care organization's legal team about the organization's IP policy early in the system evaluation phase of technology selection.

If the health care organization has an IP policy, nursing needs to ask, "Is this policy realistic in its adherence, implementation and enforcement?" Whenever IP comes into play, nurse executives would be wise to prepare themselves for a spirited negotiation where both sides have to give a little and sometimes a lot. One might be negotiating for naught if the health care industry shows limited demand for a particular product. In an attempt to predict market demand, a leader will need to conduct an objective market analysis. The results of that analysis will determine the uniqueness of the IP, a characteristic which drives its value.

The value of applied and IP rights is related to the cost associated with that IP. To commercialize IP, the market requires an infrastructure that hospitals do not have. That infrastructure includes creating and updating technical documentation, producing user guides, offering technical and user support, and delivering a full range of code stabilization and migration services. Once a leader has determined the market demand for the IP, estimated the cost associated with delivering it to the marketplace, and projected the expense of supporting that IP over time, a decision will need to be made about whether or not revenue potential warrants such an investment – both from the health care organization's perspective and the vendor viewpoint.

Once the issue of IP rights has been settled, nursing leaders need to read the vendor contract from start to finish. Even though few nursing leaders actually do this, there are valuable insights to be gained. Understanding how one's organization approaches system selection and finalizes its contractual relationship with a strategic business partner such as a technology vendor often gives nurse executives real insight into where the organization is headed and why. Many times, directional information is not discussed – at least openly – but by reading the contract in detail, you can often draw conclusions that would otherwise be veiled.

Finally, no discussion of nursing and technology would be complete without speaking about the Nursing Executive Dashboard (NID). Typically created by the nurse informatician for the CNO, the NID visually communicates the status of key performance indicators (KPIs) related to technology initiatives – from deployment to replacement. CNOs use dashboard information to bridge the gap between nursing, IT, and the organization's all-important corporate suite. Dashboard data helps the CNO demonstrate the impact and value of technology, from an individual initiative perspective as well as a collective overview standpoint.

In other operational areas, such as finance, physician utilization, patient relations, and product line management, dashboards have been used for years. Dashboards are visually oriented reporting tools that flag issues and concerns in time for intervention, pinpoint cross-disciplinary interdependencies, and identify trends that would otherwise go unnoticed. Dashboards, which can be created to monitor almost any KPI, deliver the business intelligence needed to streamline processes and boost profitability.

The disparate systems used in hospitals and health care organizations have hampered the use of dashboards until recently. Advanced technology, such as data extraction tools, middleware, and sophisticated reporting capabilities, is now in place to fuel the data needs of executive dashboards. It is high time that a nursing dashboard delivers to the CNOs' desktop the business intelligence needed to leverage technology, streamline processes and efficiencies, and improve patient care.

Finally, nurse leaders who understand and appreciate the application of technology to the profession undoubtedly value the role of public policy in supporting, funding, and advancing health care in the United States. Making nursing's platform heard on local, regional, and national levels requires the voices of all of us – not just a few selected "spokespeople."

It is simply not enough to speak to each other via professional organizations and affiliate groups. We must make our opinions known to those in our government who control the agenda and the money. Nursing can no longer afford to depend on the "good will" of lobbyists, candidates, and those in office.

Further, nurses cannot and should not expect government officials to know what the nursing profession needs. By tabling our self-interests, the profession can unite to educate, inform, and persuade office holders to become champions for our profession and the value nurses bring to patients.

> I know of no safe repository of the ultimate power of society but people. And if we think them not enlightened enough, the remedy is not to take the power from them, but to inform them by education (Thomas Jefferson).

Reference

1. Moore GA. *Crossing the Chasm*. New York: HarperCollins; 1991.

Bridging Technology: Academe and Industry

11

Pamela R. Jeffries, Krysia Hudson, Laura A. Taylor, and Steven A. Klapper

There is an identified gap between the academic preparation of nursing students and the needs/expectations of clinical agencies who hire them after graduation (Nursing Executive Center of the Advisory Board Company, 2008). Based on the results of a survey of nursing school academic leaders and frontline hospital leaders (nurse managers, directors, educators, and charge nurses), the report identifies a "preparation-practice gap" that reflects the concerns of hospital leaders about the "practice readiness" of new nursing graduates in six general areas: clinical knowledge, technical skills, critical thinking, communication, professionalism, and management of responsibilities. Only 10.4% of the 135 *nurse executives* who responded to this survey agreed that new graduates are fully prepared in these areas, while 89.9% of 362 *nursing school leaders* agreed.

Many of these outlined competencies are directly related to the ways in which nursing students gain clinical experiences during their academic program while performing technical skills, managing patients, communicating, and exercising critical thinking. The use of simulation technology with the incorporation of informatics could be one of the enabling vehicles to achieve these competencies that need to be strengthened in nursing education today. This chapter discusses the use of nursing informatics and the role of simulation in nursing education and practice. Since the American Association of College of Nurses (AACN) mandated the incorporation of informatics, simulation, and other types of required curricula essentials to help bridge the preparation–practice gap of BSN nursing graduates, nursing informatics and the use of simulation technology are driving curriculum reform and faculty development programs at different levels of academic preparation. This chapter describes examples in nursing education where nursing informatics has been blended into simulation environments and explores the implications for educators as nursing curricula are redesigned and transformed.

P.R. Jeffries (✉)
Johns Hopkins University School of Nursing, 525 North Wolfe Street, Baltimore, MD 21205, USA
e-mail: pjeffri2@son.jhmi.edu

M.J. Ball et al. (eds.), *Nursing Informatics*,
DOI: 10.1007/978-1-84996-278-0_11, © Springer-Verlag London Limited 2011

Simulations

Simulations are defined as events or situations made to resemble clinical practice as closely as possible.[1] Various types of simulations are being incorporated into the teaching–learning environment today. As educators incorporate simulations into their courses and nursing curricula, major advantages as well as challenges have been noted with these innovative pedagogies as shown in Table 11.1.

Simulations can offer nurse educators and health care providers a significant educational strategy to meet the needs of today's learners by providing interactive, practice-based instructional strategies. Implementing and testing the use of simulations have the potential to enhance the following:

- Active student involvement in the learning process. By interacting with the simulations, examples, and exercises, learners are required to use higher order thinking rather than simply mimic the teacher role model. Decision-making and critical-thinking skills are required by this teaching modality.
- More effective utilization of faculty in the teaching of clinical skills and interventions.
- More flexibility for students to practice based upon their schedules. Learners can access the simulation at their convenience and not be required to practice the skills in front of an instructor, although that option would remain available for those who needed the extra instruction or reinforcement. Learners can revisit this skill multiple times in a safe, nonthreatening environment that is conducive to learning.
- Improved student instruction; more consistent teaching of overall clinical and didactic instruction; increased learner satisfaction in the classroom and clinical setting; safer, nonthreatening practice of skills and decision making; and state-of-the-art learning environment.

Table 11.1 Advantages and challenges of incorporating simulations in curricula

Advantages	Challenges
No patient risk	Teacher-centered to student-centered pedagogical shift
Manipulated clinical situations	
Planned learning time	Performance anxieties
Controlled learning environment	Increased faculty preparation time
Harm-proof mistakes	
Enhanced psychomotor skills	Expense (resources, equipment, and assistance)
Multirole simulations	
Active student learning	Needed physical space
Immediate feedback	Nonreplicated events
	Resources
	Technical support/computer literacy required
	Few participants per simulation

- Competency check for undergraduates, new graduates, or new orientees during orientation. The simulation experience provides a competency check of the participants' knowledge, skills, and problem-solving abilities in a nonthreatening, safe environment.
- Creation of new interactive educational model for nursing education, promoting a higher order of skills set by the learner.

Figure 11.1 shows that one approach to designing simulations is to use the simulation framework[2] developed from the theoretical and empirical literature related to learning outcomes in higher education.[3,4] A framework ensures that faculty design quality simulations and implement appropriate, theoretically-based innovations in order to obtain the best outcomes expected of learners. A review of the nursing and other health care literature, including medicine and anesthesiology, as well as related literature from nonhealth care disciplines guided the development of this framework.

As shown in Fig. 11.1, the framework has five major components with their associated variables: students, teachers, educational practices in simulation, the simulation, and outcomes. All variables may not be relevant to all studies; however, the framework is intended to provide a context for relating a variety of likely variables. The first two components of the model are *teacher factors* and *student factors*. Successful learning from the use of simulations requires proper simulation design and appropriate organization of the students in the simulation with the teacher serving as a facilitator of learning

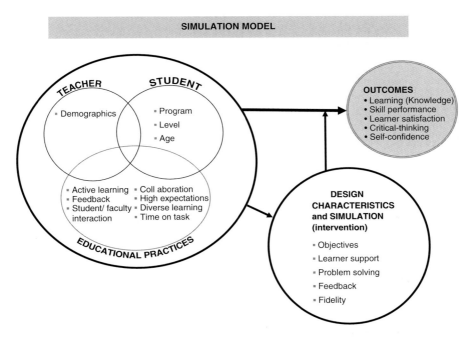

Fig. 11.1 Simulation framework.[15]National League for Nursing, *Nurs Educ Persp.* 26(2):28–35. With permission

as depicted by the theoretical model. The *educational practices in simulation* are incorporated in the design and implementation of the simulation to promote better student performance and satisfaction as evidenced in the educational literature.[4] A fourth component of the model, which serves as the intervention in teaching–learning practices, is the *simulation*. The type of simulation designed determines the *outcomes* that should be achieved by the learners. These outcomes are proposed to be influenced by the degree to which the educational practices in simulation are incorporated in the design and implementation of these simulations. Effective teaching and learning using simulations are dependent on teacher and student interactions, expectations, and roles of each during these experiences.

Simulations can serve as an important vehicle to incorporate health care informatics, particularly when the simulation encounter includes the use of a clinical information system (CIS) in the patient's room. This allows the nurse to retrieve important data to realistically inform decision-making and problem-solving in the simulated environment and activity reflecting real-life practice. Incorporating informatics into a simulation before students are required to perform the same activities and nursing assessments and interventions on real patients assists in potentially bridging the preparation–practice gap that exists today.

Healthcare Informatics

Incorporating healthcare informatics in the teaching–learning activities of clinical simulations can serve as one model of care to bridge the practice gap and to promote patient safety. Healthcare informatics is foundational to the provision of safe, quality care, performance management, and quality improvement.[5] Healthcare informatics is the intersection of information science, computer science, and health care. It integrates the resources, devices, and methods required to optimize the acquisition, storage, retrieval, and use of information in health care and biomedicine. Healthcare informatics is central to information synthesis (Williamson and Weir, 2009).

Healthcare informatics tools include not only computers, but also clinical guidelines, formal medical terminologies, and information and communication systems. Graves and Corcoran[6] provided the infamous early definition of nursing informatics: "Nursing informatics is a combination of computer science, information science and nursing science designed to assist in the management and processing of nursing data, information and knowledge to support the practice of nursing and the delivery of nursing care." Medical informatics, social work informatics, and a variety of health care disciplines have informatics woven into their care delivery methodologies.

Healthcare informatics education is designed to provide knowledge and skills in the application of information technology in the provision of health care. New care practitioners must gain knowledge and skills that will prove useful when embarking on new careers. Healthcare informatics focuses on the use of automation to improve health care. To meet the strong demand for professionals with advanced training in healthcare information systems,

New graduates to any healthcare profession need a skill set adaptable to computer technologies and EHRs to support work processes and information access experienced in the course of daily work flow. Employees at all levels and job types within today's healthcare workplace need a new set of skills and knowledge to embrace and effectively utilize computer technologies and electronic information (p. 5).[7]

Healthcare informatics focuses on the use of automation to improve health care. To meet the strong demand for professionals with advanced training in healthcare information systems, the education and competencies of faculty and graduates must be identified, structured, and guided. A variety of professional organizations are dedicated to the development of health care professionals and to "promoting the effective organization, analysis, management, and use of information in health care in support of patient care, public health, teaching, research, administration, and related policy" (www.amia.org). In 2008, The American Medical Informatics Association (AMIA) and the American Health Information Management Associations (AHIMA) formed a joint initiative to address the urgent need to support interventions necessary to guide and implement educational programs and support "investments in education and training for health informatics and health information management."[7]

Successful incorporation of healthcare informatics requires the transformation of educational directives of the multiprofessional facet of health care including clinicians, medical education, nursing education, and resident training. All new frontline providers must be directed to measure outcomes, strive for innovative improvement strategies, and apply evidence into practice (Conway and Clancy[8]; AMIA www.amia.org; AHIMA www.ahima.org). Currently, the Office for National Coordination of Healthcare Information Technology (ONCHIT) supports the implementation of informatics-focused educational programs, primarily in medical schools, to assist with training and adoption and interoperability of such functionality.[5] This is true internationally as well. AMIA and the International Medical Informatics Association (IMIA) have agreed upon five informatics competencies that drive informatics educational curricula (www.amia.org):

- Health information literacy skills
- Privacy and confidentiality of health information
- Health information/data technical security
- Basic computer literacy skills
- Health informatics skills using the electronic health record (EHR)

Technology Informatics Guiding Education Reform (TIGER)[9] is a 2005 informatics initiative whose primary purpose is the expansive health information technology (HIT) exposure among the largest group of health care providers – nursing. The TIGER initiative works to help the United States realize its 10-year goal of EHRs for all its citizens. The initiative involves over 70 professional nursing organizations, vendors, and governmental entities with the aim to enable practicing nurses and nursing students to fully engage in the unfolding digital electronic era in health care. The initiative's goal is to identify information/knowledge management best practices and effective technology capabilities for nurses. Through its Web site at www.TIGER.org, TIGER creates and disseminates local and global action plans that can be duplicated within nursing and other multidisciplinary health care training and workplace settings. Nurses have been involved in all levels of EHR standards development, testing, and integration, in addition to responsibilities that span all aspects of care delivery. Nursing professionals share a unified voice through the Alliance for Nursing Informatics (ANI), a collaboration of organizations, which plays a pivotal role of nursing in health care. As a result, ANI nurse leaders were appointed to the National eHealth Collaborative board and committees. Nurses also serve on the National Health Information Network Governance Work Group.

Informatics and Simulation in Nursing Education

In the current health care climate, preparing the future nurse provider to be adequately prepared to successfully navigate the technology-driven health care arena is paramount. Safety, quality, and information management are all "moving" targets. Patients are sicker, disease presentation and management are complex, and reimbursement is challenging. In collaboration with Department of Health and Human Services, ONCHIT has declared that the education of the frontline care provider must include substantial preparation for the development, utilization, management, and leadership of health information technologies in practice.

Computing has been used in health care for decades. As computing evolved, the use of computing in the health care arena exploded to include not only sophisticated assessment documentation systems and electronic health and medical records, but also the full incorporation of mobile devices and telemedicine. Nursing has adapted informatics to increase the safety of patients and the education of the frontline workforce in the elements of safety protocols via HIT; this requires teaching strategies and models that incorporate the newest technologies. The National League of Nursing (NLN) has called for innovation in nursing education.[10] More recently, a survey conducted by the NLNs Informatics Competencies Task Group of the Educational Technology and Information Management Advisory Council found only 50–60% of responding schools had informatics integrated into their curriculum and student experiences with information systems were only during "clinical experiences."[11]

Basic competencies were identified in a landmark study by Staggers et al.[12,13] One would argue that these competencies (such as computer competencies and information competencies) change as the technology and health care change. How can educators keep pace with the growth of technology? It is not certain that any educating body can manage to keep pace with the increasing rate of change of technology; however, for the safety of the patients, the management of information technology is a critical skill and behavior needed of today's nursing graduates. Principally, student experiences with information systems should be prior to clinical practice; one approach, therefore, is to integrate clinical simulations with health information systems to prepare students for the practice.

Nursing can look to the airline industry as an example to prepare safe practitioners for the complex health care environments integrated with healthcare information systems. Simulators have long been used for pilots in training to learn the environment, to prepare for flight conditions, to manage the flow, and assimilation of information within the cockpit and to and from the tower in order to safely pilot a plane. Nursing can also simulate aspects of the nursing care environment and the integrated health care systems via the use of clinical simulations integrated with informatics to assess, diagnosis, implement, and evaluate patient care and outcomes.

Integrating Informatics and Simulation in a BSN Nursing Program

The health care environment is changing at unprecedented rates, and concomitant changes in educational delivery are required. This chapter describes one approach to integrating healthcare information/informatics and the use of simulations in a BSN nursing program. The BSN nursing curriculum described uses the program's technology point-of-care delivery curriculum implementation and rollout in the preparation of nurses into the informatics-laced world of health care. In June 2006, faculty from a large baccalaureate program restructured the clinical and theoretical curriculum to incorporate full point-of-care technology, specifically Eclipsys SCM 4.5 and their Knowledge-Based Charting (KBC) module to support nursing documentation in a standardized EHR. The KBC module is a result of a strategic partnership between Eclipsys and the Clinical Practice Model Resource Center (CPMRC). CPMRC is the source of the evidence-based content, including evidence-based Clinical Practice Guidelines that is intentionally designed within the Eclipsys SCM software.[14] This met an important goal of integrating evidence and informatics into the JHUSON curriculum. Since the initial inception, seven clinical and/or laboratory courses across the undergraduate baccalaureate curriculum are actively engaged in point-of-care technology. Over 400 students and 70 faculty have been oriented to and actively coached and trained on Eclipsys and KBC, a curriculum tool that creates a collaborating learning community and strengthens the theory–research–practice triangle.

Assessment

Until recently, students learned assessment skills through faculty demonstration followed by practicing techniques on classmates and laboratory partners. Although the techniques of nursing assessment, for example auscultation, can be perfected through the use of practice with other students, assessment findings are those of the clients. Patients, unlike nursing students, have abnormal assessment data or symptoms. The use of simulators, like Laerdal SimMan™, allows students to observe abnormal assessment data within the environment of a controlled laboratory setting while gaining confidence in the assessment of these findings. High-fidelity simulators offer the faculty interactive ability to create adventitious lung sounds, heart sounds, elevated heart and respiratory rates, and a variety of physical findings indicating a more complex patient scenario. Wheezes, rales, and rhonchi can all be auscultated on the medium- or high-fidelity simulators. Instructors can incorporate low-fidelity interactions, such as faculty-developed patient–student scenarios, and progress to higher fidelity interactions where the student must recognize presenting symptoms before the manikin's condition worsens. Allowing the student to make "hands-on" mistakes and learn from their choices and decision making in this environment impacts clinical decision making and provider confidence during clinical *learning experiences* with real patients. Literature indicates that simulation allows for positive skill and knowledge acquisition.[15,16]

Table 11.2 Comparison of point of care and mobile decision support systems

	Point of care	Mobile (PDA)
Updates	Centrally	Via user
Licensing	Centrally	Via user
Completeness	Unabridged	Abridged
Access	Limited	Unlimited
Challenges		Convenient, small screen making the data difficult to analyze at times

Other than high-fidelity simulations, other applications can be considered simulation as well. The use of decision support systems (DSS) is a key component in patient safety. Prior to the age of computing, the Physician Desk Reference (PDR) and other written guides were DSS available in the clinical environment. Other guides that existed included the policy and procedure manual, and the pathophysiology and clinical laboratory texts. Thanks to the Institute of Medicine initiatives (2004), health care has increased the availability of DSS in the clinical environment. Systems such as Micromedex™, Lexicomp™, Up to Date™, and First Consult™ are generally available in the clinical arena. The introduction to these DSS is crucial early in the nursing education to promote the development of assessment and critical-thinking skills of the student. For instance, in First Consult, a student can evaluate a headache in several different age populations. Understanding the context, e.g., age of the client and the clinical symptom, is critical in effective treatment. For example, in First Consult, in the young adult, a headache may indicate a tension headache; whereas in an elderly population, this diagnosis may indicate malignant hypertension.

There are challenges when nurse educators introduce DSS in a clinical or classroom setting. For instance, introducing a DSS in a classroom is important. However, students need practice in using DSS prior to using these aides in a clinical setting. Nevertheless, it is well known that having DSS at the point of care is essential to the decision maker so that quicker, more efficient assessments can be conducted. Students must have access to point-of-care computers and mobile devices if educators are preparing students for "real world practice." Table 11.2 shows a comparison of point-of-care and mobile DSS.

Diagnosis

Historically, nursing has struggled to quantify the care given. Using languages has allowed nursing to quantify the quality of care given, although recent criticism includes the lack of a consistent nursing classification system. Recent efforts have attempted to unite classification systems so that all professions could use the same taxonomy. With that being said, the use of a nursing classification in nursing education is paramount. A consistent nursing classification helps students to frame and examine the patient with predetermined interventions linked to the diagnosis. Several attempts have been made to automate a

Table 11.3 American Nursing Association's recognized languages

Language	Website
NANDA	www.nanda.org
Nursing Intervention Classification	http://www.nursing.uiowa.edu/cnc/
Home Health Care Classification (HHCC)	http://www.sabacare.com/
Omaha System	http://www.con.ufl.edu/omaha
Nursing Outcomes Classification	http://www.nursing.uiowa.edu/cnc/
Nursing Management Minimum Data Set (NMMDS)	
Patient Care Data Set (PCDS)	
Perioperative Nursing Dataset	http://www.aorn.org/
Systematized Nomenclature of Medicine (clinical terms) SNOMED CT	http://www.ihtsdo.org/snomed-ct/
International Classification for Nursing Practice (ICNP®)	
ABC codes developed by ABC coding Solutions	http://www.nursingworld.org/MainMenuCategories/ThePracticeofProfessionalNursing/NursingStandards/DocInfo/NIDSEC/www.ABCcodes.com

Source: http://www.nursingworld.org/MainMenuCategories/ThePracticeofProfessionalNursing/NursingStandards/DocInfo/NIDSEC/RecognizedLanguagesforursing.aspx

nursing classification system such as the Virginia Saba's Clinical Care Classification System (http://www.sabacare.com/).

The use of taxonomies in nursing education has been hampered due to the sheer number of ANA-recognized nursing languages, as shown in Table 11.3. Adoption of one standardized language is a current goal. Currently, the International Classification for Nursing Practice (ICNP) and Systematized Nomenclature of Medicine – clinical terms (SNOMED) are the most widely used languages. It is also widely believed that ICNP encompasses all nursing specialties and may be the best foundation of a basic nursing language.[17]

Implementation

Implementing clinical interventions in a simulated environment using scenario-based simulations integrated with CISs can be a challenge. Educators are challenged to ensure that students meet clinical hour requirements while offering valid clinical experiences and real-world experiences. Students can participate in a simulated clinical environment in a variety of ways. Second Life and Micro Sim™ offer two examples of approaches that blend simulations with informatics and other technologies.

Second Life

Second Life is a virtual environment where students are able to participate in a clinical learning experience. Several virtual learning environments have been created in Second Life. One such simulation, shown in the YouTube video at http://www.youtube.com/watch?v=oLhuBNkYOsU, has the student participants to enter the Island of Evergreen (owned by the State of Washington). In this Second Life site, a student would select an avatar (a computer-generated student-chosen facsimile of the student) who would be required to work in an Emergency Department. Within the simulation, the avatar actually interacts with a patient. For faculty, Second Life can simulate the clinical environment without necessitating real estate (building space)! As with any virtual environment, orientation to the virtual world is necessary for both educators and learners. The convenience of having a virtual orientation is astounding. Conversely, this requires that students have the computing power to participate at home in this environment and the faculty to have the technical skills and support to build a realistic environment.

Micro Sim™

Laerdal Medical, Inc. also has created a virtual environment in which students can practice with specific patient cases that they may face in the clinical environment. Patient scenarios can be planned to correspond with the units where the students will practice. In this virtual environment, students can also be graded using the Micro Sim cases. The students may practice prior to grading of the cases provided.

Evaluation

Both examples of simulation software (Second Life and Micro Sim™) allow students to practice implementation of their learned skills prior to practicing in a live environment. Software utilization requires constant evaluation to ensure students are achieving the clinical, information management, and knowledge skill sets required for clinical practice today. Table 11.4 describes the advantages and disadvantages of evaluating student's clinical skills and knowledge in online vs. traditional platform.

Table 11.4 Advantages and disadvantages of online vs. traditional methods to evaluate students' clinical skills and knowledge

Advantages	Disadvantages
Quick feedback	Usually limited to objective questions
Self-assessments	Security
Convenience	Difficult to authenticate students' work
Computer-marking (e.g., grading) time savings	Usually knowledge-based and superficial

Source: McKimm et al[20]

Simulations allow for quick evaluation of skills in the laboratory. For example, setting SimMan with vital signs and specific lung sounds – such as those performed in health assessment – allows faculty to quickly reinforce positive outcomes with students and/or redirect to additional opportunities for further practice.

Integration of technologies into curricula provides multiple opportunities for active learning and mastering of informatics skills required of new nursing graduates as well as faculty. Students can establish a portfolio of EHR documentation reflecting their progressive learning and offer it as evidence of their informatics knowledge and skills with future employers. An example of incorporating an EHR in a BSN nursing curriculum includes an approach used by educators at Johns Hopkins University School of Nursing when Eclypsis™ was built into the students' clinical laboratory experiences. A core group of faculty comprises the "Eclipsys team"; their involvement was paramount to the success of technology–curriculum integration. The team supports faculty to become newly enabled by technology through the open exchange of insights, ideas, and frustrations regarding EHR and HPS. Team actions include:

- Promoting faculty "buy in" through assisting with "brain storming" regarding how to incorporate the technology into course content.
- Providing "dry runs" of technology experiences before going live with clinical courses.
- Communicating through frequent emails and meetings with faculty to determine how the project is proceeding.
- Creating well-crafted instructional aides for faculty and students (such as "How To" instructional aides designed for each course, CD ROMs, online videos, and PowerPoint presentations with streaming audio).
- Supporting faculty and students when problems occur.

These actions were crucial in fashioning an integrated technology community within the school, advancing the curriculum to provide informatics competency, and providing numerous opportunities for students to develop critical-thinking, problem-solving and team-building skills.

Incorporating a Clinical Information System (CIS) into Simulations

As health care evolves to include the EHR into all aspects of patient care, student training of EHR use should also follow. The EHR is the ultimate embodiment of defined nursing outcomes. For instance, if a nurse performs wound care but does not document his or her actions, then he or she has no data to support the actions taken. Moreover, the EHR can help to track and trend positive and negative outcomes associated with assessments, diagnoses, and interventions. The documentation in the EHR is one product that nurses create each day.

Simply put, the EHR is a shared system. The ability for nurses to produce information that is succinct and integrated into other aspects of the EHR can transform the manner in which the health care team communicates and operates within any given institution. It is within these confines that Johns Hopkins University School of Nursing (JHUSON) has implemented its own EHR system for student use.

Case Study: Johns Hopkins University School of Nursing and Eclipsys Corporation

In early 2005, JHUSON and Eclipsys Corporation entered into a partnership. Eclipsys donated its flagship EHR product, Sunrise Clinical Manager (SCM), to the JHUSON for the school to introduce SCM as an instructional tool into its curricula. Eclipsys provided servers to run the system, as well as workstations, laptops, tablets, and personal digital assistants (PDAs) for students to access the system. The partnership between Eclipsys and the JHUSON agreed that Eclipsys would donate computer equipment, software, CPMRC content, consultant time, and training in exchange for the JHUSON implementation of SCM into its curriculum, the disclosure to Eclipsys of methods used by the school, shared customized objects such as flowsheets and structured notes, and feedback regarding system improvements pertaining to both education and health care.

Eclipsys trained a core group of faculty members and IT staff, the project leader, an informaticist, a faculty advocate, and an information technology specialist. This team was trained in all basic operations of the Eclipsys system including how to configure data dictionaries and system settings, create flowsheets and structured notes, and maintain the backend databases and system software. It was essential to gain expertise in the system since the JHUSON would maintain and continue to build the SCM system within the university environment. In addition, CPMRC provided overviews and guidance on how KBC was designed and the implication of using the evidence-based content and Clinical Practice Guidelines as a way for faculty and students to develop an individualized plan of care and associated clinical documentation.

Successful implementation of any EHR system is dependent on many factors. First, end user involvement in the implementation is vital to its success. In the JHUSON, the role of the faculty advocate was crucial to the success. This faculty member represented the concerns of the faculty while helping faculty overcome the uncertainties of using a new system. Second, SCM demonstrations were greatly needed for a successful implementation. Prior to each new pilot, Eclipsys' end-user training sessions and demonstrations were held. In a study by Beiter et al.,[18] demonstrations of the EHR improved attitudes, knowledge, and needs of the patients, physicians, and staff. Third, user attitudes toward an EHR system can contribute to its success or failure.[19]

The initial goals of this system were clear. The first goal was to provide an environment where students could practice using an EHR without the risk of adversely affecting live patient data. Significantly, there was faculty concern that JHUSON was teaching the use of an EHR system (SCM) that was present in many hospitals – including The Johns Hopkins Hospital – but not necessarily all hospitals where students may be employed, and the JHUSON version of the Eclipsys system was not yet present in the hospital's clinical units, which were at that time using an older version of SCM. Second, the Eclipsys team wanted to provide a good professional practice framework for students to learn how to document correctly via KBC. The team planned to choose a first semester nursing class to pilot and implement and slowly thread the EHR system through the Baccalaureate Curriculum.

Semester One: Principles and Applications of Nursing

The first class chosen to pilot the EHR was a nursing skills class (Principles and Applications of Nursing course). In this first semester class, nursing students are taught how to perfect basic nursing skills – such as intramuscular injections, IV insertion, and wound care. This class was chosen because the faculty advocate was also the course coordinator for this class. Since this class was taught in units, it was decided that for each unit or "module," a flowsheet would be created in SCM as shown in Fig. 11.2.

a

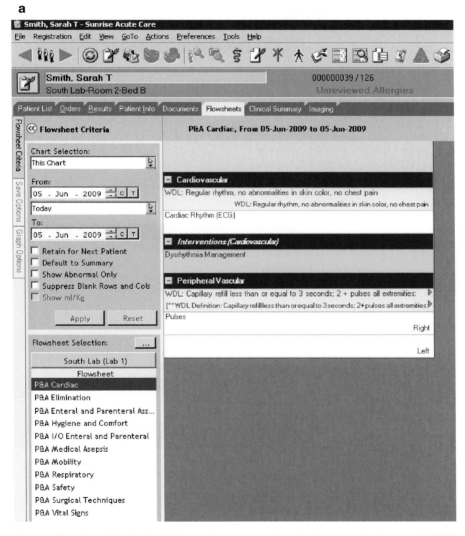

Fig. 11.2 Flowsheets for the beginning nursing course where the electronic health record (EHR) was incorporated. © Eclipsys Corporation. All rights reserved 2001–2009. Eclipsys product screen shot(s) reprinted with permission from Eclipsys Corporation

b

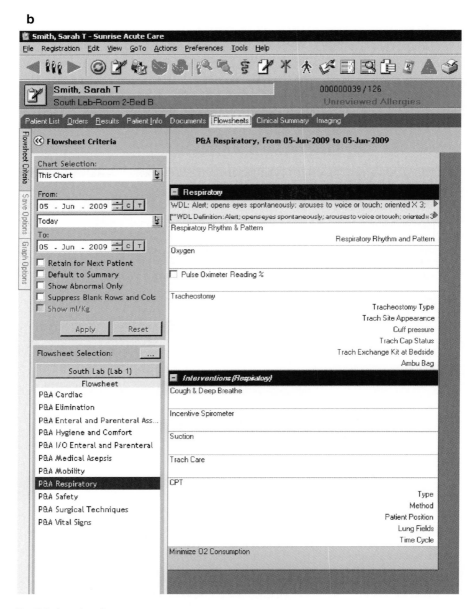

Fig. 11.2 (continued)

Each flowsheet was designed to cover "core content" that was specifically covered in that area. For instance, in the Vital Signs flowsheet, normal vital signs are covered (blood pressure, heart rate, respiratory rate, and temperature); however, not all activities or "documentable" items in the unit were covered in the flowsheet. The course coordinator decided which primary nursing skills student nurses must know how to document.

The flowsheets were designed to be small and succinct. Instructors who participated in the course needed to know fundamentals of the system. Radio buttons (Fig. 11.3), called single-select lists, indicate only one choice can be made. For example, only one type of heart rate assessment may be documented here. Check boxes (Fig. 11.4), called multi-select lists, indicate that more than one selection can be made. For instance, skin color can be mottled and red. In addition to these forms of input, the instructors needed to learn how to use a suggested text box. The suggested text box is a location to chart anything not found on the list provided (see Figs. 11.4 and 11.5). The suggested text box – or free text box – is the empty box at the bottom of Figs. 11.4 and 11.5. Spelling and correct medical terminology are paramount in this area.

Whenever possible, instructors encouraged students to select items within the list in flowsheets, instead of using the free text box. Students, as new data gatherers, were taught that using the listed items is a positive skill. Listed items are easily quantifiable – and this can only serve to help our nurse researchers to better evaluate nursing care in the future.

The first flowsheet tested in the introductory nursing course was the Surgical Techniques flowsheet. Essentially, student nurses had to evaluate wound care and the appearance of the wound provided in the nursing lab (see Fig. 11.5).

A pilot test of the initial use of the EHR was done by all involved. The results revealed three major findings. First, instructors were uneasy with a new form of documentation and consequently felt better if they had other EHR "skilled" instructors to assist. "How to" handouts were left beside the computers as guides to help answer instructors' common questions. As their confidence increased, instructors began offering case scenarios to accompany the unit on wound care. For instance, an instructor said to a student, "Please chart NORMAL findings." The second finding in the pilot revealed that when the students were presented with a long list of evidence-based options, instructors needed to discuss the possibilities of each listed item. The nursing lab was now bringing the lecture to life. A third major finding was noted by the instructors. A few students attempted to chart without

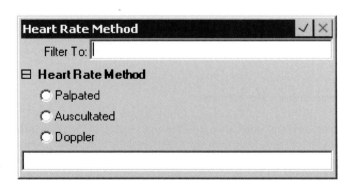

Fig. 11.3 Examples of radio buttons where the student can select only "one" choice. © Eclipsys Corporation. All rights reserved 2001–2009

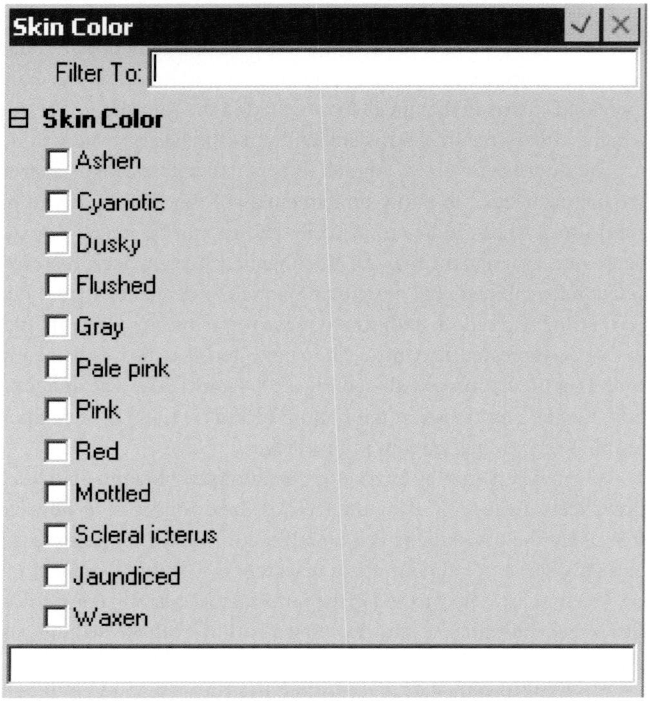

Fig. 11.4 Example of a multi-select list where more than one choice can be selected to provide information about the client. © Eclipsys Corporation. All rights reserved 2001–2009

washing their hands after a procedure; the students were readily corrected and instructed on the role computers play in medical asepsis.

In addition, the physical layout of the practice lab environment in relation to the Eclipsys SCM EHR system was significant. JHUSON has three nursing practice labs with 14 beds in each. SCM was configured to match the physical lab. It contained three Locations, one for each of the three practice labs. Each Location, or Unit, in SCM contained 14 beds, each populated by a patient configured by the Eclipsys Team. Computer workstations in the labs were wall-mounted on Ergotron® computer arms. These arms allowed the computers to be easily adjusted for each student, as well as to be folded away when not in use. This was extremely important as the practice labs can be very busy when class is in session. A bulky computer could easily become an obstruction and affect the class flow. In most cases, two beds shared one computer, which was mounted between them (see Fig. 11.6).

Semester One: Health Assessment

Another course offered in semester one which uses the EHR is Health Assessment. In this course, students learn to assess health findings in patients. Unlike the introductory nursing courses, the course coordinator chose to use one flowsheet – a comprehensive assessment flowsheet (see Fig. 11.7). The rationale was simple – one assessment sheet is optimal in clinical care and that is what students would see in clinical rotations.

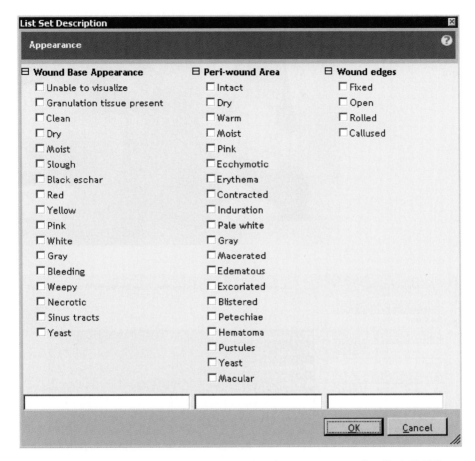

Fig. 11.5 Example of content in the EHR where wound appearance was described. © Eclipsys Corporation. All rights reserved 2001–2009

The instructors in this course were also required to understand fundamentals of documentation (single-select lists, multiselect lists, and free text boxes). However, in this class, the assessment sheet used "Charting by Parameters" or within defined limits (WDL) (see Fig. 11.8).

The students and instructors needed to recognize that the actual patient findings should be compared to identified parameters for each functional health pattern based on the evidence/consensual validation of the standard assessment parameters appropriate for that functional health pattern or system assessment. These parameters could not be the normal values of the patient individually. For instance, if a patient "normally" has an O_2 saturation of 88 – this is NOT an absolute normal finding. Hence, the patient would be considered outside the defined parameters.

In addition, the EHR system needed to be adapted to the course. Since students were expected to chart on their expected findings each week, instructors needed to track these findings as well. Hence, the Eclipsys Team devised a plan to track students. Each student

Fig. 11.6 The mounting of the computer workstations on an Ergotron computer arm

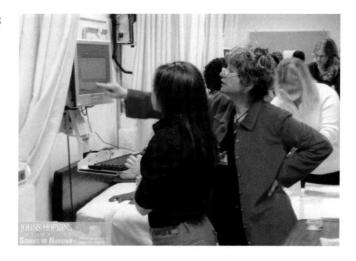

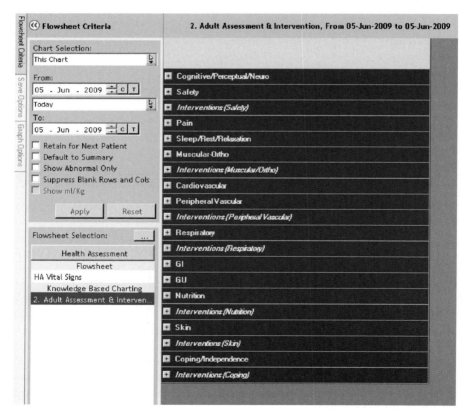

Fig. 11.7 Picture of the total assessment/intervention flowsheet. © Eclipsys Corporation. All rights reserved 2001–2009

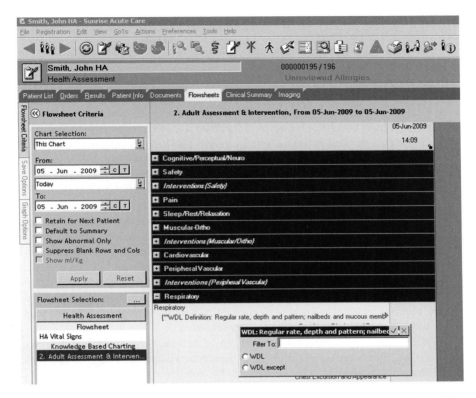

Fig. 11.8 Charting by defined parameters. © Eclipsys Corporation. All rights reserved 2001–2009

was required to register him/herself as a patient. In Health Assessment, for example, a student named John Smith would register a patient in the SCM system as John HA (for Health Assessment) Smith. This allowed faculty to track student progress in this Semester One class – and in other classes as well.

Other Technical Challenges

The JHUSON Eclipsys SCM system is currently designed to work with seven nursing courses and has a total of 27 flowsheets and six structured notes assigned among the courses. It was decided that each course would have its own location configured as a unit in the SCM system, containing its own clinical documentation and configurations. For example, the nursing for child health course has its own location in the system called the pediatric unit. Assigned to this location are the pediatric patient profile structured note, the pediatric critical care vital signs flowsheet, and the pediatric assessment and intervention flowsheet. Furthermore, each course has a security group associated with it to restrict students who are not part of a course from accessing that course's materials in SCM. In fact, security was configured so that students cannot make changes to the work of other students, only to their own work.

SCM user account creation and configuration for students also posed a challenge. The Eclipsys Team needed to figure out how to get student accounts into the Eclipsys SCM system with the appropriate access. The solution was to export student class enrollment data from the JHUSON's Active Directory system and use the SCM Express Load utility to bulk upload the data into SCM, thereby creating the student accounts. An enrollment in a class which used Eclipsys allowed for an account to be created with proper security access in the system. Student accounts in the system also had preconfigured patient lists that matched each registered course. For example, if a user was registered in Nursing for Adult Physical Health, a user account was created with membership to the Adult Health security group and a patient list was configured in the user's profile called Adult Health. Originally, student passwords were configured to match student ID badge numbers, but this had negative aspects. Student ID badge numbers were somewhat easily deciphered, which is adverse to teaching the principal that a password is a valuable resource which should be complex and not easily discernable so that others cannot gain unauthorized access to important information. Furthermore, students did not always have their student ID badges or remember their own student ID badge numbers, making it difficult for them to logon at times. Eventually, SCM was integrated into the JHUSON's Active Directory system, allowing students to logon to Eclipsys SCM with the same usernames and passwords they use to access the school's computer resources.

Another technical issue was how to "reset" the SCM system at the start of each semester so that the patients and patient information reverted to a default state and changes made during the previous semester were not present. The solution was to create a master database that was not to be used by students or instructors. The Eclipsys SCM system uses Microsoft SQL Server to store its databases. At the start of each semester, the master SCM database is copied to a new database in the SQL Server. It is in this new, copied database that students perform all of their work. This structure also allows the Eclipsys Team to perform configuration changes to the production master database, but not affect the current users of the system by allowing changes made by the team to be seen in the system during the following semesters. Of course, if an immediate change is necessary for a course currently using the system, the Eclipsys Team will make configuration changes in the current semester database as well as the master database.

To further integrate the EHR system, the Eclypsis Team also incorporated SCM with the Laerdal SimMan™ simulation manikin in the JHUSON's simulation laboratory. This combination of SimMan™ and SCM allowed faculty to truly test the assessment skills learned. Students participated in full simulations with the high-fidelity simulators. Assessments or procedures were conducted on SimMan and documentation of the tasks was entered into the EHR. Not only did students enter data, but they also used existing data, strategically placed in the EHR by instructors, to analyze and diagnose the cause of the SimMan's symptoms.

Nursing Implications and Conclusion

Nursing graduates must be prepared to create and establish safer and more efficient practice environments. Faced with many challenges today in health care education, health professionals must explore innovative ways to teach medical and nursing students real-world clinical practice in a cost-effective, productive, and high-quality manner. An overview of how educators from one baccalaureate program are incorporating the EHR, evidence-based content based on a professional practice framework, and information management into the clinical simulations offered to the students can serve as a guide for others. Incorporating the emerging evidence and technologies, as noted, involves many challenges; however, students must learn about systems they are held accountable to know when entering nursing practice upon graduation. Combining simulations that are integrated with informatics provide a real-world experience and opportunities for students to solve problem and critically think in a controlled, safe environment before working on a clinical unit where patients are involved.

Discoveries and development in educational technologies include a wide array of options such as the simulation activities integrated with healthcare informatics. Such developments and educational practices create an environment that is ripe for systematic and substantial change. No longer is it acceptable to provide students with limited clinical experiences and immerse them with lecture content and small group work in an attempt to meet the need to impart requisite, technical knowledge; this mode of instruction is *inadequate* to prepare them for the complexities of the workplace. Clinical simulation, combined with healthcare informatics and clinical experience and experiential teaching methods, is a powerful tool to prepare competent nurses for clinical practice.

References

1. Seropian M. General concepts in full scale simulation: getting started. *Anesth Analg.* 2003;97:1695-1705.
2. Jeffries PR. A framework for designing, implementing, and evaluating simulations used as teaching strategies in nursing. *Nurs Educ Persp.* 2005;26(2):28-35.
3. Bonk C, Cunningham D. *Searching for Learner-Centered, Constructivist, and Sociocultural Components of Collaborative Education Learning Tools in Electronic Collaborators.* Mahwah: Lawrence Erhlbaun Association; 1998.
4. Chickering A, Gamson Z. Seven principles of good practice in undergraduate education. *AAHE Bull.* 1987;39:3-7.
5. Blumenthal D. Stimulating the adoption of health information technology. *N Engl J Med.* 2009;360(15):1477-1479.
6. Graves JR, Corcoran S. The study of nursing informatics. *Image J Nurs Sch.* 1989;21(4): 227-231.
7. Joint Work Force Task Force. *Health Information Management and Informatics Core Competencies for Individuals Working with Electronic Health Records.* Bethesda: American Medical Informatics Association; 2008.
8. Conway PH, Clancy C. Transformation of healthcare at the front line. *JAMA.* 2009;301(7): 763-765.

9. Technology Informatics Guiding Education Reform (TIGER). The TIGER initiative: evidence and informatics transforming nursing: 3-year action steps toward a 10-year vision. www.aacn.nche.edu/education/pdf/TIGER.pdf; 2007. Accessed 29.09.09.
10. National League for Nursing. *Position Statement: Innovation in Nursing Education: A Call to Reform*. New York: NLN; 2003.
11. National League for Nursing. National league for nursing issues call for faculty development and curricular initiatives in informatics: NLN Board of Governors urges better preparation of nursing workforce. www.nln.org/newsreleases/informatics_release_052908.htm; 2008. Accessed 28.09.09.
12. Staggers N, Gassert CA, Curran C. A Delphi study to determine informatics competencies for nurses at four levels of practice. *Nurs Res*. 2002;51(6):383-390.
13. Staggers N, Gassert CA, Curran C. Informatics competencies for nurses at four levels of practice. *J Nurs Educ*. 2001;40(7):303-316.
14. Wesorick B, Troseth M, Cato J. *Intentionally Designed Automation Creates Best Places to Work and Receive Care. Healthcare Technology*, vol. 2. San Francisco: Montgomery Research; 2004.
15. Jeffries PR. *Simulations in Nursing Education: From Conceptualization to Evaluation*. New York: The National League for Nursing; 2007.
16. Ravert P. An integrative review of computer-based simulation in the education process. *Comput Inform Nurs*. 2002;20(5):203-208.
17. Hyun S, Park HA. Cross mapping the ICNP with NANDA, HHCC, Omaha System and NIC for unified nursing language system development. *Int Nurs Rev*. 2002;49(2):99-110.
18. Beiter PA, Sorscher J, Henderson CJ, et al. Do electronic medical record (EMR) demonstration change attitudes, knowledge, skills or needs? *Inform Prim Care*. 2008;16(3):221-227.
19. Beuscart-Zephir MC, Brender J, Menager-Depriester I. Cognitive evaluation: how to assess the usability of information technology in healthcare. *Comput Methods Programs Biomed*. 1997;54(1/2):19-28.
20. McKimm J, Jollie C, Cantillion P. Clinical review: ABC of learning and teaching: Web based learning. *BMJ*. 2003;326:870-873.

In the summer of 2009, all eyes were on the national scene watching the Office of the National Coordinator (ONC) to see what was happening with 'meaningful use.' There were many different perspectives and responses, from approval to concern to outright disagreement of the direction emerging from those working on its definition. Generally speaking, responses by the American Hospital Association (AHA) and the American Medical Association (AMIA) were supportive of the work being done. The nursing profession made its voice known as well.

Nursing and 'Meaningful Use'

The Alliance for Nursing Informatics (ANI) recommended "expanding 'meaningful use' to include any healthcare professional, for example registered nurses (RNs) and advanced practice registered nurses (APRNs), serving diverse and underserved populations across the continuum of care." ANI urged that the term 'meaningful use' should address and connect care across the continuum including, but not limited to: acute, ambulatory, long-term, community-based, home care, and public health based settings. Consistent with nursing's historical perspectives regarding health care, the leadership at ANI encouraged policy makers to address the "data and information necessary for managing these populations and take a broader perspective utilizing documentation from all members of the clinical team." Specific recommendations addressed patient-centered documentation, clinical performance measures, quality measures, and standards for data sharing. The complete ANI Memo and recommendations to the ONC are included as Appendix B at the back of this book.

If these recommendations are addressed at the policy level, then issues included in the definition of 'meaningful use' in 2013 and 2015 will be consistent with nursing's goals and the issues discussed in this section of the book. Examples from the latest 'meaningful use' document released by the ONC's *Health IT Policy Committee* (2009) include transmitting prescriptions, managing chronic conditions, ensuring performance on quality and safety measures, helping patients use self-management tools, accessing patient data from multiple sources, and using clinical dashboards within electronic health records (EHRs).

TIGER leadership and the broader TIGER community echoed and enriched the issues voiced by ANI and by the ONC. TIGER input highlighted the roles nursing must play in

˜ standards harmonization, usability and clinical application design, evidence-based practice (EBP), and adoption of personal health records (PHRs). Underscoring the role of health information technology in education and practice settings, TIGER recommended establishing informatics competencies for clinicians, using virtual demonstration centers to showcase best practices, encouraging partnerships between education and practice, and strengthening workforce development by integrating meaningful 'use expectations' into academic curricula. The TIGER response also identified and gave the rationale for the four key goals:

- Clinical documentation recorded in EHR
- Clinical decision support at the point of care
- Use of patient lists and decision support to manage chronic conditions
- Documentation of family medical history

The complete TIGER Memo and recommendations to the ONC appear in Appendix B in the back of the book.

To achieve the goals defined by the ONC, we must first understand the topics discussed by the authors in this section on: *Infrastructure, Adoption, and Implementation.* Chapter 12 explores how the national agenda and agencies impact policy and where nursing's voice can best be heard. Chapter 13 explains how health information standards can link and maintain application interoperability across healthcare systems. Chapter 14 drives home the message that usability and clinical design issues must be addressed in order to reach the health informatics goals set for 2011, 2013, and 2015.

Ending this section is Chapter 15, which looks at EBP and its role in improving patient safety, supporting decision-making, and responding to consumer health information and misinformation. Nurses face a steep challenge in using research as evidence for practice (Pravikoff et al. 2005). Given staffing shortages, demands on their time, and the lack of formalized evidence-based nursing, the nursing profession must overcome considerable difficulties to access and synthesize research for use in EBP (Simpson 2005).

The National Informatics Picture

In Chapter 12, "The National Informatics Picture," Carolyn Padovano and Alicia Morton lay out the issues driving healthcare reform, ranging from the burden of unsustainable spending to the promise of emerging technologies. The heart of their chapter, however, relates to the adoption of health IT and the history and structure of the federal agencies involved with IT mentioned in other chapters in this section and throughout the book. Among the federal agencies they describe are the Office of the National Coordinator (ONC), American Health Information Community (AHIC), National eHealth Collaborative (NeHC), Health Information Security and Privacy Collaborative (HISPC), National Health Information Network (NHIN), Health Information Technology Standards Panel (HITSP), and Certification Commission for Health Information Technology (CCHIT). The chapter concludes with a discussion of ONC's collaborative efforts with other federal agencies, including those addressing standards and interoperability, and usability and clinical design, topics covered in chapters 13 and 14.

Standards and Interoperability

In Chapter 13, "Standards and Interoperability," Joyce Sensmeier and Elizabeth Halley provide readable technical information. Their review of the need to adopt health IT interoperability, highlights issues addressed in 'meaningful use' dialogue, demystifies standards and harmonization, and clarifies why nurses must attend to these critical topics. Data standards organizations discussed include: Health Level 7 (HL7), Accredited Standards Committee (ASC X12), and the International Health Terminology Standards Development Organization (IHTSDO). Topics in the nursing domain include the following code sets: Nursing Minimum Data Sets (NMMDS), Nursing Terminologies Clinical Care Classification (CCC), International Classification of Nursing Practice (ICNP), North American Diagnosis Association (NANDA), Nursing Interventions Classifications (NIC), Nursing Outcomes Classification (NOC), and the Omaha System Perioperative Nursing Data Set (PNDS). The authors stress the need for nurses to understand the HITSP Interoperability Specification Roadmap and Harmonization Framework and highlight TIGER priorities and activities, and conclude by emphasizing once again nursing's role, responsibilities, and opportunities for involvement. The concerns practicing nurses express about their ability to document with nursing related data make the value of this chapter clear. Sensmeier and Halley provide nurses with the information they need to 'wise-up' and add to the profession's informed voice in health IT decisions.

Usability and Clinical Design

In Chapter 14, "Usability and Clinical Design," Nancy Staggers and Michelle Troseth assist nurses and other clinicians working to understand the significance of these two key areas and influence the changes that need to be made in health IT. Emphasizing the need for evidence-based, patient-centric technology that supports interdisciplinary collaboration at the point of care, the authors make the case that health IT systems should be informed by and/or positively transform nursing workflow. IT systems, they contend, should provide access to published literature and knowledge—and support the creation of new knowledge. The chapter examines human factors, ergonomics, human-computer interaction, and research as they relate to usability. The emphasis throughout is on the importance of design that supports nurses as they provide interdisciplinary collaborative care and gives them access to an (EBP). The chapter offers valuable guidance to nurses and other clinicians responsible for adopting and /or implementing health IT.

Evidence-Based Clinical Decision Support

In Chapter 15, "Evidence-Based Clinical Decision Support," Diane Hanson discusses EBP and its role in ensuring competency and patient safety in the context of increasingly complex patient care by supporting nurses as they assess, plan, deliver, and evaluate care. As examples of EBPs that might be overlooked, she cites the use of low dose aspirin, Braden Skin Risk Assessment, and proper positioning to prevent ventilator associated pneumonia. Stressing the importance of leadership, she relates how chief nursing officers can provide organizational support in the adoption of EBP. As sources for EBP, Hanson lists the Cochrane Collaboration, Agency for Healthcare Research and Quality (AHRQ), Public Health Agency of Canada's Canadian Best Practice Portal, and National Guideline Clearinghouse. As key groups supporting EBP, she cites the Leapfrog Group, Volunteer Hospital Association, American and Canadian Hospital Associations, Joint Commission on Accreditation of Healthcare Organizations, Gartner Group, and Institute of Medicine. The chapter describes the four basic methods of guideline development and consensual validation and highlights how they are used to disseminate best practices, achieve excellence in care delivery, meet or exceed quality standards, prevent complications, reduce omissions in care, and introduce innovation. As a guide to the reader, Hanson then introduces several guideline developers that use rigorous methodologies to generate high quality guidelines useful at the point of care.

Transformation

Written by nurses for nurses, Section 3 provides the technical information nurses need to understand and influence decisions regarding the choice, adoption, and implementation of clinical information systems across the healthcare continuum. Success in realizing the target goals of 'meaningful use' set for 2011, 2013, and 2015 will depend upon an informed nursing profession, speaking with a strong voice on behalf of all clinicians and the patients they serve.

References

Health IT Policy Committee (2009) "Meaningful Use." healthit.hhs.gov/portal/server.pt/gateway/ PTARGS _0_10741_872719_0_0_18/meaningful%20use%20matrix.pdf. Accessed 18 July 2009

Pravikoff D, Tanner A, Pierce S (2005) Readiness of U.S. nurses for evidence-based practice: Many don't understand or value research and have had little or no training to help them find evidence on which to base their practice. *Amer J Nurs* 105(9):40–51

Simpson RL (2005) Practice to evidence to practice: Closing the loop with IT. *Nurs Management* 36(9):12–17

The Evolving National Informatics Landscape

12

Carolyn Padovano and Alicia Morton

Introduction

The escalating cost of health care and the need to improve patient safety and reduce medical errors, coupled with national disasters, terrorism, and other unsustainable health care trends, have necessitated major health care reform in the United States. The focus on the adoption of electronic health records (EHRs) as a top priority within the National Health Information Technology (HIT) Agenda is the key driver toward achieving the transformation needed. This chapter reviews the industry trends, drivers, federal mandates, and initiatives influencing health care practice through the use of information systems and technology. It specifically examines the federal and private momentum and activities to date in the areas of governance, policy, technology, and adoption. The chapter concludes with recommendations to increase the engagement and visibility of the nursing profession and its influence on health care reform and HIT adoption.

Statistics and Trends Driving Health Care Transformation

Unsustainable Spending

Health care spending per person in the United States is higher than any other nation in the world. It is predicted that spending on health care in the US will double by 2017, reaching $4.3 trillion and accounting for 19.5% of the nation's gross domestic product.[1] It is also predicted that, by 2017, Medicare spending is expected to account for $884 billion, which is one fifth of all national health spending; and that Medicaid is expected to grow on an average of 7.9%

C. Padovano (✉)
Health Information Technology, Business and Future Technologies
Research Computing Division
Social Statistical & Environmental Sciences,
RTI International, 701 13th Street, N.W., Suite 750
Washington, DC, USA
e-mail: cpadovano@rti.org

M.J. Ball et al. (eds.), *Nursing Informatics*,
DOI: 10.1007/978-1-84996-278-0_12, © Springer-Verlag London Limited 2011

each year, reaching $717.3 billion or 16.8% of health spending.[1] Compounded by the statistics that nearly 46 million Americans are uninsured, all of these are unsustainable trends.

Unfortunately, the fact that US health care costs have been rising at more than 8% per year over the past 10 years has not translated into an equivalent return on investment, as US health care quality has only risen at 3.1% per year.[2] This rising cost and the quality disparity of the US healthcare system demands change. The US is in critical need of health-care system transformation, and as Leatherman and McCarthy [2] point out, this level of performance is unworthy of the wealthiest nation in the world.

Nursing Shortage

Another statistic that is driving the charge for US health care transformation is the current and impending worsening of the nursing shortage. Presently, there are close to three million practicing nurses in the US, accounting for over 55% of all health care workers. The aver-age age of a nurse in the US is 47 years old and rising.[3] It is predicted that there will be a severe shortage of nurses by 2014, with no relief in sight, due not only to this professional population retiring, but also the decline of enrollment in nursing schools and the significant increase in workforce demands in caring for the aging "baby boomer" population.

Lack of Disaster Preparedness and Planning

A discovery that has contributed to the US recognizing the critical need for health care trans-formation included the highly publicized, insufficient disaster preparedness and recovery strat-egies deployed when Hurricanes Katrina and Rita struck. Disaster preparedness and planning at the service delivery level varied considerably across the state-administered federal programs. It was noted that these programs struggled to increase capacity quickly to meet the emergent demands.[4] As a result, the White House conducted a study entitled *The Federal Response to Hurricane Katrina: Lessons Learned* (http://library.stmarytx.edu/acadlib/edocs/katrinawh. pdf), and reported several recommendations for the Department of Health and Human Services (HHS) to consider. The paramount recommendation included that HHS take a leading role in improving disaster response in delivering human services and health care for disaster victims.

Growing Health Care Consumerism

Consumers of health care are taking a more active role in making informed decisions about their health care and are actively seeking health promotion information. Thanks to wide-spread Internet access, the availability of online health care information and tools (such as clinical guidelines, treatment protocols, medical references/libraries), and user-friendly health care social networking sites, consumers can now obtain personalized health care advice and patient support services. In addition, consumers are researching medical conditions via web-based videos, employing personal health care coaches, and/or developing their own personal health records (PHRs). Empowering consumers and providing tools to manage their wellness and health care needs is a key enabler of this needed healthcare system transformation.

Emerging Telehealth

Wireless technology has become standard practice in hospital environments. As such, the use of medical devices, such as heart and respiration monitors, and blood pressure, and pulse oximetry machines, is becoming a standard practice in nonhospital and home environments. The ability of these remote devices to send information/data to the patient's health care provider and/or directly to the patient's PHR or EHR is becoming a more common occurrence. This trend will have significant impact improving patients' empowerment, health status, and access to care, especially for consumers with chronic illness and those who live in rural areas.

Transparency of Health Care Information and Cost

Another trend that is driving health care transformation in the US is the use of financial incentives to reward providers. Organizations and health plans are utilizing technology to disseminate information on health care quality measures, patient safety metrics, and health plan and product pricing. In addition to insurers and employer groups advocating and offering health IT platforms (such as PHRs) to customers, they are also providing more consumer-driven health plans by utilizing the web. For example, several private and public health plans allow patients to search on prescription drugs by their zip code in order to find the location of the pharmacy with the most cost-effective treatment. Also, online provider and organizational ratings are now available to the general public, such as www.consumersunion.org, www.angieslist.com, www.healthgrades.com, and www.hospitalcompare. hhs.gov. This movement toward transparency will continue as members of the public partner more in their health care decisions and treatment plans. Consumers will ultimately demand more accountability, as they have done in every other service industry.

Health Information Technology Adoption: A National Priority

Within the last decade, several groundbreaking health care reports have been published, and all of them concluded that it is imperative for the American health care delivery system to be overhauled. The famous report from the Institute of Medicine (IOM), *To Err is Human: Building a Safer Health System,*[5] cited that over 44,000 Americans die each year as a result of medical errors that could have been prevented. This landmark report garnered worldwide attention from health care leaders, policy makers, health care organizations, professional associations, private and public insurers, and consumers. The report recommended and proposed six aims for improving health care in America. These stated health care should be:

1. Safe – Avoid errors and injury to patients
2. Effective – Provide services based on scientific evidence
3. Patient-centered – Account for preferences and characteristics
4. Timely – Reduce waits and delays

5. Efficient – Avoid waste, provide coordination
6. Equitable – Provide same services independent of cultural, socioeconomic status, educational background, and/or geographical location.

The next IOM report, *Crossing the Quality Chasm: A New Health System for the 21st Century,*[6] focused on developing a strategy to operationalize improvement of the quality of America's healthcare system. The recommendations for health care reform that were put forth were directed at three levels of our current system: the Environmental Level, the Healthcare Organizational Level, and the Provider and Patient Level. As a result, the reports that followed focused on the reform needed at these levels of our healthcare system. All published by and available from the National Academy Press in Washington, DC, they include:

- Envisioning the National Health Care Quality Report (2001)
- Leadership by Example: Coordinating Government Roles in Improving Health Care Quality (2002)
- Fostering Rapid Advances in Health Care: Learning from System Demonstrations (2002)
- Priority Areas for National Action: Transforming Health Care Quality (2003)
- Health Professions Education: A Bridge to Quality (2003)
- Key Capabilities of an Electronic Health Record System (2003)
- Keeping Patients Safe: Transforming the Work Environment of Nurses (2003)
- Patient Safety: Achieving a New Standard for Care (2003)
- 1st Annual Crossing the Quality Chasm Summit: A Focus on Communities (2004)
- Quality Through Collaboration: The Future of Rural Health (2004)
- Health Literacy: A Prescription to Ending Confusion (2004)
- Building a Better Delivery System: A New Engineering/Healthcare Partnership (2005)
- Performance Measurement: Accelerating Improvement (2005)
- Building the Workforce for Health Information Transformation (2006)
- Preventing Medication Errors: Quality Chasm Series (2006).

Federal Momentum and Activities

The series of US health care reform reports published by IOM, other agencies, and universities concluded that utilization of information technology was key to the promise for transforming the healthcare system to achieve the IOM's foundational aims of safety, effectiveness, patient family centeredness, timeliness, efficiency, and equity. President Bush led the charge by establishing the goal that most Americans would have an EHR by 2014. In April 2004, President Bush issued Executive Order (EO) 13335, Incentives for the Use of Health Information Technology and Establishing the Position of the National Health Information Technology Coordinator, which established the position and Office of the National Coordinator for Health Information Technology (ONC) within the HHS, "to provide leadership for the development and nationwide implementation of an interoperable health information technology infrastructure to improve the quality and efficiency of health care."

Within a few months of the National Coordinator being named, a framework for strategic action focused on consumer-centric, information-rich health care was released.[7] This document launched the federal government's coordinated HIT strategic planning efforts by clearly articulating the need for change and the necessary key actions to achieve the President's adoption goal. The framework described four main goals, with several strategic actions for each which ultimately directed many of the federal and private-sector HIT efforts for several years following. These goals and their aims were:

- *Inform clinical practice* by incentivizing EHR adoption, reducing the risk of EHR investments, and promoting EHR diffusion in rural and underserved areas
- *Interconnect clinicians* by fostering regional collaborations, developing an interoperable Nationwide Health Information Network (NHIN), and coordinating federal health information systems
- *Personalize health care* by encouraging use of personal health records, enhancing informed consumer choice, and promoting the use of telehealth systems
- *Improve population health* by unifying public health surveillance architectures, streamlining quality and health status monitoring, and accelerating research and dissemination of evidence

Another key Executive Order, EO 13410, Promoting Quality and Efficient Health Care in Federal Government Administered or Sponsored Health Care Programs, was issued by President Bush in August 2006. This Executive Order focused on transforming the healthcare system and was intended to ensure that federally administered or funded health care programs promote and adhere to four principles known as the "cornerstones of value-driven health care" (http://www.hhs.gov/valuedriven/index.html). The four cornerstones identified became significant drivers for the ONC and federal HIT activities. They include:

- *Interoperable Health Information Technology* – Support and recognize common technical standards for secure and interoperable communication and data exchange
- *Measure and Publish Quality Information* – Define what constitutes quality of care and support the design of systems that collect, measure, and report on quality
- *Measure and Publish Price Information* – Enhance transparency to all Americans providing comparisons about the cost of their health care options
- *Promote Quality and Efficiency of Care* – Reward those who provide and purchase high-quality, competitively priced health care.

The Federal Government's Role in HIT Adoption

Office of the National Coordinator

With the previously noted drivers in place, HHS and ONC led the federal charge and reached out to the private sector in pursuit of the effort to achieve the President's goal of EHRs for most Americans by 2014. The ONC strategic framework[7] established several goals that led to specific public and private sector actions in the areas of governance, policy, technology, and adoption. In June 2008, ONC published a strategic plan as an update to the 2004 framework highlighting two broad goals, Patient-Focused Health Care and Population Health, each with several objectives and measurable outcomes. The Strategic Plan entitled *The ONC-Coordinated Federal Health IT Strategic Plan*: 2008-2012 plan is public-centric and focuses on the activities that ONC and its federal partners will need to take toward achieving the President's goal (http://www.dhhs.gov/healthit/resources/HITStrategicPlan.pdf).

Governance: Federal, State, and Local Activities

In order to accomplish the President's vision of widespread EHR adoption by 2014, a governance and collaboration body was created by Secretary Leavitt in July of 2005. The committee, known as the American Health Information Community (AHIC), was chaired by the HHS Secretary and originally included 17 members, nine from the public sector and eight from the private sector. This public/private collaboration was established under the Federal Advisory Committee Act (FACA) to advise the Secretary, recommend actions toward a common interoperability framework, and serve as a forum for a broad range of stakeholders providing input on HIT adoption.

During the course of the AHIC activities, workgroups were established in seven priority areas: Biosurveillance/Population Health; Consumer Empowerment; Chronic Care; Electronic Health Records; Confidentiality, Privacy, and Security; Quality; and Personalized Health Care. The detailed work performed in these workgroups involved hundreds of experts and stakeholders and yielded 200 recommendations that were advanced to the Secretary of HHS over the course of 25 meetings. Many of these recommendations were accepted by the Secretary and acted upon, such as the EHR demonstration project and the e-prescribing bonus payment incentive launched by the Centers for Medicare and Medicaid as part of the Medicare Improvements for Patients and Providers Act of 2008. Another significant component of the AHIC work consisted of developing HIT and Health Information Exchange (HIE) priorities that informed the development of use cases and a roadmap for standards development and harmonization.

As the original charter for the AHIC neared completion, efforts ensued to establish an AHIC successor in the private sector that would continue to have federal participation, but would not be a FACA committee. Therefore, the *AHIC Successor, Inc.* was founded in 2008 to transition AHIC's accomplishments and accountabilities into a new nonprofit membership organization and is now known as the National eHealth Collaborative (NeHC). The NeHC has created a national priority process based on "value cases" which evaluates the business value proposition and benefits of developing specifications for utilizing electronic health information.

As of this writing, the NeHC had met already with President Obama's transition team and was continuing with plans for promoting the use of EHRs and HIT as part of the national economic stimulus package and comprehensive health care reform plan.

Policy

In order to accomplish the privacy and security objectives necessary for widespread HIT adoption, ONC funded several contracts to examine state and organizational privacy, security, and legal barriers. The *State Alliance for e-Health*, launched by the National Governors Association for Best Practices, was formed to build state government consensus on many HIT and information exchange privacy and security issues. Another state activity, the *State-Level Health Information Exchange Consensus Project*, was chartered to uncover the statewide barriers to HIE and to have a supportive and collaborative forum for states to develop organizational policies and practices to enable data sharing and sustainability of state-level HIE organizations. Lastly, ONC funded the development of the Health Information Security and Privacy Collaborative (HISPC). This collaboration, now in its third phase, has convened up to 42 states and territories to assess the variations in privacy and security related to organizational-level business policies and state laws that affect HIE, and to develop detailed, replicable solutions for implementation.

Technology

The Nationwide Health Information Network (NHIN)

In order to accomplish the interconnectedness and interoperability objectives, ONC initially awarded four contracts to the following HIT vendors: Accenture, Computer Sciences Corporation (CSC), IBM, and Northrop Grumman in November 2005. The four vendors were challenged with developing prototype architectures for the NHIN. Then, each vendor was asked to demonstrate their prototype architectures by interconnecting three communities to exchange data based on the AHIC priority areas/use cases. The second phase of the NHIN effort consisted of these organizations demonstrating HIE by beginning trial implementations of the NHIN. As a result, these organizations and federal agencies formed the NHIN Cooperative in August 2008 to implement, test, and demonstrate core capabilities to support the NHIN. The culmination of the capabilities and the use cases was demonstrated at the fifth NHIN Forum in December 2008. Other results of the NHIN efforts have produced a number of tools (i.e., standards, services, and policies) which are freely available to enable organizations in implementing secure electronic health information exchange (see: http://healthit.hhs.gov/portal/server.pt/community/ healthit_hhs_gov_nhin_inventory/1486). The newly established FACA committee, the Health IT Policy Committee, has a NHIN Work Group and a Health IT Policy Committee and can be found at http://healthit.hhs.gov/policycommittee. Today, the NHIN operates as the NHIN Exchange with many diverse federal and private sector entities partnering to securely exchange electronic health information, and continuing to meet the evolving needs of its users in order to achieve the goals of the Health Information Technology for Economic and Clinical Health (HITECH) Act.

Additionally, a new initiative has been launched, NHIN direct, with the goal of assisting health information exchange at a more local and less complex level. For more information about the Nationwide Health Network Direct Project, please visit http://nhindirect.org.

Health Information Technology Committee (now that HITSP is no longer active) Standards Panel (HITSP)

In order to accomplish the standards in HIT objective, ONC led a contract to establish the HITSP in 2005 in accordance with President Bush's EHR initiative. The primary mission of

HITSP is to create processes to harmonize existing HIT standards. HITSP developed as a public–private partnership and includes more than 300 health-related organizations. The organization operates with an inclusive governance model established by the American National Standards Institute (ANSI). HITSP's main goals include: (1) Achieving a widely accepted and useful set of standards that enable and support widespread interoperability among health care software applications; (2) Synchronizing relevant standards in the health care industry to enable and advance the interoperability of health care applications; and (3) Interchanging health care data. As a result, the panel has developed interoperability specifications (IS) for numerous AHIC priority areas/use cases (for a full list, see www.hitsp.org).

There is a formal recognition process within HHS for these IS. Upon HHS Secretary's recognition, these standards are to be included in certified HIT products and supported by federal agencies and federal contracts pertaining to HIT. As of April 30, 2010, HITSP's contract with HHS/ONC concluded. However, with the American Recovery and Reinvestment Act (ARRA) of 2009, the Health IT Standards Committee (as a FACA) was established. The committee is charged with making recommendations to the National Coordinator for Health IT on standards, implementation specifications, and certification criteria for the electronic exchange and use of health information. It is also responsible for assessing the policy recommendations of the Health IT Policy Committee. Formal recognition of standards are now done through rule-making; the most recent being published July 28, 2010 45 CFR Part 170 - Health Information Technology: Initial Set of Standards, Implementation Specifications, and Certification Criteria for Electronic Health Record Technology: Final Rule.

Adoption

Certification Commission for Health Information Technology (CCHIT)

In order to accomplish the standards in HIT products and the adoption of interoperable HIT objectives, ONC recognized the importance of creating a certification body for EHRs and their networks. The certification of HIT products would assure the customer (i.e., providers and health care organizations) that the products that they are purchasing are reliable, valid, functional, secure, and interoperable, thereby decreasing the risk for the purchaser. With assurances like these, ONC concluded that the development of an organization such as this would ultimately be a significant catalyst for increasing the adoption of HIT in the US. In response to the 2004 HIT Strategic Framework, three leading HIT industry associations – the American Health Information Management Association (AHIMA), the Healthcare Information and Management Systems Society (HIMSS), and the National Alliance for Health Information Technology (the Alliance) – developed this independent, voluntary, private-sector certification organization. Shortly thereafter, ONC issued a contract to CCHIT to develop and evaluate certification criteria and an inspection process for ambulatory EHRs. CCHIT has been very successful and has received significant buy-in from the vendor marketplace, with the majority of ambulatory and inpatient EHR vendors being certified. To see a list of certified products and their associated vendors, go to www.cchit.org. The three main areas in which certification criteria have been developed include the following:

- Functionality – To ensure that the systems can support the activities and perform the functions for which they are intended
- Security – To ensure that systems can protect and maintain the confidentiality of data entrusted to them
- Interoperability – To ensure that system can connect to and exchange information with other systems

The criteria for certifying ambulatory, inpatient, and specialty EHR products are updated every year.

CCHIT develops its criteria for these certification programs through 12 volunteer workgroups. The workgroups include Ambulatory EHR, Behavioral Health, Cardiovascular Medicine, Child Health, Electronic Prescribing, Emergency Department, Interoperability, Inpatient EHR, PHRs, Privacy and Compliance, Security, and HIE. CCHIT disseminates all draft criteria, proposed certification expansion areas, and its strategic roadmap on its web site and urges public comment at www.cchit.org.

Other Federal Partners

With ONC responsible for ensuring the alignment of public and private sector programs and initiatives related to HIT and HIE, several governmental initiatives have been put in place. To assist federal agencies and departments in planning and implementing HIT that aligns with national initiatives, the Federal Health Architecture (FHA) serves as an organizing body consisting of more than 20 federal partners (see www.hhs.gov/fedhealtharch/). On the policy side, ONC convenes an interagency HIT Policy Council to coordinate federal HIT policy decisions across federal departments and agencies.

In addition to the formal collaborations noted above, ONC develops, maintains, and directs the implementation of a federal strategic plan to guide the nationwide implementation of interoperable HIT. In this role, ONC is in close contact with all the federal departments and agencies in relation to HIT activities. Federal agencies, such as the Department of Veterans' Affairs (VA), Department of Defense (DOD), Centers for Medicare and Medicaid Services (CMS), Agency for Healthcare Research and Quality (AHRQ), and many others, are key leaders in the drive toward the President's adoption goal.

Opportunities for Nurses to Engage

When President Bush appointed a National Coordinator for HIT back in 2004, the first step Dr. David Brailer took in this new position was to convene a national HIT summit. In July 2004, he brought together national leaders in HIT to discuss what was then termed the National Health Information Infrastructure (NHIN).

Later that year, recognizing the need to bring the nursing profession to the table in future discussions of the national HIT agenda, nurse leaders launched the Technology Informatics Guiding Education Reform (TIGER) Initiative. In late 2006, TIGER sponsored a national invitational summit for nurses. The summit's findings, published in 2007, set forth a vision and strategic action plan for nursing. Purposefully aligning its goals with ONC's strategic plan, TIGER focused on ensuring that the nursing profession's voice would be heard at the national level. For more information on TIGER and the strategic plan, go to www.tigersummit.com.

To realize its strategic plan, TIGER established a number of collaborative working groups. One of these, the National HIT Agenda Collaborative, examined policies relevant to the TIGER vision and the nursing profession's mission, pinpointing potential representation gaps on policy issues that required closure. The Collaborative identified three areas where the nursing profession required greater visibility and where their contributions would enhance and promote the National HIT agenda and the transformation of health and care in the US. The three areas where greater nursing leadership and involvement is needed are:

- In clinical, standards, and policy initiatives generated by the AHIC/NeHC and the ONC (such as participation in Workgroups and in Use Cases)
- In advancing the initial standards harmonization and interoperability efforts of ANSI-HITSP by participating in the two current HHS/ONC FACAs - the HIT Policy Committee and the HIT Standards Committee (such as working on the Committees and developing the IS).
- In the certification process for HIT products (such as volunteering for a Workgroup, and reviewing and commenting on the CCHIT Work products)

How to Get Involved

National eHealth Collaborative

The best way for nurses to become involved in NeHC is to serve on the Board and/or become a member. For those not able to serve on the board or formally join, staying abreast of the meetings and events is essential as this group will have significant impact in setting the priorities for standards development and adoption. By participating in the development of these priorities into Value Cases, nurses and nursing informaticists can then drive policies and HIT development that meet their needs and represent their practice. Visit www.nationalehealth.org to learn more about how you can get involved and to view the schedule for participation.

Health Information Technology Policy and Standards Committee

The best way for nurses to become involved in HIT policy and standards now that HITSP is inactive to stay abreast of the two HHS/ONC FACAs, the HIT Policy Committee and the HIT Standards Committee. All the meetings are open to the public and the materials are available on the www.healthit.hhs. gov website. Nurses are encouraged to reach out and become engaged with your local and state health IT initiatives, such as, the HIT Regional Extension Centers, State HIT and Health Information Exchange (HIE) programs, and Beacon

Communities. As discussed in previous sections, HITSP's work was driven by a series of priorities, set by the AHIC/NeHC. Nurses participated at that time in the development of Use Cases and by offering recommendations for IS and related constructs in their related domain expertise. Visit www.hitsp.org to learn more about HITSP's past accomplishments.

Certification Commission for Health Information Technology

The best way for nurses to get involved with CCHIT is to submit an application during "calls" for Commissioners' and Work Group Chairpersons' appointments. Another way is to volunteer to participate on one of their workgroups which aligns most closely with your clinical specialty or expertise. Reviewing draft materials and providing comments during Public Comment periods will ensure that nurses' voices are being heard. Other ways to keep current and informed include (1) attending Town Hall in-person meetings, Town Hall teleconference calls, conference presentations; (2) monitoring the Commission and Work Group activities through meeting minutes; and (3) serving as a juror for CCHIT's commercial certification program. All are effective ways to impact health and care in the US. Visit www.cchit.org to learn more about how to get involved and to view the schedule for participation.

The Recovery Act of 2009 (Public Law 111-5)

The best way for nurses to get involved in the future of the National HIT Agenda is to become aware and to understand the American Recovery and Reinvestment Act of 2009 (Recovery Act, or ARRA) and its relation to health care reform and information technology. The Act is an economic stimulus package enacted by the 111th United States Congress and was signed into law by President Barack Obama on 17 February 2009. Designed to provide a stimulus to the US economy in the wake of the economic downturn, the Act provides funding for a wide range of activities, including domestic spending in education, health care, and infrastructure. The stimulus package's worth is cited at $787 billion, with health care totaling $147.7 billion and HIT accounting for approximately $19 billion.

To address the new funding available in the Recovery Act, ONC published a new implementation plan that outlined how HIT investments would be used to improve the health of Americans the performance of the nation's health system. Nurses can take advantage of funding opportunities and participate in HIT initiatives and programs currently underway as a result of the Recovery Act. Because the legislation, the implementation plan, the funding opportunities and the associated programs are still evolving, it is important that nurses obtain up-to-date information and details by visiting ONC's website at www.healthit.hhs. gov. As of this writing, activities and HIT programs of interest to nurses include:

The HITECH (Health Information Technology for Economic and Clinical Health Act) Priority Grants Program – On 20 August 2009, the White House announced the roll-out of two critical grants program that will help health care providers and states in the selection and implementation of EHRs and the exchange of health care information. The first grant program is the HIT Regional Extension Centers (RECs) Program, developed to fund several RECs in the United States. The Centers are intended to help providers who need technical hands-on experience with the adoption of certified EHRs. A national HIT Research

Center (HITRC) will be developed to educate and enable these Centers to communicate with one another. The second grant program provides assistance to States and Qualified State Designated Entities (SDEs) charged with developing policies and implementation plans to facilitate HIE within states and across the nation. Additional information on these grant programs and others is available at Grants.gov and FedBizOpps.gov. A comprehensive summary of Launching HITECH (Blumenthal, 2010) can be found in the February 4, 2010 edition of the New England Journal of Medicine, and will be described below.

- *Regional Extension Centers Program* ONC established this program and awarded grants to approximately 70 RECs in the US in order to support ambulatory providers to adopt and become meaningful of EHRs.
- *State Health Information Exchange Cooperative Agreement Program* - ONC is supporting health information exchange (HIE) among states for providers and hospital entities.
- *Beacon Community Program* - ONC created this funding to support approximately 15 communities in building and demonstrating their HIT infrastructure and exchange capabilities. The goal of this program is to demonstrate how the meaningful use of EHRs can achieve measurable outcomes in improving the quality of care in a geographic region.
- *Strategic Health Information Technology Advanced Research Projects (SHARP)* - ONC is funding research in four areas to address the impediments to HIT adoption. These four areas include: Security of HIT; Patient-centered cognitive support; HIT applications and network/platform architectures, and secondary uses of EHR data. The outcome of these projects is to understand the impediments in adoption and to ultimately solve these issues in order to advance adoption in this country.
- *Meaningful Use Regulation* – ONC and CMS developed regulations that provide health care providers with reimbursement incentives when these clinicians successfully use EHRs (termed "meaningful users"). The incentive payments are expected to begin in 2011. The final rule was published July 28, 2010, and can be found at http://edocket.access.gpo.gov/2010/pdf/2010-17207.pdf. For a summary of the "Meaningful Use" regulation for EHRs, see the August 5, 2010 edition of the New England Journal of Medicine (Blumenthal & Tavenner, 2010).
- *Standards and Certification Criteria Regulation* - ONC published the final rule on July 10, 2010. The final rule contains the initial set of standards, implementation specifications, and certification criteria for EHRs, and can be found at http://edocket.access.gpo.gov/2010/pdf/2010-17210.pdf.
- *Workforce Programs:*
- *Curriculum Development Centers*: ONC has provided grants to institutions of higher education (or consortia thereof) to support health IT curricula development geared for preparing trainees to perform the following six workforce roles: Practice workflow and information management redesign specialists; clinician/practitioner consultants; implementation support specialists; implementation managers; and technical/software support staff and trainers.
- *Community College Consortia to Educate Health Information Technology Professionals*: ONC provided grants to more than 70 community colleges in all 50 states to rapidly create HIT education and training programs or expand existing programs. Community Colleges funded under this initiative will establish intensive, non-degree training programs that can be completed in six months or less for the six workforce roles being addressed by the Curriculum Development Centers.Community College Consortia to Educate Health

Information Technology Professionals: ONC provided grants to more than 70 community colleges in all 50 states to rapidly create HIT education and training programs or expand existing programs. Community Colleges funded under this initiative will establish intensive, non-degree training programs that can be completed in six months or less for the six workforce roles being addressed by the Curriculum Development Centers.

- *Competency Examination for Individuals Completing Non-Degree Training*: ONC awarded a grant to support the development and initial administration of a set of health IT competency examinations for the six community college workforce roles.
- *Program of Assistance for University-Based Training*: Another ONC grant program that awards nine universities to rapidly increase the availability of individuals qualified to serve in specific health information technology professional roles requiring university-level education. The six roles targeted by this program are: Clinician/Public Health Leader, Health Information Management and Exchange Specialists; Health Information Privacy and Security Specialist; Research and Development Scientist; Programmers and Software Engineer; and Health IT Sub-Specialist.

A Final Word

To transform health care in the United States, nurses must step forward to learn more, become more involved, and take leadership roles in the upcoming Recovery Programs. By raising their voices and speaking out, nurses will influence health care reform and HIT adoption – and patient advocacy and high-quality health care will be the result.

References

1. Keehan S, Sisko A, Truffer C, et al. Health spending projections through 2017: the baby-boom generation is coming to Medicare. *Health Aff.* 2008;27(2):w145-w155.
2. Leatherman S, McCarthy D. *Quality of Healthcare in the United States: A Chartbook.* New York: The Commonwealth Fund; 2002.
3. Bureau of Health Professions. *The registered nurse population: Findings from the March 2004 National Sample Survey of Registered Nurses.* Washington: Department of Health and Human Services; 2006.
4. Tait S. *Hurricanes Katrina and Rita: Federal actions could enhance preparedness of certain state-administered federal support programs.* Washington: Government Accountability Office; 2007.
5. Institute of Medicine. *To Err Is Human.* Washington: National Academy; 2000.
6. Institute of Medicine. *Crossing the Quality Chasm: A New Health System for the 21st Century.* Washington: National Academy; 2001.
7. Thompson TG, Brailer DJ. *The Decade of Health Information Technology: Delivering Consumer-Centric and Information-Rich Health Care.* Washington: US Department of Health and Human Services; 2004.
8. Blumenthal D Launching HITECH. *The New England Journal of Medicine.* 2010; 362 (5), p. 382-385.
9. Blumenthal D Tavenner M. The "Meaningful Use" Regulation for Electronic Health Records. *The New England Journal of Medicine.* 2010; 363 (6), p. 501-504.

Standards and Interoperability

13

Joyce Sensmeier and Elizabeth Casey Halley

I have an almost complete disregard of precedent, and a faith in the possibility of something better. It irritates me to be told how things have always been done. I defy the tyranny of precedent. I go for anything new that might improve the past.

Clara Barton

Why is there such an urgency to adopt health information technology (IT) interoperability standards? What does this urgency mean for nursing?

It has been well documented that our health care system is in crisis. What worked in the past is no longer viable and must be improved. Despite spending over $1.6 trillion on health care as a nation, there are still serious concerns about high costs, avoidable medical errors, administrative inefficiencies, and poor coordination – all of which are closely connected to the failure to incorporate health IT into our health care system, according to the Agency for Healthcare Research and Quality.[1] To address these concerns, numerous efforts have commenced which include setting a goal for the adoption of electronic health records (EHRs) recognition of interoperable health IT standards as part of the President's National Health IT Agenda to lower cost and drive quality improvement, and the American Recovery and Reinvestment Act of 2009 (ARRA). Through these and other public/private efforts, the importance of advancing quality care and reducing costs through adopting interoperable health IT has been brought to the forefront of the nation's efforts to improve the health care system.

Health IT standards and interoperability are complex concepts. Understanding these terms and how they impact nursing practice, and embracing the means for nurses' involvement with influencing the adoption of health IT standards and interoperable EHRs are important responsibilities of the nursing profession. This chapter sets the stage by providing definitions of standards and interoperability, reviewing the components of the National Health IT Agenda, and examining the standards adoption process. The role nurses must play and challenges they face in understanding and adopting interoperable health IT and standards are further explored.

J. Sensmeier (✉)
Vice President, Informatics, Healthcare Information and Management Systems Society,
Chicago, IL, USA
e-mail: jsensmeier@himss.org

M.J. Ball et al. (eds.), *Nursing Informatics*,
DOI: 10.1007/978-1-84996-278-0_13, © Springer-Verlag London Limited 2011

What Is a Health IT Standard?

When two or more people are in a meaningful conversation, the words they exchange are easily understood. Conformance to a standard language is inherent in the interpretation of the message content being spoken and heard in the conversation. When such a discussion occurs over a telephone line, the content is sent and received using communication standards to transmit the voices between participants.

Health IT standards work in a similar fashion. They provide structured content and formatting to ensure that a sending and receiving system accurately compiles and interprets a message. Such an example would begin with a physician entering a medication order into an EHR system. The pharmacist receives the medication order and processes it within the pharmacy information system. Finally, the nurse receives the order, administers the medication, and documents the delivery in the clinical documentation system. To ensure the proper medication order information (patient, medication, strength, form, dose, route, and schedule) is filled properly by the pharmacist and administered correctly by the nurse to the patient, terminology standards must be employed. Once a patient is discharged, ensuring that the electronic version of their medication list is securely and accurately provided to them and/or their providers requires interoperable health IT standards to be in place.

As defined by the Healthcare Information Technology Standards Panel (HITSP), the term "standard" is used to refer to Specifications, Implementation Guides, Code Sets, Terminologies, and Integration Profiles.[3] More specifically, it is a well-defined approach that supports a business process and (1) has been agreed upon by a group of experts; (2) has been publicly vetted; (3) provides rules, guidelines, or characteristics; (4) helps to ensure that materials, products, processes, and services are fit for their intended purpose; (5) is available in an accessible format; and (6) is subject to an ongoing review and revision process. Standards may be developed, maintained, and distributed through numerous venues including accredited standards development organizations (SDOs), professional associations, academic institutions, and the federal government (http://www.standardslearn.org).

Health IT standards include data standards for the clinical content, technical standards for the formatting, and security and privacy constraints surrounding the exchange. Some of the prominent health IT SDOs include Health Level Seven (HL7, http://www.hl7.org), Accredited Standards Committee (ASC X12, http://www.x12.org), and the International Health Terminology Standards Development Organization (IHTSDO, http://www.ihtsdo.org). Other prominent organizations that develop, maintain, and distribute health IT standards include the Regenstrief Institute, responsible for Logical Observation Identifiers Names and Codes (LOINC®, http://loinc.org); the World Health Organization (WHO), responsible for International Classification of Diseases (ICD, http://www.who.int/classifications/icd/en/); while the American Medical Association is responsible for the CPT codes (http://www.cap.org/apps/cap.portal?_nfpb=true&).

There are also several health IT standards that support the nursing domain and are recognized by the American Nurses Association (ANA, http://www.nursingworld.org/npii/terminologies.htm). These terminology standards represent the content of nursing language which includes the concepts or terms that are used to document nursing practice. These nursing domain content standards are developed by different organizations, are recognized by the American Nurses Association and including the following:

Code sets
    Nursing Minimum Data Set (NMDS)
    Nursing Management Minimum Data Set (NMMDS)

Nursing terminologies
    Clinical Care Classification (CCC)
    International Classification of Nursing Practice (ICNP®)
    North American Nursing Diagnosis Association (NANDA)
    Nursing Interventions Classification (NIC)
    Nursing Outcomes Classification (NOC)
    Omaha System
    Patient Care Data Set (PCDS)
    Perioperative Nursing Data Set (PNDS – Retired)

Multidisciplinary terminologies
    ABC Codes
    Logical Observation Identifiers Names & Codes (LOINC®)
    Systematized Nomenclature of Medicine (SNOMED-CT®)

Well-defined standards are the foundation for interoperability between and among systems and they can fulfill the promise of electronically enabled health care. By harmonizing standards, different information systems, networks, and software applications will be able to "speak the same language" and work together technically to support management and use of consistent, accurate, and accessible health information for providers and consumers. As defined by the federal government's health IT initiative, there are several requirements for standards to fully support health IT outcomes:

- The proper standard must be identified for a particular purpose.
- Where there are needs for new or additional standards, these standards gaps must be filled.
- Detailed specifications must be available to guide the implementation of standards in an exact and consistent way.
- There must be widespread adoption of standards by healthcare information systems and their users.

These standards, once harmonized, can:

- Allow consumer information to follow the consumer and be available to providers to support clinical decision making even if the information originates in different locations and different computer systems
- Promote security and confidentially in health IT systems by enabling approaches for information protection and access control

- Improve patient safety, promote quality improvement, and facilitate clinical research based on appropriate use of consistent data
- Protect populations by supporting public health disease detection and management

What Does Interoperability Mean?

Interoperability is the essential factor in building the infrastructure to create, transmit, store, and manage health-related information.[2] In the context of health IT interoperability, standards must be employed to meet the information sharing needs across care settings, providers, patients, and population health environments. The ability for computer systems to talk to each other, share information, and understand what is being shared is the fundamental interoperability notion. It is through the interoperable exchange of health information that expected decreases in costs (by decreasing duplicative tests, improving administrative efficiencies, increasing access to patient clinical results and information to decrease repetitive input) and increases in quality (by decreasing errors related to lack of information such as allergic reactions to medications or current medication lists and increasing a patient's access to their health information) are expected to be realized.

The complexity of adopting interoperable health IT standards is not that there are limited health IT standards, but rather that there are too vast a number of standards. In addition to overlaps in health IT standards coverage, there are also gaps. To address the fundamental need for harmonized health IT standards to enable the exchange of health information, several public and private initiatives were enacted. Among these efforts was the National Health IT Agenda initiative launched by the President of the United States in 2004.

The National Health IT Agenda

In 2004, President Bush called for widespread adoption of the EHR within 10 years, and in his State of the Union address, stated that by computerizing health records, we can avoid dangerous medical mistakes, reduce costs, and improve care. To stimulate activities toward this vision, the president signed Executive Order 13335 establishing the Office of the National Coordinator for Health IT (ONC). The President, through the National Health IT Agenda, envisioned a health care system that puts the needs of the patient first, is more efficient, and cost-effective. The President's plan was based on the following tenets:

- Health information will follow consumers so that they are at the center of their own care.
- Consumers will be able to choose physicians and hospitals based on clinical performance results made available to them.
- Clinicians will have a patient's complete medical history, accessible computerized ordering systems, and electronic reminders.

- Quality initiatives will measure performance and drive quality-based competition in the industry.
- Public health and bioterrorism surveillance will be seamlessly integrated into care
- Clinical research will be accelerated and postmarketing surveillance will be expanded.

To achieve these goals, several activities were initiated and contracts awarded by ONC. These included the development of a National Health IT strategic framework and the establishment of the American Health Information Community (AHIC) that would set the priorities for information exchange. Since 2006, AHIC identified approximately 26 priority areas associated within three perspectives. These perspectives include Consumer, Provider, and Population Health. HITSP received these priorities as value cases and harmonized, approved, and recommended interoperability standards. The Health Information Security and Privacy Collaboration (HISPC) was responsible for addressing privacy and security policy questions affecting interoperable health information exchange. The Certification Commission for Healthcare Information Technology (CCHIT) performs certification of EHR systems, and the Nationwide Health Information Network (NHIN) develops and implements requirements to provide a secure, nationwide, interoperable health information infrastructure. In 2009, President Obama signed ARRA into law, thus committing to continuing the adoption of health IT through funding in his economic stimuli plan (www.recovery.gov). AHIC has transitioned to federal advisory committees called the HIT Policy Committee and the HIT Standards Committee, and the earlier use case process used to illustrate priority areas was renamed value cases.

The Standards Adoption Process

Through the National Health IT Agenda and HITSP harmonization framework, a process for adopting health IT standards was established. As a cooperative partnership between the public and private sectors, HITSP was formed for the purpose of harmonizing and integrating standards that meet clinical and business needs for sharing information among organizations and systems (http://www.hitsp.org/). This harmonization process, as noted in Fig. 13.1, starts with identifying priority areas to be illustrated in value cases. These value cases were prioritized and provided to HITSP who engaged the appropriate technical committees for requirements analysis, standards selection, and development of interoperability specifications portrayed in Fig. 13.2.

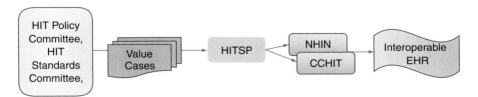

Fig. 13.1 Components of the National Health IT Agenda

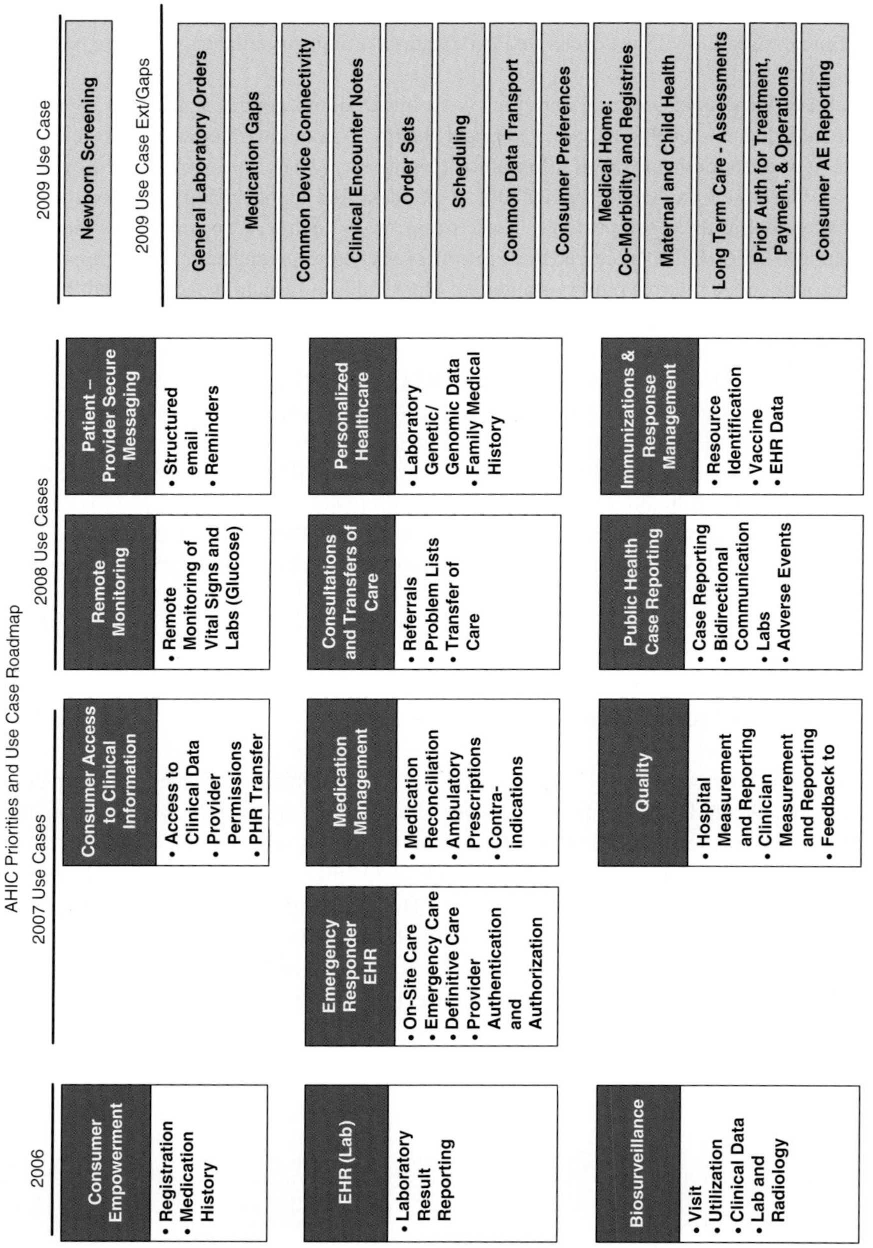

AHIC Priorities and Use Case Roadmap

2009 Use Case

Newborn Screening

2009 Use Case Ext/Gaps

General Laboratory Orders

Medication Gaps

Common Device Connectivity

Clinical Encounter Notes

Order Sets

Scheduling

Common Data Transport

Consumer Preferences

Medical Home:
Co-Morbidity and Registries

Maternal and Child Health

Long Term Care - Assessments

Prior Auth for Treatment,
Payment, & Operations

Consumer AE Reporting

2008 Use Cases

Patient – Provider Secure Messaging
- Structured email
- Reminders

Remote Monitoring
- Remote Monitoring of Vital Signs and Labs (Glucose)

Personalized Healthcare
- Laboratory Genetic/Genomic Data
- Family Medical History

Consultations and Transfers of Care
- Referrals
- Problem Lists
- Transfer of Care

Immunizations & Response Management
- Resource Identification
- Vaccine
- EHR Data

Public Health Case Reporting
- Case Reporting
- Bidirectional Communication
- Labs
- Adverse Events

2007 Use Cases

Consumer Access to Clinical Information
- Access to Clinical Data
- Provider Permissions
- PHR Transfer

Medication Management
- Medication Reconciliation
- Ambulatory Prescriptions
- Contra-indications

Quality
- Hospital Measurement and Reporting
- Clinician Measurement and Reporting
- Feedback to

Emergency Responder EHR
- On-Site Care
- Emergency Care
- Definitive Care
- Provider Authentication and Authorization

2006

Consumer Empowerment
- Registration
- Medication History

EHR (Lab)
- Laboratory Result Reporting

Biosurveillance
- Visit
- Utilization
- Clinical Data
- Lab and Radiology

Fig. 13.2 HITSP interoperability specification roadmap

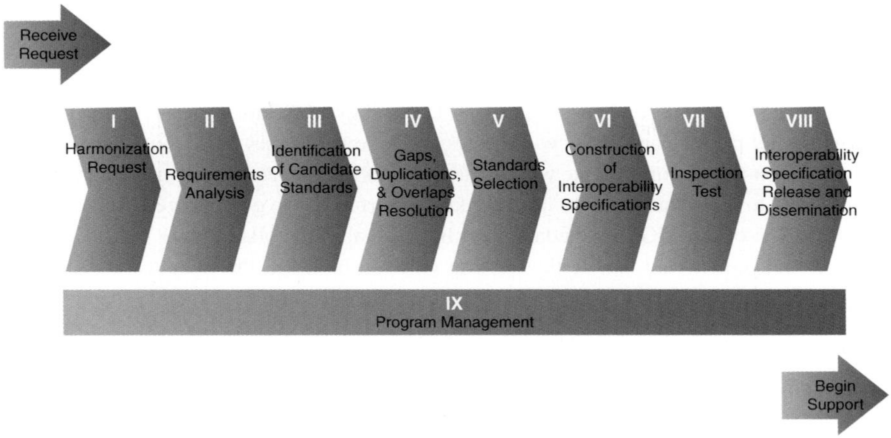

Fig. 13.3 HITSP harmonization framework

   The HITSP interoperability specifications also identify where there are standards gaps and overlaps in addressing the value case and provide suggested steps for addressing these issues if unresolved during the interoperability specification development process shown in Fig. 13.3.

   Once standards were approved by the HITSP Panel, they were presented to the U.S. Secretary of the Department of Health and Human Services (HHS) where they were accepted, and then after a year of testing and refinement, the standards were recognized by the HHS Secretary. The significance of standards recognition is that according to Executive Order 13410 signed by President Bush in August 2006, federal agencies administering or sponsoring federal health programs must implement any and all relevant recognized interoperability standards. These standards have also become part of the certification process for EHRs and networks. Progress is currently being made toward adoption of these national standards. For example, the Boston Medical Center Ambulatory Electronic Medical Record (EMR) which connects to community partners in the city of Boston and surrounding areas has four different types of EMRs with 12 of the community health care centers electronically exchanging health information. HITSP interoperability specifications are the foundation for this platform that has moved health information exchange beyond sharing lab data only to including multiple patient data components of the EHR (http://www.himss.org/ASP/himssNewsHome.asp).

The Role of Nursing

Throughout the standards development, harmonization, and adoption process, it is essential that nurses and other key stakeholders are involved to ensure that the essential data structures, concepts, and content are addressed, and that health IT is appropriately leveraged to support safe, efficient, effective patient care. Nurses' acceptance of EHR use can be affected by many factors, including system reliability, accessibility, and impact on workflow.[4] Health

IT standards and interoperability are foundational elements for enabling the effective and appropriate use of information technology across the care spectrum.[5] The TIGER Standards and Interoperability Collaborative is one of nine TIGER Collaboratives that worked to ensure that all nurses are educated in using technology and informatics to deliver safer, higher-quality patient care (http://www.tigersummit.com). Nurses need consistent training and education to feel comfortable with the use of information technology in their everyday practice and to understand how to leverage key opportunities to get involved.

The vision of the TIGER Standards and Interoperability Collaborative was to support nursing engagement and enable the nursing voice to be heard throughout the standards adoption process and national health IT activities. This vision states that:

- All nurses will understand the importance of health IT standards and interoperability on the delivery of safe, effective, efficient, and patient-centered care.
- All nurses will understand how to become engaged in the health IT standards adoption efforts to ensure the nursing voice is represented and included.

While there are many opportunities for nurses to get involved, a basic understanding of the process and importance of these activities and the mechanism for engagement is lacking. As a part of its goals, the TIGER Standards and Interoperability Collaborative set about to address these needs.[6] Through this Collaborative's efforts and those of its associated work-groups, the following activities have been addressed:

- Catalog the most relevant health IT standard adoption efforts
- Create tutorials that educate nurses on the basics and value of standards and interoperable systems
- Develop awareness campaigns
- Collect case studies and examples that illustrate the importance of health IT
- Develop a standards and interoperability collaboration website

The workgroups have created information modules, useful tools, and practical resources including tutorials and case studies that are now available to promote nursing involvement in and understanding of health IT standards and interoperability efforts.

The leadership of nurses who play key roles in national health IT standards activities was important to the success of this effort. For example, in order to mentor nurses in how to participate in the public comment periods convened by various health IT standards organizations, facilitated sessions for nurses were held using web-conferencing capability. Nurse leaders led these virtual sessions, describing the comment process and guiding the review of documents and submission of comments so that participants could more easily understand how to provide feedback, thus sharing their knowledge and experience.

Understanding the Benefits of Standards and Interoperability

Nursing was at the forefront in the development of standardized terminologies that represent the content of patient care delivery. As we move into a time of realizing the goals of an EHR that is interoperable and creates secondary data for research, the importance of

Table 13.1 Learning objectives of standards and interoperability for nurses

Definition and technology	Understand what informatics is and why technology and informatics are important to improve patient safety and the quality of health care
Standards	Understand the source for multiple health care information technology standards that are necessary for collecting, reusing, and exchanging data and information among multiple health care professionals
Interoperability	Understand the benefits of the interoperability of patient data, information, and knowledge for patient safety and quality
Data use	Be able to document coded nursing concepts and values using the international reference information model which facilitates the organized collection, association, storage, and exchange of patient information
Workflow use	Be able to document and link nursing concepts for nursing process by using the American Nurses Association's recognized reference and interface terminologies and evidence-based practices
Information use	Be able to identify when data quality and integrity have been jeopardized from altered use of valid and reliable patient assessment instruments or by missing or inaccurate documentation necessary to calculate/score a patient finding. (i.e., Glasgow Coma Scale, Children's Coma Scale, NIH Stroke Scale, Geriatric Assessment Scale, Apgar Scale, Barthel Index, Aldreti Scales, Beck II Depression Inventory, Braden Scale, Morse Fall Risk score)
Knowledge use	Be able to access the evidence-based knowledge resources for definitions of concepts, clarifying instructions on their use, currency and primary source references, and other educational or research evidence regarding population-specific details for decision making
Clinical decision support	Understand applied clinical decision support mechanisms within an interdisciplinary practice and appropriately respond to clinical decision support prompts and messages to close the loop

this foundation of standards is emphasized. While nurses may use and generate standards-based data and information in their efforts to document, research, and deliver patient care, an understanding of the benefit of standards and interoperability is frequently lacking. Through its efforts over the past several years, the TIGER Health IT Standards Tutorials Workgroup 2 set about to provide this basic understanding of standards, the benefits of interoperability, and the role of the nurse in using, promoting, and developing standards and interoperable systems. Table 13.1 provides an overview of the workgroup's objectives and identifies learning modules that will be developed over time.

Call to Action

All stakeholders must work together to ensure that health IT standards are adopted in EHR systems. Nurses should take a lead role in assuming their professional responsibility for engaging in the development and adoption of those standards needed to achieve widespread health information exchange. The TIGER Standards and Interoperability

Collaborative developed an action plan to support nursing engagement and to enable the nursing voice to be heard.[7] The Call to Action states that:

- To ensure safe, efficient, and quality care, nurses must be advocates for patient-consented, secure, and reliable exchange of health information
- Collaboration across professional disciplines, health care organizations, and society is necessary to achieve our collective goal of improving care delivery through use of interoperable electronic health records
- For the betterment of clinical practice and the profession, nurses must embrace collaboration and build a consensus agreement regarding standardization of nursing language
- Nurses have a professional responsibility to be engaged in standards development, harmonization, and implementation activities, including encouraging adoption of and patient engagement in Personal Health Records and Electronic Health Records
- Nurses should encourage collaboration to achieve interoperable health information exchange for clinical research and education
- Nurses should perform environmental scanning for lessons learned from use of emerging technologies in other industries such as communications, banking, and retail
- Nurses must ensure ongoing collaboration across all nursing specialties regarding adoption of interoperable standards for health information exchange

As we work to address the agenda of the new Administration, there are many questions ahead. However, if health care reform is at the forefront of our national conversation, it is likely that the National Health IT Agenda and the efforts of these initiatives will continue to be leveraged to provide a foundation for use of EHR systems across a nationwide network. While standards-based health information exchange is not the sole solution for broad scale health care reform, it does provide a foundation for achieving many of health care reform's largely accepted goals, such as improving access, cost, and quality of health care, while empowering consumers in their health care decisions and ensuring the privacy and security of personal health information. Nurses must be at the table to inform these discussions. This Call to Action provides a template for how nursing engagement can be achieved.

Opportunities for Involvement

The various components of the National Health IT Agenda offer numerous opportunities for involvement including participation on boards, panels, workgroups, and technical committees and by providing public comments as input to regulations and other draft documents. These opportunities are avenues for nurses to ensure that the nursing perspective is not only represented, but also addressed. Nurses should prepare themselves to contribute to these discussions by attending relevant conferences and webinars, reading journal articles and white papers, and reaching out to their peers. Seeking membership in professional organizations that provide needed resources and focus on standards and interoperability related activities is another avenue for getting involved. Participation opportunities are summarized in the Standards Catalogue, which also provides web site links to learn more (http://tigerstandards.pbworks.com/Work+Group+1).

By becoming informed, working together, and sharing their wisdom, nurses will have an impact on this unfolding vision to advance quality care and reduce costs, thereby improving upon the past through standards and interoperability.

References

1. Agency for Healthcare Research and Quality. Medical Errors: The Scope of the Problem. Fact sheet, Publication No. AHRQ 00-P037, Rockville. http://www.ahrq.gov/qual/errback.htm; 2000.
2. National Alliance for Health Information Technology. Defining Key Health Information Technology Teams. http://nahit.org/images/pdfs/HITTermsFinalReport_051508.pdf; 2008.
3. American National Standards Institute. HITSP Glossary. Reference 20080926 Version 1.2. Submitted to Health Information Technology Standards Panel. http://publicaa.ansi.org/sites/apdl/hitspadmin/Reference%20Documents/HITSP%20Glossary.pdf; 2008.
4. Kossman SP, Scheidenhelm SL. Nurses' perceptions of the impact of electronic health records on work and patient outcomes. *Comput Inform Nurs*. 2008;26(2):69-77.
5. Westra BL, Delaney CW, Konicek D, et al. Nursing standards to support the electronic health record. *Nurs Outlook*. 2008;56(5):258-266.
6. Sensmeier J, Halley EC. Standards and Interoperability Collaborative Summary Report, TIGER Initiative; 2009 www.tigersummit.com.
7. Martin KS, Sensmeier J. Participating in national standards initiatives: a call to action. *Nurs Outlook*. 2009;57(1):65-67.

Usability and Clinical Application Design

14

Nancy Staggers and Michelle R. Troseth

> *The first accountability of a great leader is to know reality*
> *Max DePree*[1]

The reality for nurses is that health information technology (HIT) is not designed to support their work or thought processes. Products with good clinical design would support nurses every day in their practices. The current HIT systems that clinicians use were originally intended for finance, laboratory, or other ancillary functions that do not support professional practice at the point of care.

More important, a compelling vision and a strong voice are absent for what nurses need most. Information technology should provide evidence-based, patient-centric technology that allows interdisciplinary collaboration at the point of care wherever the point of care is located. HIT should be an enabler vs. a barrier for care. *To redefine reality, nurses must first understand the significance of usability and clinical application design that can shape the future of the products nurses use every day.*

The significance of usability and clinical application design was identified as a top priority for nurses at the Technology Informing Education Reform (TIGER) Summit in late 2006. The TIGER Summit gathered nurses from government, service, education, and informatics to set a 10-year vision and 3-year action plan. During the TIGER Summit, the participants identified two critical and interdependent pillars to be further defined and acted upon:

Informatics design: Evidence-based, interoperable intelligent systems that support education and practice to foster quality care and safety.
Information technology: Smart, people-centered affordable technologies that are universal, usable, useful, and standards-based.

These two critical components led to the development of the TIGER Usability and Clinical Application Design Collaborative to further define key concepts, patterns and trends, and recommendations to HIT vendors and practitioners to assure usable clinical systems at the point of care. This chapter provides a summary of a year's worth of intense work by this Collaborative along with additional supporting information and urgency related to the topic.

N. Staggers (✉)
School of Nursing, University of Maryland, Baltimore, MD, USA
e-mail: staggers@son.umaryland.edu

M.J. Ball et al. (eds.), *Nursing Informatics*,
DOI: 10.1007/978-1-84996-278-0_14, © Springer-Verlag London Limited 2011

Although design is an attribute of usability, how design is applied to the clinical applications used at the point of care is key to support safe, quality care. The Collaborative studied usability, application design, and their interdependencies and integrated them into their final recommendations:

- Usability and its goals must
  - Be informed by and/or positively transform nursing workflow
  - Include systems designed using known principles and processes
  - Include work with system developers to maximize clinical system effectiveness
- Clinical application design and/or its goals must
  - Support evidence-based practice (EBP)
  - Enable collaborative and interdisciplinary care
  - Provide seamless access to published literature and knowledge
  - Support the creation of new knowledge (knowledge discovery)
  - Speed the translation of research into practice

For the TIGER Vision to be realized, the profession must educate itself on usability and key clinical application design principles. This education along with strong advocacy from nursing professionals will determine how well evidence and informatics are integrated into day-to-day practice. The need to be clear and provide strong advocacy was recently highlighted in the United States when the American Recovery and Reinvestment Act (ARRA) was signed on 17 February 2009, with significant funding to accelerate the National HIT Agenda for those that met "meaningful use" criteria. What the Tiger Initiative via this Collaborative has identified essentially is that meaningful *use* will require good *usability and clinical application design* to achieve the large scale adoption by nurses, the largest group of the health care workforce. Formal comments from TIGER were submitted to the Office of the National Coordinator for Healthcare Information Technology (ONC) on "Meaningful Use;" also several other nursing leadership groups to assure the needs of nursing as knowledge-workers and frontline care givers were heard. It is our hope that the findings and recommendations in this chapter will help nurses from education and practice speak to the role of usability and clinical application design in HIT adoption.

What Is Usability?

Medical professionals have been trained to expect that some things just do not work, and they should devise ways to work around them, rather than notifying managers to change the system. Wears and Perry[2]

The lack of user friendliness is the key barrier to user acceptance. Staggers and Kobus[3]

The origins of usability and its related concepts include psychology, engineering, and computer science. The essence of usability is to design tools and computer applications that match humans and their specific tasks (activities) for specific environments. Usability principles are applied widely outside health arenas; health care has been slow in adopting these important principles, resulting in computer applications and technology that fit poorly into nurses' work. However, more recent literature acknowledges the importance of usability in product design.[4-6]

Specific Definitions

Usability is one aspect of "human factors," (HFs) a broad term about the interrelationships among humans, their tools, tasks, and environments. Related concepts are pictured in Fig. 14.1.

HFs is the study of interactions among people, the tools people use, and the environments in which they use them. Researchers emphasize the importance of understanding human capabilities and limitations and how these fit with the design of tools for work (or play) in various environments. HFs include broad topics such as the layout of the controls in a car to match a petite driver, how the light switches in a room map to the lights they turn on, or designing an effective method to assure an accurate sponge count in an operating room.

Ergonomics is the physical design and implementation of equipment, tools, and machines related to human safety, comfort, and convenience. Ergonomics principles are used to determine where equipment is placed in an ICU patient's room, which design of a computer mouse fits your hand best, or how well a wide new ski works in powder snow.

Human–computer interaction (HCI) is the study of how people design, implement, and use interactive computer systems and how these systems affect individuals, organizations, and society.[7] HCI principles include, among other things, how to design a computer screen

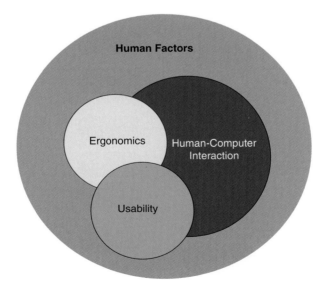

Fig. 14.1 The relationship of human factors terms. Figure adapted from Staggers[28] and reprinted with permission

(user interface) for nurses to detect adverse physiological events, the use of color consistently in an application for easier comprehension, or the flow of elements within a clinical system to support nurses' documentation.

Usability is the extent to which a product can be used by specific users in a specific context to achieve specific goals with effectiveness, efficiency, and satisfaction (adapted from ISO[8]). Usability is centered on the fit between the elements of users (nurses in this case), tasks, a context, and a product. Usability topics include how easy a product is to learn, to remember, to use in everyday work or play, and the effectiveness of a product for a specific task at hand. For example, usability can include how quickly nurses determine the fluid balance in a patient over the last 4 h using a new intake and output screen, how many errors nurses make when detecting physiological parameters in a current application or how easy a new infusion pump is to learn. Essentially, usability is about designing products that are easier to use by matching them more closely to users' (nurses') needs and requirements in particular settings.[9]

The Significance of Usability for Products and Systems

> We submit that usability is one of the major factors—possibly the most important factor— hindering widespread adoption of EMRs [Electronic Medical Records]. HIMSS[10]

Usability is crucial in the design, implementation, adoption, and use of clinical products. Good usability results in products that are effective, efficient, and satisfying to use, as Fig. 14.2 illustrates.

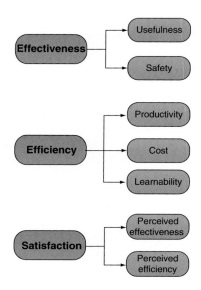

Fig. 14.2 Usability goals

More important, incorporating usability principles assists in the design of products that promote improved decision making as well as patient and practitioner safety. When product usability is poor, the outcomes can be as drastic as missed diagnoses, serious errors, patient mortality, and extreme user frustration to the point of not using a product or even clinical information systems deinstallation. A recent report on usability from the Health Information and Management Systems Society[10] bolsters these statements stating that usability has a strong, often direct relationship with clinical productivity, error rates, user fatigue, and user satisfaction.

Usability Goals

Core usability principles include:

- An early and consistent focus on users of the product
- Iterative design processes (multiple versions matched to users, tasks, and environments)
- Systematic product evaluations (with product users and metrics)

Major system users are identified early and representatives included in the design and evaluation process throughout the product's lifecycle. Including nurses early and often in system design assures that products are designed with nurses' goals, tasks (activities), and decision making in mind. Product design includes multiple versions with systematic evaluations to determine flaws in design. Usability evaluations allow nurses to give feedback to designers in a structured manner. The product is redesigned using nurses' feedback and retested. Several iterations (versions) assure that a product is effective, efficient, and satisfying to use. This process better ensures the product's fit to the users (nurses), tasks goals, and the environment at hand. As can be seen, usability and the design of clinical products are interrelated.

What Is Clinical Application Design?

Building on the sound principles of usability described above, Clinical Application Design addresses how we integrate usability principles with EBP, interdisciplinary collaboration, and knowledge discovery within a systems-thinking design, as shown in Fig. 14.3. In essence, we are applying usability and other design factors that are critical to making information technology the stethoscope of the twenty-first century.

First, EBP is an essential element of professional nursing practice today. Information technology and usability alone will not support EBP being lived at the point of care. EBP is defined as "the integration of best research evidence with clinical expertise and patient values".[11] Therefore, the HIT systems that nurses use must be able to integrate EBP into their design so nurses have the best research evidence and be able to apply their own clinical expertise as well as address the patient's values and situation at hand.

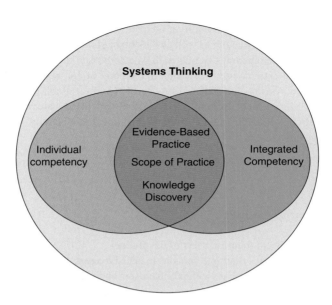

Fig. 14.3 Clinical application design essentials. Figure adapted from the CPM Resource Center (2008) and reprinted with permission

A recent report by the Institute of Medicine, *Knowing What Works in Healthcare: A Roadmap for the Nation,*[12] addresses how we must strengthen our capacity for assessing evidence on what is known and not known about "what works" in health care and calls for assessing evidence as well as developing and integrating evidence-based clinical practice guidelines into daily practice. Clinical application design supports the principles of EBP and the integration of evidence-based clinical practice guidelines and other EBP tools into the workflow and thoughtflow of the nurse and interdisciplinary team as well as speeds the translation of research into practice. Also, the integration of EBP with HIT solutions enables clinical decision support at the point of care. Nurses want decision support that is integrated into their workflow and within the context of the patient they are caring for in a way that is not disruptive, distractive, or annoying within the process of caring for patients.

The significance of this and the design of technology were highlighted in a recently published Joint Commission on Accreditation of Healthcare Organizations Sentinel Event Alert[13] on implementing health information and converging technologies. The report identifies that any form of technology may adversely affect the quality and safety of care if it is designed or implemented improperly or is misinterpreted. "Not only must the technology or device be designed to be safe, it must operate safely within a safe workflow process" (p. 1). As we design intelligent systems to support nurses as knowledge-workers by providing clinical decision support at the point of care, there are great lessons to learn from several studies on "alert fatigue" by poorly implemented computerized provider order entry (CPOE) systems that generate excessive numbers of drug safety alerts as well as unnecessary information alerts or complex documentation steps that lead to unsafe "workarounds" because they do not fit the context of the patient's situation and/or the clinician's thoughtflow and workflow.

Second, interdisciplinary collaboration must be supported by a design using systems-thinking principles. Interdisciplinary collaboration is supported by IT clinical application design that supports integrated scopes of practice. Integrated scopes of practice delineate the competencies and accountabilities of the different disciplines represented on a clinical team and can bring the highest level of interdisciplinary collaboration. Integrating scopes of practice means that clinicians from different disciplines work together as an interdisciplinary team, with each member understanding and relying on the competencies and accountabilities of the others.[14] Clarity on systems-thinking design, scope of practice, and integrated scopes of practice are all critical to leveraging IT to enable interdisciplinary collaborative care.

Last, clinical application design should foster techniques for data-mining to allow nurses to analyze and create new knowledge. This is critical in leveraging IT for advanced practice. A whole new world of knowledge discovery is waiting for nurse executives, educators, researchers, informaticists, and practitioners as we prepare the nursing workforce to have crucial conversations about usability and clinical application design to influence the future of nursing and health care IT.

Literature Review and Framework

The Collaborative completed a comprehensive literature search, collected case studies, and synthesized material into a framework comprising four areas:

- Determining clinical information requirements
- Safe and usable clinical design
- Usability evaluations
- HFs foundations

Building on work done by Gregory Alexander[15] for his dissertation research, the Collaborative updated the original literature review as part of the TIGER process. Each area of the resulting framework includes a description of the topic, its significance for nursing, key points about the subject, and recommendations for HIT vendors and point-of-care practitioners.

Literature Review and Analysis Process

In the first phase, Alexander used formal methods to perform a systematic literature review of the HFs and usability literature. Methods included article relevance assessments, data extraction, and data analysis.[16] The search included the following research databases: Cumulative Index of Nursing and Allied Health Literature (CINAHL), Ovid MEDLINE, PsycINFO, INSPEC, and the EBM Reviews: Health Technology Assessment Database (CLHTA) for the years 1980–2003. Substantial technology changes for devices and information systems before 1980 would make earlier references not pertinent. Key search terms used for the literature search included: HCI, HFs or Usability, health$ or health care or medical, and nurs$. Reference lists of publications were checked for additional references after the search was conducted. The search yielded 110 articles for analysis.

Alexander evaluated the articles meeting inclusion criteria using conceptual development methods described by Rodgers (2000). Excel spreadsheets were created to capture information describing HFs and usability in each article. The spreadsheets included concepts identified in the literature and their definitions. In all, 256 related terms were identified. Any relationships with other concepts were included to describe concepts, and origins of the concepts were extracted from the literature. Conceptual definitions were compared across different disciplines to determine if there were any conceptual differences, conflicting definitions, or if new concepts were being recognized by other professional disciplines. Theories used in HFs and usability literature were also identified. Data from Alexander's initial analysis of the literature were provided to the usability Collaborative working group for subsequent analysis.

The second phase of the literature review included updating Alexander's formal literature search, and the Collaborative performed a secondary analysis of the resulting data. Three HFs experts working with the TIGER Collaborative working group independently organized the 256 related HFs and usability terms from the literature into an existing framework derived from the Usability Engineering Lifecycle described by[17]:

- Human–Computer Interaction or Human Factors Theories
- Human Information Processing
- Information, Representation, and Visualization
- Hardware – input/output technologies
- Requirements Analysis
- Representational Analysis
- Functional Analysis
- User Analysis
- Task Analysis
- Environmental Analysis
- Usability Design
- Safety/Error prevention
- Usability Testing

The related terms were organized using an open source internet software package called Websort (http://websort.net), using a cluster analysis approach to sort and classify data. The output was a tree diagram, called a dendrogram, representing the combined input of the experts. The dendrogram represented a higher level classification schema for the related terms. Members of the Tiger Clinical Design and Usability Collaborative used the dendrogram and their related terms to further sort the literature into the usability engineering lifecycle categories.

Once the literature was classified into categories, workgroup members were assigned to the differing sections. Workgroup members identified key points from the articles in their section. These key points were then collated by workgroup leaders and used to develop the final recommendations.

Recommendations

Recommendation 1: Determine Clinical Information Requirements

Description. The purpose of analyzing clinical information requirements is to help developers understand users, their needs, and determine the demands of their work. Various analysis methods allow a complete description of the user population and their characteristics, including physical characteristics and abilities, users' goals, attributes of the work environment, typical activities or tasks, and current user experiences. Requirements analysis is important at the beginning of development activities to delineate the particular functions to be completed by the human-product-environment and tasks performed by humans to achieve their goals.[18]

Significance. Requirements analysis provides information to system designers about the users in particular, allowing the product to be developed with real users in mind. This process is known as "user-centered design." User-centered design encourages participation with users who are directly involved in the design process. An imperative exists for nurses to be codevelopers, participating in requirements analysis methods to create tools that support professional practice and can be used effectively, efficiently, and safely in our health care system.

Key points

- Requirements analysis is done by collecting data through observing the current workflow, interviewing end users (nurses and allied health) and management, and discussing the practice/business needs and desired goals to accomplish.
- Requirements are established to assure that a product will perform to certain standards. HFs research uses knowledge about the capabilities and limits of humans to guide the design of products, systems, and services.[19]
- Computers should be designed to match users' mental organization of work including internal representations including thought processes.
- The seven plus or minus two rule: The brain can process 5–9 items or chunks of information at any given moment.[20] This rule is still valid 50 years later!
- The human work environment must include not only the physical environment and the objects within it, but also psychological factors such as mental workload, stress levels, information flow, and group dynamics. Humans do not exist in isolation, but as part of an entire system.[21]
- When designing an interactive system, one of the basic problems is the allocation of tasks between the human and computer. An ingredient for solving the task allocation problem is the knowledge of the ways in which multiple tasks may interact and subsequently degrade or enhance the performance of the human or computers.[22]
- Task analysis, one way to determine requirements, quantifies complex patient care processes by recording physical activities or tasks of patient care including time measurements, information processes, communication strategies, and motion patterns. A task is an activity that includes an immediate purpose, a machine output or consequence of

action, and the human inputs, decisions, and outputs needed to accomplish the purpose. Task analysis is performed by recording the systems' response to each user action. The generated flowcharts and task descriptions can be used to document how certain actions of the system or user result in error.[23] Although task analysis can be a useful tool in understanding workflows, it may not adequately capture the complexity and the inter-relatedness of the clinical workflows and professional practice.

- Clinical decision-support tools should be integrated into workflow and clinical applications to avoid cognitive and/or task overload.

Recommendations for vendors

- Consider the requirements of different skill levels of practitioners. A novice nurse may need prompts and guidance more than an experienced nurse. Allow nurses to choose their own level of support
- Work directly with the organization's analysts and end users to validate requirements before building or customizing the product. As the product is being developed and/or customized, vendors should work with the organization to make sure that the specifications of the build are meeting their clinical and key stakeholder requirements
- Clinician representation on vendor development teams is critical. Recommend clinicians as vendor product managers to assure understanding of clinical needs and develop efficient and effective requirements
- Assure that requirements are written very clearly to avoid misinterpretation and clinical information requirements are met, particularly by developers (nonclinicians) who make hard-code designs
- Partner with strategic business partners to enhance core competencies outside of vendors' scope to meet the needs of end users and management

Recommendations for practitioners

- The requirements process should be owned by clinicians, not the information technology (IT) department or the vendor
- Clinicians must be involved in requirements development and should maintain and/or change the requirements to meet professional standards and legal requirements
- Physician, nurse, and allied health champions are critical in all phases of the project, beginning with requirements development and extending through systems maintenance
- Complete a workflow analysis for each user/department touching an electronic health record
- Workflow includes identifying who, what, where, when, and why by including specific participants, from whom information is being collected and with whom information is being shared
- Determine how systems will support evidence-based practice/research (EBP/EBR). Embed EBP into clinical screen design to access latest information at their fingertips (Clinical Decision Support) and support the continuum of novice to expert clinicians
- Include requirements for all desired reports during clinical information requirements development

- Clinicians need the ability to locate, manipulate, and aggregate documentation effectively and efficiently
- Use of text fields or "free text" should be used judiciously as will inhibit later analysis and knowledge development
- Work toward a common data dictionary if not using a standard one such as SNOMED CT®. Create an organizational policy to use one common language and standard abbreviations
- Include all areas in clinical information requirements – billing, medical records, unit secretaries, etc. – these areas are often forgotten until problems occur
- Determine the ease of customizing the system to meet clinical information needs, who should be responsible for those customizations, and the degree of simplicity required to make changes
- Include technical requirements for tools that ease the uploading and configuration required for desired results. An example from real world: "We recently had a department purchase a system with no IT input. They did not think of the technical implications, and the system did not have any kind of upload tool – all the rooms and beds, physician information, services (orders) and inventory had to be manually loaded, one at a time. One of the reasons the clinicians got the system was because the inventory and menu features were so cool – but they don't have it implemented all the way yet because of the technical work required!"
- Avoid the tendency to do a one-for-one replacement of existing paper forms. The reason is to avoid computerizing bad processes or creating poor workflow. All paper forms need to be analyzed, with a workflow analysis, and then reviewed by end users
- Consider the process for customization of the reports and the level of training/background required to write them. Vendor-only report design is likely to be redesigned later
- Interdisciplinary teams are most effective. Key players are nurses, pharmacists, physicians, social work, respiratory therapists, rehabilitation therapists (physical, occupational, and speech language), pastoral care, and dietitians for patient-centered systems
- Documentation should include a mandatory electronic signature that does not allow others to reopen and modify records
- An audit trail should allow the provider to track documentation in all areas to identify who performed what function at what time

Recommendation 2: Design Safe and Usable Clinical Information Technology

Description. Minimizing error is one of the primary goals of usability and HFs design. The majority of system errors occur due to a system flaw rather than a worker issue. Designing safer, more usable systems requires that users, developers, and subject matter experts work together throughout design processes leaving little room for interpretation about how technology should be designed and how workers/technology interact to complete work. System design processes should be based upon user characteristics, understanding problems encountered by users, human information processing abilities as users interact with products in a specific environment to complete their work at hand.

Significance. The design of safer, more usable systems is important because it facilitates error prevention and ensures that nurses provide the effective care (or other work) intended. Payoffs for using HFs approaches are fewer errors involving patients, health care personnel, and other users; decreased training cost; a better fit with the way nurses work and think; improved decision making; less time spent redesigning systems that fail to meet expectations, and greater user satisfaction. HFs approaches are very relevant to nursing today because of the penetration of advanced technologies in the clinical setting, greater complexity of patient care, the amount of information generated in settings, and the role litigation has on the cost of health care.

Key points

- Better systems must be developed to prevent errors and ensure that clinicians provide the effective care they intend to provide.[24]
- Systems should facilitate the application of scientific knowledge to practice and provide clinicians with the tools and supports necessary to deliver evidence-based care consistently and safely.[25]
- The systems approach encourages us to think about relationships between people and technology.[26]
- If the HF is taken into account, a tight fit between person and design can be achieved and the technology is more likely to fulfill its intended purpose.[26]
- Medical devices will be used safely and effectively only if the interaction of the operating environment, user capabilities, and device design is considered in the manufacturing of the device.[27]
- Health care has been slow to adopt usability techniques that have long been used by corporations outside health.[3]
- Technology designers often focus on technology alone and too little on how people perform with technology.[26]
- Incorporating HFs in the design of the clinical information systems allows for correct data entry, display, and interpretation; contributes to sound clinical decision making; and decreases the time it takes to complete tasks, training time, software rewrites, burden of support staff, and user frustration.[28]
- Users must work with designers to determine both effectiveness and efficiency of products and make redesign suggestions to enhance both of these usability goals.[28]

Key recommendations for vendors

- Clinical application development should be clinician-driven and not engineer-driven.
- Design with the end in mind: Make it easy to do the right thing and hard to do the wrong thing
- Highly usable products provide a consistent look and feel across all applications. Identify and/or develop a style guide for designers to design for consistency.
- Using a style guide consistent with industry standards to decrease development and training time. Following an industry standard makes a system appear more usable to the user.
- Consider color blindness, ergonomics, and other human capabilities and limitations in the design of end-user equipment.

- Consider the environment in which the technology will be used. Location, temperature, and surrounding objects will all affect the way technology will be used (or not) and how users create workarounds.
- Utilize evidence-based content sources and encourage clients to share best practices among each other.
- Assure that access to evidence-based information is integrated into the professional documentation in a logical, simple way that does not create multiple steps to access or document against within the context of the patient situation.
- Request information on how evidence-based information provided by a vendor/third-party sources is updated and the implications for the organization and end users.

Recommendations for practitioners

- Think about organization-wide processes: Standardize common processes such as documentation, medication times, order sets, and alerts before EHR system design.
- Consider the trade-offs for using standard templates. Templates save time, standardize assessment expectations, and allow easy documenting; however, practitioners can ignore template parameter details over time. They can easily document inaccurate information, e.g., patient comes in comatose and field saying "alert and oriented X 3" is not edited. Assure user understands their professional accountability and decision making that is not dependent on the clinical application design
- Allowing free text medication orders and/or allergies can contribute to errors. For example, drug/allergy information should be chosen from a formulary.
- Partner with engineers to assess the robustness of wireless networks and devices. Assuring adequate technical infrastructure is critical to prevent issues such as system unreliability, downtime, and "deadspace" that can interrupt patient care and clinician workflow.
- Have a back-up plan for network downtime or when devices cannot access the network.
- Failure mode effects analysis is a valuable although time-consuming exercise. It is a step-by-step process analysis to identify potential risks and mitigation steps. One facility used this technique when physicians were canceling and reordering medications, but not altering the start times. The outcome was that patients received double doses of meds for 1 day.
- Ergonomics should be evaluated for each device (e.g., carts, hand-helds, workflow fit, etc.), so that the device fits the workflow rather than dictating it.

Recommendation 3: Conduct Usability Evaluations

Description. Once users and their requirements are understood, prototypes of products can be designed or systems redesigned. Evaluations are conducted to determine if humans can interact and perform functions safely and easily.[18] A usability evaluation is the process of having users interact with the product or system to identify design flaws not noticed by designers. Evaluations are conducted early in the design cycle and throughout iterative designs of the product. Usability evaluation helps determine excessive psychological or physical loads when humans interact with the product; ease to learn the product; the impact on efficiency, productivity, error-generation and job satisfaction; and the ease to remember how to use the system over several interactions.[18]

Significance. Usability evaluations ensure that products are safe for nurses to use, efficiently designed for nursing activities and safe for patients. Evaluations can detect design flaws early in product development.

Key points

- A user-centered design process is driven by the needs and characteristics of users and involves them in feedback sessions (usability evaluations).
- Usability evaluations can be formal or informal.
- Usability evaluations include assessing factors that make work easy or hard.[2]
- The purpose of usability evaluations is to detect flaws in the fit between the product design, the user, and the environment.
- Actual users should interact with products during usability evaluations.
- Usability experts should also validate and test products at frequent intervals to identify defects and areas for improvement.
- User-centered design is an iterative process where prototypes are developed, users provide feedback, and products are improved.
- Usability experts should also validate and test products at frequent intervals to identify defect and areas for improvement. Are there too many clicks, colors?
- Evaluators should define specific goals for each usability evaluation, create a test plan, and systematically capture and analyze data from the interaction with representative users.
- Examples of evaluation objectives are: increased efficiency/productivity; increased reliability; minimum training resource costs; improved habitability; and user appeal and flexibility.[19]
- One particularly useful way to understand users' workflow and environment is through observation.
- Usability evaluations occur early and often in the development process. User feedback from evaluation is used to redesign the product to make it more effective, safe, efficient, and satisfying to use.
- Feedback sessions and focus groups should contain homogeneous users because each has unique needs and workflow.
- Usability evaluations are completed prior to the general release of the application.
- Select the amount, type, and structure of information presentation to the user under both normal and emergency conditions to optimize performance and maintain human confidence in the process.[22]
- Formal evaluation methods should be quantifiable. Note the kind of performance that must occur and how it will be measured.[19]
- Test for situational awareness in decision making. This accounts for all the interactions between a person and a system, together with the conditions that must be satisfied if the interactions are to be effective.[19]
- HFs engineering can be used as a framework for constructive thinking to help health care teams perform patient safety analyses.[23]

Recommendations for vendors

- Change introduced late in the systems development cycle is more costly than change introduced early.
- Conduct safety and error testing with every application offered. The robustness of testing depends on the application, for example, the care plan on a medical-surgical floor may not demand as much robust testing as would medication order entry for neonatal intensive care unit (NICU).
- Testing is not the sole responsibility of organizations implementing product(s). Usability testing should be a part of every vendor's processes.
- Develop a formal team to be responsible for usability evaluations of all products.
- Assess usability early in development of your product. Solid design is accomplished through user-centered design, iterative product design, and systematic evaluations. This includes observations of real users interacting with vendor products and anticipating potential user problems.
- Plan on usability evaluations being included in customer contracts.
- Prototype testing should be a line item built into every project plan and should occur at intervals as the product is being created.
- Designers should understand the reasoning beyond workflow to generate innovative designs that can better meet user needs in surprisingly delightful ways (e.g., professional practice, interdisciplinary integration, cues and information to guide care specific to patient situation, excellent patient summaries based on documentation and critical data, etc.).
- Focus most iterative design time on high-risk areas. High-risk areas include drastically new features such as computerized provider order entry (CPOE), functions that impact patient safety, or with users who might significantly impair product success and/or have high standards of acceptance.
- Iterative design can be most cost effective for high-risk areas.
- Recognize and address designer confirmation bias. Confirmation bias is where the designer seeks out views that already support their own views or design direction. Confirmation bias is more often found in feedback sessions and focus groups. Ways to prevent this are to: (1) have more than one person ask questions of the group, (2) have a team debriefing of the information presented by the focus group, (3) provide a transcript of the comments made in the focus group to discourage misinterpretation, or (4) not have the designer drive the feedback session.
- As part of the design process, analyze similar systems to understand their successes and failures and how that knowledge may impact your design.
- Once design alternatives have been identified, pick the best design with appropriate trade-offs. Trade-offs includes prioritization of the feature for the market, impact to future designs, and overall development effort.

Key recommendations for practitioners

- Have usability evaluations included in the contract with your vendor.
- Include usability evaluations in your project plan, test as you build.

- Have the vendor provide usability evaluation data for previously developed products.
- Users who defined requirements should test the product to assure that it meets their needs.
- End users need to have major role in testing along with clinical informatics specialists. Analysts can identify special situations during testing.
- Include printing the patient record as part of the test plan and test of ease to print, ease to read, ability to sequence events.
- Count the number of "clicks" and scrolling needed to complete common processes.
- Include typical scenarios to test patient safety functions, for example, scenarios that validate clinical decision-support tools are working within the appropriate workflow plan on extensive testing after the system build is "frozen" before going live to make sure one "fix" did not break something else.
- Frequently assess for ways to improve the system/reporting/staff education.

Recommendation 4: Construct the Foundations in Human Factors

Description. This field is derived from multiple disciplines including engineering, psychology, information science, and aviation. Experts emphasize the need to understand human capabilities and limitations as people perform work, the design of tools such as medical devices that fit users, and work processes that enable safer, more efficient ways of performing work.

Significance. HFs helps us understand human behavior and complex decision making, performance in high stress jobs, capabilities and limitations of the human body, resource utilization in high workload areas, and human error in the system. If HFs are taken into account, a tighter fit between people and system processes can be achieved resulting in improved decision-making capability, less stress on the job, enhanced performance including error prevention, enhanced human capability and fewer barriers to get work done, improved use of staff, and safer systems.

Key points about HFs

- The purpose of the HFs field is to promote the discovery and exchange of knowledge concerning the characteristics of human beings that are applicable to the design of systems and devices of all kinds.[29]
- HFs is the study of the interrelationships between humans, the tools they use, and the environments in which they live and work.[28,30,31]
- HF is also the application of behavioral principles to the design, development, testing, and operation of equipment and systems.[32]
- HF engineering (HFE) is directed at human behavior, human performance, human capabilities/limitations, human utilization, and human safety and health.[27,30,33]
- Ergonomics, usability engineering, and user-centered design can be considered closely related to or synonymous terms.[34]

- Three classifications of human errors include:
  - *Technical errors,* in which the action taken is not the action intended, arise from deficiencies of technical skill or from poor HFs design in the equipment or apparatus involved
  - *Judgmental errors,* in which action represents a bad decision, arise from lapses in training or poorly developed decision-making skills
  - *Monitoring and vigilance failures* in which the essence is a failure to recognize or act upon visible data requiring a response.[35]
- Usability addresses specific issues of human performance during computer interactions within a particular context. Usability goals may be expressed in terms of overall effectiveness, efficiency, and satisfaction concerning users' interactions with information systems.[28]
- Three axioms of usability: (1) an early emphasis on users in the design, development, and purchase of systems; (2) iterative design; (3) empirical usability measures or observations of users and information systems.[28]

Key recommendations for vendors

- Use International Standards Organization guidelines for usability (ISO 9241-11).
- Design to Section 503 of the Rehabilitation Act of 1973. Always have an option to enlarge text size for easier viewing by individuals.
- Consider physical and sensory capacities such as vision, hearing, and manual dexterity of the user population. Consider how design factors can impact human performance such as the differences in the sounds of different alarms, requirements for reaching controls, and legibility of the displays. The designer needs to take advantage of well-established population stereotypes such as using the color red to signal danger.
- Allow for end-user design of screen configurations. For example, have a user-definable home page that would allow the user to determine what order to enter assessment or other data so that user's preferred workflow could be facilitated.
- Create a "documentation preview" mode that allows the clinician to see a narrative version of their point and click documentation. Consider the limitations of human capability that needs to be taken into consideration when designing interfaces.
- Designers must be careful with the use of color because of color blindness and object-based proximity as shown in the Stroop test. The Stroop test shows that if there are multiple dimensions belonging to an object and one of these dimensions is irrelevant, there will be a disruption in performance. It shows that reaction time is lengthened if the wrong word for color (blue) is printed in a red card.
- Color that stands out can be processed quickly for decision making.
- Make sure colors with symbolic meanings are used consistently with their meaning. For example, red means stop or danger, amber is warning, green means go or safety.
- Each device needs to be tested by vendor to ensure that the application looks and functions properly (see Usability Testing section of this report). The devices should be tested in a clinical setting and additional adjustments may be made.

- Vendors need to come to the facility site and observe workflow. The focus is on clinician workflow with the vendor assisting the facility to meet their desired state.
- Usability of specific software is only one factor that affects the overall usability of a solution used by clinicians in a particular health care agency. Other factors include hardware, training, system set-up, interoperability, clinical decision-support tools, and usability of other software products in the solution.
- The product development team, from conceptualization to the delivery of the product, should be a cross-functional team with varied backgrounds and expertise. The cross-functional team should include software engineers, usability experts, analysts, documentation experts, education experts, quality experts, domain experts, and other clinicians who are domain experts for clinical software applications.
- Computer designers and clinicians speak different languages, are socialized in different roles, work in different environments, and have different motivators. Clinicians on the development team may be employees, consultants, product reviewers, members of focus groups, members of test teams, or clinicians working at clinical trial sites. This rich set of sources helps to provide the diversity of domain knowledge needed for usable products.
- The closer the clinicians are to the development process, the more likely it is that the software will meet the user's needs. Development time is lost if nonclinicians must spend time getting answers to clinical questions or fixing software that nonclinicians developed without appropriate user input.

Key recommendations for practitioners

- Insist that your informatics team includes a clinical informaticist or other team member with knowledge about HFs and usability principles.
- Educate yourself and your peers on HFs and usability principles; bring voice to addressing these principles in appropriate venues.
- Consider the workspace requirements for humans to complete their work.
- Be educated about ergonomics principles including how to position computers on wheels/walls or desk top to promote good posture.
- Devise methods to involve end users in product design and implementation such as focus groups or observations to promote usable products and decrease resistance.
- Advocate for "single sign on" to limit the number of password/usernames one needs to remember per user/system.
- Evaluate device attributes such as battery life, use on all shifts (dimmer displays at night), display size, and purchase a variety of devices for best fit to tasks.

Case Studies

The Collaborative collected case studies that illustrated usability and clinical application design. These examples were intended to demonstrate best practice exemplars as well as challenging cases. From the more than 30 case studies received, the Collaborative identified factors influencing their success or failure.

Best Practice Exemplars

Factor 1. Involvement of end users throughout the entire process

- System selection
- System design
- System testing
- Training end users
- System implementation
- Postimplementation optimization

Factor 2. Integration with existing systems

- Clinician acceptance and system adoption
- Accuracy (fewer transcription errors, avoids duplicate documentation)
- Patient safety due to synchronized, accurate information
- Timeliness of information collection, reporting, and use

In the successful clinical applications, user and key stakeholder involvement began early in the project with system requirements development and system selection. Throughout the entire process, clinicians worked with developers to create definitions, wording, and graphics that represented professional practice and workflow process. At the same time, vendors took the time to understand the workflow and processes of the end users, including how they see or "view" the information.

Challenging Case Studies

The case studies identified as "challenging" exhibited a number of factors that were essentially the reverse of the above:

- Lack of staff/end-user participation in selection and design
- Lack of end-user involvement in system tailoring, testing, and education
- Lack of staff involvement in identifying system requirements, including functionality and reporting
- Driven by timelines vs. what was going to best meet the clinician and organizational needs

In these cases, the resulting implementations evidenced

- More application and hardware problems
- Lower satisfaction from end users
- Excessive follow-up and fixes
- At one site, education post go-live pulled the application and is installing a different system

Nurses and their interdisciplinary colleagues need innovative technology to simplify their work and provide them clinical guidance for the safety of their patients. This kind of innovative technology includes usability and clinical application design principles.

Usability is the fit between system users, their work, and environments. Imperatives include engaging the users early and often in the clinical systems lifecycle; understanding users, their tasks, and their environments; and conducting usability testing and redesigning before implementation. These steps better assure smooth implementations and user adoption of complex clinical systems. Clinical application design meets systems-thinking requirements that are critical to the complex health care environments. Contemporary designs include EBP, interdisciplinary collaboration, and knowledge discovery.

Good usability and clinical application design are no longer choices, but a mandate to support safe, effective decision making. All nurses – practitioners, researchers, educators, and leaders – should become aware of these principles and give voice to them at every venue where it impacts end users and patient care. Nursing informatics specialists can help educate nurses about usability. Together, nurses and nursing informatics specialists can assure excellent clinical application design to meet point-of-care practice needs for the twenty-first century.

Case Study 1: A Usability and Clinical Application Design Challenge

A medical center implemented an EMR with orders, clinical documentation, and results retrieval to improve efficiencies and enhance patient safety in the perinatal units of a small medical center, including Labor and Delivery (L&D), NICU, and Newborn Nursery

Selection process

- The system was installed elsewhere in this integrated delivery network
- The executives wanted a fast 6-month installation at the maximum

Usability challenges

- Existing order sets and documents from other sites were not uploaded and tailored to this site. Clinicians were asked to input individual orders (not acceptable).
- Needed computer terminals were ordered late and arrived the day of go-live. Clinicians competed for working terminals at the nurses' stations
- Workflow among units was not considered or tested. Shared information such as mother's blood type and L&D information was not available to NICU or Newborn Nursery, causing confusion about potential patient safety issues
- Generic training was given because the site tailoring was not done. On go-live, users did not know where to locate information before it had changed in the lag between training and go-live

Outcomes

- The clinicians had to endure an unnecessarily painful implementation and its potential patient safety impacts
- Working out usability issues took months after go-live

Case Study 2: A Usability and Clinical Application Design Exemplar

Three separate acute care hospitals in a health care system in the southern United States wanted a new clinical system after having used various systems in the past.

Selection process

- A Clear Vision: The new system had to support all disciplines, CPOE, EBP, and clinical decision support at the point of care.
- An interdisciplinary team and leadership evaluated the system

Usability/design wins

- Selecting a system with a professional practice framework that was "pre-configured" to meet vision and team requirements as well as avoid cost and time requirements for design and build
- Multiple users analyzed the system: Bedside clinicians, ancillary departments; quality risk, legal, and management
- Users identified additional content needs. These were developed and tested before implementation
- The system was tested/validated for usability, design, and practice needs
- Education included practice changes along with how to use the system
- Developed a methodology to respond rapidly to end users

Outcomes

- Standardized practice in three different acute care hospitals in 15 months
- Significant improvement in core measures and nurse-sensitive outcomes

Acknowledgments   The authors wish to acknowledge the workgroup leaders and members of the Tiger Collaborative on Usability and Clinical Application Design for volunteering their time to study this important topic. Special recognition to Dr. Gregory Alexander for contributing his dissertation work and time for the rich literature review and analysis and to Donna Dulong, Executive Director of the Tiger Initiative, for her guidance, support, and tireless work.

References

1. DePree M. *Leadership is an Art*. New York: Doubleday; 1989.
2. Wears RL, Perry SJ. Human factors and ergonomics in the emergency department. *Ann Emerg Med*. 2002;40:206-212.
3. Staggers N, Kobus D. Comparing response time, errors, and satisfaction between text-based and graphical user interfaces during nursing order tasks 135. *JAMA*. 2000;7:164-176.
4. Ash JS, Sittig DF, Dykstra R, et al. The unintended consequences of computerized provider order entry: findings from a mixed methods exploration. *Int J Med Inform*. 2009;78(suppl 1): S69-S76.
5. Kushniruk A, Triola M, Stein B, et al. The relationship of usability to medical error: an evaluation of errors associated with usability problems in the use of a handheld application for prescribing medications. *Stud Health Technol Inform*. 2004;107(pt 2):1073-1076.
6. Stead W, Linn H. *Computational Technology for Effective Health Care: Immediate Steps and Strategic Directions*. Washington: National Academies; 2009.
7. Myers B, Hollan J, Cruz I. Strategic directions in human-computer interaction. *ACM Comput Surv*. 1996;28:794-809.
8. International Standards Organization. ISO, standard # 9241-11. Available at UsabilityNet http://www.usabilitynet.org/about.htm; 2006.
9. UsabilityNet. What is usability? http://www.usabilitynet.org/home.htm; 2006.
10. Health Information and Management Systems Society. Defining and Testing EMR Usability: Principles and Proposed Methods of EMR Usability Evaluation and Rating. http://www.himss.org/content/files/HIMSS_DefiningandTestingEMRUsability.pdf; 2009.
11. Sackett D, Strauss D, Richardson W, et al. *Evidence-Based Medicine: How to Practice and Teach EBM*. London: Churchill Livingstone; 2000.
12. Institute of Medicine. *Knowing What Works in Healthcare: A Roadmap for the Nation*. Washington: National Academy; 2008.
13. Joint Commission on Accreditation of Healthcare Organizations. Safely implementing health information and converging technologies. *Sentinel Event Alert*. 2008;(42):1-4.
14. Belmont C, Wesorick B, Jesse H, et al. *Clinical Documentation. Health Care Technology*, vol. 1. San Fransisco: Montgomery Research; 2003.
15. Alexander GL. *Human factors, automation, and alerting mechanisms in nursing home electronic health records*. Doctoral dissertation. Columbia: University of Missouri. http://edt.missouri.edu/Summer2005/Dissertation/AlexanderG-080105-D2928/; 2005.
16. Cochrane. *The Cochrane Manual*. Cochrane Collaboration; 2006.
17. Rodgers BL. Concept analysis: an evolutionary view. In: Knafl KA, ed. *Concept Development in Nursing*. 2nd ed. Philadelphia: Saunders; 2000.
18. Nielsen J. *Usability Engineering*. Cambridge: AP Professional; 1993.
19. Wickens CD, Lee JD, Liu Y, et al. *An Introduction to Human Factors Engineering*. 2nd ed. Upper Saddle River: Pearson Prentice Hall; 2004.
20. Nemeth CP. *Human Factors Methods for Design: Making Systems Human Centered*. Boca Raton: CRC; 2004.
21. Miller G. The magical number seven, plus or minus two: some limits on our capacity for processing information. *Psych Rev*. 1956;63:31-97.
22. Traub P. Optimising human factors integration in system design. *Engineering Manag J*. 1996;6:93-98.
23. Leveson NG. Software safety: why, what, and how. *Comput Surv*. 1986;18:125-163.
24. Potter P, Boxerman S, Wolf L, et al. Mapping the nursing process: a new approach for understanding the work of nursing. *J Nurs Admin*. 2004;34:101-109.

25. Leape LL, Berwick DM, Bates DW. What practices will most improve patient safety? Evidence based medicine meets patient safety. *JAMA*. 2002;288:501-507.
26. Institute of Medicine. *Crossing the Quality Chasm: A New Health System for the 21st Century*. Washington: National Academy; 2001.
27. Vicente K. *The Human Factor*. New York: Routledge; 2004.
28. Creedon MA, Malone TB, Dutra LA, et al. Human factors engineering approach to gerontechnology: development of an electronic medication compliance device. In: Graafmans J, Taipale V, Charness N, eds. *Gerontechnology, A Sustainable Investment in the Future*. Amsterdam: IOS; 1998.
29. Staggers N. Human factors: imperative concepts for information systems in critical care. *AACN Clin Issues*. 2003;14:310-319.
30. Bashshur RL, Lathan CE. Human factors and telemedicine. *Telemedicine J*. 1999;5:127-128.
31. Schneider PJ. Applying human factors in improving medication-use safety. *Am J Health Syst Pharm*. 2002;59:1155-1159.
32. Weinger M, Pantiskas C, Wiklund ME, et al. Incorporating human factors into the design of medical devices. *JAMA*. 1998;280:1484.
33. Meister D. *Conceptual Aspects of Human Factors*. Baltimore: Johns Hopkins University Press; 1989.
34. Foley ME, Keepnews D, Worthington K. Identifying and using tools for reducing risks to patients and health care workers: a nursing perspective. *Jt Comm J Qual Improv*. 2001;27: 494-499.
35. Stahlhut RW, Gosbee JW, Gardner-Bonneau DJ. A human centered approach to medical informatics for medical students, residents, and practicing clinicians. *Acad Med*. 1997;72:881-887.
36. Cooper JB, Newbower RS, Kitz RJ. An analysis of major errors and equipment failures in anesthesia management: considerations for prevention and detection 258. *Anesthesiology*. 1984;60:34-42.

Evidence-Based Clinical Decision Support

15

Diane Hanson

It is not enough to do your best; you must know what to do, and THEN do your best.

W. Edwards Deming

It has been stated that something can be greater than the sum of its parts. This is the case with the current synergistic advancements in both evidence-based practice (EBP) and health information technology (HIT) at the point of care. Some would claim that EBP is leading the way for more meaningful adoption of HIT. Others will credit the advancements in HIT as the reason EBP is now becoming a reality. The greater opportunity for nurses remains in the ability to thoughtfully and boldly leverage the convergence of both as a catalyst in accelerating support to advance practice and technology at the point of care.

This chapter defines EBP; examines the obstacles, opportunities, and current reality; describes the current national initiatives; and outlines the available HIT tools available to support a culture that adopts and sustains EBP principles. This chapter concludes with an examination of the vision for EBP and HIT adoption and the current reality and discusses how nurses can become involved in taking action today.

Evidence-Based Practice: More Than a Buzz Word?

EBP is not a new concept in nursing, nor is it a current "flavor of the month" buzz word to be ignored. It was founded by Professor Archibald Cochrane, evolved at McMaster University in Ontario in the early 1990s, and built on the well-known theory of research-based practice. It was built on this theory by including aspects of evidence from the literature, such as randomized controlled studies, meta-analysis, and systematic reviews, along with clinical expertise, experience, and patient preferences and values. In addition to nursing, EBP has also been a recognized priority with other clinical disciplines that make up the interdisciplinary team of caregivers at the point of care delivery.

D. Hanson
CPM Resource Center/Elsevier, Hudsonville, MI, USA
e-mail: dianehanson@cpmrc.com

M.J. Ball et al. (eds.), *Nursing Informatics*,
DOI: 10.1007/978-1-84996-278-0_15, © Springer-Verlag London Limited 2011

There are an array of opinions about how EBP is implemented and whether it is an effective approach to the delivery of patient care. Critics are worried that it is a "cook-book approach" that puts patients at risk of not having their care customized or individualized based on their unique health care needs. In reality, the EBP process is very complimentary and supportive to the nursing professional process of assessment, goal planning, intervening, and evaluating. It augments the professional workflow and thought process with a step that includes searching for, finding, and evaluating pertinent evidence to answer defined clinical questions.[1] Sackett, Strauss, Richardson, Rosenberg, and Haynes define EBP as "The integration of best research evidence with clinical expertise and patient values."[2] Even though there are other definitions and ideas presented throughout the literature, the above definition seems to be the "gold standard."[3,4] This definition helps quell the concerns of its critics by supporting standardization as well as individualization and values clinical expertise in addition to researched findings in making decisions for individual patients.

EBP concepts utilize hierarchies to indicate and evaluate the relative strength of published evidence. Medical evidence hierarchies rely heavily on research-based evidence such as meta-analysis of randomized clinical trials (RCT). This type of evidence is represented exclusively in medical evidence hierarchies and has the highest credibility while nonexperimental research has little or no credibility. This strict definition required for medical hierarchies can create too narrow of a focus in answering a broader range of patient care questions asked by nurses and allied health providers related to the provision of preventative and therapeutic evidence-based intervention and treatment options. Consequently, when nurse researchers develop hierarchies for rating the strength of evidence sources (Table 15.1), meta-analysis of RCT is still placed at the highest level along with systematic reviews; quality improvement, qualitative, experiential, and expert opinion evidence is included at the lower level in the hierarchy scale.[5] EBP in nursing critically evaluates and considers anecdotal case reports, quality improvement data, and the opinion of experts, especially when the researched evidence is nonexistent or nonconclusive.

Table 15.1 Strength of evidence from research or other sources[a]

Level I	Systematic review or metaanalysis of *multiple* controlled studies
Level II	*Individual* experimental study
Level III	Quasiexperimental study
Level IV	Nonexperimental study or qualitative study
Level V	Case report or systematically obtained, verifiable quality, or program evaluation data
Level VI	Opinion of recognized expert(s) or respected authorities

[a]The hierarchy of evidence used by the Clinical Practice Model Resource Center (CPMRC)™ is adapted from both Stetler et al.[5] and Melnyk and Fineout-Overholt[18]

Why is Evidence-Based Practice a Priority in Health care Today?

To consider why EBP is an important priority for nurses to understand and make a commitment to, we need to explore more closely the historical institutional patterns and traditional approaches that have been used for care delivery. Traditional approaches to guide clinical practice (experience, trial and error, authority, ritual and routine) are based on the assumptions that:

- Unsystematic observations from clinical experience alone are a valid method of building and maintaining one's knowledge base.
- The study of disease is a sufficient guide for clinical practice.
- New treatment modalities and tests can be evaluated effectively through traditional education approaches, experiences of authority figures, and common sense.
- Expertise and experiential learning is a sufficient base from which to generate valid answers for clinical practice.

These approaches to clinical practice put a high value on traditional scientific authority and knowledge acquisition through local experts, individual practice patterns, or written recommendations by recognized experts in the forms of policies, procedures, care paths, and standards or guidelines. The use of traditional approaches in the absence of appraisal and incorporation of the most recent evidence have historically caused wide variations in practice between providers, organizations, specialties, and regions. Care inconsistencies and lack of standardized quality measures create the differing levels of care and outcomes that patients experience when seeking health care. Traditional care approaches that rely on clinical experience, rituals, and routines quickly become out-of-date in the fast-paced and changing dynamics of health care delivery. The Institute of Medicine Report *Crossing the Quality Chasm* stated "Care should not vary illogically from clinician to clinician or from place to place."[6] The Agency for Healthcare Research and Quality's (AHRQ) website highlights research that supports the use of EBP principles to improve the quality of patient care. It has been noted that over the past 40 years, medical information has grown at an astonishing rate. MEDLINE®, as one example, contains more than 16 million citations and 670,000 references were added in 2007.[7] This volume of information makes it impossible for care providers to review, retrieve, and understand the results from all recent clinical trials and other studies. Lack of exposure to new evidence can result in consumers not receiving the latest treatment regimens from their health care providers. Some examples of new evidence recommendations that could be omitted unknowingly by a health care provider because of out-of-date knowledge include:

- Preventive therapies (e.g., pneumococcal vaccine, low-dose aspirin)
- Braden Skin Risk Assessment
- Minimally invasive heart therapies and cancer tumor treatments
- Proper positioning to prevent ventilator-associated pneumonia
- New birth control options

EBP proposes to support the key quality indicators of competency, safety, consistency, and individualization of care. Individual competency improves with appraisal and application of the latest available evidence. Because omissions in care are less likely to occur with evidence-based decision making, there is a direct correlation to improved patient safety. For example, when evidence suggests that a major complication of spinal cord injury is spinal shock, the nurse should understand the risk, provide regular assessments to identify the signs and symptoms, and intervene with appropriate interventions necessary to minimize and prevent risk. If the nurse does not possess the appropriate knowledge or have access to current evidence sources, omissions are likely to occur and appropriate interventions may not be utilized. These care omissions unknowingly increase the risk for that complication. Heater et al.[8] reported that "when healthcare providers base their practice on the best evidence from research, in combination with their clinical expertise and patient preferences, practice improves, resulting in approximately 28% better outcomes for patients and their families."

Current Reality: Understanding the Challenges

The realities and challenges facing health care organizations today are well documented and can be discouraging when trying to implement new clinical decision-making frameworks to support EBP. Health care organizations are filled with well-intended care providers who are facing multiple barriers to change. While the Institute of Medicine[6] advocates the use of EBP as a means of improving patient safety, efficiency, and the effectiveness of health care, significant challenges still exist. The current challenges fall into the categories of individual clinician practice and organizational culture and infrastructure.

Individual Clinician Practice: Time Constraints

Nurses are experiencing increased pressure in practice to improve quality at the same time as create efficiencies in service delivery. Patients are requiring more complex care and have a heightened awareness of unsafe care practices, increasing the workload expectations for nurses at the same time as shortages are on the rise. Patient care assistants and extender roles are being added to the skill mix which requires more delegation, prioritization, and teamwork efforts on licensed nurses. In addition, nurses are being expected to integrate their services within an interdisciplinary team to better coordinate care and improve patient safety. So, when do nurses find the needed time to visit the library or spend time searching the Internet for researched answers to their most pressing clinical questions about patient care? Obtaining and appraising the evidence, as the first step in the evidence integration cycle, is a very time-consuming proposition for most nurses.

Dr. Hieb from the Gartner Group made this statement in a research report,[9] "Healthcare professionals generally do not have sufficient time to perform an exhaustive search of the available literature." Research suggests that clinicians would have to read multiple articles a day to remain up to date in one specialty area of practice.[10] Information is "turning over" at a constant rate, and the Internet has created a situation that makes access and dissemination of this information easy and fast. Access is not usually the prevailing issue; it is the time constraints of searching and appraising that become one of the biggest challenges of EBP decision making at the point of care.

Individual Clinician Practice: Skill Level and Readiness

Significant gaps in practicing nurses' skills for identifying, accessing, retrieving, evaluating, or utilizing published evidence exist.[11] Greater than 60% of practicing nurses graduated from their initial education program before computer access was widely available in health care,[12] and almost two-thirds graduated from programs in which the curriculum did not require research or the use of technology.[13] National surveys have indicated that the majority of nurses have known information needs several times per week and prefer asking colleagues for answers to clinical questions over searching credible databases for information. In addition, 58% of nurses report never using journals or research and 82% report never using a hospital library.[1,11] A significant dilemma for nursing is the demand for professional nursing practice that is based on the latest evidence at the same time that challenges exist in the preparation of nurses to meet this demand.[1]

Individual Clinician Practice: Attitude Toward EBP

One of the most important steps in EBP implementation is examining and understanding the underlying attitudes toward EBP by individual nurses. In other words, ask yourself what you believe about EBP as it relates to your nursing role in health care and then ask your colleagues. What do you currently expect from your care providers? Patterns of relying on and valuing historical practice (ritual, tradition) to make clinical decisions about patient care are well engrained and difficult to change. In a recent presentation, Melnyk and Fineout-Overholt[14] outlined attributes of successful EBP clinicians.

In addition to knowledge and skill level, belief that EBP improves care outcomes and beliefs in the ability to implement EBP were listed as key attributes. Making it a priority to understand the strong viewpoints in those that value historical practice, as well as uncovering the fears that may be associated with EBP concepts, can assist in the shifting of individual attitudes toward EBP. Nurses are very much interested in providing care improvements that have a demonstrated patient outcome impact. Identifying and measuring outcomes associated with the use of EBP can also assist in attaching value to the use of research in practice.

Organizational Culture and Infrastructures

Even with the best researched evidence available to support nurses in the clinical decision-making process, organizational barriers can severely limit the infusion of this evidence into practice. Creating a culture that embraces EBP is no small task. Chief nursing leaders often

uncover barriers such as lack of funding, lack of manager support, lack of dedicated expertise, absence of widespread clinician adoption, and lengthy institutional approval processes.
Organizations also often do not have existing infrastructures such as governance models,
organizational practice councils, technology tools, and education programs to assist with
implementing EBP and changing culture for sustainable outcomes in practice.

Because health care organizations are complex, interdependent systems, creating a culture that adopts and sustains EBP requires a comprehensive implementation model that is
inclusive of a multifaceted approach.[15,16] Fragmented efforts and initiatives will likely fail
or have limited unsustainable impacts on the adoption of EBP.

Implementation Models for Evidence-Based Practice

Establishing and sustaining EBP as an essential component of health care transformation is a
significant undertaking. The role of the organization cannot be underestimated. Little exists in
the research literature demonstrating effectiveness of efforts to operationalize EBP for nursing
within organizations beyond single interventions.[17] It is generally agreed that a combination of
various approaches and interventions are most effective in demonstrating success with the
adoption of EBP. Many models exist that recommend multifaceted approaches to EBP implementation.[15,18-23] These models have common recommended components (single interventions) that in combination appear to be giving some direction toward creating a sustainable
implementation for organization-wide EBP adoption (Table 15.2).

Health Quality Initiatives and Supporting Organizations

Quality and patient safety initiatives aim to improve, statistically, the outcomes of health
care by providing guidance and to direct specific mandates. EBP is tightly connected to
many of the health quality and patient safety initiatives nationally and internationally.

- Institute of Medicine states that HIT systems should facilitate the application of scientific knowledge and provide clinicians with tools necessary to deliver evidence-based
  safe care.[6]
- Institute of Medicine addresses the need for nurses and other clinicians to strengthen
  capacity for assessing evidence on what is known and not known about "what works"
  in health care and calls for the development and daily implementation of evidence-
  based clinical practice guidelines in the workflow.[24]
- Health Canada lists as one of its strategic outcomes to strengthen the knowledge base to
  address health and health care priorities. Canada also has several provincial initiatives
  that focus on patient safety, standardization, and improved knowledge dissemination.[40]
- The Joint Commission (www.jointcommission.org) and Accreditation Canada have
  standards that evaluate hospital practice patterns with evidence-based, interdisciplinary
  care planning processes.[38]

Table 15.2 EBP adoption

Component topic	Recommended interventions
Leadership Endorsement/Systems Approach	Identify Leadership Champions Consider Leadership Teams Multisystem level leadership endorsement Create a Strategic Plan for EBP Create a value-oriented culture Plan with the end in mind Identify barriers and a plan to overcome them
Governance Committees/Clinician Involvement	Create Council/Committee Structures Consider hospital–university research partnership Clinicians involved in all aspects of the process Focus on clinical practice standards and quality
Education programs/build expertise	Assessment of Readiness Provide written and electronic resources Rapid Cycle training intensives Skill-building workshops (1–3 h) Create a Mentor Program Identify and educate system EBP experts Involve Advanced Practice Nurse roles in process Journal clubs and discussion groups Provide evidence-based practice tools Scope of Practice analysis by clinicians
Setting Organizational Expectation	Build EBP expectation into job descriptions Include EBP projects into performance goals Connect EBP to Clinical Ladder Programs Clinician involvement in research studies Create an organizational research publication plan
Systems Thinking Framework for Implementation	Implement a professional practice model Support clinical scholarship, reflective practice Make evidence-based tools readily available Track utilization of evidence-based tools Outcomes measurement and reevaluation Address deviations Interdisciplinary/Transdisciplinary Collaboration Provide practice councils for clinician dialog HIT that integrates EB knowledge

- The Institute for Healthcare Improvement (IHI) is leading improvement efforts in health care through the world (www.ihi.org). Many of their campaigns cultivate innovative concepts for improving the care given to patients. IHI supports initiatives that rely on sound evidence-based research to improve quality screening, intervention, and evaluation.
- National Quality Forum published priorities and goals in a 2008 report. The report solidly states that the vision is a system that can promise absolutely reliable care, guaranteeing that every patient, every time, receives the benefits of care based solidly in science.[25]

EBP also has an emphasis on dissemination. Sharing of supporting evidence creates a widened awareness within individual, systems, associations, and practices. Databases such as the Cochrane Collaboration, the Agency for Healthcare Research and Quality, the Public Health Agency of Canada's Canadian Best Practice Portal, and the National Guideline Clearinghouse facilitate dissemination. Diverse groups, including leaders in corporate America such as the Leapfrog Group, the Volunteer Hospital Association, the American and Canadian Hospital Associations, The Joint Commission, Gartner Group, and The Institute of Medicine, have provided us with an objective, intense, and complex description of today's realities that not only call for improvement, but also provide a sense of direction for nursing. EBP is one of the primary strategies that will help nurses answer the call for health care improvement.

Health Information Technology Advancement

Nursing clinicians have been waiting a long time for HIT that will serve them in care delivery. Historically, HIT solutions did little to support the clinical documentation and knowledge needs of the nurse. Information technology design and usability for health care has lagged behind other industries in vision, innovation, and support for professional workflow and practice. At the same time, investment in information systems in the United States alone is expected to exceed $35 billion in 2009. Health care organizations are often unable to realize a significant return on investment (clinical and financial) and there has been documented a widespread dissatisfaction with nursing clinical documentation and knowledge systems for care delivery. Belmont et al.[26] identified the following four key guiding principles for advancement with clinical documentation system intentional design that have challenged the status quo:

* *Build a coherent patient story* that is captured as the patient moves through the care delivery system as one coherent record. The story would be individualized for one patient, in partnership with them, and include important patient preferences.
* *Empower interdisciplinary care* by valuing the contributions of each interdisciplinary team member and creating clinical documentation that allows disciplines to coordinate, communicate, and integrate their services as a cohesive team to improve patient care and outcomes.
* *Support integrated scopes of practice for all clinicians* by clarifying roles, responsibilities, competencies, and EBP for which each interdisciplinary team member is accountable.
* *Provide evidence-based information at the point of care* in the form of clinical practice guidelines, risk screening tools, and clinical documentation that drive critical thinking and professional decision making at the point of care. Combine evidence-based recommendations with clinical expertise and individualize patient values to make care decisions.

Since 2003, only a select few HIT vendor systems have incorporated these principles to demonstrate advancements in software design to support a professional practice framework. There is still considerable opportunity for growth and innovation of technology solutions that are built to support nursing and allied professions integration within the clinical documentation system. Technology development is just beginning to accelerate and evolve to advance and support EBP and interdisciplinary integration. Examples of software functionality and features required to support this evolution include:

- Ability to access (solicited) evidence-based resources within the workflow tools, providing further clinical decision support without the clinicians having to access a separate system.
- Capabilities that allow information to be pushed out (nonsolicited) into the appropriate place in the workflow within context of the patient to support an evidence-based recommendation.
- Robust technology system infrastructure to handle complex data structures and provide content versioning capabilities to refresh evidence, quality initiatives, and patient safety requirements.
- Concurrent documentation capabilities within the patient forms and time columns to support "real time" documentation by the entire team. This allows a knowledge system to record and respond quicker to entries, so clinical patterns can be detected and changes in care can be initiated.
- Ability to autopopulate templates with information already collected somewhere else, providing better consistency of care, patient hand offs, and continuity in quality evidence-based decisions. Care providers should not need to start over with every encounter.
- Ability to have information flow from order to action, speeding treatment for the patient based on the latest evidence in the information system.
- Analytical capabilities that assist in the identification of care gaps and provide recommended intervention.
- Viewing capabilities so that evidence-based information can be shared, along with the patient priorities as data consolidated onto one review screen.
- Interdisciplinary care planning capabilities that interact with the other forms vs. just provide static screens or check lists.
- Care planning tools that utilize preconfigured evidence-based tools from credible sources to drive quality patient care decisions.

Technology advances show great promise in the ability to aid in the speed at which research can be disseminated into practice and EBP is adopted. Efforts will require passionate nursing leadership, intentional design, and innovative thinking to leverage this opportunity.

Evidence-Based Practice Tools and the Use of Technology

Advancements in access to the available evidence-based information and tools add to the promise that technology can now be leveraged to support the key driver of EBP in the quality care movement. Currently, there are multiple ways that nurses can access information to support evidence-based decision making.

Evidence Retrieval Systems

Used to find the evidence needed to answer clinical questions, online evidence retrieval systems have proven to be popular among health care clinicians. Substantial use by clinicians has been demonstrated at the point of care.[27] These systems provide answers to clinical questions, but often lack the speed required by the clinician in the care moment. Nurses and other care providers can grow impatient when answers do not directly pinpoint the exact information sought, require much sorting or synthesis, or are lacking in quality. Many evidence retrieval systems are oriented toward the health care library model and are organized by medical classification (disease, diagnosis, condition) or by resource type (journal, guideline, textbook). The use of search filters or structured queries can optimize and enhance the strength and applicability of the search results.[28]

More recently, evidence retrieval system technology has been enhanced to combine search filters with metasearch capabilities. This allows searching of multiple search engines simultaneously using filters (metasearch filters). This allows the user to create search profiles to support specific contexts or standard, replicated query sets of data. Using metasearch filters creates a more structured search for evidence-based information and has been researched and proven to help clinicians increase clinical decision velocity to enhance clinical decision making.[29]

Website Searches

The Internet has gained substantial popularity over the last decade as an information source. Concern over the quality of health care information available on the World Wide Web is widely acknowledged in the medical literature due to inconsistencies in rules for posting information, unclear definitions of quality, and search engine inefficiencies.[30] Nurses who are interested in using Internet searches to answer clinical questions are encouraged to develop a list of health information websites trusted for their credibility that can be used routinely. Advanced skills are required to access the internet and create a consistent method for evaluating the quality of each website. In an article by Hoss and Hanson,[30] a consistent set of questions are listed to help nurses critically appraise internet websites (Table 15.3).

Clinical Practice Guidelines

Clinical practice guidelines, also called guidelines or best practice guidelines, are collections of practical information, systematically developed based on the best available research to assist providers and patients to make health care decisions under specific clinical circumstances (Field et al. 1990).[39] One of the major barriers to EBP is the constraint of time, as discussed earlier in this chapter. Nurses who believe that EBP requires them to conduct their own integrative review for every clinical question that arises will quickly become discouraged. Fortunately, there are organizations around the world that have developed rigorous methods for integrating published research into evidence-based guidelines.[31-33] Guidelines are excellent clinical management tools used to disseminate

Table 15.3 Evaluation of websites

Question	Considerations
Is the information from a recognized authority?	Most credible organizations that have become recognized authorities have a Web site up and running to serve health care providers Examples: Sigma Theta Tau www.nursingsociety.org Centers for Disease Control www.cdc.gov
Does the Web site comply with voluntary standards?	Sites that comply voluntarily with quality standards from organizations such as Health on the Net Foundation and Institute, display easily identified icons on their homepage
Is the author biased or uncredentialed?	Objective information is presented with a variety of sources used to compile material, similar to reviewing references at the end of any published journal article. Caution when using .com commercial sites
Who is the audience?	Look for a clearly stated purpose on the website, often found in the "About Us" tab
Is the information complete and accurate?	Examine to see if website has a peer review process
Is the website current and regularly updated?	Websites should be updated on a regular basis to remain credible. Review dates of postings
Are the recommendations valid?	Recommendations are valid when they are firmly founded on scientific facts and produce the desired results. Consistency with other published evidence supports validity and credibility
Will the information help your client?	When applying recommendations from Web sources, one should consider whether it fits the patient's needs and preferences or values

best practices, achieve excellence in care delivery, meet or exceed quality standards, prevent complications, reduce omissions in care, and introduce innovation. To be a useful tool, guidelines need frequent updating to reflect the latest evidence in the researched literature. Guideline development follows four basic methods: (1) opinion, (2) consensus, (3) evidenced-based, and (4) combined evidence-based with consensual validation.[34]

Opinion guidelines represented some of the earliest efforts of key specialty experts. Consensus guidelines utilized more formal consensus methods to represent the opinions of collective domain experts. With the development of more rigorous evidence-based methodologies, opinion and consensus methods have become less utilized in guideline development. Evidence-based guideline development should include critique of the quality and evaluation of the strength of the published evidence. Guideline developers such as the Scottish Intercollegiate Guidelines Network (SIGN), the CPM Resource Center (CPMRC), and the Registered Nurses Association of Ontario (RNAO) utilize rigorous methodologies to generate high quality, useful guidelines for the point of care. The Appraisal of Guidelines for Research & Evaluation (AGREE) tool was created to be used by guideline developers

Table 15.4 AGREE tool criteria overview

Structure and content of the AGREE Instrument
AGREE consists of 23 key items organized in six domains. Each domain is intended to capture a separate dimension of guideline quality
Scope and purpose (items 1–3) is concerned with the overall aim of the guideline, the specific clinical questions, and the target patient population
Stakeholder involvement (items 4–7) focuses on the extent to which the guideline represents the views of its intended users
Rigor of development (items 8–14) relates to the process used to gather and synthesize the evidence, the methods to formulate the recommendations, and to update them
Clarity and presentation (items 15–18) deals with the language and format of the guideline
Applicability (items 19–21) pertains to the likely organizational, behavioral, and cost implications of applying the guideline
Editorial independence (items 22–23) is concerned with the independence of the recommendations and acknowledgement of possible conflict of interest from the guideline development group

Source: http://www.agreecollaboration.org/instrument/

to assure that development processes follow specified quality criteria[41] (AGREE Collaboration 2004), shown in Table 15.4.

High-quality evidence-based guidelines can be extracted and translated into information technology to provide clinical decision support as a new innovation in health care. Using guideline recommendations as the basis for care planning, assessment, intervention, goal outcome, and patient teaching in the electronic health record brings evidence-based information from the literature into the workflow and thoughtflow of the nurse. Figure 15.1 shows an example of a guideline recommendation translated into technology.

Clinical Information Systems

Clinical information systems show promise in supporting EBP by providing the technology platform in which to integrate knowledge. Evidence-based information and content for professional nursing practice lends substance to technology design that supports the knowledge worker. The interdependence of technology and EBP is evident. Bakken et al.[35] indicate that there are few reports outlining approaches for providing decision support for evidence-based nursing practice through integration of evidence into clinical information systems. Current trends for evidence integration include the use of Infobuttons and weblinks from within the technology platform. Infobuttons have been used for several years in passing context-specific patient information out to an evidence repository and having it retrieve pertinent information that fits the patient situation, with recent work showing high satisfaction among clinicians.[36]

Documentation-based clinical decision support is an emerging innovation to improve disease management, care coordination, and treatments. One example of a documentation-

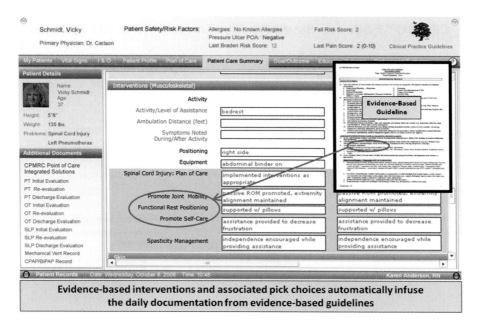

based clinical decision-support tool is an innovation at Partners Healthcare in Boston, called "Smart Forms".[37] Smart Forms are developed to not be interruptive in nature, but provide a structured process for documenting a multiproblem visit note while capturing coded information that informs further recommendations for care. Schnipper et al.[37] stated, "Documentation-based decision-support tools provide a unique opportunity to improve on the current paradigm of decision support. If designed correctly, such systems could seamlessly integrate into the current workflow of busy clinicians by suggesting actions at a time when a clinician is still in the process of clinical documentation."

Columbia University implemented EBP information for nurses in the clinical information system in the form of best practice alerts, scoring algorithms, standard measures associated with hospital policy, and risk scoring for key nursing assessment measures.[35]

Great insight on integrating practice and technology comes from an International Consortium of over 270 health care organizations that has evolved an EBP framework for over 25 years. The framework has been used to innovate within HIT solutions. Today, 122 hospital organizations are live with evidence-based, interdisciplinary documentation at the point of care. Technology was leveraged to integrate evidence-based assessments, interventions, care planning, clinical practice guidelines, and goal-outcome evaluations into the professional practice workflow of the clinicians (Fig. 15.2).

These types of approaches that use an information technology infrastructure to integrate EBP into the workflow will be the most effective in supporting advancements in both technology and EBP adoption.

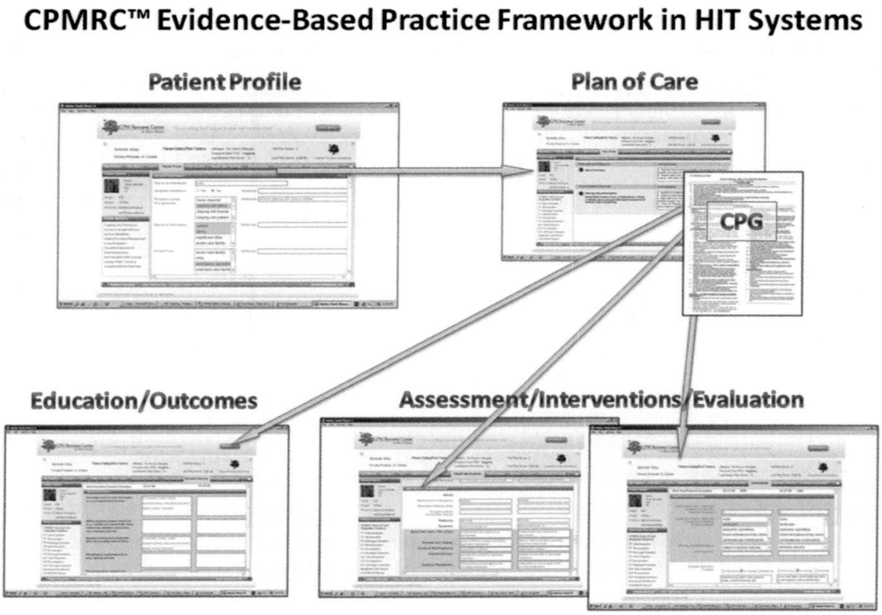

CPMRC™ Evidence-Based Practice Framework in HIT Systems

Fig. 15.2 Evidence-based practice documentation framework. Used with permission from CPM Resource Center, an Elsevier Business. All rights reserved

---

The Role of Nursing: A Call to Action

The positive convergence of technology advancements and the EBP movement in nursing provides opportunities to innovate and change the current reality. EBP is a priority in health care, but it does not just happen on its own. Nurses have an opportunity to take a leadership role in creating the needed infrastructures that will support and strengthen knowledge at the point of care. Building a future that supports EBP can be accomplished and sustained with greater efficiency when designed within a clinical documentation system and using well-defined evidence-based principles and clinical content will assist in advancing technology design.

Nursing leaders need to look for practical ways to support and sustain EBP in the midst of automation initiatives. Advances in technology have and will continue to impact nursing practice. Nurses should remember that automation can neither replace relationships, accountability, critical thinking, and communication, nor can it dictate care. Individual nurses can improve their own knowledge by exploring and becoming familiar with EBP processes, resources, and practice integration strategies. The future is full of possibilities as technology and EBP implementation continue to be developed and enhanced.

Buckminster Fuller said, "If you want to teach people a new way of thinking, don't bother trying to teach them. Instead, give them a tool, the use of which will lead to new ways of thinking." The convergence of technology advancements related to clinical documentation and care planning and the intense focus on evidence-based strategic initiatives and mandates create a wonderful opportunity for health care organizations, care clinicians, and vendors to partner to create a new reality today.

Nurses can be champions of innovation by adopting and using the technology tool of automated clinical documentation in combination with evidence-based clinical practice. The learning that takes place within every nurse and the improvement ideas that are generated could create an opportunity for nurses to achieve a long envisioned goal of building a strong future and leaving a legacy that supports EBP.

References

1. Pravikoff DS, Tanner AB, Pierce ST. Readiness of U.S. nurses for evidence-based practice. *AJN*. 2005;105(9):40-51.
2. Sackett D, Strause D, Richardson W, et al. *Evidence-Based Medicine: How to Practice and Teach EBM*. London: Churchill Livingstone; 2000.
3. Newhouse RP. Examining the support for evidence-based nursing practice. *JONA*. 2006;36(7/8):337-340.
4. Spasser MA. Evidence-based nursing resources. *Med Ref Serv Q*. 2005;24(2):71-85.
5. Stetler CB, Morsi D, Rucki S, et al. Utilization-focused integrative reviews in a nursing service. *Appl Nurs Res*. 1998;11(4):195-206.
6. Institute of Medicine. *Crossing the Quality Chasm: A New Health System for the 21st Century*. Washington: National Academy; 2001.
7. National Library of Medicine. MEDLINE® fact sheet, http://www.nlm.nih.gov/pubs/factsheets/medline.html; 2009. Accessed 8.07.09.
8. Heater B, Becker A, Olson R. Nursing interventions and patient outcomes: a meta-analysis of studies. *Nurs Res*. 1988;37:303-307.
9. Heib B. *Evidence-Based Medicine: How to Make It Real Gartner Research Notes*. Stamford: Gartner; 2001.
10. Oranta O, Routasalo P, Hupli M. Barriers to and facilitators of research utilization among Finnish registered nurses. *J Clin Nurs*. 2002;11(2):205-213.
11. Tanner A, Pierce S, Pravikoff D. Readiness for evidence-based practice: information literacy needs of nurses in the United States. *Stud Health Technol Inform*. 2004;11(pt 2):936-940.
12. US Department of Health and Human Services. The registered nurse population: findings from the 2004 sample survey of registered nurses. http://bhpr.hrsa.gov/healthworkforce/rnsurvey04/default.htm; 2004. Accessed 9.07.09.
13. National League for Nursing Accrediting Commission. *Accreditation Manual with Interpretive Guidelines by Program Type forPostsecondary and Higher Degree Programs in Nursing*. 2006 ed. New York: NLNAC; 2006:125-128.
14. Melnyk BM, Fineout-Overholt E. Igniting evidence-based practice in clinical settings: basics & beyond. In: *Program and abstracts of the 39th Biennial Convention of Sigma Theta Tau International, the Honor Society of Nursing*, Baltimore, MD; 3–7 Nov 2007.
15. Stetler C. Role of the organization in translating research into evidence-based practice. *Outcomes Manage*. 2003;3:97-103.
16. Timmermans S, Mauck A. The promises and pitfalls of evidence-based medicine. *Health Aff*. 2005;24(1):18-28.
17. Foxcroft DR. Organizational infrastructures to promote evidence based nursing practice: the Cochrane Collaboration. http://www.medscape.com/viewarticle/486107; 2007. Accessed 28.01.09.
18. Melnyk B, Fineout-Overholt E. *Evidence-Based Practice in Nursing and Healthcare: A Guide to Best Practice*. Philadelphia: Lippincott Williams & Wilkins; 2005.

19. Newhouse R, Dearbolt S, Poe S, et al. Evidence-based practice: a practical approach to implementation. *J Nurs Admin*. 2005;35(1):35-40.
20. Rycroft-Malone J, Kitson A, Harvey G, et al. Ingredients for change: revisiting a conceptual framework. *Qual Saf Health Care*. 2002;11:174-180.
21. Titler MG, Kleiber C, Steelman VJ, et al. The Iowa model of evidence-based practice to promote quality care. *Crit Care Nurs Clin North Am*. 2001;13:497-509.
22. Turkel M et al. An essential component of the magnet journey: fostering an environment for evidence-based practice and nursing research. *Nurs Adm Q*. 2005;29(3):254-262.
23. Wesorick B. *Standards of Nursing Care: A Model for Clinical Practice*. Philadelphia: J.B. Lippincott; 1990.
24. Institute of Medicine. *Knowing What Works in Healthcare: A Roadmap for the Nation*. Washington: National Academy; 2008.
25. National Quality Forum. Aligning our efforts to transform America's healthcare national goals and priorities. http://www.nationalprioritiespartnership.org/AboutNPP.aspx; 2008.
26. Belmont RL, Wesorick B, Jesse H, et al. *Clinical Documentation. Health Care Technology Volume 1*. San Fransisco: Montgomery Research; 2003.
27. Westbrook J, Gosling A, Coiera E. Do clinicians use online evidence to support patient care? A study of 55,000 clinicians. *J Am Med Inform Assoc*. 2004;11(2):113-120.
28. Haynes RB, Wilczynski NL. Optimal search strategies for retrieving scientifically strong studies of diagnosis from Medline analytical survey. *BMJ*. 2004;328(7447):1040.
29. Coiera E, Westbrook J, Rogers K. Clinical decision velocity is increased when meta-research filters enhance an evidence retrieval system. *J Am Med Inform Assoc*. 2008;15(5):638-646.
30. Hoss B, Hanson D. Evaluating the evidence: web sites. *AORN J*. 2008;87(1):124-141.
31. Grinspun D, Virani T, Bajnok I. Nursing best practice guidelines: the RNAO project. *Hosp Q*. 2001/2002;Winter 5(2):56-60.
32. Twaddle S. Clinical practice guidelines. *Singapore Med J*. 2005;46(12):681-686.
33. Wesorick B, Hanson D. *Clinical Practice Guidelines*. Grand Rapids: Practice Field; 2000.
34. Hanson D, Hoss B, Wesorick B. Evaluating the evidence: guidelines. *AORN J*. 2008;88(2): 184-196.
35. Bakken S, Currie L, Lee N, et al. Integrating evidence into clinician information systems for nursing decision support. *Intl J Med Inform*. 2008;77:413-420.
36. Collins S, Currie L, Bakken S, et al. Information needs, infobutton manager use, and satisfaction by clinician type: a case study. *J Am Med Inform Assoc*. 2009;16(1):140-142.
37. Schnipper J, Linder J, Palchuk M, et al. "Smart forms" in an electronic medical record: documentation-based clinical decision support to improve disease management. *J Am Med Inform Assoc*. 2008;15(4):513-523.
38. Accreditation Canada. 2008 Canadian Health Accreditation report. www.accreditation-canada.ca; 2007.
39. Field MJ, Lohr KN. *Guidelines for Clinical Practice: Directions for a New Program*. Washington: National Academy; 1990.
40. Health Canada. http://www.hc-sc.gc.ca/ahc-asc/activit/about-apropos/index-eng.php#strat; 2009. Accessed 8.07.09.
41. The Agree Collaboration. Introduction to the AGREE Collaboration. http//www.agreecollaboration.org; 2009. Accessed 9.07.09.

In times of change, learners inherit the Earth, while the learned find themselves beautifully equipped to deal with a world that no longer exists.

Eric Hoffer

What does the future hold? No one really knows, but what we do know is that we get glimpses of the future from words, events, and symbols; from the promises of leaders and of innovation, and from the awareness of social trends. All of these lend perspective to the topics covered in this section. The chapters we have chosen to include in this section reflect our belief that science fiction writer William Gibson was right when he observed, "The future is here. It's just not widely distributed yet."

Today technology and informatics topics appear not only in the traditional print and broadcast media but also on the World Wide Web on websites for federal Health and Human Services agencies and other policy arenas. They have even found their way to the social media, including twittering.

Technology and use of the electronic record have been touted having a significant impact on patient safety, on reducing cost, and improving communication across systems and between and among patients/consumers, providers, and families. Discussions in the media and at national conferences, including one in May 2009 sponsored by the National Library of Medicine, have focused on the personal health record (PHR) and consumer involvement.

Personal Health Record and Management of Personal Health

Chapter 16, "Personal Health Record (PHR): Managing Personal Health," draws upon the work of one of the two future-oriented TIGER collaborative. Authors Charlotte Weaver and Rita Zeilsdorf examine the growing involvement of consumers in their own care through their use of the PHR. With medical information no longer limited to healthcare professionals but easily accessible in the public domain, nurses and other clinicians must take into account the impact of the new phenomenon of the 'informed' patient. The same is true for nursing educators and health services researchers.

In the future, Weaver and Zeilsdorf explain, nurses will need the knowledge and experience to use health enabling technologies, health information sites, emailing and document exchange, social networks, and wireless monitoring, not only in healthcare settings but also in the home. Health literacy will be a major issue. In addition to educating individuals, families, and communities, about specific conditions, nurses will need to be ready to improve health literacy. They will need to teach consumers how to use health-enabling technologies like the PHR, how to access trusted health information sites, and how to use tools interactively to communicate with primary care providers. And this means overcoming the technology and informatics gap that exists today—not just among patients, but also among nurses, nursing faculty, and other healthcare providers.

Innovation at the Point of Care: Smart Systems

Healthcare took center stage on Capitol Hill in 2009, with contentious debate on how best to provide coverage to the nearly 50 million Americans with no health insurance. Earlier in the year, as part of the American Recovery and Reinvestment Act (ARRA), Congress allocated funding for innovative technology to improve outcomes at the point of care.

John Silva, Nancy Seybold, and Marion Ball address this topic in chapter 17, "Disruptive Innovation: Point of Care," and offer their vision for a 'smart' health information technology system. Challenging many of the current point of care technologies, they provide a contemporary view of how technology should provide support to clinicians, including nurses. The system they describe would support nursing users by reclaiming time spent on administrative tasks while providing relevant clinical information and knowledge at the point of care. Today's end-users, the authors believe, expect to access relevant information and execute useful transactions with little or *no* learning curve. The smart system they envision would provide better monitoring and transmitting of data, improving disease management for consumers and clinicians in home and healthcare settings.

Innovation at the Point of Care: Extending Care

Of course, innovation requires a 'rethinking' of technological tools and informatics. In chapter 18, "Extending Care: Voice Technology," Debra Wolf, Amar Kapadia, and Pam Selker Rak report on one futuristic innovation that effectively extends nursing's hands and feet while maintaining a high level of knowledge- and science-based practice. They describe how voice-assisted technology is being used in long-term and acute care setting. A wearable, wireless device allows mobile nursing staff to communicate and interact with a 'smart' machine, something like Hal in *2001: A Space Odyssey*. When deployed in conjunction with a speech recognition engine, electronic medical record applications can be more effective, supporting real-time documentation, communication with other clinicians, and paging and text message functions—all at the point of care. The authors report initial findings suggesting that this innovative new technology improves efficiency and has high user satisfaction in both long-term care and acute care settings.

Nursing Leadership: Critical to Success

In chapter 19, "Nursing's Contribution: An External Viewpoint," healthcare writer Mark Hagland urges nurses to claim their rightful place as leaders in nursing informatics and technology. A champion of the nursing profession, he challenges nurses, especially those in the growing fields of nursing informatics, to take on new roles in the interdisciplinary, consumer-driven healthcare of the future. The insights he has drawn from interviewing and observing executive level healthcare managers and nursing leaders have led him to conclude that clinical and nurse informaticists will be the ones largely responsible for making changes in clinical workflow and at the point of care. They will provide the framework for integrating technology into care and for diffusing innovation across all healthcare settings. Echoing Roy Simpson in chapter 10, "Nursing Leadership: Challenging the Status Quo," Hagland charges chief nursing officers with ensuring that nurse informaticists are at the table when key decisions are made regarding the purchase, adoption, and implementation of health information technology.

Personalized Medicine and Comparative Effectiveness Research

The Institute of Medicine and the Agency for Healthcare Research and Quality are continuing efforts to define and conduct comparative effectiveness research (CER) as an approach to managing care. At the same time, the 2009 Presidential appointment and Senate confirmation of Dr. Frances Collins as Director of the National Institutes of Health have generated renewed interest in personalized medicine with a focus on genetics.

These emerging topics—CER and personalized medicine—are addressed in chapter 20, "Transforming Care: Discovery Enabled by Health Information Technology." Authors Barbara Frink and Asif Dhar discuss how these two important and sometimes controversial topics inform practice, research, and health reform. In the past, the translation of scientific evidence into clinical practice conformed to strict guidelines. CER will change this, challenging traditional approaches to evidence-based practice. By using information technology to reuse clinical data as a new source of information, CER will disrupt the hierarchy of evidence. New sources of scientific information available at the point of care will make it possible to tailor treatment to individual characteristics of each patient, improving the personalized medicine approach. The authors describe how this process will work, how it will impact practice, education, and research, and what roles specialized federal initiatives addressing genetics will play. Although the personalized medicine approach is relatively new globally, CER has been used for some time in many countries where clinical data has been more available and interoperable, as chapters in Section 5 describe. Nonetheless, obtaining, tracking, and conducting scientific exploration of nursing-related data and information will pose significant challenges for the United States and the international community.

TIGER Virtual Learning Environment

In chapter 21, "Local Global Access: Virtual Learning Environment," Teresa McCasky, Beth Elias, Jacqueline Moss, and Christel Anderson paint a futuristic picture of a high-tech Virtual Demonstration Center. As conceptualized by one of the TIGER collaboratives, the Center will address education and training of health professionals locally and globally, concerns that are also the target of ARRA funding for investment by the Office of the National Coordinator and the Health Resources and Service Administration. The authors lay out a path to the future, they describe and make the case for a future virtual learning environment to demonstrate the use of technologies to improve practice and education and thereby speed the diffusion of innovations, including those mentioned in this book, into practice. They describe four approaches that facilitate learning by customizing the learning environment: (1) observable, for example, videos, powerpoint; (2) trialable, as provided by interactive multimedia opportunities; (3) learn-while-doing, such as training during technology implementations as well as continuing education; and (4) simulations that allow for user feedback and experimentation. As this chapter concludes, creation of a Virtual Demonstration Center will play a key role in easing the adoption of health IT by nurses and the rest of the healthcare community. Virtual learning based on partnerships between and among healthcare settings, educational institutions, and industry will be required for access to electronic records and other up-to-date health IT and innovative technologies.

TIGER Phase III

In late 2009, TIGER Phase III activities were already in process. While Phase III leadership was being formed, a small group of TIGERs began to develop a proposal for grant funding to support a second invitational symposium. Planned to disseminate the work of TIGER Phase II beyond nursing professional groups to include interdisciplinary and allied health colleagues, this second symposium will:

- Highlight the application and integration of relevant TIGER Collaborative accomplishments to other disciplines and care providers
- Flesh out disciplinary and interdisciplinary elements of the virtual demonstration center that will become a new virtual learning environment for technology and informatics
- Explore next steps for the nursing profession's health IT journey related to technology and informatics.

To disseminate its work even more broadly, TIGER Phase III will address the digital divide that now exists within minority communities and rural settings. It will also focus on establishing partnerships and acquiring the funding needed to set up the Virtual Learning Environment that will serve as a repository for competency-based learning activities.

Creating this environment will be the first outcome of Phase III and will support the following anticipated outcomes in TIGER Phase III:

- Developing a U.S. nursing workforce capable of using electronic health records to improve the delivery of healthcare
- Engaging more nurses in the development of a nationwide health information technology infrastructure
- Accelerating adoption of smart, standards-based, interoperable, patient-centered technology that will make healthcare delivery safer, more efficient, timely, accessible, and efficient
- Applying and integrating of relevant TIGER accomplishments for interdisciplinary and allied health colleagues in order to assist them in their work
- Developing a U.S. healthcare workforce capable of using electronic health records to improve the delivery of healthcare
- Accelerating adoption of smart, standards-based, interoperable, patient-centered technology that will make healthcare delivery safer, more efficient, timely, accessible, and efficient.

In the context of culture change, Patricia Hinton Walker, who will lead TIGER throughout Phase III, calls upon the historic voices of Nightingale, Dix, Wald, and Breckenridge, to renew our focus on what nursing is and has always been about – improving patient-centered care and patient safety.

More information on TIGER appears at the back of this book. Appendices provide the TIGER Executive Summary Report and lists of the committed individuals who helped to advance the TIGER agenda, including leaders of Phase I, Collaborative Leaders and Leadership for Phase II, and members of the Phase III Executive Committee and the newly formed Collaborative Leadership (TLC) group.

> *"The critical responsibility for the generation you're in is to help provide the shoulders, the direction, and the support for those generations who come behind."*

> *Gloria Dean Randle Scott*

Personal Health Record: Managing Personal Health

16

Charlotte Weaver and Rita Zielstorff

This chapter presents the work of the TIGER Collaborative on Consumer Empowerment and the Personal Health Record (PHR). The entire body of work for the TIGER Collaborative Team #9 is available at http://tigerphr.pbworks.com/ The first part of this chapter will review the state of the science on the potential of health consumerism as seen through the lens of health literacy and nursing's role as an advocate, educator, and facilitator for using health-enabling technologies. The second half of the chapter focuses on the domain of the PHR – state of the art, adoption, public policy, and nursing's role in care delivery and enabling individuals to self-manage and to be active participants in their care decisions.

Consumer Empowerment and Technology

Consumer empowerment in the United States developed in direct response to the availability of product testing and quality evaluation information. Starting in the 1930s with the publication of the now famous *Consumer Reports*, consumerism continued to emerge as a force throughout the twentieth century.[1] As new transformative technologies came into the marketplace in the early 1990s, most notably personal computers, the internet, and broadband combined with health policy activism,[2-4] these forces extended consumer empowerment into healthcare. The explosive growth of the internet with health information sites that offered disease specific to general health information put direct access to health information into the hands of lay consumers.[5,6] Over the past two decades, consumer empowerment in healthcare has continued to grow, fueled by increased access to expert knowledge and the latest clinical science. Medical knowledge and science, heretofore only available to health professionals, quickly became public domain as powerful search engine tools, such as Yahoo and Google,[7,8] entered the marketplace. Concurrently, government-funded research and its publications were placed on the Web and made available to the public.[5,9]

C. Weaver (✉)
Gentiva® Health Services, Atlanta, GA, USA
e-mail: charlotte.weaver@gentiva.com

M.J. Ball et al. (eds.), *Nursing Informatics*,
DOI: 10.1007/978-1-84996-278-0_16, © Springer-Verlag London Limited 2011

Additionally, some universities have taken the step to convert their libraries to be online and to be available to the public;[10,11]and by the turn of the century, most professional and scientific journals have placed their publications on the Web with availability to the general public for a fee ([12] (Health Affairs 2009). Indeed, this phenomenon of pervasive information availability in which the "informed" consumer may have as much knowledge for a particular health concern as the general practitioner or specialist has caused major cultural change in the traditional "patient" role and flattened the power dynamic between provider and patient.[13-15]

The transition in our society from a "patient" to a "consumer" orientation has ramifications in terms of what people want from their providers, health organizations, and health plans.[14] For nurses, we will want to be aware of health policy that advocates for informed and participatory consumerism, as well as the latest trends in consumer behaviors and expectations so that we can appropriately tailor our care delivery approaches to these culturally different consumer populations.

Consumer Trends, Behaviors, and Expectations

Two recent surveys by Deloitte and the California HealthCare Foundation (CHCF) looked at consumer behaviors and expectations. The results from these two survey studies give a view into the extent that the American public wants more technology tools and access to information that will help them manage their health.[14,16] The findings from both surveys indicate a strong pragmatic mindset in the United States (US) public on current use or inclination to use technology tools for self-management and active participation in their health decisions.

The Deloitte survey, based on a nationally representative sample of 3,031 adults conducted in September 2007, aggregated their consumers based on behaviors, attitudes, and beliefs about how the health system performs.[14] Deloitte clustered their survey population into six consumer segments that resulted in demographics, socioeconomic, ethnicity, age, and education being blended across all six groups. As the Deloitte authors noted, "the healthcare consumer market is clearly not homogenous." By avoiding the usual sociodemographic stratification of survey respondents, the Deloitte survey results give us insight into the variance of consumers' choices and behaviors that are lost within the traditional survey groupings. The five areas of consumer activity examined were self-directed care, traditional health services, information seeking, alternative and nonconventional health service, and financing.

Findings from the Deloitte survey on the "self-directed care" and "information seeking" categories show that consumers want programs and tools to help them improve their health. Over 60% of these consumers wanted tools that would provide personalized recommendations to improve their health. And specifically, 55% of the survey respondents indicated that they wanted tools that would help them assess, monitor, or manage their health. Specifically, the requested tools related to in-home monitoring devices, PHRs, electronic same day appointment scheduling, test and lab results, access to their medical records, and trusted information sites for their medications, treatments, and disease conditions. The Deloitte study authors summarize that these consumers were delivering the message of wanting more information, control, and partnership. The report concludes that their findings "point to clear signals that consumerism is a significant trend that all industry stakeholders must consider."[14]

The CHCF 2008 study basically reports a similar level of consumerism as found in the Deloitte study. Three out of four consumers surveyed in the CHCF study expressed interest in being able to view their medical records and lab results, to schedule appointments and to exchange e-mails with their physicians.[16] However, the CHCF study noted that there is significant disparity between what patients want to do online and what they are able or allowed to do. CHCF found that the barriers come from the uneven use of patient-centered health information technology. Their survey looked at physician practices and healthcare organizations in five types of medical practices located in different states across the country. The CHCF survey concludes that "consumers are clamoring for PHRs that will give them access to clinical data linked to health information targeted to their needs."[16] Furthermore, in organizations that have this patient-centered approach, such as Kaiser Permanente, their PHR adoption has shown a steep adoption curve with rates doubling annually.[17] The CHCF survey findings also agreed with the Deloitte's 2008 study in which both found that insured and uninsured consumers were equally keen to have broader use of technology to do online appointments scheduling, e-mail access, and electronic access to medical records and test results.

Under the Pew Research Center, the Pew Internet and American Life Project has provided running statistics on adoption of the internet, types of use, daily use, and usage patterns from 2000 to 2009.[18] The Pew survey data show that in the years between 2000 and 2009, internet use grew from 46 to about 75% of all US adults. Over this 9-year period, searching for health information stayed as a major reason for use of the internet. In 2009, 61% of adults indicated that they used the internet to look up health information.[18] In terms of the social nature of health information seeking on the internet, a 2008 Pew study documents the extent to which information is exchanged in social networks.[19] The finding that half of all online inquiries performed are done so on behalf of another person is important in understanding the difference between direct online seeking of information and getting others to do it for you. This social aspect of indirect internet use and health literacy levels needs to be considered as we evaluate the literature discussed later in this chapter.

Of all US adults who seek out health information, about 60% say that the information that they obtain affect their decisions about how to treat an illness or their approach to maintaining their health or as a caretaker for someone else. Importantly, there has been a shift in percentage of "e-patients" reporting that the health information obtained had helped them from 31% in 2006 to 60% in 2008.[19] The term "e-patient" has been adopted in the literature to designate those individuals who use technology to seek information, manage their health, and make decisions.[20]

In terms of demographic descriptors, lower income communities use the internet less than middle or higher income groups, but more than 53% report having internet access.[21] While only one third of Spanish speaking (no English) individuals use the internet, over 55% of Latinos in the American population go online.[22] The highest internet use is in the under 18 age group, with numerous surveys reporting fewer than 17% use of the internet in the over 75 age group.[23-25] However, the "baby boomer" generation, the 50–64 age group, are heavy users of the internet at 75% reporting frequent to daily use Jones and

Fox.[23] Projections are for internet use among older adults to increase greatly in the next decade, as will its usage as a resource for health information and disease management for our elderly with chronic diseases.[16,25]

An increasing array of health-enabling technologies is being introduced to support consumer empowerment and self-management of wellness and disease. Policymakers define these enabling technologies as providing the potential to improve clinical excellence, the care experience, and the continuity and affordability of care[3,26,27] (Deloitte 2009a). A key technology in this exploration is the PHR. The electronic PHR and its related technologies are seen as a tool that gives people more control over their care and allows them to be participants in their care management decisions[3,17] (Harris 2009; Deloitte 2009).

Health Literacy in the U.S. Population

Paradoxically, in the face of this information age and a culture of consumer empowerment, the evidence shows that great disparities exist in our population's ability to access, understand, and act on health information.[3,24,25] As we will review, these levels of "health literacy" have consequences for health outcomes, quality of care, and healthcare costs, as well as for adoption and use of health-enabling technologies, such as the PHR.[26,28-30] For nurses, the relevancy of this area of health literacy goes to the core nursing value of enabling our patients to do for themselves that which they would if they were able.[31] This value is also at the heart of consumer empowerment, and nurses have an important role to play in helping to develop and deliver appropriately tailored instructions, guidance, and health information. Traditional concepts of "patient education" also need to be converted to one of "participating consumer." In this framework, the nurse's role is that of a "facilitator," as nurses teach and enable self-sufficiency by showing individuals how to improve their health literacy skills and to use health-enabling technologies.

Major Literature Resources and Milestone Contributors

Over the past decade, the Department of Health and Human Services (HHS) has sponsored a number of major projects and studies on health literacy that report literacy levels, variations by demographic, cultural and socioeconomic factors, health outcomes, and costs.[3,24,26,27,30,32,33] The National Library of Medicine's (NLM's) bibliography of 2000 provided our standard definition of "health literacy" and in the updated 2004 version offers 651 citations on work published in the field between 1998 and 2003.[33] A cornerstone in this literature is the 2003 National Assessment of Adult Literacy (NAAL) survey that represents the first national assessment of health literacy.[24] The U.S. Department of Education (DOE) conducted the NAAL, and the Office of Disease Prevention and Health Promotion (ODPHP) within HHS collaborated with DOE to develop the health literacy component in the NAAL.

Two health literacy evidence reviews stand out in the literature. Both published in 2004, one from the Institute of Medicine (IOM) and the other from the Agency of Healthcare and

Quality Research (AHRQ), these reviews pulled together the evidence that linked health literacy levels to health outcomes, quality of care, and cost.[29,30] The IOM Health Literacy Committee's report was entitled *Health Literacy: A Prescription to End Confusion*; and AHRQ's review, *Literacy and Health Outcomes,* served as important guides to policymakers' strategies going forward. In 2008, AHRQ published an in-depth look at populations shown to have the lowest health literacy levels and internet use entitled, *Barriers and Drivers of Health Information Technology Use for the Elderly, Chronically Ill and Underserved.*[34]

Health Literacy Defined

Health literacy was defined in the NLM 2000 Bibliography as the degree to which individuals have the "capacity to *obtain, process,* and *understand* basic health information and services needed to make appropriate health decisions."[33] Both Healthy People 2010 and the IOM's Committee on Health Literacy adopted this definition.[27,30] Generally, the key concepts applied in government health literacy initiatives relate to an individual's ability to obtain information, to process it in a way that enables the person to understand it in his/her context, and to decide appropriate actions to take.[24] The NAAL study measured health literacy as a component within a general literacy study using a nationally representative sample of more than 19,000 adults. NAAL assessed ability to use and understand prose, documents, and quantitative health information and defined four literacy levels that are now used as a standard:

1. Proficient: Can perform complex and challenging literacy activities
2. Intermediate: Can perform moderately challenging literacy activities
3. Basic: Can perform simple everyday literacy activities
4. Below Basic: Can perform no more than the most simple and concrete literacy activities.

The percentages shown in Table 16.1 mean that 30 million persons have *Below Basic* health literacy skills; 47 million persons have *Basic* health literacy skills; 114 million persons have *Intermediate* skills; 25 million persons have *Proficient* skills; and 5% of the population or 11 million persons are nonliterate in English and are unable to test. In terms of health choices and use of resources, these proficiency levels are linked to the following behaviors for those 30 million adults in the *Below Basic* health literacy category:

Table 16.1 Percentage and number of adults in each level[24] (Whitehurst 2006)

Health literacy level	Percentage of adults in each health literacy level	Number of corresponding adults in millions
Below basic	14	30
Basic	22	47
Intermediate	53	114
Proficient	12	25

- Thirty-seven percent or 11 million obtain no information from newspapers
- Forty-one percent or 12 million obtain no information from magazines
- Forty-one percent or 12 million obtain no information from books or brochures
- Eighty percent or 24 million obtain no information from the Internet[24,35]

Those most likely to have *Basic* or *Below Basic* health literacy levels in our general population were racial and ethnic minorities except Asian/Pacific Islanders; people who did not speak English prior to starting school; people over 65 years; people with less than high school education; people living under the poverty level; and, people who do not use the internet for health information. As shown in Table 16.1, the NAAL survey also found that only 12% of US adults had *Proficient* health literacy. While there was a strong relationship between education levels and health literacy, the survey also found that 44% of high school graduates and 12% of college graduates had *Below Basic* or *Basic* health literacy. Health literacy was found to be an issue for all ethnic groups, and for our elderly, two thirds of those over 75 years of age had *Below Basic* or *Basic* health literacy.

The 2004 IOM evidence review report noted that the NAAL results mean that over half of all American adults – 90 million people – have difficulty understanding and using health information. The IOM's evidence review found that these literacy levels in communities within the American population were related to healthcare outcomes, quality of care, and healthcare costs.[30] And most directly, the 2004 IOM evidence review included a number of studies that linked higher rates of hospitalization and use of emergency services among people with limited health literacy.[36-41] In light of these findings, the IOM Committee on Health Literacy called for widespread, innovative educational programs and improvement in the development of patient education materials that starts at kindergarten and continues through life to transform America to a health literate society. The IOM Committee on Health Literacy concludes that allowing current literacy levels to continue is costly in wasted services, resources, and billions of avoidable costs. The IOM Committee's summary recommendation calls for healthcare providers and organizations to develop and make accessible health information that matches the health literacy skills of the American public.[30]

Health policy leaders have explored the significance of the NAAL's survey findings for PHR adoption in a number of projects.[3,26,28,32] These study initiatives conclude that there is a projected link of literacy to PHR use because adults with limited health literacy skills show that they are not accustomed to using the Internet as a health resource. Indeed, as referenced above, the NAAL survey found that those with *Basic* or *Limited Basic* proficiency levels prefer mass media or interpersonal sources of health information over other sources. Hence, the health policymakers project that those with lower health literacy levels will not be able to handle many of the multiple and complex tasks in electronic PHR offerings.[3]

Health Policy to Promote Health Literacy

Starting at the beginning of this decade, health policy began advocating for patient-centered care, wellness/disease prevention, and self-management in chronic disease in a very vocal way.[4,27] In 2001, the IOM released its recommendations for transforming the

US healthcare system.[4] The 2001 IOM report linked evidence that outcomes improved when patients had the opportunity to participate in their care decisions as a full partner in decision-making. Thus, the IOM recommended "patient-centered care" and the use of health information technology to enable this transformation in care delivery. The Healthy People 2010 initiative is a wide-reaching effort on the part of HHS to improve the health and quality of life of Americans and builds on *Healthy People* initiatives pursued over the past two decades.[3,27] The Healthy People 2010 program is based on two goals: increase quality and years of healthy life; eliminate health disparities. Started in 2000, progress has been monitored through 467 objectives in 28 focus area. Focus area #11, "Health Communication" relates to health literacy, use of technology, adoption patterns, broadband availability, health communication and education materials, programs, and resources. Under the Focus Area #11's umbrella, other HHS divisions have tackled specific programs using evidence and research. These Programs have addressed use of broadband internet access, proficiency levels of health literacy, and HHS-sponsored health communication campaigns using research in their program development and providing health information web sites.

In response to survey and evidence reviews findings on low health literacy levels in American society and its linkage to health outcomes and costs, there has been a concerted effort in health policy programs to address the gaps. Numerous calls have been made for innovative approaches to make health information more accessible across all segments of the American society. Some of the most notable of these HHS supportive programs have become available just recently.[32,42,43] The HHS Administration on Aging and ODPHP have collaborated to provide federal, state, tribal, and local partners in the Aging Network with a health literacy resource, *Tools for Improving Health Literacy*, which is available online and in CD format.[3] It is designed to help professionals in aging care communicate with older adults at all literacy levels on issues such as long-term care and evidence-based disease prevention programs. The HHS Health Resources and Services Administration is developing an interactive, Web-based *Health Literacy Training Program* for its grantees. The Federal Communications Commission has the congressionally mandated goal to promote affordable access to robust and reliable broadband products and services for all Americans. In September 2006, the Surgeon General and ODPHP co-sponsored the *Surgeon General's Workshop on Improving Health Literacy*. Based on evidence provided during the Surgeon General's workshop, a plan to raise awareness and identify promising practices is in development by the HHS Health Literacy Working Group.[26]

The development of programs to promote the areas evaluated in these major health policy studies focuses on an individual's ability to perform the following:

- Navigate the healthcare system, including locating providers and services and filling out forms
- Share personal and health information with providers
- Engage in self-care and chronic disease management
- Adopt health-promoting behaviors, such as exercising and eating a healthy diet
- Act on health-related news and announcements[28]

In March 2002, The Joint Commission, together with the Centers for Medicare and Medicaid Services, launched a national campaign to promote health literacy. Named the *Speak Up™* program, they developed brochures, posters, and buttons to urge patients to take a role in preventing healthcare errors by becoming active, involved, and informed participants on the healthcare team. Their brochure, "Understanding Your Doctor and Other Caregivers," was released in 2008 in both English and Spanish and is available online.[44] This guide gives directions and tips to consumers on how to navigate the healthcare system, how to gain information, and how to interact with caregivers as a partner in their care decisions.

The ODPHP has published a health literacy action plan and a Quick Guide to Health Literacy, both of which are based on research.[32] In May 2008, the Office of Civil Rights published two HIPAA brochures in eight languages to educate healthcare consumers about the HIPAA privacy rule and their rights under this act. The brochure, *Privacy and Your Health Information,* walks the consumer through what information is protected and how it can be shared. From the perspective of the individual's rights, the second brochure, *Your Health Information Privacy Rights,* details how to access one's medical records, to request an accounting of disclosures, and to file a complaint.[45]

Business and Service Provider Collaborative Programs

In the mid-1990s, Kaiser Permanente, the nation's largest, nonprofit health maintenance organization, began offering its members the ability to ask health questions to nurses over the Web. In the last few years, it has gone much further with its Web-based *My Health Manager* PHR, which enables patients to make appointments, send e-mail questions to doctors, and place prescription orders online. In June 2008, Kaiser announced a partnership with Microsoft to use its Microsoft's Health Vault PHR service to offer it 156,000 employees and 8.7 million members a consumer-controlled PHR.[17]

Entering the PHR market just a few months after Microsoft, Google introduced its *Google Health* solution. *Google Health* is a consumer-controlled PHR with functions that allow a person to build a health profile; import medical records from physicians, hospitals, and pharmacies; and share their record and online health service directory. (*Google Health* is available at: http://www.google.com/intl/en-US/health/about/) In addition to Kaiser, Microsoft has partnered with the Mayo Clinic and New York-Presbyterian Hospital; Google is working with the Cleveland Clinic and Beth Israel Deaconess Medical Center. While there are many companies offering a PHR solution on the Web, the entry of Microsoft and Google into this space in partnership with leading healthcare organizations is seen as potentially hastening the adoption of electronic health records (EHRs).

Nurses' Role in Health Literacy and Consumer Empowerment

Nurses have a key role to play in health literacy and consumer empowerment. Included in the American Nurses Association's scope and standards of practice are the traditional functions of serving as an advocate for the patient, an educator, and an enabler of an individual's efforts to gain optimum self-management of their health and/or disease management.[46] As this literature review emphasizes, the importance of patient education in the realm of consumerism and technology must take on the added nuance of health literacy – teaching people how and where to find information, how to use this information for their own health management, and how to navigate the health system. While all care settings carry responsibility for teaching and education, we know that individuals have the least ability to learn in acute care settings, ambulatory somewhat better, with the person's home being the most optimum setting.[47] Therefore, as nurses consider how best to tailor teaching and materials to fit the individual's ability to learn, acute care discharge planning should include transitioning to community and home healthcare for patient teaching and to support learning skills that increase their health literacy proficiency.

Long-term, patient-centered relationships are mostly developed in the context of primary care in the community and in the home. And this presents a great opportunity for nurses at all levels of practice. The extent to which an individual is "empowered" to be fully engaged in their healthcare and management of the health and disease condition is largely in the domain of professional nursing. It is a challenge for us to accept, but the question is, "Will we?" As patient advocates, if nursing can accept this challenge, we will help raise awareness of the gap that exists between health information currently available and address it in our practice.

The significance of health literacy levels for nurses working in community primary care and home healthcare, therefore, is that teaching and patient education need to be a major part of the nurse's plan of care for every individual. As referenced above, eventually at some point, most individuals encounter challenges in their ability to understand information and to take action on that information, regardless of their education or proficiency levels.[30] Importantly, the nurse's ability to teach effectively requires assessment skills based on a solid knowledge and understanding of the skills that make up health literacy proficiency levels. As the primary source of patient and family education and instructions in self-management, nurses are key resources in helping make the United States a health literate society. Now and going forward, nurses will need to be able to assess the "health literacy" levels of an individual to establish the appropriate education and supports needed. As the studies reviewed here demonstrate that these critical education interventions are as important to include in the plan of care as any procedure or medication.[30]

While advocacy, education, and support of the patient are nursing functions that cross all care settings, consumer empowerment in healthcare also carries a requirement for nurses to know about an array of technologies and learning modalities. Nurses' efforts to improve health literacy levels will extend to instructing individuals on how to use the technology resources available to them in their home and community. Nurses will need to be able to show individuals how to use health-enabling technologies, such as a PHR, how to access trusted health information sites, and how to use tools interactively to communicate with their primary care team. Knowledge of health-enabling technologies, health information sites, emailing and document exchange, social networks, and wireless monitoring will be as basic for nurses to know as is handwriting with a pen.

Emergence of the PHR in Health Policy

Somewhat parallel to health policy initiatives like Healthy People 2010, the Markle Foundation has been a consistent leader throughout this decade in championing the consumer's perspective in effective use of the PHR. Known for its seminal surveys and the work of its PHR Working Group, the Markle Foundation has contributed significantly to moving the consumer-based, ePHR discussion forward. On 11 October 2005, the Markle Foundation published the results of a large national survey on PHRs, reporting that a large majority of Americans favor having interoperable health records that they themselves control.[48] The importance of the PHR being "person-centric," portable, and under the control of the individual emanated from the Markle Foundation's work and has informed health policy.

Starting with the work of the Healthy People 2010 initiative in 2000, HHS has promoted the PHR as the cornerstone of its health-enabling technology strategies.[3,27] As reviewed earlier, HHS' health strategy goals over this past decade have been to transform the US healthcare system having as its base an informed consumer with sufficient health literacy skills to enable their self-management and active participation in their healthcare decisions.[4,27] The PHR has come to be seen by health policymakers as an essential tool to accomplishing this goal of an empowered and informed consumer society. Since the beginning of this twenty-first century, the evolution of both EHR and PHRs offerings in the marketplace has been fast, furious, and fueled by direct grant funding, policy guidance, and most notably by HHS's intervention through the creation of the Office of the National Coordinator in 2004 (Thompson and Brailer 2004). The PHR has evolved over the last 10 years to such an extent that today most healthcare organizations, health plans, and EHR vendors offer a PHR. This explosion of offerings is evidenced in an (NLM/AHIMA) National Library of Medicine/American Health Informatics Management Association collaborative survey in which they counted more than 200 PHR solutions available in the market in 2007 (Sweet 2008).

While there has been no agreed-upon industry standard for what constitutes a PHR, there are two notable definitions often referenced. As one of the earliest consumer foundations to work in the PHR field, the Markle Foundation, through their *Connecting for Health: A Public-Private Collaborative*, published its definition in 2003.[49] The Markle Foundation's PHR Working Group generated this vision and definition of the PHR as "an Internet-based set of tools that allow people to access and coordinate their lifelong health information and make appropriate parts of it available to those who need it."[49] Two years later, the AHIMA published a more detailed definition that addressed the key areas of contention – record ownership, control, and sources:

> PHR is an electronic, lifelong resource of health information needed by individuals to make health decisions. Individuals own and manage the information in the PHR, which comes from healthcare providers and the individual. The PHR is maintained in a secure and private environment, with the individual determining rights of access. The PHR does not replace the legal record of any provider.[50]

The points that the AHIMA PHR Working Group were addressing in their definition that the individual owned their PHR as well as access to it. A second dimension that was not in practice in most of the PHRs available at the time was that the PHR should be a lifelong record populated by all sources that generated health information about an individual. Accessibility was to be from anyplace at anytime with privacy and security and guarantee supported by audit trail and transparency capabilities that allowed the individual to monitor security. And finally, stated is the expectation that the information within a PHR could be exchanged with health providers.

To address this lack of consensus on the PHR definition, in 2007, the Office of the National Coordinator for Health Information Technology (ONC) issued a contract for definitional work to the National Alliance for Health Information Technology (NAHIT). In April 2008, the NAHIT concluded a year-long process to create a consensus-based PHR definition based on literature reviews and public comment. Incorporating many of the concepts put forward by the Markel Foundation and AHIMA, this ONC-sanctioned definition describes an electronic record wholly managed by the consumer, conforming to nationally recognized standards, and capable of exchanging information with multiple sources:

> An electronic record of health-related information on an individual that conforms to nationally recognized interoperability standards and that can be drawn from multiple sources while being managed, shared, and controlled by the individual.[51]

PHR's Historical Evolution

Early health policy initiatives are reflected in the work coming from HHS through a myriad of governmental undertakings. Notable among these is the ODPHP. The work this department has produced through the Healthy People 2010, Focus #11 team has concentrated on the development and adoption of information and communication technologies (ICT) for improving health in our US society.[3,27] The body of work from the Health People 2010 project has served to launch other efforts from HHS departments including, the IOM, ARHQ, and ONC. This ICT health policy has also been pushed from the White House itself. In 2004, President Bush expressed his vision for an electronic health network linking doctors, hospitals, and patients. One element of his plan included the creation and adoption of lifelong electronic PHRs for patients.

In early 2005, the Secretary of HHS established the Commission on Systemic Interoperability. The members of this commission were appointed by the President and Congress and charged with developing a strategy to make healthcare information instantly accessible to consumers and healthcare providers. The Commission's report entitled *Ending the Document Game: Connecting and Transforming Your Healthcare through Information Technology* provided detailed and specific recommendations that have served to guide policy initiatives through to current day. Noting what it costs in terms of human lives not to have patient healthcare information available to doctors, the Commission called for the needed regulatory, reimbursement, and technical work to be done to make it possible for every consumer to have an interoperable electronic PHR by 2015.[52] Also in 2005, the Centers for Medicare & Medicaid Services (CMS) released a report on its

Request for Information regarding its role with PHRs. In June 2006, it awarded contracts to two vendors to pilot user-friendly PHRs to be generated from its claims data. In its third pilot series, it will select four vendors to test downloading Medicare claims data into commercial PHRs. Recently, it announced a 1-year pilot in two states, where Medicare recipients will voluntarily sign up to receive a PHR from one of the four vendors.[53]

The NLM has been an active participant in consumer empowerment and use of health-enabling technology. In 2006, the NLM released its Long Range Plan for 2006–2016. It included a strategic vision of patient health records as evolving toward "multimedia personal health knowledge bases."[54] Similarly, the Office of the National Coordinator of HIT (ONC) made several references to PHRs in its ONC-Coordinated Federal Health IT Strategic Plan: 2008–2012.[55] Specifically, to achieve the goal of patient-focused health care, the strategic plan calls for promoting "the nationwide adoption of interoperable EHRs by providers, and the adoption of PHRs and other consumer health IT tools by consumers and their designees"[55] (p. 19).

PHR Advocacy by Foundations and Consumer Groups

Other major health professional organizations, foundations, and consumer groups have also engaged in promoting the adoption of PHRs systems. In April 2006, as a service to the public, the American Association of Retired People (AARP) Public Policy Institute published a report describing PHR applications available to consumers and posted this information and their report on the AARP web site.[56] Another consumer advocacy body, the National Health Council (NHC), has promoted use of electronic PHRs as part of its "Putting Patients First®" initiative. In October 2005, the NHC announced a project, *Engaging Communities to Promote Electronic Personal Health Records (EPHRs)*. This NHC project will pilot initiatives in three states to educate the public about the benefits of PHRs, in the belief that greater adoption of PHR's would ultimately benefit the health and safety of those who use them.[57]

Believing that current-generation PHRs fail to live up to the promise of helping patients to be more engaged in maintaining their own health, the Robert Wood Johnson Foundation formed Project Health Design.[58] After soliciting applications to design innovations in PHR technology, Project Health Design awarded 18-month grants to nine interdisciplinary teams to develop prototype systems with advanced functionality for specific populations of users.[59] The resulting work is described in the 2009 final report of the Round 1 grantees.[60]

Health payers have also joined in the advocacy for PHR adoption. America's Health Insurance Plans (AHIP) and Blue Cross Blue Shield Association announced in May 2006 that they were forming a coalition to develop standards for an interoperable PHR. These insurers recognized that lack of portability acted as a major barrier to use of the PHRs supplied to their members, potentially representing 200 million Americans.[61] The resulting standards for electronic data interchange were published in June 2007.[62]

From a business perspective, the Continua Health Alliance serves as an example of activities in this sector of the marketplace. Continua Health Alliance came together as a group of technology, healthcare, and fitness companies looking to establish an ecosystem for their employees that connected personal health, fitness products, and technology services. The aim of the Alliance was to make it possible for patients, caregivers, and healthcare providers to more proactively address ongoing healthcare needs.[63,64]

Why ePHRs Are an Empowering Technology

At the simplest level, a PHR is an aggregation of one's health-related information obtained from many sources over the course of one's life. The content of a person's PHR varies widely. A 2006 survey by the Forrester Research group found that the five most common types of information that people kept in a PHR were (1) insurance information, such as policy numbers; (2) physician/specialist contact information; (3) personal information, such as contact information, social security number; (4) currently prescribed medications; and (5) history of insurance claims, payments, and health expenses. The next three categories were the list of illnesses and surgeries, followed by immunization records and past lab results.[65]

Our TIGER Collaborative team's work focused on electronic PHRs (or ePHRs). While it is certainly not necessary to use technology to record and store one's PHR, there are many benefits to using technology for this task. For example, software applications that support the gathering of data for one's PHR can also use that information to provide customized information about one's diagnoses or medications, or personalized reminders for preventive tests and treatments such as flu shots. Indeed, the Robert Wood Johnson's Project Health Design sees the record and its associated tools as a PHR "system" that enables consumers to "help people lead healthy lives and become engaged participants in their care."[66,67] Specifically, PHRs help empower consumers through the following: improved patient safety; access to their personal health information and general health information; communication with healthcare providers; and informed decision-making about their own care.

Patient Safety

Consumers are only too aware of the fragmentation of the current healthcare system. According to a 2007 Wall Street Journal/Harris Interactive poll, "only one third (33%) of adults are very confident in their physicians and other healthcare providers having a complete and accurate picture of their medical history."[68] In fact, many errors occur because individual professionals are not fully aware of all the therapies that the patient is receiving or has received.[69] A comprehensive PHR maintained and made accessible by the patient is one defense in a fragmented healthcare system.[70,71] In addition, in an emergency situation where the patient is unable to communicate, a personally carried PHR abstract that describes allergies, current diagnoses, and medications can make the difference between life and death.[72]

Education and Decision Support

Many PHR systems offer vetted educational information about diagnoses, medications, drug interactions, tests, and procedures written in a language that is appropriate for non-medical consumers and linked to the user's own record. Some also provide access to health-related news services, often tailored to the consumer's stated interests. The Harris Poll shows that over 80% of people who are online use the internet for retrieving health information, and on average, they do so almost five times per month.[73] When a PHR system offers vetted information in consumer-oriented language, tailored to the consumer's health interests, improvements in health literacy and personal engagement in one's health may result. Other educational and decision-support features that may be provided in a PHR system include the following:

- Decision support tools such as smoking cessation, decisions trees for when to see doctor for a problem, etc.
- Ability to enroll in online educational programs based on medical history/current conditions
- Information about local healthcare providers or insurers
- Health risk assessments and personalized suggestions for lifestyle changes
- Health tips for foreign countries and diplomatic contacts
- Medical glossary (with translation to vernacular)
- Clinical trials information with eligibility information and links to contacts for enrollment

Assistive Reminders

Some PHR systems allow the user to specify reminder times for medications or for recording findings such as blood pressure or spirometry readings. These reminders can be routed to the user's pager or cell phone. Some systems remind users when it is time to get a flu shot or other appropriate preventive tests and procedures such as mammogram, colonoscopy, etc. If such calls to action result in greater compliance, they could theoretically lead to prevention or earlier detection of disease and improved personal and population health.

Communication and Support Services

A Harris Interactive Poll found that the majority of patients (74%) would like to be able to communicate directly with their physician, and similar majorities would like to have access to other communication services such as test results via email, ability to schedule appointments, and ability to upload home-based medical information such as blood pressure, blood sugar, etc.[74] The Deloitte and CHCF surveys reviewed earlier in this chapter found very similar results[14] (CHCF 2008). Yet these surveys also report that fewer than 25% of physician practices offer such services to their patients. In some instances, support services that might be offered (particularly in an HMO environment) include access to a 24-h nursing line or access to a health coach to set personal health goals.

Integration with the Electronic Health Record

Many believe that the most benefit of a PHR is gained when the PHR is "tethered," or integrated with a healthcare system or physician's EHR.[70] The reason for this is that while the patient is the best source for history, symptoms, and data recorded in the home, information generated by professionals is best recorded by professionals and more likely to be accepted by other professionals. In this "tethered" model, one additional benefit is that the patient can view the information recorded by his or her professional caregivers and can request the provider to correct information when that is necessary.

Currently Available ePHR Products

Just as there are many definitions of ePHRs, there are many types of products available to the consumer. One common way of characterizing ePHRs is by describing whether it is "tethered," "interconnected," or "standalone."[70] As noted earlier, a tethered PHR is one that is offered by the consumer's healthcare provider, insurer, or employer. Information may be pre-populated with data generated by the sponsor (such as lab test results, claims, etc.) and supplemented by the consumer. An interconnected PHR is one where a service provider gathers data (with permission of the subscriber) from all various sources and stores it in a central location, with the subscriber granting access as appropriate to family and healthcare providers.[75] The standalone PHR is one where only the subscriber enters information. Privileges can be extended to others to see the record, or the record can be printed for others to see. Kaelber and colleagues envision a "hub and spoke" system where the patient-controlled record is the hub, with information exchanged as appropriate between the PHR and the records of healthcare providers, payers, laboratories, pharmacies, radiology services, and personal devices.[76,77] Such a system does not yet exist, due to many issues including interoperability of automated systems, lack of a clear business case, cost, and security and privacy concerns.

Costs to the Consumer

Costs also vary widely, ranging from nothing (for most tethered applications) to several hundred dollars per year for subscription services that gather information from various sources to populate the central record. Some offerings charge only for certain services, such as "online visits" with the physician. In a first of its kind, the Center for Information Technology Leadership (CITL) performed a cost-benefit analysis of four architecture types of PHRs to determine actual cost over a 10-year period if 80% of the US population were to adopt it usage. The four architecture PHRs evaluated were as follows: provider-tethered; payer-tethered; third party, and interoperable PHR (described above). Their model held constant eight PHR functions across these four types. From their model, CITL's estimates showed that it would cost more than 130 billion to install the *provider-tethered* PHR, but only five billion for *payer-tethered* and *third party*. Ongoing, annual maintenance costs were estimated at two billion for *payer-tethered* and *third party*; but *provider-tethered* came in at 43 billion. The *interoperable PHR* had the lowest cost to install and highest net value in cost savings of $19 billion annually. In marked contrast, the *provider-tethered* presented a loss of $29 billion annually; and *payer-tethered* and *third party* allowed for a net cost savings of $11 billion annually.[76,77]

Use and Usage

Though hundreds of thousands of consumers have access to an ePHR through their physician, health system, insurer, or payer,[75] most polls reveal that when asked, consumers think that the idea of a personally controlled, longitudinal PHR is a good thing,[14,48] actual usage of ePHRs is very low. A 2007 poll by Harris Interactive showed that only three percent of respondents said they used an ePHR either on their own computer or on the internet.[68] The Markle Foundation's *Connecting For Health* survey of June 2008 found that only 2.7% of respondents said they had a PHR, though nearly half-expressed interest in using one, and the majority agreed with each of several benefits cited.[78] Even with aggressive marketing, some health systems and HMOs report a usage rate of their sponsored ePHR only in the vicinity of 15% or so.[75]

Barriers to Use and Acceptance

Since the majority of persons believe that a personally controlled PHR is a good idea, and a very large number of people have access to an ePHR, why is actual usage so low? Many reasons have been proposed[70] (Green 2008), including the following:

Lack of awareness: Many people are not aware that they have access to an ePHR, and even if they are aware, they do not see the benefit of using it. Often, the most motivated users of a PHR are those who have a chronic condition or have multiple conditions and complex regimens.[65,79] This may be because people who fall into this category have greater need for information and for communication and coordination with their family and their healthcare providers. Noting that lack of awareness is a significant barrier to adoption, the NHC began an initiative in 2006 to develop messages educating consumers about the benefits of ePHRs and promoting use of the technology.[57]

Privacy and security concerns: As was the case early in the use of online banking, consumer wariness over privacy and security are significant barriers to adoption. Connecting for Health found that of the people who said they were not interested in having a PHR, over half cited concerns over privacy.[78] Harris Interactive polls show similar results, with 40% saying that privacy risks outweigh the benefits of using an ePHR.[68] Recognizing the need to address the issue, many public and private organizations have promulgated policy statements and guidelines. The Markle Foundation's Connecting for Health recently released its Common Framework for Networked Personal Health Information, proposing policy and technology principles that enhance the protection of privacy of information contained in ePHRs.[80] The framework was officially endorsed by a large number of prominent organizations, including very large healthcare systems, technology developers, consumer advocacy groups, and payers.[78] The Office of the National Coordinator of Health Information Technology released its own Nationwide Privacy and Security Framework for Electronic Exchange of Individually Identifiable Health Information, outlining principles that "are expected to guide the actions of all healthcare-related persons and entities that participate in a network for the purpose of electronic exchange of individually identifiable health information."[81] The Certification Commission for Healthcare Information Technology[82] is developing standards for certification of ePHRs that will include criteria for safeguarding privacy of information stored in ePHR products.

Lack of interoperability and portability: For many, a major disincentive to use a PHR is the amount of time needed to enter detailed information about diagnoses, medications, and test results, especially when the language is technical and difficult to comprehend.[70] Interoperability, that is, the ability for disparate systems to convey information to each other in computer-recognizable format, would greatly increase the convenience and efficiency of a personally controlled record. However, very few physicians use an electronic record to begin with, and even when they do, they rarely are able to convey information to a patient's separate (i.e., "untethered") record system. Even when insurers, employers, or health systems do populate the user's tethered record with information generated from within (such as claims data and laboratory test results), the information is constrained to only what is generated by that system, making the record incomplete. Furthermore, it is usually not then portable when the user moves to another health system, insurer, or employer. AHIP has developed standards for portability of insurer-generated claims data, a positive step for users of insurer-tethered PHRs.[61,62]

Lack of required features: In 2007, the NHC sponsored several meetings of representatives of patient organizations, health plan representatives, and patients. In those meetings, it became clear that the functionality described by the providers of ePHRs did not match the requirements of patients, many of whom had chronic diseases. Five major deficiencies were identified: disease-management tools that cover multiple co-morbidities; ability to track medication dosage in greater detail; ability to create end-of-life directives; ability to offer personal data for research; and ability to grant access to family members and professional caregivers.[83] Yet, research has shown that persons with chronic diseases are among the most motivated to use an ePHR.[65,79] The Robert Wood Johnson Foundation's Project Health Design asserts that today's ePHRs are only in their first generation, and that in order to truly assist people to manage their health, second-generation systems must evolve to meet the diverse needs of a population with varying levels of self-efficacy, health literacy, technical capability, and family and social supports.[66]

Innovations

A number of innovations, real, planned, and envisioned, show the promise of how PHRs can evolve to become a more valuable tool for consumer activation in their own health.

In late 2006, the Robert Wood Johnson Foundation's Project Health Design awarded 18-month grants to nine interdisciplinary teams to develop prototype systems with advanced functionality for specific populations of users. One of the requirements was that the prototype must be interoperable with the other grantees' applications. Among the innovations: a "conversational assistant" that engages patients with heart disease to record symptoms in natural language and to interpret the findings; a child-focused personal medication management system with customizable, age-appropriate "skins"; and a system that enables monitoring the physical activity of sedentary adults and generates a customized plan that increases activity levels consistent with their lifestyle.[59,60]

Yasnoff[84] has described a concept that is gaining traction: the "health record bank." In this system, each person would be provided with an "electronic account" where all providers of health services to an individual would "deposit" copies of their transactions with that person into a central repository. Account holders would grant access to appropriate people

to make "withdrawals," as the consumer sees fit. At this time, a few states are experiment-
ing with the concept, including Louisiana, Washington, and Oregon states.[85]

In Washington State, patients themselves designed a PHR called the "Shared Care Plan"
that enables them to engage fully with their care providers in managing chronic illness for
themselves and for their family members.[86] Readers who are interested in touring the
application can visit www.sharedcareplan.org. The system supports a conceptual model of
delivering care that is patient-centered. The Chronic Care Model was first developed by
Wagner et al.[87] with funding from the Robert Wood Johnson Foundation. Its major elements are the community, the health system, self-management support, delivery system
design, decision support, and importantly, clinical information systems[87] (Improving
Chronic Illness Care 2008).

Continua Health Alliance, after two years of developing guidelines for interoperability
of home-care devices, PHRs and EHRs, demonstrated the sharing of data among a variety
of pre-certified products and solutions at a conference in October, 2008. With dozens of
companies spanning the spectrum of healthcare, the Alliance claims as its mission to
"establish an ecosystem of connected personal health products and services."[64]

Standards and Usability Principles for ePHRs

According to the Forrester Research group, "Usability and design drive customer satisfaction, word of mouth, and ultimately, growth."[88] One complaint made by people who are
unenthusiastic about ePHRs is that they can be difficult to use. Applications developed by
technical experts, and even those designed by healthcare professionals, do not always take
into account the needs and sensibilities of consumers, who may suffer from disabilities,
lack of computer expertise, and poor health literacy. According to Forrester Research,
technical products will be adopted when consumers "can identify the *benefits* of those
products and believe those benefits are worth the effort and cost."[88] Tang and colleagues
assert that in order to achieve adoption, "the developers and users of EHRs and PHRs must
understand individuals' and clinicians' mental models of healthcare processes, and the
related workflows."[70] Similarly, Project Health Design asserts that PHR systems "ought to
be grounded in an understanding of the daily lives and health challenges of the individuals
they are designed to support," and that "PHRs must begin with an in-depth look at what
patients need and then find ways to collect, analyze, and deliver tailored information that
supports those objectives and fits easily into the user's daily life" [60] (p. 4). There is a rich
literature in usability principles for information systems, and some research has been
done specifically on usability principles of patient-focused applications.

Sources on ePHR Standards and Certification

Earlier, we discussed that some of the barriers to greater adoption of ePHRs are concerns
over privacy and security, lack of interoperability and portability, and lack of needed features. Several government, quasigovernment, and private organizations are addressing

these concerns by developing guidelines and standards for ePHRs that are intended both to guide the consumer in selecting a product and to spur developers to create products that meet minimum criteria. For examples of these standards and criteria, the reader is referred to these entities and their publications listed here:

1. Office of the National Coordinator for Health Information Technology.[81,89] Nationwide Privacy and Security Framework for Electronic Exchange of Individually Identifiable Health Information. http://www.hhs.gov/healthit/documents/NationwidePS_Framework. pdf
2. Certification Commission for Healthcare Information Technology.[82] Consumer's Guide to Certification of Personal Health Records. http://cchit.org/files/CCHITPHRConsumerGuide08. pdf
3. Connecting for Health.[80] Common Framework for Networked Personal Health Information: Overview and Principles. http://www.connectingforhealth.org/phti/reports/ overview.html
4. Health Level Seven, Inc. PHR-System Functional Model, Release 1, DSTU. Available for download from http://www.hl7.org
5. Continua Health Alliance, Use Cases for Interoperability of Devices and Solutions.[64] Available for viewing at http://www.continuaalliance.org/use_cases/

Nurses' Role in Promoting Use of ePHRs

If the ePHR is a tool that promotes patient empowerment and supports the patient's engagement in their own healthcare, then nurses as healthcare professionals and patient advocates are obligated to become familiar with the technology and to promote its use when the technology is available and the patient is amenable. Tang and colleagues assert that education in the health professions for all disciplines should include information about ePHRs as well as methods for teaching patients how to use them.[70] Nurses who specialize in informatics should have advanced education about ePHRs, including elements of design, usability, interoperability, available tools and products, implementation, maintenance, integration with EHRs, privacy, security, and authentication.[70] The Scope and Standards of Nursing Informatics Practice were augmented by the American Nurses Association to include patient use of technology for decision-making.[90] The revised Scope and Standards make several explicit references to patients' use of technology for managing their health and the role of nursing informatics specialists in supporting that function. For example, the patient is now included as a focus of education about effective and ethical uses of technology, and the patient's use of information tools and resources for health information is included as a focus for nursing informatics research. Certainly, it is a major objective of TIGER's Collaborative 9 Team to make information available to all nurses about ePHRs and to encourage inclusion of this content into nursing curricula. Nurses who enjoy using the technology to support nursing care can find new niche roles for themselves in telehealth, home care, case management, and population health using ePHR and communication technologies.

Nursing Informatics and Consumer Health Informatics

While the content areas just described are legitimate concerns for nursing informatics, there is a broader, multidisciplinary field that deals with technologies that support individual's knowledge and participation in their healthcare. Consumer Health Informatics is defined as use of communication and information technologies "to support consumers in obtaining information, analyzing their unique healthcare needs, and helping them make decisions about their own health."[91] Nurses have a vital role to play in this multidisciplinary field, with their clinical knowledge as well as their unique focus on patient education, patient empowerment, and patient advocacy.

Summary

The Markel Foundation's *Connecting for Health* PHR Work Group concluded in its 2006 report that to achieve healthcare transformation, our strategies must include a means to create a networked environment for PHRs and the aggregations of different types of data streams. These data include health claims data, pharmacy data, diagnostic images, and lab data. In the expectations that interoperability will be increasingly a reality, it is projected that providers will gradually form and join networks as their systems gain the ability to exchange information.

Implied in the AHIMA's 2005 PHR definition is a state of interoperable standardization, portability, and standardized terminology. This vision is still in the making to be a reality, but much closer with the standardization work that is being done under the direction of the Office of the National Coordinator for Health Information Technology and its numerous standards development bodies, such as HITSP (Health Information Technology Standards Panel), AHIC (American Health Information Community), and CCHIT (Certification Commission for Healthcare Information Technology). In 2009, the additional step has been taken under the Obama administration, as part of the American Recovery and Reinvestment Act (ARRA), to form a policy committee to oversee such a nationwide infrastructure. Formed by the Government Accountability Office (GAO) in April 2009, the Health Information Technology Policy Committee was charged with creating a framework for the development and adoption of a standard national infrastructure that would enable health data exchanges and transactions across organizations, stakeholders, and geographic areas (GAO 2009). It is exactly this interoperable standard that the major players in the marketplace, such as Microsoft Health Vault, *Google Health*, and Revolution Health, are banking on as they enter into this potentially lucrative niche market (AHIMA[92] at http://tigerphr.pbworks.com/).

Included in this review are a plethora of public and private entities that are actively engaged in all aspects of electronic PHRs, from policy statements to guidelines to standards to active development of applications for consumer use. Many of the references already cited in the report provide evidence of this. In addition, the Strategic Plan for Health IT from the Office of the National Coordinator for HIT not only describes an approach to HIT planning but includes a wide-ranging description across all government agencies of current initiatives dealing with health information technology.[89] That President Obama has also declared his intention to promote greater use of technology in healthcare only bodes well for the field.[93] The environment has never been more promising for the prospect of achieving electronic PHRs that are complete, accessible, affordable, easy to use, feature-rich, interoperable, and secure.

References

1. Saxon W. Frederich J. Schlink, writer and pioneer in consumerism (obituary). New York Times January 20. http://www.nytimes.com/1995/01/20/obituaries/frederick-j-schlink-writer-and-pioneer-in-consumerism-103.html?scp=9&sq=healthpercent20consumerismpercent20&st=cse; 1995.
2. Franklin D. The consumer, patient power: making sure your doctor really hears you. New York Times 15 August 2006. http://query.nytimes.com/gst/fullpage.html?res=9C06E4DB173EF936A2575BC0A9609C8B63&sec=health&spon=&scp=21&sq=health20consumerpercent20empowerment&st=cse; 2006.
3. Office of Disease Prevention and Health Promotion. Department of Health and Human Services. Healthy people 2010. Progress review on focus 11. www.healthypeople.gov/data/2010prog/focus11; 2007.
4. Institute of Medicine. Crossing the Quality Chasm. A New Health System for the 21st Century. Washington: National Academy; 2001.
5. New York Times. About Google. http://topics.nytimes.com/top/news/business/companies/google_inc/index.html?inline=nyt-org; 2009.
6. New York Times. About Yahoo. http://topics.nytimes.com/top/news/business/companies/yahoo_inc/index.html; 2009.
7. Broder C. Consumer demand will drive healthcare change, speakers say. Healthcare IT News. http://www.healthcareitnews.com/news/consumer-demand-will-drive-healthcare-change-speakers-say; 2005. Accessed 8.09.09.
8. Harris MC. Physicians need IT to succeed in consumer-driven Healthcare environment. Online presentation, HIMSS Virtual Conference, November. http://www.healthcareitnews.com/news/physicians-need-it-succeed-consumer-driven-healthcare-environment; 2007.
9. National Cancer Institute. National Institutes of Health. Clinical trial results. http://www.cancer.gov/clinicaltrials/ct-types-list; 2009.
10. Harvard Libraries Online. http://lib.harvard.edu/; 2009
11. Yale University Library. http://sfx.library.yale.edu/sfx_local/azlist; 2009. Accessed 11.07.09.
12. Nursing Outlook. Official Journal of the American Academy of Nursing. http://www.elsevier.com/wps/find/journaldescription.cws_home/623105/description#description; 2009.
13. Balint M. The Doctor, His Patient and the Illness. New York: International Universities Press; 1957.
14. Deloitte. Many consumers want major changes in health care design, delivery. Deloitte LLP. http://www.deloitte.com/dtt/article/0,1002,cid%253D192717,00.html; 2008.
15. Dickerson SS, Brennan PF. The Internet as a catalyst for shifting power in provider-patient relationship. Nurs Outlook. 2002;50:195-203.
16. Seidman J, Eytan T. Helping patients plug in: lessons in the adoption of online consumer tools. California Healthcare Foundation. www.chcf.org/documents/chronicdisease/HelpingPatientsPlugIn.pdf; 2008.
17. Lohr S. Kaiser backs Microsoft patient-data plan. NY Times, June 10. http://www.nytimes.com/2008/06/10/business/10kaiser.html; 2008.

18. Pew Internet & American Life Project. Online activities, 2000–2009. http://www.pewinternet. org/Static-Pages/Trend-Data/Online-Activities-20002009.aspx; 2009.
19. Pew Internet Online. Demographics of internet users; 2008.
20. Ferguson T, Frydman G. The first generation of e-patients. *BMJ*. 2004;328:1148-1149.
21. Madden M. Internet penetration and impact. Pew Internet & American Life Project. http:// www.pewinternet.org/Reports/2006/Internet-Penetration-and-Impact.aspx; 2006.
22. Fox S, Livingston G. Latinos online. Pew Internet & American Life Project. http://www.pewinternet.org/~/media//Files/Reports/2007/Latinos_Online_March_14_2007.pdf.pdf; 2007.
23. Jones S. Fox S. Generations online in 2009. Pew Internet & American Life Project. http:// www.pewinternet.org/Reports/2009/Generations-Online-in-2009.aspx; 2009.
24. Kutner M, Greenberg E, Jin Y, et al. The Health Literacy of America's Adults: results from the 2003 National Assessment of Adult Literacy (NCES2006-483). U.S. Department of Education. Washington, DC: National Center for Education Statistics. http://nces.ed.gov/pubsearch/pubsinfo.asp?pubid=2006483; 2006.
25. Rideout V, Neuman T, Kitchman M, et al. *E-health and the Elderly: How Seniors Use the Internet for Health Information*. Menlo Park: The Henry J. Kaiser Family Foundation; 2005.
26. Office of the Surgeon General. Proceedings of Surgeon General's Workshop on Improving Health Literacy. National Institutes of Health, Bethesda, MD. http://www.surgeongeneral. gov/topics/healthliteracy/pdf/proceedings120607.pdf; 2006.
27. Office of Disease Prevention and Health Promotion. Department of Health and Human Services. Healthy people 2010, Chapter 11, Health Communication 2000. http://www.healthypeople.gov/document/html/volume1/11healthcom.htm; 2000.
28. Baur C. Health literacy as a factor in the adoption and use of Personal Health Records. Deparment of Health and Human Services. Presentation for US Surgeon General's Office. http://tigerphr.pbworks.com/Work+Group+3 or contact at Cynthia.Baur@hhs.gov; 2006. Accessed 2.08.09.
29. Berkman ND, DeWalt DA, Pignone MP, et al. Literacy and health outcomes. Evidence report/technology assessment #87. AHRQ Publication No 04-E007-1. www.ahrq.gov/clinic/epcsums/litsum.pdf; 2004. Accessed 3.07.09.
30. Lynn NB, Panzer AM, Kindig DA, eds. *Committee on Health Literacy, Institute of Medicine. Health Literacy: A Prescription to End Confusion*. Washington: National Academies; 2004.
31. Henderson V. *The Nature of Nursing: A Definition and Its Implications for Practice, Research, and Education*. New York: Macmillan; 1966.
32. Office of Disease Prevention and Health Promotion. Department of Health and Human Services. Quick guide to health literacy. www.health.gov/communication/literacy/quickguide/; 2006a.
33. Zorn M, Allen MP, Horowitz AC. National Library of Medicine, NIH. Understanding health literacy and its barriers. Current bibliographies in medicine 2004–1 (2000) and (2004). http:// www.nlm.nih.gov/pubs/cbm/healthliteracybarriers.html; 2004. Accessed 11.07.09.
34. Agency for Health Research and Quality. Barriers and drivers of health information technology use for the elderly, chronically ill, and underserved, Rockville, MD. http://www.ahrq.gov/ clinic/tp/hitbartp.htm; 2008. Accessed 8.07.09.
35. Whitehurst GJ. Director, Institute of Education Sciences, U.S. Department of Education. Presentation at the Surgeon General's Workshop on Improving Health Literacy, Bethesda, MD. http://www.surgeongeneral.gov/topics/healthliteracy/panel1.htm; 7 Sep 2009. Accessed 11.07.09.
36. Baker DW, Gazmararian JA, Williams MV, et al. Functional health literacy and the risk of hospital admission among Medicare managed care enrollees. *Am J Public Health*. 2002;92(8):1278-1283.
37. Baker DW, Parker RM, Williams MV, Clark WS. The relationship of patient reading ability to self-reported health and use of health services. *Am J Public Health*. 1997;87(6):1027-1030.
38. Baker DW, Parker RM, Williams MV, Clark WS. Health literacy and the risk of hospital admission. *J Gen Intern Med*. 1998;13(12):791-798. Comment in: *J Gen Intern Med*. 1998;13(12):850-851.

39. Friedland R. New estimates of the high costs of inadequate health literacy. In: *Proceedings of Pfizer Conference Promoting Health Literacy: A Call to Action*. Washington: Pfizer; 7–8 Oct 1998:6-10.

40. Scott TL, Gazmararian JA, Williams MV, et al. Health literacy and preventive health care use among Medicare enrollees in a managed care organization. *Med Care*. 2002;40(5):395-404.

41. Williams M, Parker R, Baker D, et al. Inadequate functional health literacy among patients at two public hospitals. *JAMA*. 1995;274(21):1677-1682.

42. Office of Disease Prevention and Health Promotion. Department of Health and Human Services. Expanding the reach and impact of consumer e-Health tools. www.health.gov/communication/ehealth/ehealthTools/default.htm; 2006.

43. Office of Disease Prevention and Health Promotion. Department of Health and Human Services. America's health literacy: why we need accessible health information. www.health.gov/communication/literacy/issuebrief; 2008.

44. Joint Commission. Understanding your doctors and other caregivers, Chicago. http://www.jointcommission.org/PatientSafety/SpeakUp/sp_understanding.htm; 2008.

45. Office of Civil Rights. Health information privacy. http://www.hhs.gov/ocr/hipaa/; 2008.

46. American Nurses Association. *Nursing: Scope and Standards of Practice*. Washington: American Nurses Publishing; 2004.

47. Institute of Medicine. *Retooling for An Aging America. Building the Healthcare Workforce*. Washington: National Academies; 2008.

48. Markle Foundation. Americans support online personal health records: patient privacy and control over their own information are crucial to acceptance. http://www.markle.org/resources/press_center/press_releases/2005/press_release_10112005.php; 2005.

49. Markle Foundation. Connecting for health. The Personal Health Working Group final report. http://www.connectingforhealth.org/resources/final_phwg_report1.pdf; 2003. Accessed 8.09.09.

50. AHIMA e-HIM Personal Health Record Work Group. Defining the personal health record. *J AHIMA* 2005;76(6): 24-25. http://library.ahima.org/xpedio/groups/public/documents/ahima/bok1_027351.hcsp?dDocName=bok1_027351. Accessed 16.07.08.

51. National Alliance for Health Information Technology. Defining key health information technology terms. Report to Office of the National Coordinator for Health Information Technology. http://www.nahit.org/images/pdfs/HITTermsFinalReport_051508.pdf; 2008.

52. Commission on Systemic Interoperability. Ending the Document Game. U.S. National Library of Medicine, National Institutes of Health, Department of Health and Human Services. http://endingthedocumentgame.gov/; 2005.

53. Government Health IT. Medicare test of PHRs gets under way in two states. http://www.govhealthit.com/newsitem.aspx?tid=72&nid=69548; 2009.

54. National Library of Medicine. Charting a course for the 21st century – NLM's long range plan 2006–2016. National Library of Medicine. http://www.nlm.nih.gov/pubs/plan/lrp06/NLM_LRP2006_WEB.pdf; 2006.

55. Department of Health and Human Services. ONC-coordinated federal health it strategic plan: 2008–2012. http://healthit.hhs.gov/portal/server.pt/gateway/PTARGS_0_10741_848083_0_0_18/HITStrategicPlan508.pdf; 2008.

56. Cronin C. Personal health records: an overview of what is available to the public. AARP Public Policy Institute. http://www.aarp.org/research/health/carequality/2006_11_phr.html; 2006.

57. National Health Council. Putting patients First® – progress toward action pilot projects. Council currents. http://www.nationalhealthcouncil.org; 2006.

58. Project Health Design. Expert teams to design new solutions for personal health records to help consumers manage their health. http://www.projecthealthdesign.org/news/5535; 2006. Accessed 16.07.09.

59. Project Health Design. Grantee projects. http://www.projecthealthdesign.org/projects; 2007.

60. Project Health Design. Round one final report. http://www.projecthealthdesign.org/media/file/Round%20Onepercent20PHD%20Final%20Report6.17.09.pdf; 2009.
61. America's Health Insurance Plans. Industry leaders announce personal health record model; collaborate with consumers to speed adoption. http://www.ahip.org/content/pressrelease.aspx?docid=18328&pf=true; 2006. Accessed 16.07.09.
62. America's Health Insurance Plans. Standards for electronic data interchange: personal health record data transfer between health plans (275). Version 3.1.4. http://www.ahip.org/content/default.aspx?bc=39|341|18427|20076; 2007. Accessed 16.07.09.
63. Continua Health Alliance. Continua Health Alliance takes next step in offering connectivity to better manage health and wellness. http://www.continuaalliance.org/news_events/press_room/FINAL_Continua_Press_Release_09_11_07.pdf; 2007.
64. Continua Health Alliance. Continua Health Alliance advances mission to create connected personal health ecosystem. http://www.continuaalliance.org/static/binary/cms_workspace/Continua_Update_release_v_FINAL_2_.pdf; 2008.
65. Bishop L. Are personal health records breaking out? Forrester Research. http://www.forrester.com/Research/Document/Excerpt/0,7211,39415,00.html; 2006. Accessed 8.09.09.
66. Project Health Design. Personal health records – current landscape and future visions. http://www.projecthealthdesign.org/about/overview; 2007. Accessed 16.07.09.
67. Project Health Design. Project health design: rethinking the power and potential of personal health records. http://www.projecthealthdesign.org/; 2007.
68. Harris Interactive. U.S. adults not very confident that physicians have the complete picture, according to a New WSJ.com/Harris interactive survey. http://www.harrisinteractive.com/news/printerfriend/index.asp?NewsID=1264; 2007. Accessed 8.09.09.
69. Ghandi TK, Weingart SN, Borus J, et al. Adverse drug events in ambulatory care. *N Engl J Med*. 2003;348:1556-1564.
70. Tang P, Ash J, Bates DW, et al. Personal health records: definitions, benefits, and strategies for overcoming barriers to adoption. *JAMIA*. 2006;13(2):121-126.
71. Cain C, Clancy C. Commentary: patient-centered health information technology. *Am J Med Qual*. 2005;20(3):164-165.
72. Wolter J, Friedman B. Health records for the people: touting the benefits of the consumer-based personal health record. *J Am Health Info Manage Assoc*. 2005;76(10):28-32.
73. Harris Poll®. Number of "cyberchondriacs" – adults going online for health information – has plateaued or declined. Rochester: Harris Interactive. http://www.harrisinteractive.com/harris_poll/index.asp?PID=686; 2008.
74. Wall Street Journal Online/Harris Interactive Health-Care Poll. Few patients have access to online services for communicating with their doctors, but most would like to. http://www.harrisinteractive.com/news/newsletters/wsjhealthnews/WSJOnline_HI_Health-CarePoll2006vol5_iss16.pdf; 2006.
75. Jossi F. Personal health records. Healthcare informatics. http://www.healthcare-informatics.com; 2006.
76. Kaelber DC, Jha AK, Johnston D, et al. A research agenda for personal health records (PHRs). *JAMIA*. 2008;15(6):729-736.
77. Kaelber DC, Shah S, Vincent A, et al. The value of personal health records. Center for Information Technology Leadership (CITL), Partners HealthCare System. Chicago: HIMSS http://www.citl.org/_pdf/CITL_PHR_Report.pdf; 2008.
78. Connecting for Health. Technology companies, providers, health insurers and consumer groups agree on framework for increasing privacy and consumer control over PHRs. http://www.connectingforhealth.org/news/pressrelease_062508.html; 2008.
79. Carrell D, Ralston JD. Variation in adoption rates of a patient web portal with a shared medical record by age, gender, and morbidity level. AMIA Symp Proc 2006:871.
80. Connecting for Health. Common framework for networked personal health information: overview and principles. http://www.connectingforhealth.org/phti/reports/overview.html; 2008.

81. Office of the National Coordinator for Health Information Technology. Nationwide privacy and security framework for electronic exchange of individually identifiable health information. Department of Health and Human Services. http://healthit.hhs.gov/portal/server.pt/ gateway/PTARGS_0_10731_848088_0_0_18/NationwidePS_Framework-5.pdf; 2008.

82. Certification Commission for Healthcare Information Technology. Consumer's guide to certification of personal health records. http://www.cchit.org/sites/all/files/20080604IntroPH RAdvisoryTaskForce.pdf; 2008.

83. National Health Council. Prototype EPHR challenges revealed, next steps planned. Council currents. http://www.nationalhealthcouncil.org/forms/newsletters/dec-07.pdf; 2007.

84. Yasnoff WA. Electronic records are key to health-care reform. Business Week, December 19. http://www.businessweek.com/print/bwdaily/dnflash/content/dec2008/ db20081218_385824.htm; 2008. Accessed 16.07.09.

85. Robinson B. Banking on health IT. Government health IT; 30 July 2008.

86. Pierson M. Pursuing perfection (P2) in chronic and complex conditions. Presentation to the Governor's Long Term Care Task Force. http://www.governor.wa.gov/LTCTF/ac_ ccm/060614/Marc_Pierson_CCM.pdf; 14 June 2006.

87. Wagner EH, Austin BT, Davis C, et al. Improving chronic illness care: translating evidence into action. *Health Aff (Millwood)*. 2001;20:64-78.

88. Bernoff J. TechPotential: predicting technology success. Forrester Big Idea. http://www.for-rester.com/Research/Document/Excerpt/0,7211,37510,00.html; 2006. Accessed 8.09.09.

89. Office of the National Coordinator for Health Information Technology. The ONC-Coordinated Federal Health IT strategic plan: 2008–2012. Department of Health and Human Services. http://healthit.hhs.gov/portal/server.pt?open=512&objID=1211&parentname=CommunityPa ge&parentid=5&mode=2&in_hi_userid=10732&cached=true; 2008. Accessed 16.07.09.

90. American Nurses Association. *Scope and Standards of Nursing Informatics Practice.* Washington: American Nurses Publishing; 2008.

91. McDaniel AM, Schutte DL, Keller LO. Consumer health informatics: from genomics to population health. *Nur Outlook.* 2008;56:216-223.

92. AHIMA Personal Health Record Practice Council. Defining the personal health information management role. *J AHIMA.* 2008;79(6):59-63.

93. Brewer B. Obama pledges to pursue health it, despite economic woes. http://www.nextgov. com/nextgov/ng_20081212_8804.php; 2008. Accessed 8.09.09.

94. Connecting for Health. A common framework for networked personal health information. www.connectingforhealth.org/commonframework/docs/P9_NetworkedPHRs.pdf; 2006.

95. Health Affairs. Founded by project HOPE in 1981. http://www.healthaffairs.org/1500_ about_journal.php; 1981.

96. Health Level Seven. PHR-system functional model, release 1, DSTU. Health Level 7; 2007.

97. Health Level Seven. Health Level Seven publishes personal health record system functional model (PHR-S FM as a draft standard for trial use. http://www.hl7.org/documentcenter/ public/pressreleases/HL7_PRESS_20081215.pdf; 2008.

98. Fox S, Jones S. The social life of health information. Pew Internet & American Life Project. http://www.pewinternet.org/~/media//Files/Reports/2009/PIP_Health_2009.pdf; 2009.

99. U.S. Department of Veterans Affairs. VA improves "My Health eVet" Web Site. http://www. washingtondc.va.gov/news/healthyvet.asp; 2003.

100. U.S. Department of Veterans Affairs. What's new on my health eVet. https://www.myhealth. va.gov/mhv-portal-web/anonymous.portal?_nfpb=true&_pageLabel=whatsNew&_ nfls=false; 2009.

101. Wall Street Journal Online/Harris Interactive Health-Care Poll. New poll shows U.S. adults strongly favor and value new medical technologies in their doctor's office. http://www.har-risinteractive.com/news/newsletters/wsjhealthnews/WSJOnline_HI_Health-CarePoll2005vol4_iss20.pdf; 2005. Accessed 16.07.09.

Disruptive Innovation: Point of Care

17

John S. Silva, Nancy Seybold, and Marion J. Ball

Insanity, doing the same thing and expecting different results
Albert Einstein

This fourth edition of *Nursing Informatics* is replete with examples of how information technology (IT) can help nurses work safer and provide "better" care. One section in this volume contains a detailed description of the TIGER initiative that lays out a set of core informatics competencies for nurses and a roadmap of how to infuse nursing with the capacity to use IT to its fullest extent. The vision of the TIGER initiative is to: "enable nurses to use informatics tools, principles, theories and practices... making information technology the stethoscope for the twenty-first century." This TIGER initiative even recommends an "IT driver's license" to certify that a nurse knows how to drive the IT systems he or she will use. No one would get a driver's license, however, if driving a car was of little use in everyday life. In order for IT to become an integral part of the practice of nursing, it must be fundamentally *useful*.

The analogy of driving a car is an apt one. Driving enables us to get from one point to another more quickly, unless we are stuck in a major traffic jam. Most car drivers know very little and care less about the intricacies of how the car works or what the engine does when it burns gasoline. All we are interested in is inserting the key, starting the car, and driving to our next location. In this context our "transportation technology" provides significant *value* and enables us to accomplish something that we could not do without it. A relevant IT analogy is depicted in a recent TV commercial for the Apple iPhone. A couple is finishing dinner and decides to go to the movies. With a few quick finger flicks, the couple identifies a movie they want to see, locate a nearby theater, and buy the tickets, all in less than a minute. The iPhone delivers immediately useful information, minimal effort by the user; and by implication, almost no training with minimal learning curve. Apple's high value for minimal cost computing paradigm has disrupted the smart phone industry. We need just this kind of disruptive paradigm in health care.

Authors' note: It is important for the reader to understand that these essential elements of a PCMH were defined exclusively by physician organizations. The authors have used the term Medical Home to be more inclusive of all health practitioners.

J.S. Silva (✉)
Silva Consulting Services, 2055 Conan Doyle Way, Eldersburg, MD 21784, USA
e-mail: jc-silva-md@att.net

M.J. Ball et al. (eds.), *Nursing Informatics*,
DOI: 10.1007/978-1-84996-278-0_17, © Springer-Verlag London Limited 2011

Our health IT systems must make it easier for us, and hopefully safer, to accomplish the key job of a clinician, which is to provide better care for patients. The major objective of health IT should be to subtract work, not to add work or make our work harder. This lack of value and utility for clinicians is the principal reason why most health professionals do not use their health IT systems (See also the Chapter "The Role of Usability and Clinical Application Design in Health Information Technology Adoption" by Staggers and Troseth). In 2001, the Institute of Medicine (IOM)[1] issued a landmark report that stated "to improve quality in health care health care professionals (HCP) needed to interact effectively and efficiently with the health IT systems." Unfortunately, the report's corollary, that health IT systems effectively and efficiently support clinical users, is not substantiated by the preponderance of evidence. Clinical IT systems have adoption rates that are typically less than 15%. A recent report from the Health Information and Management Systems Society's EHR Usability Task Force[2] concluded:

> Electronic medical record (EMR) adoption rates have been slower than expected in the United States, especially in comparison to other industry sectors and other developed countries. A key reason, aside from initial costs and lost productivity during EMR implementation, is lack of efficiency and usability of EMRs currently availableThe recent National Academy of Science (NAS) study *Computational Technology for Effective Health Care: Immediate Steps and Strategic Directions* agreed that current health IT systems do not support clinical users and are not designed for usability. It concluded that the current health IT efforts may even set back the vision of twenty-first century health care.[3]

The above reports and studies do not address the fundamental relationship between value and usability; that is, the usability of a system is intimately related to the immediate value that the system provides to its users. The iPhone's rapid and pervasive success is a clear example of how value and usability are inextricably intertwined. A recent report[4] described the value proposition to clinical users thus:

> If technology eases their [clinical users] work in compelling ways, they will adopt it, just as they have adopted cell phones and personal digital assistants. Clinicians will adapt, if they see the value of doing so. Clinicians want systems that support and enhance their work – in short, that ease it, not complicate itThe next section describes the conceptual architecture for a Smart Point of Care (POC) system that is designed to specifically address value and utility for clinicians.

Vision and Value of Clinician Support via a Smart POC System

Imagine a "Nursing Support system" at the POC that

- Knows and uses your context; where you are, what patient you are seeing, what set of tasks you need to perform – based on locally relevant outcomes and measures
- Supports all the coordination and scheduling tasks that you must "orchestrate" for your patients
- Is customized based on what you enter, what you need to see, and what you do – to closely replicate the way you think

- Moves from device to device – installing automatically on whatever device you are using, scaling to the display, hardware capacity, operating system
- Connects securely to whatever source of information is required by you – electronic records, results, reference literature, and more[5,]

The fusion of efficient, best clinical practices, and patient information at the POC will directly support improved quality of care and produce cost savings that have not been realized by current health IT systems. "Savings" and "improved quality of care" can never be realized if clinicians would not put the data in. Contrary to some conventional wisdom, they are avid adopters of *useful* information technology and just want a product that can "help them do everything they need to do at the point of care."[7] Thus, a clinician's work environment that actively supports intelligent provision of clinical data and information to and from its clinical users could become a "highly leveraged" interface to health and other systems that are needed to support the full spectrum of health services delivery. Such a system could transform the health care sector and realize the true potential of useful IT as shown in Fig. 17.1.

This work environment would support its nursing users by reducing the time it takes for purely administrative tasks while providing relevant clinical information and knowledge to the POC, thus increasing the time available for a nurse to think about all the data and information about a patient and then, thoughtfully, address the patient's problem. It is *not* intended to increase the number of patients a nurse can manage per hour, per shift, or other measure of "productivity." Although the overall timeline is shortened, the time "saved" is now available for listening to and talking with the patient!

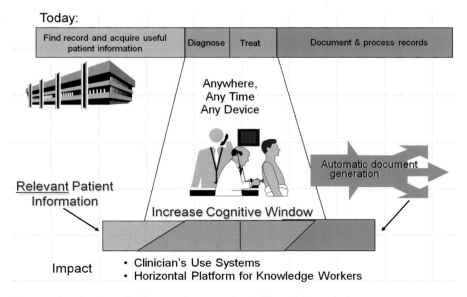

Fig. 17.1 Changing how clinicians work. From John S. Silva, with permission

The Smart POC system described above has other key attributes, namely:

- It anticipates your needs – have data/information you need before you need it
- It understands your context-dependent workflows
- It waits on you
- It hides all the complexity of underlying health IT systems with simplicity ("magical" IT)
- It is built to bring immediate value to you

A conceptual architecture for Smart POC support is shown below in Fig. 17.2.[6] The three components operate within a services-oriented architecture and exchange data within the Smart POC and to external information sources (such as local HIS, health information exchanges (HIE), and knowledge sources) using standardized messages.

The Context/Task Manager (C/TM) is the "heart" of the architecture. It monitors user's activity to determine context, uses models of user's tasks and current/expected context to anticipate activities, tasks, and necessary data exchanges with the User Interface Manager (UIM) and the Information Broker (IB) components, and maps user activities and tasks to the most appropriate support application for a true extensible software-as-a-service framework. The IB component is the data/information cache for its users as well as the connection point to external systems. The set of services required by the IB are available in many commercial HIE or SOA offerings from vendors. Both the C/TM and IB have analytic engines that monitor the efficacy and efficiency of user and system tasks vs. outcomes to continuously enhance best practices and system performance. The UIM component presents relevant data, information, and medical knowledge to clinicians and gathers data from them. It has presentation strategies to achieve communication goals that depend upon

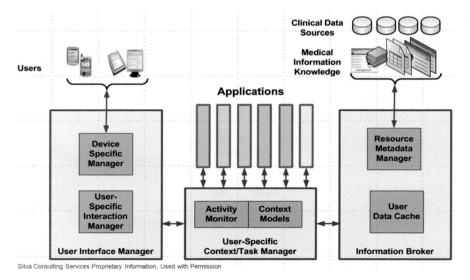

Silva Consulting Services Proprietary Information, Used with Permission

Fig. 17.2 Conceptual architecture of the smart point of care (POC) environment. From John S. Silva, with permission

current context, criticality of message and device being used; adapt to the unique style of the clinician; and provide a consistent set of metaphors regardless of the clinician's location.

The Smart POC system is designed to:

- Automatically present relevant clinical data and information via prefilled "Clinical Widgets"
- Offer "Executable" patient care plans
- Unobtrusively collect patient data
- Generate relevant charge or billing information as a by-product
- Adapt to the nurse's and communities' best practices

The value proposition to nurses and other clinical users is that they would have an IT designed for them that implements a systems engineering approach for the collection, distribution, and maintenance of best practices, clinical data, and system performance. This context-aware Smart POC uses clinician-specific and continuously adapting practice patterns that have the potential to dramatically enhance the quality and efficiency of health service delivery. The systems approach addresses the very thorny and expensive issue of how to make practice guidelines/best practices relevant to local context and, at the same time, solves the "how can we maintain and evolve the practices that we have implemented" question. The built-in business intelligence and analytic tools provide clinicians and managers the "What's Been Done" vs. "What Should Be Done" based on context and outcomes. This near real-time feedback loop simultaneously provides analyses for informed decisions about

- What is best for "my" patients
- What is best for our community, our state, and our nation (population-level)
- Best practicesand is described more fully in the "A Model for Health Care Success" section below. The following section identifies major IT innovations that are in place or coming soon that will make such a Smart POC system as just described feasible to develop and implement.

The Future of Information Technology

The Internet has transformed information availability. Agile companies are realizing reduced costs, increased revenue, faster time-to-market, and increased customer satisfaction. They are capitalizing on Internet-enabled applications such as dynamic supply chains, customer relationship management, and emerging web services opportunities. Concurrent with the above trend, cloud computing, which are vast girds of always-on computing resources, is fundamentally changing how companies purchase these IT components and services. No longer are businesses being held "captive" by expensive and very proprietary hardware and software. They can access inexpensive, best-of-breed systems and services that are priced as commodities in the fast pace of Internet time.[8] In many cases, fairly robust versions of software products are free, like Google Analytics and many web conferencing systems, or the international phone service Skype. As a result, today's users expect to access whatever information one needs, wherever and however one needs, and execute useful transactions with *no* learning curve. The gold standard at publication time is instant access to online banking services, from your iPhone, in a seamless interface that just works to pay your bills and manage your finances. Health IT needs to play in the same sandbox.

Much more powerful, lightweight, and low-power computers and advances in user interfaces and human–computer interaction approaches are bringing computers to the point where they interact with humans in a way that is natural to us ("intimate computing"). The Smart Room project at the University of Pittsburgh Medical Center is using these technologies and ubiquitous computing to fully integrate clinical information systems and clinical workflows directly in the patient's room. For example, a nurse enters the Smart Hospital Room wearing aWiFi tag. The sensor in the room automatically recognizes her and retrieves relevant patient information from the UPMC electronic medical record and task information from the nursing system. The room then displays the information to both the nurse and patient to enhance patient safety as alerts and reminders are displayed in real time (Sharbaugh and Ball, 2009 personal communication).

Manufacturing approaches used for computers are finally shrinking medical devices and making them significantly more affordable and pervasive. These devices, which require a fraction of the maintenance, supplies, and technical support of their counterparts even a decade ago, will be commonly available in doctor's offices. They will also usher in a new age in monitoring disease states. Devices specifically crafted to monitor diseases and medications will be used daily within the home and will transmit data and analyses directly to monitoring systems and/or physicians' mobile devices and office systems.[9]

These technologies and the resultant influx of data, analyses, and alerts will further exacerbate the need for a new family of applications like the Smart POC system. Without these intelligent systems and their feedback loops, it will be impossible for nurses and other clinicians to stay abreast of all that is happening to their patients without being overwhelmed by information overload.

Can health care exploit these new IT opportunities? Not with current IT systems, nor with the focus on "sick" care. The next section explores a new model for the delivery of consumer-centered holistic health services and the emerging role of health practitioners to focus on coordinating and optimizing these services as opposed to only doing sick care. It also identifies the opportunity for nursing to participate in and define a new health practice through the design and use of usable health IT.

A Model for Health Care Success

Our healthcare system is a very large $2+ trillion enterprise with many diverse "business units." Each of these business units is firmly entrenched within the system and has a vested interest in ensuring that its portion of revenue increases or, at worst, does not change. There is therefore significant pressure to keep the status quo and continue to focus on treating disease in patients (i.e., delivering sick care).

Other industrialized countries have found that delivering a majority of health services through primary care physician practices and focusing on health by keeping people healthy work quite well. These systems do not require over 15% of their gross domestic product (GDP) as our system in the United States does. Since wholesale changes to our healthcare system are not feasible in the current climate, is it possible to use the above principles in pilots of a new model that just might become the measure of success for our *health*care system?

In the United States, the Medical Home is unique in that it focuses, like systems in many other industrialized countries, on primary care physician practices and on keeping its participants healthy. The Medical Home model has already developed substantial traction in both the private and public sectors:

- Centers for Medicare and Medicaid Services (CMS) have started demonstration projects to test the concept of a medical home as part of the Tax Relief and Health Care Act of 2006.
- There were 20 bills in 10 states that provide for a medical home demonstration project.[10]
- A number of Fortune 100 companies and other organizations have formed the Patient-Centered Primary Care Collaborative to promote the model and foster implementation.

The Medical Home model, as defined by the "Joint Principles of the Patient-Centered Medical Home,"[11] is a physician-directed practice that provides accessible, continuous, comprehensive, and coordinated care that is delivered in the context of family and community (the seven essential elements: (1) Each participant has an ongoing relationship with a personal physician trained to provide first-contact, continuous, and comprehensive care. (2) The personal physician leads a team of people at the practice level who collectively take responsibility for patient care. (3) That physician is responsible for providing for all of the patient's health care needs or arranging care with other qualified professionals for all stages of life. (4) Care is coordinated and integrated across all elements of the complex health care system and the patient's community. This is facilitated by the deployment of information technology and health information exchange. (5) Care is based on quality and safety, including the use of evidence-based decision support, IT, performance feedback to physicians, active engagement in quality improvement activities, patient education, and incorporating feedback from patients in decision making. (6) Access to care is timely and supported by improved methods of communication between patients and the health care team. (7) Payments appropriately recognize the added value provided to patients who have a PCMH). Geisinger reported that it had a 20% reduction in hospital admissions, a 7% reduction in overall medical costs, and significant improvements in more than 20,000 diabetic patients that were managed in Medical Home.[12]

Berenson et al. recently identified challenges to adoption of the Medical Home model that included: physician preferences and attitudes, practice size, target population, and new management responsibilities. Regarding the management challenge, Berenson states:

> It [a full-featured medical home] requires developing processes and systems (including IT) to support high levels of access for and communications with patients, coordination of patients' care within and outside the practice, capturing and using data for care of patients and populations and evaluation of performance, and support for evidence-based decision-making[13]

In addition, there is no uniformity regarding what constitutes a "good" Medical Home. There exist numerous flavors of the model: some practices focus on coordination of care, some are patient-centered, and yet others focus on chronic disease management. Importantly, few have undertaken a "clean sheet" approach to the design of the new practice to optimize the activities of all Medical Home staff. Since nursing staff already coordinate clinical activities for many of their patients, it would seem to be a natural fit for nursing to play a major role in the coordination of health services in these environments. Nurses are often the case managers in companies that provide chronic disease management support.

There is a strong expectation that the member's Medical Home will be the connection point for all interactions between the health consumer and their required medications, specialists, diagnostic studies, and the like. It is envisioned that the health consumer, in a Medical Home environment, will transition from a passive "patient" that is told what to do to a fully engaged and active partner in his/her care. Thus, a successful Medical Home must engage and reward all participants, including the end user: the health care consumer. Much work has been done on the adoption and use of patient-driven tools for the management of chronic conditions, and consumers in general have come to expect a high level of transparency and access to critical information in other aspects of their lives (in particular financial). Capitalizing on both of these trends through an intuitive, web-based "Medical Home" will support the desired outcomes; healthier people receiving efficient, targeted, and appropriate health services. The online Medical Home should allow users to access their own information, understand the choices they have for care, actively manage their own chronic conditions, and participate as a partner in the healthcare "system," rather than being at the mercy of it, as is commonly found in traditional environments.

This is a key opportunity for nursing to step forward and ensure that the business practices and IT are done right. The Medical Home needs to support the primary mission of nurses; that is, to provide coordinated, patient-centric care without a lot of distraction from administrative and other "peripheral" tasks. A well-designed Medical Home, and its underlying IT systems, should allow nurses to do their job and reap the benefit from more effective delivery of care, and satisfied and healthy patients. Integration of in-home monitoring and a new emphasis on wellness care in the Medical Home model will allow nurses to alter the fundamental health care equation from fixing people ("sick care") to nurturing people in health and in sickness. Unfortunately, these new business practices, the information exchanges, and the capabilities to support consumer engagement have yet to be defined. Most of these capabilities are not available in any existing EHR system. Given its track record to date, it is unlikely that the health IT community can provide the technology to fix this problem. Nor have health IT providers demonstrated an ability or a willingness to successfully import technologies from other industry sectors. Unfortunately, in the absence of appropriate and useful IT support for these critical components, it is unlikely that Medical Home efforts will achieve the anticipated benefits or that these efforts can be sustained without ongoing public and private investments. The last section in this chapter describes a roadmap to build out the IT infrastructure needed for a successful Medical Home.

Roadmap to the Successful Medical Home

There are several examples of exploiting existing technologies for success. Most recently, the Obama campaign exploited the "Net Effect" and social networking to engage and enable Americans to participate directly and actively in the campaign. As has been well-documented, Wal-Mart dominates the consumer marketplace by exploiting IT that links their partners to a high performance virtual enterprise and that delivers real-time business intelligence to all participants. In both situations, a transparent IT infrastructure provides strong value to participants.

Our approach recommends that we:

- Establish a Medical Home project that focuses on bringing world class IT infrastructure with measurement tools to participating Medical Home practices so that
  - Each one can provide the most effective and efficient health services to its members
  - Each one can continuously improve those health services based on immediate feedback from its outcomes
- Foster diverse implementations of the PCMH model across a variety of health care practices (small to large) and settings (rural to urban)
- Enable Americans (members) to participate directly and actively in their Medical Home using the best of social networking and customer relationship management tools

The different implementations need to range from groups of small primary care practices and outsourced Medical Home services networked together (collaborating partnerships) to large multidisciplinary practices. Each implementation would provide a "sufficient" or complete set of Medical Home services. Measuring progress and assessing successful or unsuccessful outcomes (for the entire program, i.e., participants, the Medical Home practice, and the IT infrastructure) is fundamental to this approach. Results would be fed back frequently to all involved parties for their evaluation; successful ones would be accelerated and Medical Home sites could adopt best clinical and management practices while avoiding IT solutions or practices that do not work. Analyses of the differing implementations will likely show which Medical Home services are necessary for specific conditions and how various implementations (collaborating partnerships to large practices) can or cannot be successful as a Medical Home. However, in the absence of an agreed-upon and common set of performance data collected from each Medical Home, it will be very difficult to draw meaningful inferences about individual implementations or how the Medical Home model could be sustained or scale nationally.

The Medical Home Project would aggressively exploit existing infrastructure tools, software, and know-how. The Project begins with a clear definition of the clinical and business needs of the Medical Home and its functions and data requirements (see Fig. 17.3). Project staff would then match the requirements with the best of the ONC Health Information Exchange approaches and technologies from other industry sectors. For example, customer relations management and supply chain management systems might,

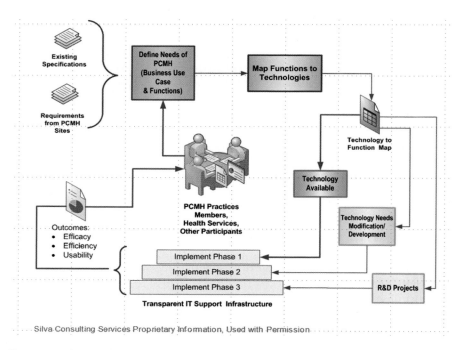

Fig. 17.3 Roadmap of the PCMH project. From John S. Silva, with permission

with modification, support some of the service-related functions of the Medical Home. Some technologies may need to be developed, while other ones that are not sufficiently mature may require research and development (R&D) efforts. A Smart POC would be piloted from available commercial technologies to support the various new coordination tasks and scheduling. It would then evolve over time to become the Medical Home staff's primary system, sitting between the "back end" computer systems and data and knowledge sources and the "front end" clinical users and customers.

Phase 1 implementation efforts should start as soon as possible, but no later than 6 months after Project start. The demonstration sites would be required to identify specific Medical Home business objectives that they will address, have measurable performance metrics for clinical, business, and IT processes, and report their metrics monthly. The Project staff would aggressively manage tasks, determine the accomplishments relative to the program schedule and funding, assess what is working and not working, and replan as new information/technologies are identified or required or to mitigate risks that invariably arise during program execution. The Medical Home Project also needs to build a support and training infrastructure so that Medical Home staff can become expert users quickly and that lessons learned and best practices can be disseminated among Medical Home sites.

As needed technologies are modified or developed and pass internal testing, they would be scheduled for Phase 2 implementation in several "test bed" Medical Home sites.

Following successful results in the test bed sites, the technology would be rolled out to the rest of the demonstration sites. Lessons learned, Medical Home outcomes and IT utility assessments will feed back into defining new or modified Medical Home needs and flow through the above cycle in successive 3–6 month iterations. The R&D projects follow the same path described above, internal testing, test bed pilot implementations and, if successful, roll out to all demonstration sites.

Importantly, the Smart POC system and the IT infrastructure would enable the Medical Home to collect appropriate clinical, administrative, and patient outcome information as a by-product of providing and orchestrating health services. The customer portion of the Medical Home web collects relevant information from individual participants as well as patient monitoring data from instrumentation in the consumer' home. As a result, best practices, local clinical guidelines, and clinical decisions could be linked directly to patient outcomes. These data, the HIE infrastructure, and associated clinical and business intelligence tools come together as a disruptive technology platform that could revolutionize evaluation processes and research. Medical Home clinical staff, management, and clients will know: what are the best practices, what practices are not effective or not safe, and what practices are more expensive without added value.

This approach seems to be just what the IOM[14] has outlined in its recent report on comparative effectiveness research (CER):

> CER is the generation and synthesis of evidence that compares the benefits and harms of alternative methods to prevent, diagnose, treat, and monitor a clinical condition or to improve the delivery of care. The purpose of CER is to assist consumers, clinicians, purchasers, and policy makers to make informed decisions that will improve health care at both the individual and population levelsThe report goes on to describe a robust CER enterprise that "consumers, patients and caregivers as well as their health care providers must be involved in all aspects of CER to ensure its relevance to everyday health care delivery." Since the diffusion of clinical practice guidelines into clinical practice has been notoriously slow and updating and evolving them very difficult, the authors believe that CER functions must be embedded into the daily functioning of a Medical Home.

The fully integrated evaluation framework is fundamental not only to the design of the IT infrastructure, but also to the design of the business and clinical practices of the Medical Home. That is, the Medical Home IT system is designed to provide immediate feedback of performance, metrics, KPIs, and other analyses, directly and transparently to local participants, clinicians, and consumers. This information continuously informs decisions by all participants so they can adjust their local practices and behaviors to continuously improve their Medical Home's performance. Thus, Medical Home would become a key model for implementing local and national CER data at the POC when decisions are made. In the absence of readily available CER data at the nexus of decision making, the CER enterprise will not achieve its stated goal of "better decision making by patients and providers."[14]

Lastly, this approach for the Medical Home is designed to address the maintainability and sustainability of guidelines. Guidelines are implemented within the Smart POC system, then continuously adapted, evolved, and communicated to the local practice setting by feeding back the Medical Home's outcomes, costs, and utilization data and new biomedical knowledge onto the guideline itself. It should be a fascinating story for the science of CER to observe and analyze the time-oriented adaption and evolution of guidelines, both within and across communities and special populations. After all, as Sir William Osler stated: "It is much more important to know what sort of patient has a disease than what sort of disease a patient has."

References

1. Institute of Medicine. *Crossing the Quality Chasm: A New Health System for the 21st Century.* Washington, DC: National Academy Press; 2001.
2. Health Information and Management Systems Society. Defining and testing EMR usability: principles and proposed methods of EMR usability evaluation and rating. www.himss.org/content/files/HIMSS_DefiningandTestingEMRUsability.pdf; 2009.
3. Stead W, Linn H. *Computational Technology for Effective Health Care: Immediate Steps and Strategic Directions.* Washington, DC: National Academies Press; 2009.
4. Ball MJ, Silva JS, et al. Failure to provide clinicians useful IT systems: opportunities to leapfrog current technologies. *Methods Inf Med.* 2008; 47: 4-7.
5. Silva JS, Ball MJ. The professional workstation as enabler: conference recommendations. *Int J Biomed Comp.* 1994;34:3-10.
6. Silva JS, Ball MJ. *Next Generation Health Professional Workstations. Yearbook of Med Inform 1994: Advanced Communications in Health Care.* Stuttgart: Schattauer; 1994:78-84.
7. Schuerenberg BK. Technology integration at the point of care. *Health Data Manag.* 2007;15(7):28-30, 32, 34. www.healthdatamanagement.com/htlm/current/CurrentIssueStory.
8. Gordon B, Gray J. What's next in high performance computing? *Commun ACM.* 2002;45: 91-95.
9. Silva JS, Ball MJ. Prognosis for year 2013. *Int J Med Inform.* 2002;66:45-49.
10. Iglehart JK. No place like home – testing a new model of care delivery. *N Engl J Med.* 2008;359:1200-1203.
11. AAFP, American Academy of Pediatrics, American College of Physicians, and American Osteopathic Association. Joint principles of the patient-centered medical home. http://www.medicalhomeinfo.org/Joint%20Statement.pdf; 2007.
12. Paulus RA, Davis K, Steele GD. Continuous innovation in health care: implications of the Geisinger experience. *Health Aff.* 2008;27(5):1235-1245.
13. Berenson RA et al. A house is not a home: keeping patients at the center of practice redesign. *Health Aff.* 2008;27:1219-1230.
14. Institute of Medicine. *Initial National Priorities for Comparative Effectiveness Research Report Brief.* Washington, DC: National Academy Press; 2009.

Extending Care: Voice Technology

18

Debra M. Wolf, Amar Kapadia, and Pam Selker Rak

Since the beginning of time, communication has revolutionized our lives and molded our future. Individuals have always possessed a natural desire to bridge the gaps between each other to communicate more efficiently and effectively than ever before. From pre-history to the twenty-first century, the human race has used its voice to convey thoughts, to inspire, and to imagine. With each passing generation, speech has facilitated the transmission of information and knowledge. Experiences passed on through speech have become increasingly sophisticated over time, allowing humans to adapt to new environments with greater speed and ease.

The 1968 Stanley Kubrick film *2001: A Space Odyssey* features an intelligent onboard computer system called HAL (*H*euristically programmed *AL*gorithmic) upon the spaceship *Discovery*. Not only did HAL maintain all of the spaceship systems on an interplanetary voyage, but also it did appear to be capable of a host of human characteristics, including art appreciation and the interpretation and expression of emotion. But perhaps HAL's most fascinating feature was advanced speech recognition, which provided the ability for man to communicate – and interact – with machine. What seemed like pure science fiction to most individuals in 1968 is today a reality. But getting here has been a journey of both communication and innovation.

Through the ages, speech has enabled easier coordination and cooperation, technological progress, and the development of complex, abstract concepts such as science and medicine. Advances in science have enabled us to communicate in new ways, each one more "immediate" than the last: from the telegraph to the telephone; from radio to television; from fax machines to email; from online message boards to text messaging on cell phones. But no matter how much the science and technology advances, the core human desires remain the same: to communicate, to document, to retrieve, and to share in a faster, more efficient manner.

D.M. Wolf (✉)
Department of Nursing, Slippery Rock University, 2370 Trimble Road,
Pittsburgh, PA 15237, USA
e-mail: debra.wolf@sru.edu, 6wolfs@comcast.net.

M.J. Ball et al. (eds.), *Nursing Informatics*,
DOI: 10.1007/978-1-84996-278-0_18, © Springer-Verlag London Limited 2011

Speech-Based Applications in Health Care

As the journey continues into the future of health care technologies, voice-assisted care applications are likely to become as commonplace as that original, age-old form of communication: the human voice.[19]

Front-End and Back-End Speech Recognition

In fact, a variety of speech-based applications are being used today in a variety of health care settings. For example, speech recognition has been implemented in both the front-end and back-end of the medical transcription process. Front-end speech recognition is where a health care provider dictates into a speech-recognition engine, the recognized words are displayed right after they are spoken, and the person dictating is responsible for editing and signing off on the document. Back-end speech recognition, also referred to as deferred speech recognition, is where the provider dictates into a digital dictation system, the voice is routed through a speech-recognition machine, and the recognized draft document is routed along with the original voice file to a medical transcriptionist who edits the draft and finalizes the report.

Speech Recognition and Electronic Medical Records

Many electronic medical records (EMRs) applications can be more effective and may perform more efficiently when deployed in conjunction with a speech-recognition engine.[13] Conducting searches and queries and filling out forms may be faster if performed by voice rather than by using a keyboard. Dragon Medical® speech-recognition software from Nuance is an example of how a voice-assisted care can work in conjunction with EMRs. Dragon Medical comes already installed with medical vocabularies covering nearly 80 medical specialties and subspecialties. To use the system, clinicians use their own words to dictate into their EMR in real time. They are then able to instantly review and sign their notes, making them available for other clinicians in real time. Dragon Medical also enables users to navigate and dictate inside EMR software by using voice commands.

Wireless Call Systems

Nurse call systems provide another example of modern voice technology that is prevalent in health care settings today. Vocera® is a wearable, wireless call system designed for mobile workers within the same building. By making the traditional nurse call system wireless and virtually hands-free, the system eliminates the need for traditional telephone communication and overhead paging systems, providing the patient a quiet environment in which to recover. The Vocera system also incorporates text messaging features and the ability to call both onsite and offsite phone numbers from the wireless unit.

Documentation, Information Retrieval, and Paging All in One

The most recent application of speech recognition in health care today is the combined use of speech recognition and synthesis for charting and communication. AccuNurse® voice-assisted care by Vocollect Healthcare Systems, Inc. combines documentation, information retrieval, and paging functions into one system. The documentation function converts spoken information to written data, reducing the amount of time staff spend creating and reviewing charts. The information retrieval and task guidance function helps reduce the number of mistakes made due to forgotten or incorrect information. Clinicians wear lightweight headsets and small wireless devices that enable them to hear personalized care plans or active orders, deliver care appropriately in a timely manner, document care in real time, and communicate with other clinicians more quickly in response to patients' and/or residents' needs. Essentially, the clinicians can page other staff members for help and chart while multitasking – all by using their voice.

Benefits of Voice-Assisted Care

While voice-assisted care helps health care facilities achieve better communication, better documentation, and better quality of care, it also provides specific benefits to those involved in the health care process, whether the technology is used within an acute care hospital or a long-term care (LTC) facility. For example:

- *Patients in hospitals or residents in nursing facilities* can benefit from faster, more accurate delivery of the personalized services they need, faster response to nurse call requests, and access to caregivers during shift changes.
- *Hospital or nursing facility administrators* can experience or visualize better care through reporting mechanisms at lower operating costs, better communication across staff, ease of responding to state regulatory surveys or inspections and other quality management initiatives, elimination of overhead paging for quieter environments, and more accountability.
- *Directors of nursing (acute care or skilled nursing)* will have instant access to staff through automated paging, spend less time in preparing end-of-shift reports, be able to respond more quickly to state regulatory surveys or inspections required in LTC settings with on-demand reports, and take a more proactive approach to managing and assessing patient/resident care.
- *General staff nurses, specialized nurses, and other clinicians* will experience faster access to patient and unit reports, identify changes in patient status before they become adverse events, and customize care information.
- *Nursing aides* will have instant access to the most recent care information, notification of changes to active orders, ability to get help without searching, elimination of flow sheets to complete and hopefully an increased amount of time to spend with patients or residents.
- *Assessment coordinators in long-term care settings* will benefit from instant, accurate, legible, and complete information on activities of daily living (ADLs) and other

minimum data set (MDS) items, complete documentation with end-of-shift reports, and improved MDS accuracy.

- *Senior administrators or executives* should experience improved reimbursements or case mix index (CMI) values (where applicable), reduction of operating costs through increased staffing efficiency and lower risk.

From an imaginary spaceship computer system to actual hospital patients and nursing facilities, technology not only shapes the way individuals view the world but also increasingly shapes the way individuals live in the world today. Over the past 20 years, voice-assisted care has become a proven way to drive better performance in the supply chain.[30] Today, that same technology is now integrating into health care environments in an accelerated fashion. With the recent advances in voice technology, first launched in the LTC sector and now being used in acute care health systems, voice-assisted care is making it possible to use human voice or speech as a method of capturing and retrieving data in real time at the point of care.

What's Driving the Move Toward Voice Technology at the Point of Care?

The need for voice technology at the point of care reaches across all areas of health care to address various needs or initiatives. Four key drivers are increasing the need for voice-assisted care across the health care sector: the trend-of transitioning healthcare away from paper to electronic records; the drive toward person-centered care and associated culture changes; the need to support governmental and regulatory demands such as eliminating hospital acquired conditions (HACs); and the need to improve patient and/or consumer perception of health care delivery. 14-16: by assisting healthcare organizations to improve measures outlined by the Hospital Consumer Assessment of Healthcare Provider and Systems (HCAHPS).

Driver 1: The Trend to Electronic Records

Within health care's complex workflow environment, developing efficient mechanisms to obtain documentation that drives clinical, financial, and operational improvements is a constant challenge. The term "documentation" can have many meanings, depending on the setting and context of the existing environment. Merriam-Webster (2009) defines "documentation" as "1: the act or instance of furnishing or authenticating with documents." Merriam-Webster (2009) further defines "documents" as "1b: an original or official paper relied on as the basis, proof, or support of something; 1c: something (as a photograph or record) that serves as evidence or proof; 2a: a writing conveying information; 2b: a material substance (as a coin or stone) having on it a representation of thoughts by means of some conventional mark or symbol."

Within health care, documentation has traditionally been viewed or anticipated as consisting of various forms of paper material with data transposed via handwritten language, computer-generated printed language, or preprinted paper with a series of checkmarks or signatures. Today, documentation is beginning to make a major transformation from traditional views within most health care organizations.[17]

With the emergence of innovative technology such as keyboard entry and voice-assisted entry, documentation may only be completed or viewed via a system that utilizes computerized technology; meaning the paper trail of documents may no longer exist. In order to transform one's practice to a new method of documenting, such as voice technology, there are numerous resources one should consider using to guide this change. In 2005, the American Nurses Association (ANA)[1] published *Principles for Documentation* in an effort to support and guide nurses in how to document, what to document, and when to document. The document provides five policy statements and eight principles for professional nurses.

The Role of Nurses and Nursing Informatics

As clinicians, nurses need to actively participate in guiding, designing, and evaluating various methods of documentation that result in documents that are viewed by many to make critical decisions. Using some form of standardized language or terminology will be critical to the future success of nurses having interoperable data available from a variety of sources. Although there are several standardized languages mentioned within this book, the focus of this chapter is to begin introducing how the spoken word can be translated into written text, while supporting policies or principles outlined so clearly by the ANA, as well as policies within the organization in which voice technology is used.

Most recently through the ANA, the *Nursing Informatics: Scope and Standards of Practice* (2008)[2] was revised and published for public viewing. This revised document sees nursing informatics (NI) as a specialty that blends the sciences of nursing, computers, and information in an effort to support the professional nurse. The key to the NI role is to assist in communicating data and information to various clinicians in order for critical decisions to be made regarding patient care. In an effort to have nurses begin using voice as a method of documenting patient care, NI specialists are needed to assist in the design, development, testing, and integration of the modern technology. As with the conversion to computerized processes, these specialists will play an instrumental role in moving to voice technology.[18]

The Needs of Nurses

The conversion from paper to computerized (keyboard) documentation has been well received by multiple health care systems and government organizations and has been generally accepted by most end users. Similarly, implementing a process that uses voice will require end users to accept another change in how they view documentation. Changing the manner one documents not only requires the individual clinicians to change but also requires a certain level of cultural change.

A study using 25 national facilities and representing over 200 units and approximately 100 participants explored what nurses believed to be technical solutions to address inefficiencies within a medical surgical unit. The study revealed that the most desired technological solutions included wireless devices that provided voice activation systems, available at point of care, while integrated into other systems with global accessibility.[3]

In order to meet the needs of nurses requesting voice technology to document patient care, an immense cultural change must occur – a change that requires collaboration and integration from all clinicians, information technology experts and vendors, as well as health policy regulations such as Health Insurance Portability and Accountability Act (HIPAA). Several change theories have studied and assessed how to initiate and create change.[4-6] One method of changing culture uses a formula of four critical elements: inspiration, infrastructure, education, and evidence.[4]

The vision that leads to the inspiration of changing to wireless voice documentation has been demonstrated through the work of the Robert Woods Johnson Foundation (RWJF) and the American Academy of Nurses. In December 2005, RWJF awarded a grant to the American Academy of Nursing for a project called "Technology Targets: A Synthesized Approach for Identifying and Fostering Technological Solutions to Workflow Inefficiencies on Medical/Surgical Units." A major component of Technology Targets is a process called Technology Drill-Down (TD2), which represents an opportunity to develop an improved process for identifying technological solutions to medical/surgical unit workflow inefficiencies.[3]

While physicians have experimented with voice in the past, nursing and allied clinicians have typically not had this opportunity. However, the RWJF-funded study found that nurses do not want to be passive consumers of technology and are disappointed with current technologies that lead to "workarounds" and take time away from their patients. Nurses indicated the need for hospital executives and technology vendors to "listen to the voice of the staff." Overall, several major themes emerged in terms of what nurses want from technology solutions[3]:

- Devices that are "smart," voice-activated, portable, and/or wireless
- Systems that provide tracking, documentation, and communication functions
- Interoperability of systems

Nurses in the study listed the following as desired outcomes of technology solutions, all of which voice-assisted care can provide: elimination of work such as documentation, charting, inventory, and duplicate communication; access to resources such as doctors, pharmacists, and interpreters; accomplishment of regulatory work such as identification and documentation; and efficient use of space. Overall, the study demonstrates that there is a significant opportunity for nurses, health care executives, and voice-assisted care vendors to partner around better functionality of electronic systems and devices used to deliver care.[3]

While nurses have clearly voiced their interest and concern in adopting innovative technology to better support current processes, this request also changes current processes and policies, as well as the manner in which staff are educated and trained to document accurately while following established guidelines. This type of change may be supported through the organization's infrastructure, which would require the support of executive administration through strategic planning and financial support.

Working with nurse clinicians to utilize technology at the point of care requires a carefully orchestrated approach that further supports the adoption of technology. Educating staff in using voice-assisted care can be seamlessly conducted within the organization in which the technology will be used. Having an educational plan that outlines a timeframe needed to introduce staff to new equipment and new processes and having a strong group of super users will be essential to successful integration of voice-assisted care.

Keys to Adoption of Innovations

Rogers[6] outlines five key attributes that if used during diffusion of an innovation will most likely lead to the adoption of the innovation by end users. The attributes include relative advantage, compatibility, trialability, observability, and complexity. Informatics nurses or general staff nurses need to demonstrate or highlight the advantages of using voice to document patient care; share how compatible the voice-assisted technology and processes are with existing systems; allow staff to play with the equipment, gaining experience on how the system operates; have staff visualize how other clinicians are using the technology within their current organization or within other health care organizations that have similar services; and show how the voice-driven technology is easy to use and manipulate.

A trial conducted at Butler Memorial Hospital, an acute care hospital in Butler, Pennsylvania, came to a similar conclusion.[7] The trial, conducted in conjunction with Vocollect Healthcare Systems, Inc. and with beta testing prior to the trial from the University of Maryland's School of Nursing, assessed the impact of voice-assisted care within an acute care environment.[8] The trial's approach demonstrated an impact that supports the findings of TD2, in which nurses welcome the opportunity to guide product development and use the product prior to activation at the point of care. The model used in the trial created an atmosphere of collaboration in which technology was seen as a positive tool to support clinicians.[31]

Driver 2: Person-Centered Care and Associated Culture Change

The second driver that is fueling the need for voice-assisted care at point of care comprises the dual forces of "culture change" and the shift to a person-centered model of care in both acute care and LTC settings. Many facilities in the LTC industry are dramatically transforming communities through culture change movements. An example is the Eden Alternative, a not-for-profit organization dedicated to remaking the experience of aging and disability across America and around the world. According to the Eden Alternative website, "Aging should be a continued stage of development and growth, rather than a period of decline."[9]

Culture change advocates have made strides in reshaping consumer attitudes toward the industry, and they are now turning to technology to help develop their charter even further. One of the technologies culture change advocates are embracing is voice-powered communication and documentation systems.[22] In the LTC sector, voice-assisted care has been shown to impact the following areas of culture change:

- Empower caregivers with the personalized information that they need, when and where they need it, on how to care for residents
- Foster teamwork while creating a homelike environment with no overhead noise[21]

- Drive higher levels of family and staff satisfaction
- Create higher cash flows from greater efficiency and maximized reimbursements.[10]
- Free up to 66% more time for direct resident care

Voice-enabled technologies play an important role because the technology has been found to require staff to spend less time on administrative duties such as charting and offer staff additional time, which can be spent with patients and residents.[32]

Driver 3: Governmental and Regulatory Demands

Another initiative that is fueling the need for voice technology at the point of care emerges from regulatory bodies and health care institutions such as the Centers for Medicare and Medicaid Services (CMS). Examples of initiatives from regulatory bodies include the mandate for electronic health records by 2014 and more automation in documentation and higher levels of data transparency.[20] With the development and publication of new quality rating systems such as the Five-Star Quality Rating System for nursing homes and consumer-facing databases such as Nursing Home Compare, Hospital Compare, and Dialysis Facility Compare, CMS has provided additional incentives for health care providers to use technology that enhances patient and/or resident care, streamlines workflow, and improves documentation, all of which can result in higher reimbursements for the health care facilities.

In an effort to begin addressing quality/safety initiatives and support clinicians at the point of care, two innovative voice-based systems have been developed to support clinician documentation and task management. The first system supports intravenous nurses when caring for peripheral and central IV lines. The voice system incorporated rules and logic that alerted nurses of the number of days a central line was inserted and if central line dressings needed changed in an attempt to decrease potential for central blood stream infections. The second system supports the daily functions of patient care assistants (PCA) within acute care settings when documenting and completing routine tasks such as ADL, vital signs, weights, and intake and output. Again, rules and logic alert caregivers to exceptions. For instance, if a weight change beyond a predefined limit is recorded, the caregiver is asked to confirm the change or to re-record the entry. The result is much higher data integrity.

By using voice-assisted care technology, health care organizations have the opportunity to address and hopefully reduce the amount of errors and total cost accumulations they may be experiencing. For example, a PCA can receive reminders to turn or reposition patients who are prone to skin breakdown or who have medical conditions that require frequent turning in an effort to reduce the occurrence of ulcers, which cost on average $40k per occurrence.

A second effort to address quality/safety initiatives and support clinicians at the point of care is through CMS. In 2008, the CMS announced a proposed rule that would update payment policies and rates under the hospital inpatient prospective payment system for fiscal year (FY) 2009, beginning with discharges on or after 1 Oct 2008. For FY 2009, CMS has proposed nine new categories of HACs, as shown in Table 18.1.

Voice-assisted care technology offers health care organizations the capabilities they need to address the conditions identified by CMS, as suggested in the three examples that follow.

Table 18.1 Hospital acquired conditions (HACs) proposed by the Centers for Medicare and Medicaid Services (CMS) for fiscal years 2008 and 2009

2008 HACs with average cost per occurrence

Foreign objects post-OR at $63,631
Air embolism at $71,636
Blood incompatibility at $50,455
Stage 3–4 ulcers at $43,180
Falls/trauma at $33,894
Catheter-associated infections (UTI), at $44,043
Surgical site infections (chest post CABG) at $299,237
Vascular catheter-associated infections at $103,027

2009 HACs with average cost per occurrence

Surgical site infections (following elective procedures)
   Total knee replacement at $63,000
   Laparoscopic gastric bypass and or gastroenterostomy at $180,142
   Ligation and stripping of varicose veins at $66,355
Legionnaires' disease at $86,014
Glycemic control
   Diabetic ketoacidosis at $42,974
   Nonketotic hyperosmolar coma at $35,215
   Diabetic coma at $45,989
   Hypoglycemic coma at $36,581
Iatrogenic pneumothorax at $75,089
Delirium at $23,290
Ventilator-associated pneumonia (VAP) at $135,795
Deep vein thrombosis (DVT)/pulmonary embolism (PE) at $50,937
Staphylococcus aureus septicemia at $84,976
Clostridium difficile-associated disease at $59,153

Average cost per occurrence taken from CMS (2008)

Glycemic Control

This is achieved through better task management and documentation of blood sugar test using glucometers or testing urine for ketones. If personal care attendants (PCAs) have a voice-assisted process that guides them through a prioritized list of tasks that must be completed by certain timeframes (such as the glucose checks using a glucometer), then they would be better able to complete the task in a timely manner, allowing the registered nurse (RN) to access the result through voice assessing the need for insulin coverage. Glucometers can be downloaded through a phone line and interfaced into an electronic health record. The challenge focuses on having the PCA complete the task on time with a reachable result for the nurse when needed. If a PCA has five to eight patients and an RN oversees medications for 8–12 patients on a daylight shift (hypothetically, if the RN covered IV meds for an LPN and all meds for two PCAs), the accessibility of information in a timely manner is critical. Glucose checks typically occur three to four times a day requiring insulin coverage early morning, noon, and at dinner time. Hypothetically on average, if a hospital prevents five cases in 1 year, this provides a return on investment (ROI) of $200,000 a year for the organization (5 at $42,974 as outlined above in CMS HACs).

Reduction in Falls/Trauma

This is achieved through better communication of fall prevention for known candidates, task management for side rail/restraint applications/toileting checks. The Joint Commission and other bodies require the documentation of restraint usage every 1–2 h to address how a patient was monitored/observed/cared for during that time. If an RN or a PCA has not documented within the required timeframe, the voice-assisted care system will remind them, or prompt them, to do so. This prompt can assist organizations in meeting documentation compliance and patient safety, by securing restraints are on, checking on patient, offering toileting, etc. When initiating documentation or seeking information on a patient who is a fall candidate (noted by fall score during initial assessment), a PCA or an RN can be alerted to this caution alert/cautionary measure and validate that side rails are up and items placed in reach of patient or confirm patient is safe to the best of their ability. If five falls are prevented within 1 year, hypothetically this averages a cost savings of $165,000 (5 at $33,894 as outlined above in CMS HACs).

Decrease in Catheter-Associated Urinary Tract Infections (UTIs)

Reduction in these infections may be achieved through better task management; documentation of catheter care and accurate temperatures; and by alerting clinicians of the number of catheter days that Foley has been inserted. The overall goal is to prevent UTIs by decreasing the number of days any Foley/catheter is in place for patients, as catheters are highly associated with urinary infections. If a system is in place that alerts an RN of the number of days a catheter has been inserted, or a PCA or an RN to compete Foley catheter care during routine ADLs, document the care and how catheter was secured (documentation compliance), the chances for UTI may be decreased. Hypothetically if five cases are prevented, this averages to a cost savings of $200,000 per year (5 at $44,043 as outlined above in CMS HACs).

These scenarios illustrate the multitude of opportunities to work with acute care organizations in identifying and addressing multiple outcome measures that will ultimately impact the organization's ROI. Other outcome considerations that may be considered are the time difference in documenting traditional method to voice-assisted care (possibly cost savings in overtime) and, importantly, compliance in documenting assisting in meeting standards set by the Joint Commission or other regulatory bodies for such areas as restraint documentation, dressing change, wound care, skin care, and interdisciplinary plan of care.

Driver 4: Patient/Consumer Perception of Health Care

The need to improve patient and/or consumer perception of health care delivery by assisting health care organizations to improve measures such as outlined by the Hospital Consumer Assessment of Healthcare Provider and Systems (HCAHPS) is an essential consideration when integrating technology. Using speech-enabled conditional logic and rules to remind clinicians to educate patients upon administration of any new medication, to offer assistance for toileting needs, or to provide genuine courtesy/respect while listening carefully may strongly support or improve an organization's survey results.

When a health care organization is considering voice technology for its nurses or clinicians, care should be taken to understand and incorporate the needs of the individuals on several fronts. Ergonomics and design considerations are important aspects when integrating voice technology.

Form Factor

An important requirement for any device, nurses will most likely request, is that the device is lightweight and comfortable. Efforts should be taken to ensure that devices do not get in the way of providing quality care. For instance, for safety reasons, it is important that devices are not easily reachable by patients and that the devices do not cause harm to caregivers who frequently work in environments that are difficult or may include spillage. Clinicians' pockets or secure belt straps may be used to hold various types of equipment. For ultimate hygiene, equipment should be operated using devices that require voice commands, so human touch is rarely required to manipulate the devices, especially in sterile environments. Headsets, if needed, should be nonintrusive and comfortable for extended use. Headsets should be able to fit a variety of head sizes, shapes, eye-wear and head-gear, such as sterile head covers. Headsets should be physically separable from devices, so that each caregiver has his/her own headset for hygienic reasons, even if the computer component of the devices is shared. Consideration must be given to batteries, which should last at least a full shift before needing to be re-charged. In addition, re-charging of batteries should be quick and easy.

Recognition Accuracy

The second need that should be considered when evaluating voice technology is accuracy. Unlike physicians, nurses often do not have the luxury of having someone else transcribe their notes and correct errors. Therefore, it is important that the quality of speech recognition be very high, and that nurses have the ability to catch and correct errors with the least amount of effort, at the point of care. For instance, a voice-recorded weight change of say over 3 lb can trigger an alert to the clinicians asking them if they are sure of their measurement and provide the ability to correct the measurement if they so desire, by using voice at point of care or at point of documentation.

Workflow

Most caregivers will likely appreciate the ability to instantly access patient records and daily task lists via voice, and careful design can ensure that the system does not become cumbersome for the caregiver. For instance, at the start of a shift, caregivers should be able to log on and find their shift assignments without having to go through a lot of steps, while staying within the norms of security standards. If they log off or put the device to sleep (hibernating state), they should be able to easily re-start their work from the point where they left off. An experienced caregiver may have different needs for task assistance from a novice, and the system should give the caregiver the ability to customize his/her interaction based on his/her needs. Caregivers should also have the ability to respond to communication requests as they desire and not have to immediately respond to every request if they are busy.

Connectivity

The ability to work offline is another important consideration. Wireless systems have become increasingly reliable. However, in the complex environment of a hospital or an LTC facility, there is still often inconsistent wireless coverage. It is important that caregivers are able to function – get their tasks and continue their charting – even with limited coverage. Ideally, the system should automatically synchronize tasks and documentation as wireless coverage improves, making technical issues completely transparent to the caregiver.

Privacy

HIPAA regulations require that key patient identifiers not be publicly disclosed. Therefore, an information system should provide the caregiver the ability to listen and document without violating any privacy rules. This level of privacy can be achieved through voice-assisted technology, by conveying key patient information to the caregiver only via a headset, and not requiring the caregiver to speak patient names.

Standards and Integration

In today's complex health IT environment, almost no system can work as an independent or standalone system. However, given the variety of systems out in the market, it is unreasonable to expect a voice solution to integrate out-of-the-box with every other possible application or system. Therefore, it is important that any voice solution be compliant with standards such as HL7 and has at least some of the common interfaces, such as admissions-discharge-transfer (ADT) available out-of-the-box.

Voice in Action: Case Studies

Voice-assisted care is becoming more prevalent in health care applications, as seen in its widespread usage in LTC and, more recently, in acute care environments.[23-24, 29]

The Boston Home[11]

The Boston Home, a 125-year-old long-term acute care organization based in Boston, Massachusetts, is one of the 18 facilities in the United States and the only one in New England that specializes in the care of middle-aged or younger adults with a progressive neurological disease, usually multiple sclerosis.

The Boston Home's staff found the regulatory language of its paper charts and care plans cumbersome and difficult to use. As a result, they looked at automated EMR systems, but could not find a system that met their needs. The staff considered a voice-activated call system, but passed on it when they realized that it did not provide a documentation feature. The director and staff finally selected voice-assisted care because it provided both voice-powered documentation and "Silent Paging" functionality, features they considered central to a user-friendly tool that could solve their documentation and communication problems.

A focus group of residents and their family members revealed the need to improve several things at The Boston Home: care planning communication; staff's access to updated resident information; and the amount of time staff devoted to patient care without being interrupted by end-of-shift reporting duties or overhead pages.

Voice-assisted care answered 90% of the issues raised in the focus group[11] and has increased productivity at The Boston Home by eliminating end-of-shift charting time and staff interruptions. Announcements now go out over the headsets, so staff can multitask while they receive important information and instructions.

With the increased productivity and time savings came streamlined documentation and improved accuracy. The Boston Home has future plans to use the voice system as part of the residents' nurse call system, so residents can page their aides from anywhere in the facility.

St. John Specialty Care Center[28]

St. John Specialty Care Center in Mars, Pennsylvania, is a skilled nursing facility with approximately 320 beds and is part of Lutheran SeniorLife's senior living and health care communities. This facility is an example of an LTC sector that is using voice-assisted care as part of its Culture Change goals.

The facility implemented voice-assisted care in 2008 in an effort to enable staff members to spend more time with residents. The LTC program at St. John Specialty Care Center focuses on serving residents with the "abundant life" model, which goes beyond traditional approaches to nursing care and concentrates on restoration and achievement. This model is the impetus of St. John Specialty Care Center's brand and Culture Change movement.

Nurses reported spending up to 70% of their day on paperwork and struggling to maintain the integrity of charts and care plans. By implementing voice, St. John Specialty Care Center eliminated 45–60 min of paperwork and 45–60 min of time spent searching for others per Certified Nursing Assistant (CNA), per shift, and directed this time back to resident care (Prickett, 2009). As a result, care plans can be much more detailed, which supports St. John

Specialty Care Center's goal to provide restorative nursing care. In addition, the paging function allows staff members to stay with residents in need and eliminates the need for disruptive overhead pages. This enhances the quality of life for residents as well as the work environment for staff members.

St. John Specialty Care Center utilized the voice-assisted care to retrieve data to determine acuity levels and subsequent staffing requirements. Using voice has increased St. John Specialty Care Center's reimbursements by improving the facility's documentation and reporting capability. Voice has also helped address quality indicators for falls, weight, wound care, and incontinence. As a result of voice-assisted care, internal controls, and professional training initiatives, St. John Specialty Care Center has seen its CMI increase by 0.11, which translates to more than $500,000 in additional reimbursement per year (Prickett, 2009).

Butler Memorial Hospital

After collaborating with Vocollect Healthcare Systems to co-develop a new real-time point of care documentation system that uses speech recognition technology, Butler Memorial Hospital in Butler, Pennsylvania, won the 2009 *CARING and Health Data Management Award* for Nursing Innovation.[17] The hospital worked with Vocollect Healthcare Systems to customize Vocollect's AccuNurse voice-assisted care system to help IV nurses deal with repetitive documentation tasks.[12]

By using the AccuNurse voice-assisted care, Butler Memorial IV nurses completely documented their tasks in the clinical information system 100% of the time, compared with 40% of the time when using the old, more manual process.[12] Using the voice-assisted care streamlined the documentation system and replaced pagers, phones, computers, and paper charts with headsets and simple dictation. The time that nurses saved on these administrative tasks resulted in their having more time with patients.[12]

Summary

Voice-assisted care delivers hands-free, on-demand data retrieval, documentation, and communication that have been proven to improve the accuracy and quality of care provided by nurses and nursing assistants. The technology has also positively impacted reimbursements and helped achieve regulatory compliance in the LTC sector. The technology allows staff to hear detailed resident care needs, document their completed tasks on demand, and instantly get help from others at any time and any place. As such, voice-assisted care is becoming a norm in LTC settings, with implementation prevalent throughout the U.S. in both for-profit and not-for-profit nursing facilities

The integration into acute care has just begun to explode. The initial trial conducted at Butler Memorial Hospital was one of the first to be completed. Although the benefits in terms of workflow efficiencies were visible and measurable, variables that need to be measured include time in documenting; changes in efficiencies related to various processes;

and level of accuracy or percentage of required documentation completed in order to meet existing standards and regulations imposed by governing bodies (imposed in order for accreditation or reimburse institutions for their services).

While more research is required in acute care environments, it is clear that the impact of voice-assisted care in the health care industry is more than "just talk." For example, in his keynote address at the 2006 Healthcare Information and Management Systems Society (HIMSS) conference, Craig R. Barrett, Chairman of the Board of Intel Corporation, included voice-assisted care among nine cutting-edge technologies that will improve health care quality while reducing costs. Similarly, the technology is also already addressing the core needs of nurses as documented in the aforementioned TD2 study funded by the Robert J. Woods Foundation and continues to capture the media's attention, as well as that of organizations such as *CARING* and *Health Data Management* that encourage the innovation of technologies that fuel NI.[26]

From caregivers empowered to deliver more personalized care, to the ability to provide a homelike environment free of overhead paging, to having additional time for more direct care in skilled nursing facilities, voice-assisted care is impacting the health care industry like no other technology.[25, 27]

But the journey still continues for most clinicians. The coming decade is certain to spur more wide and varied applications of voice-assisted care in health care, including more integration directly with nurse call systems, as well as the trend for nurses to become increasingly involved in more collaborative initiatives, studies, trials, and deployments that serve to develop voice in key applications that impact their daily work lives – not to mention the lives of their patients in hospitals and/or residents in LTC facilities.

References

1. American Nurses Association. *Principles for Documentation*. Silver Spring: ANA; 2005.
2. American Nurses Association. *Nursing Informatics: Scope and Standards of Practice*. Silver Spring: ANA; 2008.
3. Cipriano P. Technological solutions to workflow inefficiencies on medical/surgical units [powerpoint slides]. American Academy of Nursing Website. www.aannet.org/i4a/pages/index.cfm?pageid=3318; May, 2009.
4. Felgen J. *I2E2: Leading Lasting Change*. Minneapolis: Creative Health Care Management; 2007.
5. Kotter J. *Leading Change*. Boston: Harvard Business School Press; 1996.
6. Rogers E. *Diffusion of Innovations*. 4th ed. New York: Free Press; 1995.
7. McGill T, Wilson M, Wolf DM, et al. Partnership in InnovationInnovative Partnering in Implementing Voice-Assisted Care in Acute Care Settings: Moving from Vision to Testing to Reality ByLucila Ohno-Machado, MD, PhDChair, AMIA 2009 Scientific Program Committee In: *Proceedings of the Annual 2009 AMIA Symposium*; 2009.
8. Blackburn M. A beta test bridge to better care. Nursing: University of Maryland 3(1):8. http://nursing.umaryland.edu/docs/publications/UMD_NursingSp09.pdf; 2009.
9. Eden Alternative. http://www.edenalt.org; n.d. Retrieved 18.05.09 May, 2009.
10. Shearon J. Vocollect healthcare systems sound advice: how voice-assisted care creates community and accelerates culture change. http://healthcare.vocollect.com/index.php/accunurse/

318

white-paper/how-voice-assisted-care-creates-community-and-accelerates-culture-change; 2009. Accessed 16.09.09.

11. Walsh C. The Boston Home. Personal interview conducted by Pam Selker Rak; March 2009.

12. Anderson H. The 2009 nursing IT innovation awards. *Health Data Manag.* www.healthdata-management.com/news/nursing_informatics-27972-1.html; Retrieved June 2009.

13. Andrews J. Keeping record. *McKnight's Long Term Care News & Assisted Living.* www.mcknights.com/Keeping-record/article/126159/; Retrieved July 2009.

14. Centers for Medicare and Medicaid Services. *CMS Proposes Additions to List of Hospital-Acquired Conditions for Fiscal Year 2009.* www.cms.hhs.gov/apps/media/press/factsheet.asp?Counter=3042; Retrieved July 2009.

15. Curry J. Headset gives nurses head start on paperwork, improves accuracy. *Pittsburgh Business Times.* http://pittsburgh.bizjournals.com/pittsburgh/stories/2007/04/30/focus3.html?jst=s_cn_hl; 2007.

16. Hayunga M. "E"-harmony. *McKnight's Long Term Care News & Assisted Living.* www.mcknights.com/E-harmony/article/122972/; Retrieved August 2009.

17. Health Data Management. The 2009 nursing IT innovation awards. Nurses replace clipboards with headsets to document their work [pdf]. http://healthcare.vocollect.com/downloads/9188.pdf; 2009.

18. Hutlock T. Bridging the voice communication gap – without a wire. *Long-Term Living Magazine.* www.ltlmagazine.com/ME2/dirmod.asp?sid=&nm=&type=Publishing&mod=Publications%3A%3AArticle&mid=8F3A7027421841978F18BE895F87F791&tier=4&id=9E497515D4174ABFAC91398AEE312E3F; 2005. Accessed 16.09.09.

19. Klie L. The 2007 implementation awards. *Speech Technology Magazine.* www.speechtechmag.com/Articles/Editorial~Feature~The-2007-Implementation-Awards-37432.aspx; 2007. Accessed 16.09.09.

20. Klusch L. Are you ready for the new survey? The QIS [Quality Indicator Survey] is coming – and now is a good time to start gearing up. *Long-Term Living Magazine* 57(12). www.ltlmagazine.com/ME2/dirmod.asp?sid=&nm=&type=Publishing&mod=Publications%3A%3AArticle&mid=8F3A7027421841978F18BE895F87F791&tier=4&id=77E715AB713E4D1AA911C482923EE5EA; 2008. Accessed 16.09.09.

21. Moen MD. Faster & quieter communication: integrating voice-assisted care with your existing nursing call system can benefit residents and staff. *Advance for Long-Term Care Management* 11(6). http://long-term-care.advanceweb.com/Editorial/Content/Editorial.aspx?CC=188358; 2008.

22. Peck RL. Voice-activated documentation comes into its own. *Long-Term Living Magazine.* www.ltlmagazine.com/ME2/dirmod.asp?sid=&nm=&type=Publishing&mod=Publications%3A%3AArticle&mid=8F3A7027421841978F18BE895F87F791&tier=4&id=6DD9A5D829744A29957100F9A38B7D22; Retrieved June 2009.

23. Radaker J. UPMC Cranberry Place. http://healthcare.vocollect.com/index.php/accunurse/case-study/upmc-cranberry-place. Accessed 16.09.09.

24. River Ridge Nursing Center in Amsterdam, New York. AccuNurse voice-assisted care featured in a video highlighting the facility's amenities. www.riverridgelc.com/Virtual_Tour.html; 2009. Retrieved 24.05.09.

25. Stouffer R. AccuNurse gives nursing home workers a technological edge. *Pittsburgh Tribune Review.* www.pittsburghlive.com/x/pittsburghtrib/s_306943.html; Retrieved August 2009.

26. Taulli T. VoIP on speed dial. *Forbes.* http://www.forbes.com/2005/12/13/voip-skype-ebay-cx_tt_1214straightup.html; Retrieved June 2009.

27. Twedt S. Vocollect's device has health care workers talking. *Pittsburgh Post-Gazette.* Retrieved from http://www.post-gazette.com/pg/09076/955925-334.stm; Retrieved June 2009.

28. Voice of success: Vocollect Healthcare Systems case study – St. John Specialty Care Center. http://healthcare.vocollect.com/index.php/accunurse/case-study/st-john; 2009.

29. Voice of success: Vocollect Healthcare Systems case study – The Church of God Home, Inc. http://healthcare.vocollect.com/index.php/accunurse/case-study/church-of-god-home; 2008.
30. Voice-powered results: Vocollect Healthcare Systems case study – Giant Eagle. Giant Eagle: How voice picking is helping Giant Eagle make every day taste better. http://vocollect.com/en/successes/gianteagle.php; 2008.
31. Walshak H. Butler Memorial Hospital streamlines IV nursing team with voice-assisted care. *Western Pennsylvania Hospital News.* www.wpahospitalnews.com/pdf/PHN_04_09.pdf; Retrieved May 2009.
32. Wood D. More time for people, not penmanship. *FutureAge.* www.aahsa.org/article.aspx?id=2006; "Retrieved May 2009.

Nursing's Contribution: An External Viewpoint

19

Mark Hagland

Across the United States, more and more hospital organizations are becoming pioneers in performance improvement, making significant progress in improving patient safety, clinical care quality, clinician workflow and effectiveness, and operational efficiency. The leaders of these organizations are pursuing highly different strategies and initiating programs in widely different patient care areas.

But one thing that all the pioneer organizations have in common is this: all those hospital-based organizations that are in the forefront of change are also leveraging the power of clinical information systems in order to move with alacrity towards performance optimization. And they are using a combination of information technology (IT) and performance improvement methodologies to effect clinical transformation – the strategic and systematic optimization of patient care delivery and operational processes.

And, within that context, nursing informatics has assumed increasing importance, as the realization among all stakeholders has taken hold that nursing informatics is a critical component of overall clinical informatics. Indeed, while the lion's share of attention in both the trade press and the mainstream media regarding clinical informatics has focused on physicians' gradual shift towards using, and benefiting from, clinical information systems, those in the know are finding that the planning and implementation of clinical information systems cannot ultimately be successful without the strong integration of good nursing informatics and nursing components as part of those overall clinical IS implementations.

As a healthcare journalist who has been following the evolution and development of performance optimization and IT use in the industry for 20 years, it is clear to me that the present moment is a pivotal time in nursing informatics specifically and in clinical informatics more generally. As pioneering patient care organizations move forward to leverage clinical information systems to dramatically improve their care quality, patient safety, clinician effectiveness, and operational efficiency, nurse leaders, nurse informaticists, and nurses in general have the opportunity to help improve not only the practice of nursing across all patient care settings but also the healthcare delivery system itself.

M. Hagland
440 West Barry Ave. #701, Chicago, IL 60657, USA
e-mail: mhagland@aol.com

M.J. Ball et al. (eds.), *Nursing Informatics*,
DOI: 10.1007/978-1-84996-278-0_19, © Springer-Verlag London Limited 2011

At the Core of Performance Improvement

In February 2009, I had the opportunity to spend a day at the Detroit Medical Center (DMC) in downtown Detroit, Michigan. Clinician, IT, and executive leaders there had just been informed that their organization had placed first in the first annual *Healthcare Informatics* Innovator Awards program, which involved the evaluation on the part of *Healthcare Informatics* editorial team members (including myself) of submissions by hospital organizations, and ultimately, the voting of their readers on the top three winners from a list of finalist entries.

And the DMC folks had a great story to share with *Healthcare Informatics* readers. Not only had they successfully rolled out a system-wide electronic medical record (EMR) across all eight hospitals in their 2,000-bed urban system, in a noteworthy 13 months (and at a cost of $31 million); but they had also done something that very few U.S. hospitals have done to date; and that is to fully leverage the implementation of their EMR, computerized physician order entry (CPOE), electronic medication administration record (eMAR), and advanced pharmacy systems, in one of the most challenging operational environments within the inpatient hospital – the neonatal intensive care unit (NICU) at Harper-Hutzel Hospitals (a twinned facility on the core DMC campus), to strong results.

There are many aspects to the DMC organization's achievement, but it is worth noting that nursing informaticists and nursing informatics are at the core of the success of the clinical IS implementation in the NICU, and particularly of the success of barcoding-facilitated closed-loop medication administration in the NICU. As at NICUs nationwide, clinicians faced multiple obstacles in attempting to implement barcode scanning-based meds administration for their smallest patients. At Hutzel, neonates weighing less than 500 g (in other words, less than one pound) now regularly survive, meaning that trying to work with standard-sized barcode labels becomes impossible, in terms of size, the curvature of the barcode around the wrist (or, more likely, the ankle, in the case of most of these neonates). But nurses, nurse leaders, and members of DMC's IT department spent weeks intensively working to develop specialized patient bands that worked in the unusual physical environment of the NICU. Equally importantly, pharmacists and nurses worked very closely together on advanced medication ordering and administration protocols, which among other things have ensured that nurses virtually never mix liquid medications any longer (a common source of medication administration errors in the NICU).

In addition, nurses and nurse informaticists at DMC were deeply involved in working out the details of the eMAR that is used in the NICU as throughout the organization. Indeed, NICU nurses at Harper-Hutzel Hospitals strongly credit bedside eMAR charting/documentation with the reduction in medication errors that has taken place since implementation.

Most of all, as I learned when I visited, the deliberately multidisciplinary, collaborative team culture that exists at Harper-Hutzel Hospitals and more broadly at the DMC has created the environment in which nurse informaticists, nurse leaders, and staff nurses regularly contribute to IT, clinician workflow, and clinical performance improvement advancement; the advancement in all those areas has been directly responsible for the success of the DMC-wide barcoded meds administration rollout and the implementation of the EMR, CPOE, eMAR, and advanced pharmacy systems across the entire organization. Thus, once I had experienced the DMC culture, it became clear to me why *Healthcare Informatics* readers voted their team achievement worthy of first place in the magazine's first annual, team-based, innovation awards program (http://healthcare-informatics.com).

Broad Industry Trends Converging: Nursing Informatics at the Nexus

My experience of reporting on the innovations taking place at the DMC speaks to broader trends compelling the healthcare industry forward, and to the centrality of clinical informatics (including, very critically, nursing informatics) in the industry's evolution. Among the key trends:

- Driven by purchaser and payer demands, hospital organizations most of all (and, more gradually and on a smaller scale, physician organizations) are moving rapidly to systematically overhaul unsatisfactory levels of patient safety, clinical care quality, patient satisfaction, and operational efficiency.
- As hospital and other organizations seek to strongly improve performance in these clinical and operational areas, they are finding that clinical IT is an inescapable and critical success factor moving forward; put bluntly, massive improvement in patient safety, care quality, clinician workflow, and operational efficiency are impossible without clinical IT facilitation.
- As a result, implementation of core electronic medical record/electronic health record (EMR/EHR) systems, long lagging in the healthcare industry, is surging; closely behind core EMR implementation is implementation of nursing and physician documentation, CPOE, advanced pharmacy, electronic medication administration (eMAR), and other critical clinical information systems, as well as the installation of stronger and more comprehensive IT infrastructure, and mobile infrastructure, to support such systems.

And those trends, in turn, are helping to fuel the following trends:

- A rapid evolution in clinical informaticist roles and hiring, including nurse informaticist development. More and more hospital organizations are hiring whole teams of nursing professionals, some without any experience, but more commonly, with at least some clinical IT implementation experience, to work full- or part-time as clinical IT implementers and advisers for their organizations.
- The gradual creation of ladders of advancement for nursing informaticists, from frontline implementer positions and data analysis positions, up through director and vice-president positions. In addition, growing numbers of chief information officers (CIOs) are coming to their positions with
- Registered nurse (RN) backgrounds, as clinical IT becomes an intense focus for hospital organizations.
- An ongoing evolution in the development of formal educational programs for nursing informatics specifically, and clinical informatics more broadly.

Qualitatively speaking, senior executives and boards of directors of hospital-based organizations are quickly coming to the realization that nurse informaticists are a crucial component to an effective IT implementation team. What's more, they are actively professionally developing nursing professionals to take on increasing levels of responsibility for clinical IT projects, implementations, and ongoing development and management. At the same time, CIOs and other IT executives and IT leaders in organizations are pushing nursing informaticists towards ever-increased levels of formalism and professionalism. Nurse informaticists are also being hired and developed by health insurers and especially by clinical software vendors.

What is most qualitatively important is not the obvious elements of these trends, such as that, for instance, the deployment of nurse informaticists is necessary for the sound implementation of nursing documentation software implementations. Rather, it is the extent to which hospital-based and other healthcare organizations are beginning to bring nurse informaticists into the core of performance improvement efforts nationwide in healthcare. In that trend lies a spectrum of opportunities for professional growth and development for nurse informaticists in the coming decade and beyond.

Within that context, nursing informaticists are becoming key members of the multidisciplinary teams that are implementing and refining EMR, CPOE, clinical decision support, advanced pharmacy, and eMAR systems. Put negatively, organizations (and I have come across a number of them in my research and reporting) that "forget" to proactively ensure nurse informaticists' place at the table when all of these systems are being planned, implemented, and refined find that their implementations have been sub-optimized, with end-users of all types (physicians, nurses, etc.) rebelling, and full adoption put at risk. Just as only physician informaticists can help design solutions to certain aspects of clinical computing, so, too, nurse informaticists are uniquely positioned to understand and work with certain aspects of clinical computing, including certain elements of clinician workflow, documentation, and patient safety protocols. What will be essential going forward is for nurse informaticists to optimize their skills and experience in order to provide their organizations with maximal levels of expertise in clinical IT implementations and improvement, while their organizations give them the support and resources they will need to produce the highest levels of output and service quality.

When EMR Use Facilitates Care Quality Improvement

In my first book, *Paradox and Imperatives in Health Care* (2007), co-authored with Jeffrey C. Bauer, Ph.D., I described an initiative to reduce central-line infection rates at Virginia Mason Medical Center in Seattle. Infection rates there were typical of most hospitals; but clinician leaders were determined to strongly improve them. And, interestingly, the ultimately successful work on central-line infections there was facilitated by nursing informatics.

What happened? As Cathie Furman, R.N., M.H.A., Senior Vice-President, quality and compliance, at the 336-bed teaching hospital, explained to me, first, clinicians spent some time analyzing what was causing bloodstream infections at the hospital. What became clear were two things. First, no standardized, systematized way to perform a central-line insertion had been implemented. And second, validation and documentation were unsatisfactory. As to the first, Charleen Tachibana, R.N., Virginia Mason's Senior Vice-President and Chief Nursing Officer (CNO), reported that she and her clinician leader colleagues established a protocol that is now strictly followed; among its elements: the clinician who inserts a central-line catheter must fully gown up, as if for surgery, including gown, mask, and gloves; the patient to be inserted must be draped with sterile drapes as in an operating room; the clinician must follow a very specific clinic protocol with regard to which vessels are acceptable for insertion, and all clinicians who might perform a central-line insertion must pass a specific test ensuring that they can insert a line into the correct vessel. And indeed, only 10% of the hospital's 600 nurses are permitted to insert a peripheral line.

Very importantly, the hospital's EMR requires that the nurse attending to any patient with a central line that has already been inserted determine each day whether the patient still needs to have that line in place. Nurse leaders at Virginia Mason agree that the fact that the EMR requires nurses to document the ongoing necessity for insertion into a patient's record each day has been helpful in compelling more careful oversight of central lines already inserted.

As a result of the systematization rigor of these processes, the central-line-associated BSI rate per 1,000 device days at Virginia Mason has declined dramatically in the hospital's critical care units, from 7.73 in 2002 to 2.81 in 2006.

Meanwhile, in my second book, *Transformative Quality: The Emerging Revolution in Health Care Performance* (2008), I described how clinician and IT leaders at the 897-bed Northwestern Memorial Hospital in downtown Chicago have been initiating literally dozens of quality improvement projects in recent years. Among these has been their implementation of so-called "smart" infusion pumps – intravenous infusion pumps that have microchips built into them and can be programmed to set use and dosage parameters, and emit warnings when those parameters are exceeded. Numerous studies in the clinical literature have found that the proper use of smart pumps can dramatically reduce medication administration errors involving IV pumps.

At Northwestern, Carol Payson, R.N., M.S.N., director of surgical patient care, and Karen Cabansag, R.N., manager of surgical patient care, have helped lead smart-pump implementation and have worked with clinical IT professionals to optimize that implementation, which went live in May 2007. Among the goals: to obtain real-time utilization data for quality improvement use; and to build a drug library, to facilitate the keying in of needed IV medications by nurses on the floors. As Cabansag told me, "It was all about delivering safer patient care."

The initial-state situation at Northwestern Memorial was very similar to that at the vast majority of U.S. hospitals, which still lack "smart-pump" technology. The problem was that staff nurses on the floors were manually entering the rate and volume to be infused in a particular IV bag. The process was riddled with potential errors and missteps, especially with key-in errors. So Northwestern Memorial clinicians and IT professionals went ahead and evaluated vendors, and selected a vendor. Then pharmacists from the hospital developed a core template for the product chosen, which was customized by the nurses and nurse managers to meet the needs of specific units at the hospital. Standardization was achieved generally and then within each of the clinical service areas (ICU, general med-surg, etc.). In this process, nurse informaticists helped facilitate processes and optimization.

Once the new system was implemented, with manual keying in eliminated, IV medication administration errors dropped dramatically. Cabansag and Payson noted that even very experienced nurses found that they were triggering alerts, a sign that the system was indeed improving the patient safety environment at the hospital.

Performance Improvement Methodologies and IT: Hand-in-Glove

The above examples, taken from my two previous books, underscore the interrelationship between patient safety and clinical care quality improvement on the one hand, and clinical IT implementation on the other. Obviously, all these concepts are highly dependent on the involvement in nursing and, within the context of IT as a facilitating agent, particularly on the involvement of nurse informaticists for success.

But in order for any discussion of the interrelationship of clinical performance improvement and clinical IT implementation to be concluded, it is essential to add in a third concept, and one that has seen intensive nurse and nurse informaticist involvement in recent years, and that is the use of formalized performance improvement methodologies in patient care settings and across healthcare organizations.

Indeed, it is far from coincidental that the hospitals and other patient care organizations that have made the most dramatic strides in improving patient safety and clinical care quality have also been those that have also used performance improvement methodologies, including Lean management, Six Sigma, and Toyota Production System (TPS) principles, to improve their clinical performance, with all their activity being facilitated strongly by excellent clinical information systems.

One important observation I made in Chap. 6 of *Paradox and Imperatives*, and one that can sometimes get lost in discussions of performance improvement, is that the hospital and patient care organizations that have successfully applied performance improvement methodologies to their clinical operations have done so strategically rather than in the typically fragmented, "micro-focus" way in which total quality management (TQM) and continuous quality improvement (CQI) strategies were applied in healthcare in the 1980s and 1990s. Of course, the application of performance improvement principles inevitably becomes expressed down to very detailed levels in practice; that is where the drill-down of general principles is made effective in specific care contexts. As Christina Saint Martin, then Vice-President for governance and administration at Seattle's Virginia Mason Medical Center, so aptly stated with regard to Virginia Mason's passionate adoption of the TPS for patient care improvement and, indeed, all operational improvement at the hospital, "VMMCs full embrace of TPS went far beyond the use of a toolkit," and became all-encompassing, a philosophy and strategy of how to deliver care and operate a hospital, not simply a box of tactics to be applied to small-bore situations.

Indeed, nurse informaticists and clinical informaticists in general at organizations like Virginia Mason are learning Six Sigma, Lean, and TPS methods and skill sets in order to effectively lead change and apply IT to the issues facing their organizations.

As I wrote about Virginia Mason's experience (p. 113)[2]:

> [I]n the process of using TPS to respond to market trends and to improve its bottom line, Saint Martin and her colleagues discovered that the methodology had produced many other improvements, from reworking nurse staffing to reducing central-line infections and ventilator-acquired pneumonia. They found that the entire way of doing things at Virginia Mason was transformed by the Toyota methodology. "The TPS paradigm is really changing the culture," Martin says.

The linkage here between performance improvement and IT is extremely clear. All the performance improvement methodologies are highly data-driven and help foster data-rich and data-intensive cultures, and obviously, obtaining all that data requires the implementation of strong, and over time, optimized, clinical information systems. And that is where clinical informaticists, including nurse informaticists, once again are exceptionally important as change leaders and innovation pioneers in their organizations. No truly successful, broad-based performance improvement can take place without data facilitation; and no useful data facilitation is possible without the intensive involvement of nurse and other clinical informaticists in architecting and implementing excellent information systems, including both clinical information systems that assist clinician end-users in their daily tasks and processes and the data warehouses, data marts, data reports, and other tools for analysis and feedback for further change-based activity.

Organizations with a Strong Clinical Leadership–IT Leadership Link

In organizations with strong nursing and clinical IT leadership, such things are understood. Take for example Methodist Hospital of Southern California, a 460-bed independent community hospital in Arcadia, a Los Angeles suburb. I interviewed three senior executives there – all RNs by background – for the November 2008 *Healthcare Informatics* cover story on nursing and IT (http://healthcare-informatics.com). Those interviewed were Kara Marx, R.N., M.H.S., the hospital's CIO; Jason Aranda, R.N., the organization's Chief Clinical Informatics Officer; and Carolyn Tadeja, R.N., its Vice-President and CNO.

The hiring of Marx as Methodist's CIO was no accident. As Marx told me for the *Healthcare Informatics* cover story, "I am very lucky to work for an organization that values our roles and our clinical perspective. In June 2006, when the hospital's senior executives decided to fund our EMR, and make that huge financial investment, they also made sure to invest in a clinical informatics department and a CIO." Indeed, just 6 months prior to Marx's hire, Methodist had hired Aranda to be its chief clinical informatics officer (his technical title is Manager, Clinical Informatics). Also, Aranda has a direct reporting relationship to Tadeja, with a dotted-line relationship to Marx, an arrangement that underscores the centrality of nursing informatics and clinical informatics to the organization's goals and objectives, as well as the level to which its chief nursing informatics officer (Aranda) is, and is seen as being, clinically embedded.

For his part, Aranda, who leads an entire team of nurse informaticists, told me that transparency of his role is absolutely critical to his team's success. And, he said, "Part of being transparent is taking the time to educate. I and my nursing informaticists have a mantra that we have to talk both about features and benefits (of any IT), not just features. What will be the benefit of a new technology? The nurse at the bedside is very task-oriented. I have a patient who has a temperature and who needs antibiotics. And I have a patient who needs heart meds. Which task do you want me to do first? So when you put something on top of that that adds another task, which becomes the priority?"

And while Methodist of Southern California is still relatively early on its journey towards clinical transformation, some organizations are already farther along the path. Another organization whose leaders I interviewed for that *Healthcare Informatics* cover story was Fletcher Allen Health Care, an integrated system in Burlington, Vermont. There, Senior Vice-President and CIO, Chuck Podesta, and Senior Vice-President and CNO, Sandi Dalton, R.N., told me that they are firmly committed to making dramatic improvements in patient safety and care quality at their 562-bed academic medical center organization. In fact, in the informatics sphere, they are working in the context of an umbrella initiative called PRISM (Patient Record and Information System Management). "Part of the goal of this whole clinical transformation initiative is to change the way we deliver care to the patient," Podesta told me. "And to me, that gets towards issues around adopting this system and making sure the people will be using the technology to change the way they deliver care, to be conscious care deliverers. Anybody can do an implementation and go live, but what is that technology actually doing for you?"

In making such leaps, the Fletcher Allen folks will doubtless be hiring more clinical, including nursing, informaticists, as time goes by. And, in that same *Healthcare Informatics* cover story, I explored the question of what makes for a strong nurse informaticist. Jackie Willis, R.N., M.S., Vice-President of Clinical Systems and Chief Clinical Information Officer at the 37-hospital Adventist Health System, based in Winter Park, Florida, told me, "I'm a translator and interpreter." Willis, who spent 20 years in clinical practical before transitioning into clinical informatics full-time, added that a strong clinical background is important in her job, linked fundamentally to a broader interest in and understanding of informatics.

Into the Future

With society in general and the healthcare industry and technology in particular evolving forward at warp speed, it is always dangerous to lay out very specific predictions. That said, some very clear trends will certainly continue to play out broadly across healthcare, among them:

- The aging of society and the massive increase taking place in chronic illness (partly driven by increasing obesity and other lifestyle-oriented problems) can be expected to proceed apace. As a result, even without other challenges impinging on healthcare costs, cost increases can be expected to be an ongoing (and very likely increasing) problem in the foreseeable future.
- Regardless of the specific shape that potential healthcare policy reform efforts might take, there will be very strong pressure on policymakers to try to rein in healthcare

costs, while expanding health insurance access. The dynamic tension between those policy objectives will most certainly add further pressure on cost-control efforts.

- Clinical IT continues to improve – if not consistently and evenly, then at least, by regular leaps and jumps – and clinical IT solutions can be expected to become more effective and user-friendly over time.
- The pace of clinical IT implementation continues to accelerate. While a large plurality of hospital organizations could reasonably be said to be "behind the adoption curve" in comparison with clinical IT pioneer organizations at press time, the adoption curve can be expected to tighten over time, as most hospital and other patient care organizations will soon be required to implement at least core EMR and other clinical information systems relatively quickly.
- Pressures on hospital and other patient care organizations toward accountability and transparency, with regard to such phenomena as pay-for-performance and value-based purchasing, clinical outcomes reporting, and cost-effectiveness, will all increase and accelerate.
- Market-based competition, encompassing consumer and purchaser selection based on technology differentiation, will certainly increase and accelerate.

Given all of the above, hospital and other patient care organizations will have their work cut out for them in the next decade. As I argued in both *Paradox and Imperatives in Health Care* and *Transformative Quality*, purchasers and payers will ensure that performance improvement – clinical and operational, of all varieties – will soon no longer be optional in healthcare. And provider organizations will only be able to make the leaps in care quality, patient safety, effectiveness, and efficiency that they will need to make through the intelligent and wise use of IT to help facilitate performance improvement.

And who will be at the nexus of all these requirements, especially when it comes to clinical performance improvement? Clinical informaticists. It is clinical informaticists, including nurse informaticists, who will be tasked with making the key changes at the level of clinician workflow and the point of care that can really transform care – in other words, with leading the charge towards clinical transformation on the ground.

As a result, the nurse informaticists of the next decade will need the following skill sets and characteristics:

- A broad understanding of the policy and operational, clinical, and technological context of their work.
- A strong clinical care background, allied to at least some degree of technical/technological knowledge or understanding.
- Good leadership and management skills.
- A good grounding in performance improvement methodologies, at some level of specificity.
- Some level of implementational experience, depending on the specific job position, organization, and particular situation.
- The personal characteristics required to work in a multidisciplinary, team-based, collaborative environment and an environment of constant innovation and change.
- The capability and desire to engage in lifelong and career-long learning and professional and personal development.

Based on my reporting and research for my books and for periodicals in the past several years, and on 20 years' experience in healthcare journalism more generally, I believe that those nurse informaticists who have the requisite experience, skill sets, and personal and professional characteristics to succeed in the emerging patient care and operational environment, one of the constant changes and multiple pressures, have tremendous opportunities ahead of them. They will also have to shoulder a great deal of responsibility, as clinical transformation – the appropriate and intelligent use of IT and performance improvement strategies to dramatically improve clinical care performance – will be an essential element in transforming our challenged healthcare system into the system of the future, one that works for all of healthcare's stakeholders.

But as recent industry history has shown, for every challenge U.S. healthcare has faced, there have been individuals and organizations up to that challenge, and more. For the nurse informaticists of today and tomorrow, opportunity will necessarily equate with challenge – and vice-versa.

References

1. Hagland M, Bauer JC. *Paradox and Imperatives in Health Care: How Efficiency, Effectiveness, and E-Transformation Can Conquer Waste and Optimize Quality.* New York: Productivity Press; 2008, p.113.
2. Hagland M. *Transformative Quality: The Emerging Revolution in Health Care Performance.* New York: Productivity Press; 2008.

Barbara B. Frink and Asif Dhar

Engraved on two of the steps leading to the University of Pennsylvania School of Nursing are these words (The first quotation is attributed to Claire Fagin, PhD, RN, FAAN. Dean of the University of Pennsylvania School of Nursing, 1977–1991, the second to Tracey White, as quoted in Benner and Wrubel[1]):

> *Knowledge will bring you the opportunity to make a difference.*
> *Caring is a profound act of hope.*

These two phrases characterize the vision of this book: *nursing informatics: where technology and caring meet.* In this chapter, we profile two areas of scientific discovery that have potential for profound effect on future healthcare delivery, quality, cost, and value. The first area we explore is personalized medicine, and the second is comparative effectiveness. The development of both of these areas will be profoundly affected by health information and health system reform. Both are subjects of national interest and attention amidst the healthcare reform discussion; both are also examples of complex relationships among science, translational systems, information technology, and stakeholder groups. Significant funding in the American Recovery and Reinvestment Act of 2009 (ARRA) has been allocated to health information technology and to comparative effectiveness research (CER) (Health Information and Management Systems Society 2009).

These discoveries offer new hope to individuals and populations for predicting risk of disease, individualized targeted treatment of disease, and avoidance of potentially harmful or inappropriate care. Advances in technology and care systems combined with the discoveries of personalized medicine and comparative effectiveness will profoundly change healthcare.

Background

Developments in information technology and knowledge dissemination are a key to the realization of the potential benefits of both personalized medicine and CER. The conver-

B.B. Frink (✉)
Vice President for Clinical Excellence and Informatics Main Line Health System 130 S. Bryn Mawr Ave. 1st Floor Gerhard Building Bryn Mawr, PA 19010
e-mail: frinkb@mlhs.org

M.J. Ball et al. (eds.), *Nursing Informatics*,
DOI: 10.1007/978-1-84996-278-0_20, © Springer-Verlag London Limited 2011

gence of these areas of discovery creates a unique opportunity to transform care. Dr. Elias Zerhouni, former Director of the National Institutes of Health (NIH), has characterized this convergence as the healthcare era of the 4 Ps: predictive, personalized, preemptive, and participatory medicine.[2] Until recently, healthcare providers were the consumers of evidence-based knowledge on behalf of patients; in an era of more personalized and preemptive care, patients will also be consumers of evidence and will become actively involved in proactively managing their health. This will require fundamental changes in the way providers and patients interact around healthcare knowledge and decision-making; and it will require innovative methods for increasing health literacy and communication mechanisms on behalf of patients and consumers.

The translation of scientific evidence into clinical practice is a fundamental issue in the generation and application of knowledge in healthcare. That translation process has traditionally followed specific guidelines and conformed to an evidence hierarchy. It is becoming increasingly clear that practice-related questions cannot always be answered effectively with current methods of inquiry. For example, questions about the effectiveness of combinations of interventions and treatments, or questions about the best treatment decisions for individual patients, are not generally answered by the "gold standard" of evidence, the randomized clinical trial. Observational studies have the potential to supplement evidence derived from controlled trials.[3,4] However, new data sources will be required to support these studies. Through the use of integrated data networks and data repositories of clinical care transactions, health information technology provides an opportunity to answer such questions in a more timely and cost-effective manner.

Until recently, the use of information technology in observational studies of clinical effectiveness and variation has been limited to the use of administrative data. With the advent of considerable electronic health record (EHR) investment, several new possibilities exist. According to Dr. Carolyn Clancy, Director of the Agency for Healthcare Research and Quality (AHRQ), "anticipated growth in investments in health IT across the healthcare sector now offers an unprecedented opportunity for redefining the possibilities of observational studies, accelerating and targeting the uptake of relevant information, and providing feedback to the biomedical enterprise itself."[5]

Leveraging healthcare information technology and reusing the associated clinical data will produce a new source of study information that will likely disrupt the hierarchy of evidence. Nevertheless the scale and the richness of these data sets will become a powerful aid in new discovery. This approach will allow patients to be looked at individually and provide a sophisticated response to fears, from patients and providers, that comparative effectiveness will lead to cookbook medicine. Indeed, research will be focused on the individual's benefit as opposed to the current "one size fits all" state of the science. The reuse of clinical data, as a non-homogeneous data source, may yield unique insights, as yet unknown.

What Is Personalized Medicine?

Individualized healthcare, often referred to as personalized medicine, refers to "the tailoring of medical treatment to the individual characteristics of each patient. It does not literally mean the creation of drugs or medical devices that are unique to a patient, but rather the ability to classify individuals into subpopulations that differ in their susceptibility to a particular disease or their response to a specific treatment. Preventive or therapeutic interventions can then be concentrated on those who will benefit from them, sparing expense and side effects for those who will not."[6] The construct of individualized healthcare is an approach to healthcare delivery that is enabled by the scientific discovery of genomics and molecular determinants of disease. Access to molecular level research, when translated into practice, has increased the knowledge base of disease detection at an earlier point in the disease trajectory, prior to symptom expression and disease progression. In addition, it has provided knowledge about disease prognosis and potential individual responses to treatment, leading to more effective therapy, and in some cases, avoidance of harm. Upon his 2009 appointment as Director of NIH, Dr. Francis Collins stated that one of his primary goals for the NIH is faster translation of science into care, including an emphasis on the field of personalized medicine.[7]

Personalized medicine is a synthesis of many areas of scientific study. Although the discovery of the human genome is fundamental to personalized medicine, advances in a number of scientific fields have enabled the translation of that science into practice. In addition to genomics (including evolving-related disciplines of pharmacogenomics and proteomics), advances in biotechnology, health information technology, and computational biology all contribute to what we refer to as personalized medicine.[8] Not unlike other scientific endeavors, the translation of genomic research findings into clinical practice presents challenges. One of these challenges is the systematic development of an evidence base that underlies practice. Evans and Khoury[9] suggest several reasons for what has been perceived as a slow pace of development of the evidence base for genetic medicine. First, genetic medicine has traditionally focused on rare diseases, which presents significant sample size issues for adequately powered and funded studies. Second, medical genetics has focused more on diagnosis than treatment and interventions, where evidence-based medicine is more active. However, as genomic interventions continue to be developed, their value must be demonstrable through the translation of the evidence base. The additional challenge is to expedite the translation into useful and useable information.

Genetic tests and genomic technology contribute to our understanding of risk and the role of genes in disease and health. With the exponential growth in genetic/genomic knowledge, there are now (as of this writing) genetic tests clinically available for 1,500 diseases, and 300 more tests are in active research (http://www.cdc.gov/genomics/gtesting/index.htm. Data cited in text current as of 30 Aug 2009). Establishing the effectiveness of this rapidly expanding knowledge base is critically important. Currently, there is only one group in the U.S. that is consistently focused on building the evidence base for genetic tests and genomic technology: the Center for Disease Control and Prevention's (CDC) EGAPP initiative – Evaluation of Genomic Applications in Practice and Prevention (Totals updated on a regular basis. See http://www.egappreviews.org/about.htm. Accessed 27.08.09). EGAPP "supports the development and implantation of a rigorous evidence-based process for evaluating genetic tests and other genomic applications for clinical and public health practice in the U.S."[10]

Another complementary effort is the Secretary's Advisory Committee on Genetics Health and Society (SACGHS). The SACGHS identified four (of five) priorities related to establishing evidence of effectiveness of genetic tests: "oversight of the clinical validity of genetic tests; transparency of genetic testing; the level of current knowledge about the clinical usefulness of genetic tests; and the ability of health professionals, the public health community, patients, and consumers to use these new tests effectively."[11]

How is Genomic Science Translated to Practice?

Khoury et al[12] describe a specific multidisciplinary translational process to develop evidence-based guidelines for genomic medicine applications. Figure 20.1 depicts their four-phase translational research process for genomic medicine discoveries and applications. By making the phases of translation research both transparent and explicit, the strength of the evidence base for use in practice is established and may generate further research.

Questions remain about the threshold of evidence for moving promising genomic applications into clinical practice. Clinical and analytic validity as well as clinical utility of genomic applications needs to be established. The issue of clinical utility in genomic applications is of particular interest. Unlike traditional medical diagnostic knowledge, with clinical utility defined in terms of the "patient," genomic applications may hold considerable benefit – or risk – beyond the patient, to other family members, and the population. Because of this, "the value of the information alone is often seen as adequate justification for (genetic) testing."[12]

Making research evidence accessible and available to researchers and clinicians is a critical link in the translation process. In the case of the human genome project (HGP), information technology was not only a key to the discovery of the human genome, but also to the daily dissemination of research findings via the internet. Dr. Francis Collins, current Director of the NIH, states that the "continuing commitment by genome scientists to global accessibility to genomic information by placing a wide variety of genome databases on public websites" is an important factor in achieving rapid scientific advances.[13] The National Center for Biotechnology Information (NCBI) maintains a regularly updated site, primarily for the scientific and provider community, on molecular and genomic technologies (http:www.ncbi.nlm.nih.gov/sites/GeneTests/?db=GeneTests). For consumers, the translation of the science must include not only information, but products and tools that enable the use of the information that promotes understanding of risk and likelihood of disease.

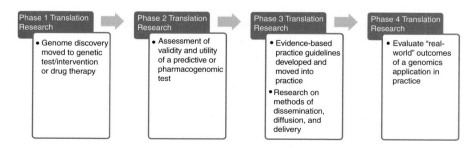

Fig. 20.1 Research translation process for genomic medicine. Adapted from Khoury et al[12]

Information technology, because of its ability to connect researchers, scientists, patients, and providers, may provide a unique solution to address the challenge presented by rapidly developing discoveries, which yield new evidence and clinical knowledge. As consumers understand more about predictive risk of disease, they can indeed become the center of their care. The aphorism "knowledge is power" is applicable in individualized healthcare. Molecular level information will clarify risk associated with both likelihood of disease and individual response to interventions. The challenge will be to provide both healthcare providers and consumers with information and decision tools that will enable more effective prevention and management of disease, and the avoidance of costly complications and ineffective or unnecessary interventions.

Some Key Stakeholders in Personalized Medicine

Indentifying the stakeholders serves to underscore the potential power of personalized medicine to transform the paradigm for healthcare. Consumers, both as individuals and as advocacy groups, are key stakeholders. Healthcare providers represent the primary link between evidence and clinical decision-making for patients and consumers. They are consumers themselves, as it pertains to the adoption and use of genomic evidence and diagnostic and therapeutic technologies.

Payers, both public and commercial, will determine reimbursement policy in the face of rapidly advancing science and be challenged with issues of member selection in the context of health management vs. disease management. No small item is the transformation and expansion of payer databases that will be required to accommodate individual clinical biomarker data.

The Life Science industry, including biotechnology, pharmaceutical, and diagnostic companies, plays a key role in personalized medicine. They have both much to gain and much to lose. For example, for the Pharmaceutical and Biotechnology industry, drugs once prescribed for all individuals with a specific disease may have a far smaller market if information is known about individual variability in drug responsiveness. Thus, the industry may experience a shift from the "blockbuster" market to the niche market, with accompanying change in the business model for drug development and testing. New partnerships may form between these stakeholder groups, in addition to the potential for establishing research collaboratives to support the highly expensive patient recruitment and multicenter trials required to bring drugs and tests to market.[8]

Policy makers are confronted with the challenges of understanding the interplay between science and translating learning from science into clinical practice and care. In addition, as they deal with healthcare priorities and funding issues, they must incorporate a new knowledge base that enables truly individual care, as opposed to "one size fits all" population-based healthcare that is the basis of today's healthcare model.

Nurses and other care providers, with their extensive contacts and educational roles with patients, families, and communities, must engage in the study of new methods of information dissemination and promotion of health literacy. Assisting patients and families as they become more active consumers of knowledge about individual healthcare risks will provide new areas for nursing research and practice.

What is Comparative Effectiveness?

Comparative effectiveness is the process of determining the relative clinical effectiveness among a number of diagnostic and intervention choices, when multiple options exist. It includes head-to-head comparisons through direct clinical trials or through the synthesis of multiple head-to-head studies.[14] Healthcare providers, consumers, and policymakers all require information about the safety and efficacy of diagnostic and treatment options employed in healthcare delivery. Such information is provided through the conduct, translation, and dissemination of biomedical research. However, there are several gaps in the process. First, the time gap between discovery and clinical application is protracted, and sometimes, the translation to practice is uneven or ineffective.[15] Second, there is a gap between what is known about individual diagnostics and treatments (compared to a placebo or no treatment) vs. comparison to multiple tests and treatments developed and used for the same conditions. Third, there is geographic variation in both the costs of interventions and access to treatment options, with increased variation in treatments supported by more limited evidence.[16]

The U.S. is not alone in the challenge of dealing with the knowledge/evidence/practice gap and the uncertainty and variation in treatment options. Several countries have established formal agencies to evaluate healthcare technologies and strategies. Some of the agency programs, such as Britain and Australia, are directly linked to a national health policy decision-making process for benefit determination; others, such as the programs of Germany and Canada, are advisory to the decision-making process for benefit determination.[17,18] All of the programs, however, have an overt link to reimbursement policy. Such is not the case in the U.S., where CER studies cannot be used to determine coverage or reimbursement policies.[17] This is an important distinction for the U.S. Critics of the program view it as a first step to rationing healthcare; proponents view CER as critical to determining relative effectiveness among treatment options, and one means of determining value. Studying the experiences, policies, and infrastructures of these agencies in countries such as Canada, Germany, Britain, France, and Australia may provide some helpful insights as the U.S. program becomes established.[19]

What Is Comparative Effectiveness Research?

CER is "the generation and synthesis of evidence that compares the benefits and harms of alternative methods to prevent, diagnose, treat, and monitor a clinical condition or to improve the delivery of care. The purpose of CER is to assist consumers, clinicians, purchasers, and policy makers to make informed decisions that will improve healthcare at both the individual and population levels."[20] The state of the science, however, is such that information is either unavailable or incomplete for decision-makers at the point of care. The institute of medicine (IOM) estimates that this lack of available information results in no clear evidence of effectiveness in more than half of the treatments delivered in the U.S.[20]

The evidence base to support CER comes from several methodologies. No different from studies of clinical effectiveness, the concept of levels of evidence underlies CER. Figure 20.2 presents a summary of the types of evidence that support CER.

CER is a subset of health services research. The biomedical research enterprise in the U.S. currently invests only 1.5% of the total research expenditure on all of health services research.[21] When the ARRA of 2009 was enacted, provision was made to increase funding for CER; $1.1B was included for CER, distributed among departments and agencies of HHS, including the Office of the National Coordinator (ONC), the NIH, and AHRQ. A Federal Coordinating Council for CER was appointed by the Department of HHS to oversee the coordination of CER conducted by the federal government. Both the Coordinating Council and the National Academy of Science's IOM were charged with recommending priorities for organization and research within CER.

The Coordinating Council recommended that the primary investment for CER be devoted to data infrastructure. This includes "development of distributed electronic data networks, patient registries, or partnerships with the private sector."[22] In addition, they recommended linking already available data sources to provide researchers with a resource to address CER questions. The IOM recommendations for priority areas of research included 29 research areas with a total of 100 research topics, 49 of which are clinical trial topics. In addition, the IOM also recognized the infrastructure requirements of a sound

Type of Research Evidence	Description	Considerations
Randomized Controlled Trials	Gold standard	Extremely costly, Multi-year duration
Observational Studies	Prospective registries, Cohort studies, cross-sectional surveys	Observed outcomes cannot be directly linked to interventions
Systematic Reviews and Syntheses	Summarize strength of existing evidence, generate new research questions, and identify gaps in knowledge. Practice Guidelines.	May lead to further RCTs. Require timely systematic review for update. May be used as basis for decision-support in EHRs.
Large Databases	Electronic Health Records, Clinical Data Repositories.	May demonstrate current practice and outcomes, but not rationale for decisions
Practice-Based Evidence *	Naturalistic view of variation in data collected from routine clinical practice	Used in situations of comparative effectiveness not appropriate for clinical trials

Fig. 20.2 Types of evidence supporting comparative effective research (CER). Adapted from Institute of Medicine[20]

CER program. To that end, they envision public–private partnerships and strategies, capacity for the support of high-efficiency randomized clinical trials, and large scale clinical and administrative data networks that are sufficient to support observational studies of patient care.[20] Each of these infrastructure recommendations underscores the importance of information technology to the achievement of a sound CER program. Such emphasis serves as further evidence of the direct link between national health policy priorities and the practice environment of both researchers and clinicians.

Some Key Stakeholders in Comparative Effectiveness

There are important stakeholder considerations in CER. Healthcare consumers require timely information from healthcare providers as they jointly consider treatment options and make decisions about courses of therapy. Educating consumers about principles that underlie strength of evidence and the prediction of treatment outcomes is an important component of an effective CER program. A comprehensive CER program should also provide tools for decision-making, not currently available, for healthcare providers. Provider access to knowledge about the relative merits of competing diagnostic and treatment options will improve clinical decision-making for individual patients. The accompanying emphasis on EHR investments in the ARRA of 2009 should have a direct effect on the availability of decision support tools for healthcare providers. Access to robust EHRs should enable access to guidelines, standards, patient profiles, and outcomes data, all of which are required for an effective CER program. Stakeholder considerations will continue to evolve as the CER program priorities and infrastructure are implemented.

The Critical Importance of Health Information Technology

As we have discussed, healthcare information technology is one of the primary enablers for realizing an individualized healthcare delivery system. To fulfill a vision of truly individualized healthcare, several new and developing health information technology solutions are required. Collecting, organizing, and analyzing individual genetic and health information and comparing those data to population-based health outcomes data will illuminate subpopulations with patterns of risk and disease that have not as yet been evident. Establishing large scale data repositories of actual clinical outcomes will enable observational studies for clinical interventions not necessarily appropriate for randomized trials.

Although there is a national and industry awareness of the need for interoperability among systems, there is considerable work to be accomplished in this area. Too often, clinical data are collected but are not able to be retrieved at even a local level, for analysis. Clinical systems designed for transactional use require alteration, so that data can be used in analyses. Interoperability between systems as well as the design of robust integrated data networks will enable differentiated communication among broad audiences, who have different needs and uses for clinical and scientific data. These changes to the infrastructure must occur with simultaneous application of data standards and standards that safeguard both the privacy and security of healthcare information.

Information technology is being used to transform research processes and is rapidly increasing the availability of knowledge and discovery to scientific and healthcare provider communities. As evidence increases for both the comparative effectiveness of interventions and the effectiveness of individualized applications of genomic science, the need for converting the evidence for use in automated decision support tools will increase. Decision support for clinicians requires ongoing research and development for the most effective use of automated alerts, reminders, and guidelines used in the process of care.[23,24]

Further challenge lies ahead in developing new methods of disseminating knowledge to consumers, patients, and families. New information tools and products will need to be developed that assist consumers in evaluating the individual health information that will be available to them: the personal risk of disease, individual response to available interventions and management of chronic disease, and the knowledge of the most effective interventions, when several similar options are available.

Semantically interoperable health information technology will provide both the researcher and healthcare provider with a powerful asset to deploy care in this new paradigm. For the researcher, large scale non-homogenous data sets will become available and will serve as a perpetual discovery tool or if you will, a test sandbox, in which the researcher will be able to test initial hypotheses, as opposed to directly testing human subjects. As knowledge is accrued "in silico" as opposed to "in vivo," the pace of discovery will be increased, and knowledge will be accrued more expeditiously, while minimizing risks to human subjects. This will make it easier for researchers to spend more time investigating the specific comparative benefits of therapeutic interventions on subpopulations and will likewise allow practitioners to understand the relative impact of therapeutic alternatives.

Information sharing solutions, akin to the World Wide Web, will accelerate the diffusion of lessons learned to a broader audience and provide new knowledge, through decision support tools, to the daily practice of clinicians.

The areas of inquiry such as personalized medicine and comparative effectiveness have the potential for transforming care as we know it. Health information technology is a critical enabler of realizing that transformation, and with it, enabling individuals to receive care, most effective for their particular risk of disease and individual response to therapy. Nurses and other healthcare providers have a unique opportunity to design, use, and evaluate information technology in the context of applying evidence-based decision-making to care. As they work with both scientists and patients, nurses and other healthcare providers will develop and test new models of care delivery best suited to the information, education, and decision-making needs of patients, families, and communities in an era of individualized care.

New questions will arise from the use of these scientific discoveries in practice. Nurses, physicians, and other healthcare providers are on the front lines of clinical practice, closely involved with critical health decisions of patients and families. The thoughtful adoption and use of new knowledge arising from both personalized medicine and CER will help realize the benefits and value of individualized care. Critical thinking about the clinical outcomes arising from the use of this knowledge in practice will give rise to new areas for research and as yet undiscovered methods of participating with patients in personalized, preemptive healthcare.

Acknowledgments   The authors thank Dr. Suzanne Feetham and Dr. Anne Wake for review of earlier drafts of this chapter. The authors acknowledge Dr. Paul Keckley, Director, and the work of the Deloitte Center for Health Solutions for policy perspectives related to targeted therapies and comparative effectiveness.

References

1. Benner P, Wrubel J. Caring comes first. *Am J Nurs*. 1988;88(8):1072-1075.
2. Zerhouni E. The promise of personalized medicine. NIH Medline Plus 2007 (Winter):1–3. http://www.nih.gov/about/director/interviews/NLMmagazinewinter2007.pdf; 2007 Accessed 29.08.09.
3. Atkins D. Creating and synthesizing evidence with decision makers in mind: Integrating evidence from clinical trials and other study designs. *Med Care*. 2007;45(10 suppl 2):S16-S22.
4. Horn SD, Gassaway JR. Practice-based evidence study design for comparative effectiveness research. *Med Care*. 2007;45(10 suppl 2):S50-S57.
5. Clancy CM. Getting to 'smart' health care. *Health Aff*. 2006;25(6):w589-w592.
6. President's Council of Advisors on Science and Technology. Priorities for Personalized Medicine. Report of The President's Council of Advisors on Science and Technology. http://www.ostp.gov/galleries/PCAST/pcast_report_v2.pdf; 2008 Accessed 20.08.09.
7. This Assoc Press article is c. 2009 and last updated at 3:44 pm EDT on 8/17/2009. The url is: http://www.msnbc.msn.com/id/32449295, accessed on 08/16/2010. Healthcare on MSNBC.com
8. Keckley P, Dhar A, Underwood H. The ROI for Targeted Therapies: A Strategic Perspective. Assessing the Barriers and Incentives for Adopting Personalized Medicine. Deloitte Center for Health Solutions (February):1–32 http://www.deloitte.com/assets/Dcom-UnitedStates/Local%20Assets/Documents/us_chs_ROIforTargetedTherapies_January2009%281%29.pdf; 2009 Accessed 16.09.09.
9. Evans J, Khoury MJ. Evidence based medicine meets genomic medicine. *Genet Med*. 2007;9(12):2.
10. Teutsch S, Bradley LA, et al. The evaluation of genomic applications in practice and prevention (EGAPP) initiative: methods of the EGAPP working group. *Genet Med*. 2009;11 (1):3-14.
11. Secretary's Advisory Committee on Genetics, Health, and Society. The Integration of Genetic Technologies into Health Care and Public Health. A Progress Report and Future Directions of the Secretary's Advisory Committee on Genetics, Health, and Society: 1–44. http://oba.od.nih.gov/oba/SACGHS/SACGHS%20Progress%20and%20Priorities%20Report%20to%20HHS%20Secretary%20Jan%202009.pdf; 2009 Accessed 30.08.09.
12. Khoury MJ, Berg A, et al. The evidence dilemma in genomic medicine. *Health Aff*. 2008;27(6):1600-1611.
13. Collins F. Foreword. In: Miller SM, McDaniel SH, et al., ed. *Individuals, Families and the New Era of Genetics: Biopsychosocial Perspectives*. New York, New York: W.W. Norton & Company. Norton; 2006.
14. Institute of Medicine. Learning What Works Best: The Nation's Need for Evidence on Comparative Effectiveness in Health Care. http://www.iom.edu/cerpriorities; 2007 Accessed 27.08.09.
15. McGlynn EA, Asch SM, et al. The quality of health care delivered to adults in the United States. *N Engl J Med*. 2003;348(26):2635-2645.
16. Fisher ES, Wennberg DE, et al. The implications of regional variations in Medicare spending. Part 1: the content, quality, and accessibility of care. *Ann Intern Med*. 2003;138(4):273-287.

17. Chalkidou K, Tunis S, Lopert R, et al. Comparative effectiveness research and evidence-based health policy: experience from four countries. *Milbank Q.* 2009;87(2):339-367.

18. Keckley P, Frink BB. Comparative Effectiveness: Perspectives for Consideration. Deloitte Center for Health Solutions, 1–36. http://www.deloitte.com/dtt/cda/doc/content/us_chs_ ComparisoneffectivenessStudy_may2009%281%29.pdf; 2009 Accessed 16.09.09.

19. Keckley, PH, Frink, BB, Comparative Effectiveness: A strategic perspective on what it is and what it may mean for the United States. *Journal of Health and Life Sciences Law.* 2009;3(1): 53-90.

20. Institute of Medicine. Initial National Priorities for Comparative Effectiveness Research. Report Brief; 2009: 1-12.

21. Moses H, Dorsey ER, et al. Financial anatomy of biomedical research. *JAMA.* 2005;294(11): 1333-1342.

22. Conway PH, Clancy C. Comparative-effectiveness research: implications of the federal Coordinating Council's report. *N Engl J Med.* 2009;361(4):328-330.

23. Lang NM. The promise of simultaneous transformation of practice and research with the use of clinical information systems. *Nurs Outlook.* 2008;56(5):232-236.

24. Lang NM, Akre ME, et al. Translating knowledge-based nursing into referential and executable applications in an intelligent clinical information system. In: Weaver C, Webber P, Carr R, eds. *Nursing and Informatics for the 21st Century: An International Look at the Trends, Cases, and the Future.* Chicago: Healthcare Information and Management Systems Society (HIMSS); 2006:291-304.

25. HIMSS. (2009). Healthcare Reform Update: Key federal leaders participate in HIMSS09. http://www.himss.org/Advocacy/ContentRedirector.asp?ContentId=69120 Accessed 08/16/2010.

Local Global Access: Virtual Learning Environment

21

Beth L. Elias, Jacqueline A. Moss, Christel Anderson, and Teresa McCasky

Introduction

A few years ago, during the American Informatics Medical Association's annual conference keynote address, Dr. David Brailer spoke about the importance of integrating information technology (IT) in healthcare. His remarks included the old saying about how a rising tide floats all boats. This adage prompted a discussion between nursing informatics leaders at the conference on the kind of nursing boats that could be launched on this rising tide. Nurses have long embraced the use of technology in practice and have been leaders in the use of technology in education.[1] However, there are some gaps in the informatics and information literacy competencies we teach in nursing education that are needed for effective nursing practice (Pravikoff et al 2005 and Jensen 2009). The nurses hearing Dr. Brailer saw the need to organize a concerted effort to integrate the use of IT into practice and education in the future. It is this rising tide of nursing practice incorporating new technologies that will "float the boat" of healthcare information technology (HIT) adoption.

To address this need for advancing the use of IT in nursing education, the Technology Informatics Guiding Educational Reform (TIGER) was formed and convened its first national summit in 2006. In order to transform nursing practice and education to better prepare nurses to practice in an increasingly automated, informatics-rich, and consumer-driven healthcare environment, TIGER concluded that the following recommendations must move forward[2]:

- Provide visibility to the 10-year TIGER vision of IT-enabled nursing practice and education to broader healthcare audience
- Demonstrate the breadth and depth of IT resources in use by nurses to enhance their practice and educational environments
- Demonstrate collaboration between industry, healthcare organizations academic institutions, and professional organizations to create educational modules for nurses that are based upon informatics competencies

B.L. Elias (✉)
The University of Alabama at Birmingham, School of Nursing Department of Community Health, Outcomes and Systems, NB 340, 1530 3rd Ave. South, Birmingham, Al 35294
e-mail: blelias@uab.edu

M.J. Ball et al. (eds.), *Nursing Informatics*,
DOI: 10.1007/978-1-84996-278-0_21, © Springer-Verlag London Limited 2011

- Provide universal accessibility to this demonstration for all nursing stakeholder groups
- Use practice examples from different practice environments that can demonstrate best practices, results of research, case studies, and lessons learned by partnering with nursing professional organizations
- Demonstrate how integrated IT systems impact nurses and the quality and safety of patient care

Demonstrating the use and utility of technology for improving practice and education can be an effective facilitator of the rapid diffusion and adoption of educational and practice technologies.[3-5] In this chapter, we describe several demonstrations of technology designed to improve nursing practice and education.

Diffusion theory, as described by Rogers,[6] informs us that the innovation adoption decision process "is essentially an information-seeking and information-processing activity." Within the industry today, a wide variety of innovative solutions offered to address this information-seeking need demonstrates the usability of technology in the delivery of patient-centered care. To persuade the nursing profession and all stakeholders to adopt these solutions, we must identify solid examples, demonstrations, and outcomes. Demonstrations should be designed on four levels, moving from minimal to extensive participant interaction and involvement. Adopters may need to move through each of these phases prior to innovation adoption or can choose to adopt at any level. However, the more engaged an individual is with the innovation, the more likely that individual is to view the innovation positively.

1. Observable demonstrations (watching a video or powerpoint) are an important first step in the information-gathering phase of the adoption decision process.
2. Trialable (interactive multimedia) demonstrations are more complex, allowing for participant-directed experimentation in a safe environment. This hands-on process can answer specific questions a nurse may have, reducing uncertainty.
3. Learn-while-doing demonstrations move closer to goals like training and allow for initial and continuing education, again in a safe environment, particularly important for patient care devices or systems.
4. Simulations move from simple demonstrations to more involved scripted educational experiences and can also allow for user feedback on needed changes to support real-world use and better ideas for development and experimentation with customization.

Demonstration Exemplars

While these examples are not exhaustive, educators, providers, and vendors are currently partnering to provide sustainable educational models that leverage technology in care practices and education. It is essential to incorporate technology in the education of current and future nurses and other healthcare professionals, both to support the integration of IT in healthcare and to prepare tomorrow's nurses.[7] There are solutions available today that support this goal and do not require large financial commitments or large human resource requirements. The benefit to nursing education, and ultimately to patient care, from these low-cost solutions is clear.

The exemplars that follow are just a few of the creative ways educators and vendors are using new technology and evolving media in order to educate and get important information out to those who need it.

Observable Exemplars

Healthcare organizations and IT vendors have partnered to create demonstration videos and multimedia to educate caregivers and purchasers of HIT. The goal of these demonstrations is to allow for the observation of a new technology in the actual care delivery setting. One exemplar, created by Siemens Corporation, is a Nursing Thought Leadership Web Cast Series, Information Technology Supporting Clinical Excellence www.siemens.com/clinicalgateway [8]. In this series, nursing professionals can see technology being integrated into actual care delivery through scenarios and can also hear from other executives and industry leaders regarding what they feel are some of the benefits of HIT.

A lighthearted observable demonstration is the emergency room (ER) Rap, a creative musical video created by ER nurses at the University of Alabama at Birmingham (UAB) as part of their observance of National Nurses Week.[9] The video uses humor and music to provide lay persons and potential future nurses a window into the world of an emergency nurse. You can find this delightful example at http://uabhealthtv.photobooks.com/default.a sp?ChannelID=6&ProgramID=93%22.

Trialable Exemplars

Trialable demonstrations engage the nurse in an interactive manner. An exemplar for this level of demonstration is the Microsoft Patient Journey Demonstrator (MPJD). The MPJD uses clinical scenarios to demonstrate their patient-centered care record. From their website launch page, you can interact with a patient record for tasks such as managing appointments, entering and reviewing patient data, and creating notes.[10] As an interactive demonstration, the nurse/participant can explore in a self-directed manner, experiencing the demonstration at their own pace and in an order that makes sense to them. The MPJD website launch page can be found at http://www.mscui.net/PatientJourneyDemonstrator.

A second exemplar for interactive demonstrations is the University of Tennessee Health Sciences Center's "The Listen Project." A YouTube video was designed and made available as an introduction to the project to help promote nurse assessment skills as well as evidence-based practice. The project extends to interactive demonstrations to stress the importance of developing "information literacy competencies of student and professional nurse."[11] You can access The Listen Project video at http://www.youtube.com/watch?v=XHVqLliBgdo.

Learn-While-Doing Exemplars: Academic Education Solutions

Moving to the next level of complexity, some schools of nursing have collaborated with HIT vendors to produce academic education solutions containing portals, interactive experiences, and hands-on simulation where students actually use the vendor's IT tools, via a vendor-based demonstration solution. Ball State University and Cardinal Health System and the McKesson Corporation created an environment to provide documentation experience with an electronic health record (EHR) used in clinical rotation.[12] Students are able to assess their patients and then document their findings in the vendor-based electronic nursing documentation system, minimizing workflow disruptions for the hospital staff. This partnership supports student access to an EHR without the costs of having an in-house school of nursing EHR system.

Another advance in transforming health education is being undertaken by the University of Kansas Center for Healthcare Informatics and the Cerner Corporation. In this collaboration model, these organizations have created an academic education solution, the simulated E-health delivery system (SEEDS). This solution is designed to provide teaching and learning tools to assist health professional students to develop competencies to harness the power of IT, thus improving the quality, efficiency, and effectiveness of healthcare.[12] More information on identifying best practices for implementing an academic education solution can be found at http://www2.kumc.edu/health-informatics/video.html.

Simulation Exemplars

The highest level of virtual demonstration is found in simulation centers. There are several exemplars of simulation and below are just a few examples.

The Garfield Innovation Center is a simulation care delivery environment where healthcare professionals can have a complex immersion experience based on realistic scenarios.[13] The Center also allows for experimentation, prototyping, and trouble-shooting in this hands-on mocked-up clinical environment. An additional strength of the Center is the collaborative nature of the simulations, bringing together professionals from different areas as participants. A description of the Garfield Center is available at http://xnet.kp.org/innovationcenter/about.html.

Simulations can also be based in virtual worlds like Second Life. In 2006, IBM developed a Virtual Healthcare Island (VHI) in the virtual world Second Life. The VHI was designed to be a unique, virtual world simulation of the challenges facing today's healthcare industry and the role IT will play in transforming global healthcare delivery to meet patient needs. The island is modeled to have "patients" go to their home on the VHI, enter information into a personal health record (PHR), visit the laboratory to have blood drawn, the clinic to discuss the results with a physician and then to the pharmacy if medications are prescribed. One possible evolution of the healthcare islands like the VHI would be to provide a virtual platform for vendors to demonstrate new devices. A short, narrated video on the VHI can be found at http://www-03.ibm.com/press/us/en/pressrelease/23580.wss.

Current Trends in Technology Demonstration

The TIGER Virtual Demonstration Center Pilot

One of the recognized barriers to improving informatics education for all nurses remains the limited access to information systems and technology that could improve healthcare delivery.[14,15] Often times, access is limited to the systems that are currently deployed in a given location. Nursing schools often rely on the clinical practicum site to provide access and education on EHRs. Nurses in practice are limited to the currently deployed technology solutions at their organization and have limited exposure to new technologies that could be applied in innovative ways to their environment to improve healthcare delivery. The TIGER Virtual Demonstration Center Collaborative team was created to develop a Virtual Demonstration Center Pilot that could address these needs.

The purpose of the Virtual Demonstration Center Pilot is to explode current thinking about what healthcare is, by engaging visitors in the demonstration of potential healthcare futures that demonstrate innovative, high quality, and maximally efficient care scenarios in compelling ways. Visitors to the Virtual Demonstration Center Pilot were able to participate in building improved healthcare future states. The Virtual Demonstration Center Pilot is intended to provide a virtual "Gallery Walk" to all nurses, nursing faculty, and nursing students via web access to nurse-focused technology applications. The Virtual Demonstration Center Pilot provided exemplars of best practice for technology utilization, contact resources, and virtual networking opportunities.

Using the innovative Healthcare Information and Management Systems Society (HIMSS) Virtual Conference & Expo Platform, http://www.himssvirtual.org/, we were able to test a variety of different themes and concepts in order to determine how best to engage our audience in the nursing practice and academic communities.[16] We provided access to over 30 resources that demonstrate how technology can be used to *enable* nursing education and nursing practice, resulting in safer, more efficient, equitable, effective, timely, and patient-centered healthcare. This timely event engaged over 300 nurses in the current issues that are the focus of the TIGER Initiative: interoperability, the national HIT agenda, competency-based education, improving the usability of clinical application design, and empowering consumers. It is envisioned that this pilot and other emerging programs will support nursing professionals as they adopt IT in their practice environments and also support nursing education as curricula change to prepare nurses for the future.

Guidelines and example scenarios were developed for industry partners to reinforce the TIGER Initiative message. The scenarios provided were used with permission from the HIMSS 2008 Interoperability Showcase IHE USA, Integrating the Healthcare Enterprise. These clinical scenarios demonstrated interoperability, focusing on clinician and patient access and information sharing across the continuum of care, and were designed to provide examples of current, short-term, and long-term future use of HIT.

The content, guidelines, and scenarios have also been made available for viewing at the TIGER Initiative Virtual Demonstration Center Collaborative Wiki http://tigervirtual-demo.pbwiki.com/.

Using Technology in Nursing Education

The level of technology use in the clinical setting is growing by leaps and bounds. In order for practicing nurses to be competent and comfortable with these technologies, they must be engaged in the application of technology during their nursing education. Using technology tools to support decision-making, guide clinical practice, retrieve information, and simulate practice has become very effective for both teaching and learning. Although the types and uses of educational technology are changing every day, their intent remains the same: to engage students in exploring educational content in a manner that (1) suits their learning style and learning needs and (2) provides informational access where and when it is needed.

Accomplishing this goal requires a change in the way nursing is now generally taught and will involve educating faculty as well as students in using the technology. Educating faculty to recognize the value and necessity of using technology in nursing education will lead to its becoming an institutional priority. Goals related to the integration of informatics and technological competencies need to be explicitly included in the organizational strategic plan. Doing this keeps these objectives in the foreground, while focusing on the allocation of resources and effort.[17]

In nursing education, we now use a myriad of technologies to enhance teaching and learning. Although there are some that might be used in several settings, these technologies can be generally viewed as those that are used in a face-to-face classroom, those that are used in an online or virtual environment, those that are used in simulation laboratories, and those that are used in the clinical setting.

Classroom Setting

For effective teaching of today's students, we must move past the instructor "talking at the class" accompanied by a powerpoint slide presentation.[18] Current students expect and need direct interaction with the content and each other. We now have the technology to allow students to interact with content experts across the country or across the world via distance conferencing. This same technology can enable students in the classroom to interview patients with congestive heart failure regarding how they manage their illness at home or work on a collaborative project with students from another school of nursing.

Another method for engaging students with the technology and the information is the use of online reference material in the classroom. The use of online reference materials through a laptop computer or personal digital assistant (PDA) enables students to create their own learning content on the fly.[19] For example, students may be given a case study regarding a particular patient and asked to collaboratively develop a plan of individualized care for that patient. Then the case can be presented to others in the class, providing practice in finding, compiling, and synthesizing key information as well as presenting information in an organized and understandable manner.

Other simple tools such as audience response clickers (these allow the student to respond to questions or surveys via radio frequencies to a main unit) provide another method of technology integration (Jensen 2008). Responses are automatically compiled and organized in a database by the instructor unit allowing immediate aggregate display of the response for feedback and interaction. These units keep the learner involved in an interactive format and allow instructors to get an immediate assessment of the class' level of understanding. These assessments can be immediately shared with students in the form of a graph or text display. They can also be used to rapidly validate preclass preparation while eliminating the need for busy work on the part of students or instructors completing other lengthier types of assignments.

Virtual Setting

Virtual instruction can supplement face-to-face instruction, or entire educational offerings can be provided online. The virtual environment allows students to access course materials when and where they choose, allowing many more to further their education than ever before.[20] Effective online instruction presents material in multiple formats that addresses different student learning styles. Students dislike listening to narrated powerpoint lectures in an online course as much as they do in a regular classroom. Meaningful course content allows the student to clearly see the relevance of learning and its application in the real world. The use of case studies and the development of products that can be used in clinical practice show clear relevance to educational goals. Student interaction with the content, course instructor, and each other is a vital component to an engaging course. We now have easy-to-use tools to accomplish these objectives.

Originally, online course content was provided through the use of the World Wide Web in an html format that looked like most other web pages we are familiar with. Now most virtual instruction is organized into courses and modules through the use of learning plat-form software.[21] These applications allow instructors to build courses and content with minimal technical expertise and can limit access to these courses to those who are officially enrolled. Tools available for use in most online course platforms include secure testing, asynchronous discussion boards, synchronous verbal and text discussion, desktop sharing, pod casts, streaming video, narrated lectures, and simulations.

Simulation Laboratory Setting

The use of the simulators must start with the development of relevant simulations that are designed to integrate with current practice or educational curriculum. Very often, students and practitioners learn procedural skills in isolation of their application in actual practice. For example, they may be highly proficient in inserting an intravenous (IV) catheter, but when faced with a patient with a plummeting blood pressure, they do not always think to initiate insertion of the IV. A number of studies have provided evidence of the successful use of simulation models in health education and practice. Indeed, the use of human simulators for nursing and medical education has been shown to enhance preparation for clinical practice across cognitive, affective, and psychomotor learning domains.

For example, a study recently compared the use of a pencil-and-paper patient scenario, a static manikin scenario, and a patient simulator scenario.[22] Students who were assigned to complete the scenario using a human simulator were more satisfied with the learning experience, perceived more diversity of learning modes, and were more confident about their ability to care for an actual client. Similarly, nursing students in England who were taught using a human simulator had significantly higher scores on an Objective Structured Clinical Examination (OSCE) than students who received traditional instruction.[23] A comparison of use of problem-based learning and simulation with medical students showed that simulation was superior for the acquisition of critical assessment and management skills.[24]

Simulators used in current simulation laboratories can be classified by how realistically they represent real patient situations on three levels: task trainers, low-fidelity, and high-fidelity simulators. Task trainers are those pieces of equipment that help the student acquire a particular skill, such as IV catheter arms or computerized catheter insertion applications. An example of a virtual task trainer is the Virtual IV manufactured by the Laerdal Company (http://www.laerdal.com/doc/6473945/Virtual-I-V.html). This task trainer combines self-directed computer-based scenarios with a haptic device that allows the student to "feel" an IV catheter being inserted into a virtual patient. The virtual patient responds to the student's actions both physically (by bleeding) and verbally (by speaking to the student regarding technique).

Low-fidelity simulators are those that mimic aspects of reality, but at a level that is not highly realistic. An example of this type of simulator is a mannequin that allows the student to practice IV catheter insertion, tracheal suctioning, and bathing but does not respond interactively to the student's intervention. One such mannequin is Susie Simon manufactured by the Gaumard Company (http://www.gaumard.com/viewproducts.asp?idproduct=23&idcategorie=47&idsubcategorie=48). In addition to allowing practice with basic skills, Susie allows students to practice giving an enema, urethral catheter insertion, or fitting a patient with an ostomy bag. Low-fidelity mannequins have the advantage of being easy to use and are relatively inexpensive compared to more interactive mannequins.

High-fidelity simulators respond to the student's intervention in a dynamic and interactive fashion. These simulators are programmed to respond in a realistic manner based on what they are "experiencing." For example, a high-fidelity mannequin might exhibit a drop in their oxygen level if a student does not apply oxygen when this is an appropriate intervention within the specified scenario. High-fidelity mannequins now exist for a variety of types of patients. Noelle is a mannequin that simulates the birth of a baby (http://www.gaumard.com/viewproducts.asp?idproduct=271&idcategorie=14&idsubcategorie=62), Stan (http://meti.com/products_ps_istan.htm) and SimMan (http://www.laerdal.com/doc/33202760/SimMan-3G.html) are adult male mannequins, and baby Hal (http://www.gaumard.com/viewproducts.asp?idproduct=283&idcategorie=6&idsubcategorie=77) can be purchased as a neonate or premature infant.

The use of low- or high-fidelity mannequins can be married to their representation in a simulated information system. Students can then access information on the simulated patient's history, allergies, drugs, and previous assessment data and laboratory values. The use of simulated information systems also helps the student to learn to navigate computerized clinical information systems and the electronic records they will encounter in practice. Not only will they gain technical skills, but also will they learn to determine what data are necessary for clinical decision-making and where these may be found.

Clinical Setting

Early exposure to online resources and reference applications in the nursing curriculum enables students to develop critical competencies in utilizing information to make decisions. As competencies in processing information are developed, the use of interactive computer programs or applications can be incorporated to support clinical practice. They may present algorithms for guiding clinical practice decision such as managing a patient in heart failure, assisting with developing nursing diagnoses or care planning, and testing clinical knowledge before it is applied to the live patient, thus promoting safety in patient care. There are three major types of applications: books and references; compilations of journals, books, and online references organized for easy search within the application; and procedure reference applications. Compilations of journals, guidelines, and procedural references are generally produced by the major nursing textbook and journal publishers in such a way that nurses can easily search for the information they need from any location that has computer access. Some applications, such as online books, can be purchased once, while others are sold as yearly subscriptions. Organizations can choose to allow access through intranets or password-protected internet sites. More and more of these applications can be downloaded or accessed through internet wireless PDAs. These applications can be used by students and staff in preparation for managing patient care, performing skills in the clinical setting, and as a quick reference for determining best practice.

Future of Virtual Demonstrations

Creation of internet-based 3-D virtual world experience could be used to demonstrate interactive, patient-centered scenarios that are technology-enabled and likely to be best practices over the next three to 10 years. Selected patient scenarios could be simulated and demonstrated in this Virtual World Demonstration Center, so that students, clinicians, and others would have a real-world immersive experience, from wherever they are. The scenarios represent what could be accomplished using current technology, short-term future technology, and long-term future technology. The same scenario used for each period of time can highlight how virtual demonstrations would change as the tools evolve.

Scenario 1: Current Technology

The Current Technology scenario is intended to demonstrate how a nursing educational experience could be designed using technology that is available today. This scenario describes a learning environment using these tools. A virtual classroom is built for nursing students to view the scenario and interact with an EHR during group lecture, "live" demonstration, and individual activities to allow for experimentation. Learning objectives and lecture material are developed to teach students the basic concepts of a PHR, EHR, and HIT in general. The lecture would be delivered in the virtual classroom, prior to group or individual activities.

After the virtual classroom lecture, the students break into groups moving into virtual patient homes for their first group exercise. One nursing student assumes the role of a patient Avatar, another student the role of a nurse Avatar. Together they complete a patient PHR, with the nurse guiding the patient. The other students act as references, advising the nurse and the patient. In a second group exercise, in a clinician's office, the patient Avatar is examined by a nurse practitioner (NP) Avatar, after review of the PHR. The NP Avatar documents the patient visit in the EHR using a tablet computer during the patient exam.

Once the group exercises are completed, students would move to a virtual lab where EHR and PHR screens would be provided for individual students to explore and interact with. Students would be able to interact with all components of a PHR and EHR at their own pace. The virtual lab would also have a reference avatar that would serve as a "help" function, designed to respond to student questions about a particular PHR or EHR component.

Scenario 2: Short-Term Future Technology

The individual pieces of technology proposed for this virtual demonstration scenario exist today but have not been developed to work together in an integrated manner. The purpose of this scenario is to show how today's tools could be developed and integrated to support learning.

Using a combination of the previously described virtual classroom, a second tool, like the Nintendo Wii, would be integrated into the group and individual exercises to provide a physical sense of being present in Second Life rather than relying on the strictly computer keyboard/display method of interaction. By giving the students a "physical" presence in the virtual classroom, the avatars' bodies move as they move their physical bodies, through the virtual space interacting as they would in the physical world. This interaction would provide a truer experiential learning environment involving more of the students' senses.

In the group exercises, the nurse, NP, and patient would have the added dimension of physically moving as they talk to each other, hand each other objects, use devices, as the NP examines the patient. For example, the patient would actually sit on the exam table, and as the NP examines her, they would both be moving in their physical world to move their avatars. Learning how to physically manage to document with a tablet personal computer while examining a patient in a virtual space would allow for more confident interactions with real-world patients as students move out of the classroom.

In individual exercises, students could interact with devices in the virtual lab such as tablet PCs and patient testing devices, using them as they would in the physical world. Hands-on experience could be simulated in a more realistic manner both for manipulating devices used during the patient visit as well as EHR and PHR tools. It would be an exciting challenge to develop this demonstration ability to closely simulate the physical world.

Scenario 3: Future Technology

We can only imagine what technology will be available and used in the future, both for healthcare and for demonstrations. In this scenario, we hypothesize what technology and learning environments may exist in the future. Perhaps a virtual computer display and keyboard would be holographically projected in front of students who role-play as a patient or nurse to enter PHR and EHR data and display it for review.

Students could learn how to use wearable (such as fabric or band-aids) home-care medical devices to collect data such as blood glucose level, blood pressure, heart rate, etc. They could have the experience of a virtual home visit to a patient, moving around the home as a 3-D hologram to help the patient with home care. Devices that give physical resistance could be developed to incorporate into a Wii-like device and virtual demonstration to help the student learn how to lift a patient without injury.

Adding the dimension of physical feedback to virtual learning and demonstrations could be valuable in preventing injury to the student once they move into the clinical environment. The benefit to students could also extend to an improved understanding of the patient experience, perhaps by putting the student in the role of a cancer patient who has severe fatigue as a result of chemotherapy. Physical feedback pressuring the student's legs and body would simulate the walking-through-water feeling that a fatigued patient can experience during simple movements. This learning can enhance students' clinical practice by providing them with a clearer understanding of their patients.

Conclusion

We believe that demonstrating the utility of technology for improving practice and education can speed its diffusion and adoption, highlight its benefits and outcomes, and support nursing professionals as they adopt IT in their practice environments.

For these reasons, we support the development of nursing curricula that include educational modules based upon informatics competencies. To the same end, we support the nursing profession and other key stakeholders who embrace the integration of technology demonstrations into practice.

Through the effective use of IT, we can transform nursing practice and prepare a workforce that can improve patient outcomes in an increasingly automated, informatics-rich, and consumer-driven healthcare environment.

References

1. Weiner E. Technology: the interface to nursing educational informatics. *Nurs Clin North Am.* 2008;43(4):ix-x.
2. TIGER. TIGER Report Evidence and Informatics Transforming Nursing: 3-Year Action Steps toward a 10-Year Vision. http://www.tigersummit.com/uploads/TIGERInitiative_Report2007_Color.pdf; 2007 Accessed 08.07.09.

3. Russell CK, Burchum JR, Likes WM, et al. WebQuests: creating engaging, student-centered, constructivist learning activities. *Comput Inform Nurs*. 2008;26:78-87; quiz 88-79.

4. Sockolow P, Bowles KH. Including information technology project management in the nursing informatics curriculum. *Comput Inform Nurs*. 2008;26:14-20.

5. Tarrant M, Dodgson JE, Law BV. A curricular approach to improve the information literacy and academic writing skills of part-time post-registration nursing students in Hong Kong. *Nurse Educ Today*. 2008;28:458-468.

6. Rogers EM. *Diffusion of Innovations*. New York: The Free; 2003.

7. Gassert CA. Technology and informatics competencies. *Nurs Clin North Am*. 2008;43: 507-521.

8. Siemens AG. Clinical Gateway. Available from URL: www.siemens.com/clinicalgateway; 2009 Accessed 05.07.09.

9. University of Alabama at Birmingham Health System (n.d.) http://uabhealthtv.photobooks. com/default.asp?ChannelID=6&ProgramID=93%22; 2009 Accessed 05.07.09.

10. Microsoft Patient Journey Demonstrator. Available from URL http://www.mscui.net/ PatientJourneyDemonstrator; 2009 Accessed 05.07.09.

11. The LISTEN Project. Available from URL http://www.listenuphealth.org/home/; 2009 Accessed 05.07.09.

12. TIGER. Virtual Demonstration Collaborative. http://tigervirtualdemo.pbworks.com/; 2009 Accessed 08.07.09.

13. Kaiser Permanente. Available from URL http://xnet.kp.org/innovationcenter/about.html; 2009 Accessed 05.07.09.

14. Melo D, Carlton KH. A collaborative model to ensure graduating nurses are ready to use electronic health records. *Comput Inform Nurs*. 2003;26:8-12.

15. Vestal V, Krautwurst N, Hack R. A model for incorporating technology into student nurse clinical. *Comput Inform Nurs*. 2008;26:2-4.

16. HIMSS Virtual Conference & Expo. http://www.himssvirtual.org/; 2009 Accessed 08.07.09.

17. Struck C, Moss J. Focus on Technology: What can you do to move the vision forward? *Comput Inform Nurs*. 2009;27(3):192-194.

18. Jensen R, Meyer L, Sternberger C. Three technological enhancements in nursing education: Informatics instruction, personal response systems, and human patient simulation. *Nurse Educ Pract*. 2009;9:86-90.

19. Barrett JR, Strayer SM, Schubart JR. Assessing medical residents' usage and perceived needs for personal digital assistants. *Int J Med Inform*. 2004;73:25-34.

20. Simpson RL. Welcome to the virtual classroom. How technology is transforming nursing education in the 21st century. *Nurs Adm Q*. 2003;27:83-86.

21. Green SM, Weaver M, Voegeli D, et al. The development and evaluation of the use of a virtual learning environment (Blackboard 5) to support the learning of pre-qualifying nursing students undertaking a human anatomy and physiology module. *Nurse Educ Today*. 2006;26: 388-395.

22. Jeffries P, Rizzolo M. Designing and implementing models for innovative use of simulation to teach nursing care of ill adults and children: A national, multi-site, multi-method study. Summary Report: National League for Nursing; 2006.

23. Alinier G, Hunt W, Gordon R. Determining the value of simulation in nurse education: study design and initial results. *Nurse Educ Pract*. 2004;4:200-207.

24. Steadman R, Coates W, Huang YM, et al. Simulation-based training is superior to problem-based learning for the acquisition of critical assessment and management skills. *Crit Care Med*. 2006;34(1):151-157.

25. Pravikoff DS, Tanner AB, Pierce ST. Readiness of U.S. nurses for evidence-based practice. *Am J Nurs*. 2005;105(9):40-51.

In 2009, when much of this 4th Edition of *Nursing Informatics: Where Technology and Caring Meet* was written, the United States was in the midst of a vigorous debate on healthcare reform. Among the issues discussed were how healthcare is delivered and outcomes measured, in the US and internationally. Whatever the final decision may be regarding health insurance reform in the US, earlier legislation provides for significant changes in health informatics and technology. The 2009 stimulus package set aside dollars for the implementation of the electronic health record and the personal health record as well as comparative effectiveness research within the stimulus package. Still more funding has been set aside for the education and training of healthcare professionals in the use of technology and informatics through programs launched by the Office of the National Coordinator for Health Care Information Technology and the Health Resources and Services Administration.

For insights in the heat of debate, many in the US have looked into recent studies comparing access, outcomes, and other key healthcare indicators. Two such studies sponsored by the Common Wealth Fund looked at six countries, Australia, Canada, Germany, the Netherlands, New Zealand, the United Kingdom, and the United States.

The first, by Davis et al. (2007), queried primary care physicians about the adoption of health information technology. Their conclusion was clear: "other countries are further along than the US in using information technology and a team approach to manage chronic conditions and coordinate care." They reported that, in Germany, New Zealand, and the UK, information systems enhanced the management of chronic conditions and medication use. It is particularly compelling that these countries scoring higher in chronic care management routinely use nurses to deliver that care.

The second, by Schoen et al. (2007), concluded that "achieving better care coordination will likely require designs that include a mix of formally integrated organizations, colocating or sharing services, and connecting through information systems." According to their findings, US adults reported problems with obtaining lab test results, billing issues, more errors, less access to physicians and care on nights, weekends or holidays than adults in the other five countries studied.

A third study, by Health Canada (2006), questioned primary healthcare providers to help lay the groundwork for culture change. Their findings underscored the need for the following:

- Accurate and timely access to clinical information to enable shared decision making by providers and patients or clients

- Ongoing communication and education with and between care partners and patients or clients
- The ability to collect and manage data to support evidence-based decision making
- Tracking information on the population being served and its specific needs, allowing for more direct and effective responses
- Standardized care practices and access to higher levels of care (specialists) regardless of geographic barriers
- The development and use of automated protocols and tools (e.g. chronic disease management) to improve efficiency and effectiveness in service delivery
- Ready access to current clinical literature, recognized best practices, and performance indicators
- The enhanced ability of patients or clients to access information and resources to assist them in the management of their own health, a key tenet of the new culture (Health-Canada 2006)

More recently, the International Medical Informatics Association's Special Interest Group on Nursing Informatics highlighted the need for international standards and international health terminology. Reporting on the International Standards Organization (ISO) Reference Terminology Model, Bakken et al. (2009) focused on its implications for delivery, evaluation, and secondary uses of nursing data in practice-based evidence and clinical research.

Like healthcare and information technology, nursing informatics is becoming more international and more standards-driven. These changes, we firmly believe, can be a positive force for the nursing profession and for patients. In the United States and in the countries around the world, nurses in the United States and around the world have more to learn—and more to teach. The four chapters in this international section, from authors across four continents, are only the appetizers for what promises to be food for thought.

Terminology Development in Canada and Beyond

Anchoring this section is the chapter by Kathryn J. Hannah and Margaret Kennedy. In chapter 22, "Invisibility to Visibility: Capturing Essential Nursing Information," the authors acknowledge the role of ISOs in identifying interoperability standards for data exchange that will, ultimately, support comparative effectiveness research around the globe. In addition to describing the evolution of the International Classification for Nursing Practice (ICNP), the authors discuss nursing data elements and minimum data sets in the Canada and the United States and offer a glimpse at work being done in the United Kingdom as part of the Association of Common European Nursing Diagnosis, Interventions and Outcomes (ACENDO). Throughout the chapter, Hannah and Kennedy emphasize the ongoing need for nursing data to document nursing's contributions to healthcare and concerns about the "invisibility" of nursing data in health services research, policy, and healthcare reform initiatives. After discussing types of language – such as natural language, controlled language, and formal language – and classification systems, they highlight the ICNP, defined as a "unified nursing language systems and a compositional terminology," citing support in Canada, research in Europe, Asia, and South America, and upcoming launch of version 2 in South Africa at the 2009 ICN Congress. This chapter carries forth the groundbreaking work Hannah reported in the 3rd edition of *Nursing Informatics*.

View of Europe from Germany

In the chapter 23 in Section 5, "Health Telematics Europe" by Ursula Hübner gives an overview of health and nursing informatics across Europe, going into greater depth for Germany. Hübner describes three types of models of care (the public integrated model, the public contract model, and the private insurance model) and discusses how these models are realized in Scandinavia, Italy, Greece, Portugal, Switzerland, the Netherlands, and the United Kingdom. She then discusses the "Bologna Process" begun in Italy in 1999 in an effort to foster harmonization in education across the European Union (EU). Using the term "health telematics" as a synonym for the convergence of telecommunication and information technologies, Hübner describes efforts supporting interoperability of patient data across the EU, including the European patient Smart Open Services project (epSOS), the use of nursing terminology and standards for documentation, and national efforts in Germany, France, and Austria to implement a type of electronic smartcard. Her discussion of how EU countries have included nurses in national eHealth programs provides food for thought for nurses in the United States.

Nursing Informatics Evolution in Brazil

In chapter 24, "Evolution: Nursing Informatics in Brazil," Heimar Marin, Denise Silveira, Grace Dal Sasso, and Heloisa Helena C. Perez present the history and evolution of nursing informatics in Brazil and states within that country. The educational initiatives they discuss include Nursing Informatics Research Groups, the Nursing Informatics Working Group of the Brazilian Health Informatics Society, and efforts to define and develop nursing informatics competencies. They describe the network now being deployed across Brazil to facilitate data sharing of data across its states and provide health care to rural hard-to-reach populations, and highlight the use of tele-health and tele-nursing and the need for progress toward interoperability. In a final section on nursing language and terminology, Marin and colleagues review five systems that have been translated and applied in the development of computerized systems in Brazil, and note that some states in the country have adopted the ICNP as the basic terminology for nursing documentation.

Training in Taiwan

In chapter 25, "A Taiwan Model: Nursing Informatics Training," the final chapter in this section, Polun Chang and Ming-Chuan Kuo lay out the concept of End-User Computing (EUC) and discuss the learning model used in Taiwan since 2003 to improve nurses' competencies in Taiwan. These authors explain how the model connects nurses and IT professionals and how it places nurses in a leadership role in designing IT applications. Serving as a detailed map, the model has been used to train more than 400 nurses and other healthcare providers in medical informatics concepts. Training has included the design of practical solutions for clinical documentation and information management, provision of communication tools among clinical nurses and IT people, and the creation of innovative personal solutions. The authors provide information and guidance for replication of a six-day learning course and the five stages that are integrated into this learning system. Throughout the chapter, Chang and Kuo emphasize the importance of nursing informatics competencies to increased user input as well as enhanced performance.

With this 4th Edition of *Nursing Informatics: Where Technology and Caring Meet* scheduled to be unveiled at the 2010 MedInfo meeting in South Africa, this international section is particularly relevant. Then, and again in 2012, when MedInfo is scheduled to be held in Canada, will be the right time to extend the TIGER diffusion in a more complete way to the international nursing informatics community.

References

Bakken S, Goossen W, Hovenga E, et al. (2009) Health Informatics Standards of Relevance to Nursing: Update from the IMIA-NI Health Informatics Standards Work Group, July 7, 2009. www.imia.org/working_groups/WG
Health Canada (2006) Canadian Health Care System Report and Publication: "Laying the Groundwork for Culture Change." http://www.hc-sc.gc.ca/hcs-sss/pubs/prim/2006-synth-legacy-fondements/2006-synth-legacy-fondements-1-eng.php
Davis K, Schoen MS, Schoenbaum SC et al., eds. (2007) Mirror, Mirror on the Wall: An International Update on the Comparative Performance of American Health Care. May 15, 2007: Volume 59. Commonwealth Fund. http://www.commonwealthfund.org/Content/Publications/Fund
Schoen MS, Osborn R, Doty MM, et al. (2007) Toward Higher-Performance Health Systems: Adults' Health Care Experiences in Seven Countries. November 1, 2007; Volume 92. Commonwealth Fund. http://www.commonwealthfund.org/Content/Publications/In-the-literature

Kathryn J. Hannah and Margaret Ann J. Kennedy

Managing vast amounts of diverse information necessitates that nurses synthesize data from diverse sources into a coherent profile of each patient and generate an effective plan of care to achieve the desired health outcomes. This chapter explores how the evolution of minimum health data sets, identification of essential nursing data elements, and controlled clinical vocabularies contribute to the identification of critical nursing information and the documentation of nursing contributions to healthcare.

Introduction

Issues related to information and information management resonate with all nurses, with challenges arising from the acceptance of core nursing data elements and the establishment of nursing data standards (controlled clinical vocabularies) for use within those data elements. Resolution and convergence on these two topics are essential for collection and storage of nursing data in national health databases. Ozbolt[1] maintains that standard terms and codes are needed to record problems and issues that nurses and other caregivers address as structured data. Such data could be used to increase the effectiveness of care and control costs in the following ways:

- Care plans or pathways for patient assignments, constructed of coded "building blocks" of known complexity and time requirements, could be used to project clinical workload requirements, so that managers could make appropriate staffing decisions, reducing redundancy and inefficiencies.
- Relevant clinical decision support and supplementary information could be linked to statements of patient problems, care actions, and goals to provide assistance integrated into the workflow at the moment of need. For example, nurses could point and click for detailed instructions on how to carry out an unfamiliar procedure. Or the diagnosis of

K.J. Hannah (✉)
Health Informatics Advisor, Canadian Nurses Association, Toronto, ON M5H 1J9, USA

M.J. Ball et al. (eds.), *Nursing Informatics*,
DOI: 10.1007/978-1-84996-278-0_22, © Springer-Verlag London Limited 2011

one problem, such as impaired mobility, could be linked to related problems, such as risk of falls, to assure that all relevant problems were included in the plan of care.

- Patient care data could be stored in relational or object-oriented databases for subsequent aggregation and analysis. This facilitates the discovery of variance from expected care or outcomes and identifying places where corrective action is needed or reveals best practices that produce the optimal balance of goal achievement and cost.
- More sensitive measures of quality and effectiveness could be provided for government and other regulators and purchasers of healthcare to consider in addition to cost when making purchasing decisions, establishing regulations, and mandating or refusing to authorize certain services.

Determining Nursing Data

For some time, the technological aspect of information management has distracted nurses at the expense of ignoring the data. Today, however, technology is found ubiquitously throughout healthcare settings and is part of the everyday practice of many nurses. Health information vendors offer integrated suites of application software (which may include patient scheduling and transfer, billing and financial management, diagnostic imaging, lab reporting, order entry applications, pharmacy, patient documentation systems, clinical support tools, and resource management applications). These suites incorporate a variety of documentation tools with variable usability but often lack the sensitivity to effectively capture essential nursing data.

Despite advances in technological applications and recommendations for improved healthcare data, nursing contributions to healthcare are *still* not included on patient discharge abstracts or in provincial or national data repositories.[2] Discharge Abstract Databases[3] are prepared by health information professionals (medical records) across Canada (with comparable documents in the United States), which contain *no* nursing care delivery information. This issue has persisted for decades and continues to ignore the substantive contributions nurses make to healthcare and health outcomes, resulting in decisions of fiscal allocation being made without calculating the contributions of the largest sector of healthcare providers.[4] Clark's (p. 42)[5] observation that "nursing is invisible in health policy decisions, in descriptions of healthcare, in contracts and service specifications" continues to reflect current practices. Extrapolating Clark's observation, this invisibility potentially further excludes nursing data from contributing to health research and health system reform.[6]

Nurses and policy makers have developed a heightened awareness of the importance of collection, storage, and retrieval of nursing data as a consequence of numerous reports and commissions, such as the Lalonde,[7] Kirby,[8] and Romanow[9] reports, all of which recommended improved data collection to support effective and appropriate decision-making.[2,4] Attention is now being directed at developing the processes and means by which the nursing profession will begin to address the essential data needs of nurses in all practice settings.

The nursing profession must provide decisive leadership in defining appropriate nursing data elements to be included in national health databases specifically through patient discharge abstracts or summaries. In the United States, the unique nursing elements are included in the nursing minimum data set (NMDS). The purposes of the NMDS are "to establish comparability of nursing data across clinical populations, settings, geographic areas, and time to describe the nursing care of patients and their families in both inpatient and outpatient settings, to show or project trends regarding nursing care needs and allocation of nursing resources according to nursing diagnoses, and to simulate nursing research (p. 1652)."[10] Such data are essential because they allow description of the health status of individuals, groups, and populations in terms of nursing care needs, establish outcome measures related to nursing care, and investigate the use and cost of nursing resources.

The Canadian NMDS is known as health information: nursing components (HI:NC) and enjoys consensus on client status, nursing interventions, client outcomes, nursing intensity, and nurse identifier.[2,11] The Canadian Nurses Association describes HI:NC as the "most important pieces of data about the nursing care provided to the client during a healthcare episode (p. 5)."[11] As Hannah (p. 49)[2] notes, it is "essential in Canada that the nursing data elements constitute one component of a fully integrated health information system (Table 22.1)."

In 2006, the Royal College of Nursing in the United Kingdom (UK) began work on identifying the key nursing data elements in the patient record to create a conceptual model.[12] The four countries encompassed by the UK (including England, Wales, Scotland, and Northern Ireland) grounded their conceptual model in the previous efforts of the Association for Common European Nursing Diagnosis, Interventions, and Outcomes (ACENDIO) and subsequently formed the North Wales Nursing Terminology Group (NSNTG) to increase momentum toward the acceptance of standardized languages. At present, the conceptual model continues to be based around the nursing process – assessment, nursing diagnosis, identifying objectives, interventions, implementation, and

Table 22.1 Definitions of health information: nursing components

Client status is broadly defined as a label for the set of indicators that reflect the phenomena for which nurses provide care, relative to the health status of clients[48]. Although client status is similar to nursing diagnosis, the term client status was preferred because it represents a broader spectrum of health and illness. The common label "client status" is inclusive of input from all disciplines. The summative statements referring to the phenomena for which nurses provide care (i.e., nursing diagnosis) are merely one aspect of client status at a point in time, in the same way as medical diagnosis
Nursing interventions refer to purposeful and deliberate health affecting interventions (direct and indirect), based on assessment of client status, which are designed to bring about results that benefit clients[45]
Client outcome is defined as a "clients' status at a defined point(s) following healthcare [affecting] intervention."[46] It is influenced to varying degrees by the interventions of all care providers
Nursing intensity "refers to the amount and type of nursing resource used to [provide] care"[47]
Primary nurse identifier is a single unique lifetime identification number for each individual nurse. This identifier is independent of geographic location (province or territory), practice sector (e.g., acute care, community care, public health), or employer

Source: Hannah (p. 49)[2]

evaluation. Referred to as the maximum nursing data set, the authors anticipate further refinement of this data set toward a minimum nursing data set, consequent to the advancement of technology in the UK.

Appropriate nursing data standards must be established for use within each of the unique nursing data elements. Thus, the two priorities in information management for nurses are identification of nursing data elements and establishment of nursing data standards for use within those data elements. Resolution and convergence on these two topics are essential for collection and storage of nursing data in national health databases.

Environmental Forces Impacting Health Information Development

Many factors influence the drive towards the development of unique nursing data elements of health information. These include the following:

- Initiatives to facilitate the evolution of national electronic health records (EHRs), built on essential and comparable data, available in a timely manner to support evidence-based care delivery.
- Healthcare system transformation resulting from soaring costs of health services, drugs, new technologies, and treatment modalities.
- Innovative models of managing and funding healthcare organizations.
- Changing demographics resulting from an aging population.
- Health services evaluation in terms of patient outcomes.
- Efforts to eliminate duplication of services and functions.
- Consumer health and increased self management of healthcare.

Although many current suites of application software offer some capability to document clinician narratives, most data are recorded in a standardized fashion, and narratives are discouraged. Most clinicians use natural language in narrative notes, which is challenging to retrieve and aggregate – potentially resulting in the loss of critical information. A number of controlled clinical vocabularies have been developed in order to address the problem of standardized textual data in the computerized client record.

Current data aggregation usually begins with coding of medical records abstracts in hospitals and coding of billing diagnosis and service encounter data in office practice. Such coding is performed by coders who usually extract data from paper-based clinical records using standardized codes for clinical data. The healthcare system of the future will permit sharing of EHRs among health professionals independent of discipline, location, time, or sector of the health system. This requires that data be entered in a standardized way, using standardized technologies. It is impractical for caregivers to do the coding of data elements in the course of delivering care because the process of coding accurately is time-consuming and interferes with the usual clinical work processes and procedures. Simply stated, the only data that will be accurate at the point of service (PoS) are those that are crucial to the provision of care by the clinician, and therefore, data for management, if it is to be reliable, can come only from an aggregation of this clinical information.

The terminologies in healthcare need to serve different purposes and end users. Clinicians need granularity at the same time as they need usability, whereas managers need classification of clinical data to support analysis. Broad classifications are therefore to be preferred for health management, but rich terminologies are needed at the point of care. Information and information management will continue to become increasingly important in the future. Nurses must demonstrate that nursing makes a difference to patient outcome and must provide quantitative evidence to support this claim. We need nursing information to facilitate articulation of our professional scope of practice and of our authority and responsibility within the healthcare system. We must determine the essential data elements required for inclusion in national, multidisciplinary patient-focused health data sets.

The absence of nursing data elements in national health information sets has been recognized by nurses in many countries as evidenced by the activities in countries outside the United States. European nurses recognized that their health systems need to include nursing data elements that are significant in the nursing decision-making process. They launched a seminal European project known as TELENURSING with special emphasis on Patient Problems/Nursing Diagnosis, Nursing Intervention, and Outcomes. Australian nurses also recognized and supported the need for integration and standardization of data from all disciplines involved in the provision of healthcare. To this end, Australian nurses participated in the development of a National Health Care Data Dictionary of standard definitions and the nursing data element identification and classifications based on these standard definitions. In Canada, many nurses recognized the need to identify the Nursing Components of Health Information to facilitate development of a national health information system during the restructuring of provincial health information systems. These examples clearly illustrate a consensus among nurses internationally that the unique nursing data elements to be included in national health data sets are nursing diagnosis (also known in some countries as client status or nursing problem), nursing intervention, patient/client outcome, and nursing intensity.

Data Standards

Although data exchange among health professionals and institutions occurs constantly, there is no single common language through which health information can be shared. In the use of terms to identify client health status, interventions, or outcomes, there is no consistency, either within a health profession, among various health professions, or across the continuum of care.

Documenting care in a consistent and retrievable way requires the use of structured clinical vocabularies. Interpretability is one of the greatest challenges regarding useful information exchange. Technology itself is not a barrier. Standardizing the terminologies used in communicating health data is essential to improve the quality of shared information, especially in electronic format. It is estimated that over 150 health-related classification and code systems exist in the world today. Hence, there is a real problem in communicating effectively and producing integrated individual health records and health databases.

Effective standard "languages" for creating intelligible data, coupled with the tools for effective and secure data exchange, are essential for effective health information sharing, retrieval, analysis, and use. Creating standardized vocabularies for healthcare not only allows different health professionals and organizations to "speak" to one another, but may also facilitate more efficient and effective data capturing.

Ideally, data entry should be a by-product of clinical activity, captured as close to the PoS or data source as possible. Such entries support data availability much closer to "real time" and allow information sharing among different and dispersed potential users. Also, the ability to consistently interpret health concepts enables their consistent retrieval and further categorization of data for the purposes of knowledge base searches (e.g., literature) or statistical analysis at group and population levels (e.g., for resource management, planning, outcomes measurement, and evaluation).

There are three main categories of language, which differ in freedom of expression. All three can be, and have been, used in electronic data and health information systems. Each has its own definition, relative advantages, and disadvantages.

Natural language (or free text) is the way in which people "naturally" speak everyday language. Natural language is the least inhibited type of language and includes a multitude of ambiguities that require contextual understanding for correct interpretation. Although it is the easiest language to deal with at the PoS, it is the most difficult for the next reader to precisely interpret or translate into different languages and conceptual classification structures. Unfortunately, natural language (or free text) does not allow for the re-use or systematic interpretation of data within electronic records. Only in codes can clinical data be transmitted in shared care and be analyzed systematically.

A controlled language (or controlled vocabulary) is a subset of a natural language. In controlled languages, data are coded and possibly organized into one or more hierarchies. Coding places explicit restrictions on terminology, grammatical rules, and/or description formats. These restrictions result in fewer ambiguous statements, a greater assurance of information reliability, and an increased potential for shared understanding. On the other hand, controlled languages necessarily restrict the richness of clinical detail and require that the person using the language be skilled in its use.

In *formal language*, all terms and relations between terms are strictly and explicitly predefined. Computer programming languages are a type of formal language. Although it is the most reliable type of language, it is the least flexible and the most difficult to learn and use.

Types of Controlled Languages

Nomenclature is a list of all the approved terms for describing and recording observations, or an agreed-upon naming convention. Simpson (p. 18)[13] defines nomenclature as an objective process for deciding the correct name for procedures given a number of alternatives in the literature. Terms used to document the planning, delivery, and outcomes of care would be part of a nomenclature of healthcare. The purpose of a nomenclature of nursing for instance is to have a dictionary of approved nursing terms, so that all data are recorded in a standardized way. A nomenclature of healthcare would contain all the terms relevant to healthcare, including but not limited to

- Client status, demographics, needs, risks, and problems.
- Diagnostic examination, physical findings, and symptoms.
- Reason for encounter.
- Treatment, interventions, and therapeutic procedures.
- Treatment objectives and treatment endpoints.
- Outcome measures.
- Functional/health status.
- Laboratory tests and results.

Classification system is a means of giving order to a group of disconnected facts by assignment to predetermined classes on the basis of perceived common characteristics. Ideally, a classification should be characterized by (1) naturalness – the classes correspond to the nature of the thing being classified, (2) exhaustiveness – every member of the group will fit into one (and only one) class in the system, and (3) constructability – the set of classes can be constructed by a demonstrably systematic procedure. Although some classifications aim to cover aspects of care broadly (e.g., SNOMED), many focus on specific areas. For example, the Nursing Interventions Classification (NIC) was created to provide a coherent inventory of direct and indirect nursing interventions. Classification systems are not meant to fully describe the health and health service needs of an individual; rather, they are more often intended to drive the statistical analysis of the health and health service needs of a population. For this reason, classification categories are not ambiguous; indeed the determinants of each "class" must be mutually exclusive in order to enable statistical analysis. The "trade-off" for this lack of ambiguity, however, is a lessening of the clinical specificity of each record or concept represented.

Controlled Clinical Vocabulary or Controlled Clinical Terminology (CCT) is a structured and limited dictionary of clinical terms used at the PoS. A CCT is intended to overcome the difficulty of term selection, with the lack of reliable classification when using large nomenclatures; and the clinicians' aversion to the formalistic and arcane nature of disease classifications.[14] As defined by the Canadian Institute for Health Information, "Controlled clinical vocabularies are standardized sets of encoded terms that allow clinical data to be captured 'the source' (i.e., entered directly into an electronic record by a health service practitioner)."[15]

Unlike classifications, the detail represented in controlled clinical vocabularies is meant to be comparable to that which is currently included in clinical records (e.g., textual summaries, reports, and progress notes). Controlled clinical vocabularies seek to represent concepts in as much detail as is commonly useful for clinicians and other health professionals in describing health-related concepts. These concepts include both specific attributes (of the client and the service being provided) and modifiers or qualifiers of those attributes. Modifiers indicate degree, time, stage, etc. of a condition or characteristic. Qualifiers indicate negation or uncertainty in a detail or condition.

Some level of categorization may occur internally in controlled vocabulary systems in order to group terms that are clinically related, usually in hierarchies according to concept and level of detail. These hierarchies are useful as a means to structure or conceptually frame the knowledge represented in the clinical domain for presentation, maintenance, and updating. They are also useful in automated implementations as the basis for data structure to enable intelligent prompting or alerting of the user to clinical events, and to facilitate database searching and relating. Ideally, controlled clinical vocabularies should balance the needs of natural language in individual documentation with the needs of shared interpretation (i.e., with less ambiguity than natural language).

Thesaurus is a type of controlled vocabulary arranged so that relationships among terms are displayed clearly and identified by standardized relationship indicators. Synonym identification may also be included. The Unified Medical Language System (UMLS) is the best known medical thesaurus. The primary purposes of a thesaurus are as follows:

- Translation: a means for translating the natural language of authors, indexers, and users into a controlled vocabulary used for indexing and retrieval.
- Consistency: to promote consistency in the assignment of index terms.
- Indication of relationships: to indicate semantic relationships among terms.
- Retrieval: to serve as a searching aid in retrieval of documents.[16]

Confusion regarding the distinction between controlled clinical vocabularies, nomenclatures, and classification systems arises when these terms are used indiscriminately both in literature and in discourse. This confusion is likely due to the fact that all three encode health information and also tend to involve some amount of concept representation. However, the fundamental difference lies in the types of concepts being represented and categorized.[15]

Both controlled clinical vocabularies and nomenclatures standardize the terms to describe health and health service-related concepts. The purpose is to create a shared "language of health" to enable the exchange of basic clinical data among different individuals, agencies, and institutions. Ideally, both should be easy to use at the PoS, and the data they create should be easily and reliably interpreted. Such data, although primarily designed to support clinical decision-making, should also support the aggregation of basic clinical data for research and administrative purposes.

The distinction between nomenclatures, controlled clinical vocabularies, and classifications can be conceptualized as points along a continuum of increasing aggregation and decreasing richness:

natural language → nomenclature → controlled clinical vocabularies → classification

Determining Nursing Data Standards

Considerable work has been invested in the identification and achievement of consensus on essential nursing data elements for inclusion in national health data sets. Work on an international nursing minimum data set (i-NMDS) started in 2006, with current efforts directed toward developing measurement indices.[17,18] Additionally, considerable effort has been invested in developing nursing data standards.[19-22] Research activity has been directed at the development and evaluation of standardized nomenclatures for nursing diagnosis, interventions, and outcomes to be used in describing the nursing care elements in a data set.[1,6,23-32]

In the United States, the American Nurses Association has recognized eight terminologies as appropriate to support clinical practice. These are as follows:

1. Home Health Care Classification: developed by Dr. Virginia Saba.
2. NANDA: developed by North American Nursing Diagnosis Association.
3. NIC: developed by Dr. Joanne McCloskey and Dr. Gloria Bulechek.
4. Nursing Interventions Lexicon and Taxonomy: developed by Dr. Susan Grobe.
5. Nursing Outcomes Classification: developed by Dr. Marion Johnson.
6. Omaha System: developed by Omaha Visiting Nurses Association.
7. Patient Care Data Set: developed by Dr. Judy Ozbolt.
8. The Clinical Care Classification system (formerly known as the Home Health Care Classification): developed by Dr. Virginia Saba.

The eight terminologies differ in purpose, scope, form, content, and process of development. As shown in Fig. 22.1, some are nomenclatures, some are controlled nursing languages, and some are classifications.

No one nursing terminology has emerged as a de facto standard, and together they do not constitute a standard or even a unified language. In an effort to unify the representation of nursing, the International Council of Nurses (ICN) commenced development of the International Classification for Nursing Practice® (ICNP®).[33] The scope of ICNP® is what nurses do (interventions) to address specific needs (diagnoses) to achieve specific results (outcomes).[33] Today, ICNP® is defined as a "unified nursing language system and a compositional terminology (p. 21)."[33] ICNP® has evolved through various iterations, and Version 1 was created in order to address the complexities of developing a fully functional and robust tool that could document nursing practice, eliminate redundancy between terms, and avoid hierarchical coding structures. The various versions have been tested and piloted

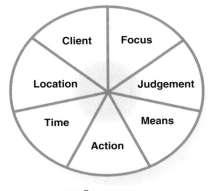

ICNP® 7 Axis Model

Fig. 22.1 Seven-axis model of ICNP® version 1 (p. 29).[33] Copyright required

extensively across Europe, Asia, and South America. Version 2 is scheduled to be launched in Durban, South Africa at the June 2009 ICN Congress.[34]

ICNP® Version 1 is structured in a single 7-axis model used to create statements containing nursing diagnoses, nursing actions, or outcomes in nursing practice. Version 1 also contains catalogs of terms or of subsets of diagnoses, actions, and outcomes specific to various practice areas or specialties.[33]

ICNP® presents nurses with a tool that functions as a cross-mapping tool to accommodate existing vocabularies, assist in developing new vocabularies (compositional vocabulary), and identify relationships (reference terminology) (p. 19).[33] This tool enables nurses to document their practice, regardless of geographical location, practice setting, or language, and allows for comparison of standardized data.

In 2000, the Canadian Nurses Association developed a discussion paper supporting the ICNP®. Strong support from nurses led to the endorsement of ICNP® for use in representing nursing data in Canada.[35-37] Nurses have further recognized the need for standards governing nursing data and have participated in the development of the ISO 18104 Reference Terminology Model for Nursing and its subsequent adoption in Canada (p. 50).[2] ISO 18204 is an international standard created by the International Standards Organization (ISO) to "establish a nursing reference terminology model consistent with the goals and objectives of other specific health terminology models in order to provide a more unified reference health model. This International Standard includes the development of reference terminology models for nursing diagnoses and nursing actions and relevant terminology and definitions for its implementation."[38] This standard recently completed a final public review and is currently awaiting formal publication as an International Standard."[38]

ICNP® research in Canada began in 1999, with Lowen's[29] examination of ICNP® Alpha Version in community-based nursing practice. In Lowen's research, ICNP® captured approximately two thirds of the nursing data. Kennedy's[6] research extended the Canadian application of ICNP® Beta 2 Version across multiple practice settings, including acute care, mental health, home-based care, and long-term care. ICNP® Beta 2 was effective in capturing the majority of nursing assessments and nursing actions across all practice domains, although nursing documentation was incomplete in a high percentage of nursing records.[6] Nursing outcomes were conspicuously absent in the nursing documentation from every domain, and although ICNP® could not be evaluated on outcomes measurements, this absence illustrated a significant gap in the loss of nursing data.[6,27] Doran's work[20] (Doran, 2006) in nursing-sensitive outcomes measurement has significant potential to contribute to ICNP® evolution and guide future research.

A landmark Canadian initiative was launched in 2006. The Canadian Health Outcomes for Better Information and Care (C-HOBIC) is an innovative model for large scale capture of standardized nursing-sensitive clinical outcomes data for inclusion in the EHR.[39] With funding from Canada Health Infoway (www.Infoway.org), the Canadian Nurses Association[40] is partnering to implement the initiative in three Canadian provinces, with a fourth joining recently. The use of the ICNP® facilitates extraction of information into relevant secure jurisdictional EHRs, data repositories, or databases.[39] From these repositories, data are made available to nurses for use in patient care in acute care, complex continuing care, long-term care, and home care. By comparing serial data on a patient across multiple time points, the C-HOBIC model can generate nursing-sensitive patient outcome reports. One of the leading benefits of the C-HOBIC model is that it provides nurses with information critical to planning for and evaluating patient care.

While the C-HOBIC implementation effort currently focuses on embedding the standardized data elements into existing systems postfacto,[39] there is a recognize the opportunity to influence the design of next generation clinical information systems. The growing array of implemented C-HOBIC sites, and national attention garnered by the C-HOBIC project, has caught the attention of system vendors, who have participated in dialogs to facilitate inclusion of C-HOBIC data elements as standard components of their future clinical documentation modules.

Issues

The first issue is the need to utilize and develop existing controlled clinical vocabularies in nursing and work towards convergence. Nursing must avoid continually "reinventing the wheel." The second issue is the need to ensure integration of all unique nursing elements of national health data sets. Additionally, with the emphasis on a multidisciplinary approach to client care, the overlapping of professional boundaries with respect to interventions must be acknowledged.

Several issues germane to the development and use of minimum data sets emerge including data integrity and the scope of data to include in a minimum data set, for example, what does "minimum" really mean. Other technical issues of relevance relate to aspects of data linkage. Once the unique nursing data elements of health information are developed, three additional issues emerge:

- Promoting the concept to ensure consensus and widespread use among nurses and all other users of health information.
- Educating nurses to ensure the quality of the data that are collected.
- Establishing mechanisms for ongoing review and revision of the controlled clinical vocabularies to ensure their currency and relevance.

Implications of Nursing Data

In the absence of a system for collection, storage, and retrieval of nursing data, the loss of valuable information is evident. The trend in healthcare is away from discipline-specific models of patient care delivery to patient-focused models that emphasize collaboration of disciplines, multi-skilling of healthcare providers, standardization of care, and streamlining of documentation through charting by exception. In this environment, it is imperative that nurses be able to articulate what is and is not nursing's role. Furthermore, nurses will be asked to demonstrate nursing's contribution to patient care in terms of outcome measures that are objective and measurable. Nurses require nursing data to identify nursing's contribution to the outcomes of care, defend resource allocation to nursing, and justify new roles for nursing in the healthcare delivery system. Similarly, nurses need to understand and value nursing data so that, in the selection and implementation of information systems for their organizations, they insist that nurses play a major role and that nursing data needs are incorporated into the selection and implementation criteria. For greater detail on the selection and implementation of information systems, see Hannah et al.[41]

Although nursing must preserve its professional identity, this must be balanced against professional compartmentalization and marginalization. Collection and storage of essential nursing data elements that are not integrated as components of national health data sets will undermine recognition of nursing contributions. This is perilous at a time when significant emphasis is being placed on multidisciplinary collaboration, patient-focused care, and patient outcomes. In view of priorities such as these in healthcare, the need for integration of data elements could not be clearer.

Nurse clinicians need to know what nursing elements are essential for archival purposes, so that nursing documentation includes data related to these elements. With the move toward standardization of care through the use of care maps, it is essential that outcomes of nursing care are determined and included. As healthcare organizations embrace the concept of charting by exception in an effort to decrease the valuable hours spent by healthcare workers in documentation, nurses must actively ensure that the tools that outline the inherent patient care delivered are not devoid of nursing's contributions and nursing data. If there are no data that reflect nursing activities, there will be no archival record of what nurses do, what difference nursing care makes, or why nurses are required. In times of fiscal restraint, such objective and quantifiable nursing data are necessary to substantiate the role of nurses and the nurse–patient ratios required in the clinical setting.

Nurse researchers need a database composed of essential data elements: first, to facilitate the identification of trends related to the data elements for specific patient groups, institutions, or regions and, second, to assess variables on multiple levels including institutional, local, regional, and national.[10,42] Collection and storage of essential nursing data elements will facilitate the advancement of nursing as a research-based discipline.[43] Nurse educators need these essential nursing data to develop nursing knowledge for use in educating nurses and to facilitate the definition of the scope of nursing practice.[44]

Finally, definition of nursing elements of health information and controlled clinical vocabularies for nursing are essential to influence health policy decision-making. Historically, health policy has been created in the absence of nursing data. At the time of profound healthcare transformation internationally, it is essential that nurses clearly articulate the central role of nursing services in the restructuring of the healthcare delivery system.

Clearly, a priority for nursing is the identification of the nursing components of health information – those essential nursing data elements that must be collected, stored, and retrieved from a national health information database. There is much work to be done that is available to ensure that nursing data elements are included in national health data bases and to achieve consensus and convergence on a common controlled clinical vocabulary for nursing. The challenge for all nurses is to identify their role in helping define the nursing elements essential for inclusion in such a database and to achieve international consensus and convergence on a common controlled clinical vocabulary for nursing. The time to respond to this challenge is now for, if we do not, the essential nursing data elements, and a common controlled clinical vocabulary for nursing will either be defined by somebody else, or will remain absent from national health databases.

References

1. Ozbolt J. *Testimony to the National Committee on Vital and Health Statistics (NCVHS) Hearings on Medical Terminology and Code Development*. Washington: NCVHS; 1999.
2. Hannah KJ. Health informatics and nursing in Canada. *HCIM&C*. 2005;19(3):45-51.
3. Canadian Institute of Health Information. *Discharge Abstract Databases*. http://secure.cihi.ca/cihiweb/dispPage.jsp?cw_page=services_dad_e; 2008. Accessed 13.06.09.
4. Hannah KJ. The state of nursing informatics in Canada. *Can Nurse*. 2007;103(5):18-22.
5. Clark DJ. A language for nursing. *Nurs Stand*. 1999;13(31):42.
6. Kennedy MA. *Packaging nursing as politically potent: a critical reflexive cultural studies approach to nursing informatics*. Unpublished Doctoral Dissertation, University of South Australia, Adelaide, Australia; 2005.
7. Lalonde M. *A New Perspective on the Health of Canadians*. Ottawa: Queen's Printer; 1974.
8. Standing Senate Committee on Social Affairs Science and Technology (Chair: The Honourable Michael J.L. Kirby). *Final Report: The Health of Canadians – The Federal Role (Volume Six: Recommendations for Reform)*. Ottawa: Queen's Printer; 2002.
9. Romanow RJ. *Building on Values: The Future of Health Care in Canada*. Ottawa: Queen's Printer; 2002.
10. Werley HH, Devine EC, Zorn CR. Nursing needs its own minimum data set. *Am J Nurs*. 1988;88:1651-1653.
11. Canadian Nurses Association. *Collecting Data to Reflect Nursing Impact: Discussion Paper*. Ottawa: Canadian Nurses Association; 2000.
12. Hughes R, Lloyd D. A conceptual model for nursing information. *Int J Nurs Terminol Classif*. 2008;19(2):48-67.
13. Simpson RL. What's in a name? The taxonomy and nomenclature puzzle, Part 1. *Nurs Manage*. 2003;34(6):14.
14. COACH. Something old, something new, something borrowed: a review of standardized data collection in primary care. In: *COACH Conference 23, Scientific Program Proceedings*. www.coach.org; 1998.
15. Canadian Institute of Health Information. *Controlled Clinical Vocabularies: Background Document*. Ontario: Canadian Institute of Health Information; 1997.
16. American National Standards Institute (ANSI). *ANSI/NISO Z39.19-1993*. Bethesda: NISO Press; 1993.
17. Goosen W, Westra B, Delaney C, et al. Working towards deployment of the i-NMDS. In: *Workshop Presented at the NI2009 Congress*. Helenski, Finland; 2009.
18. Goossen W, Delaney C, Coenen AM, et al. The international nursing minimum data set: i-NMDS. In: Weaver C, Delaney C, eds. *Nursing and Informatics for the 21st Century: An International Look at the Trends, Cases, and the Future*. Chicago: HIMSS Press; 2006.
19. Delaney C, Mehmert M, Prophet C, et al. Establishment of the research value of nursing minimum data sets. In: Grobe SJ, Pluyter-Wenting ESP, eds. *Nursing Informatics: An International Overview for Nursing in a Technological Era*. Amsterdam: Elsevier; 1994:169-173.
20. Doran D. Enhancing continuity of care through outcomes measurement. *Can J Nurs Res*. 2004;36(2):83-87.
21. Doran D, Harrison M, Laschinger H, et al. Relationship between nursing interventions and outcomes achievement in acute care settings. *Res Nurs Health*. 2006;29(1):61-70.

22. Werley HH, Lang NM. The consensually derived nursing minimum data set: elements and definitions. In: Werley HH, Lang NM, eds. *Identification of the Nursing Minimum Data Set.* New York: Springer; 1988:402-411.

23. Anderson BJ, Hannah KJ. A Canadian nursing minimum data set: a major priority. *Can J Nurs Adm.* 1993;6(2):7-13.

24. Bulechek GM, McCloskey JC. Nursing interventions: taxonomy development. In: McCloskey JC, Grace HK, eds. *Current Issues in Nursing.* 3rd ed. Mosby: St. Louis; 1990:23-28.

25. Grobe SJ. Nursing intervention lexicon and taxonomy study: language and classification methods. *ANS Adv Nurs Sci.* 1990;13(2):22-33.

26. Jenny J. Classifying nursing diagnoses: a self care approach. *Nurs Health Care.* 1989;10(2): |82-88.

27. Kennedy MA, Hannah KJ. Representing nursing practice: evaluating the effectiveness of a nursing classification system. *Can J Nurs Res.* 2007;39(7):58-79.

28. Lang NM, Marek KD. The classification of patient outcomes. *J Prof Nurs.* 1990;6:158-163.

29. Lowen E. *The use of the International Classification for Nursing Practice® for capturing community-based nursing practice.* Unpublished Master's Thesis. University of Manitoba, Winnipeg, Manitoba; 1999.

30. McCloskey JC, Bulechek GM, Cohen MZ, et al. Classifications of nursing interventions. *J Prof Nurs.* 1990;6:151-157.

31. McLane AM. Measurement and validation of diagnostic concepts: a decade of progress. *Heart Lung.* 1987;16(pt 1):616-624.

32. North American Nursing Diagnosis Association. *North American Nursing Diagnosis Association: Taxonomy I: Revised 1989.* St. Louis: North American Nursing Diagnosis Association; 1989.

33. International Council of Nurses. *International Classification for Nursing Practice®, Version 1.* Geneva: International Council of Nurses; 2005.

34. International Council of Nurses. *International Classification for Nursing Practice®, Version 2.* http://www.icn.ch/icnp_v2countdown.htm; 2009. Accessed 6.06.09.

35. Canadian Nurses Association. *Nursing Information and Knowledge Management.* Ontario: Canadian Nurses Association. http://cna-aiic.ca/CNA/documents/pdf/publications/PS87-Nursing-info-knowledge-e.pdf; 2006. Accessed 2.06.09.

36. Canadian Nurses Association. International classification for nursing practice: documenting nursing care and client outcomes. *Nurs Now.* 14. http://www.cna-nurses.ca/CNA/documents/pdf/publications/NN_IntlClassNrgPract_e.pdf; 2003. Accessed 2.06.09.

37. Canadian Nurses Association. *Position Statement: Collecting Data to Reflect the Impact of Nursing Practice.* Ontario: Canadian Nurses Association; 2001.

38. International Organization for Standardization (ISO). ISO 18104:2003. http://www.iso.org/iso/catalogue_detail.htm?csnumber=33309; 2009. Accessed 20.06.09.

39. Hannah KJ, White PA, Nagle LN, et al. Standardizing nursing information in Canada for inclusion in electronics health records: C-HOBIC. *J Am Med Inform Assoc.* 2009;10(1197).

40. Canadian Nurses Association. *Mapping Canadian Clinical Outcomes in ICNP®.* http://www.cna-aiic.ca/c-hobic/presentations/default_e.aspx; 2008. Accessed 1.06.09.

41. Hannah KJ, Ball MJ, Edwards MJ. *Introduction to Nursing Informatics,* vol. 3. New York: Springer; 2006.

42. Werley HH, Devine EC, Zorn CR, et al. The nursing minimum data set: abstraction tool for standardized, comparable, essential data. *Am J Public Health.* 1991;81:421-426.

43. Werley HH, Zorn CR. The nursing minimum data set: benefits and implications. In: National League for Nursing – 1987–1989, ed. *Perspectives in Nursing.* New York: National League for Nursing; 1988:105-114.

44. McCloskey JC. The nursing minimum data set: benefits and implications for nurse educators. In: National League for Nursing, ed. *Perspectives in Nursing 1987–1989.* New York: National League for Nursing; 1988:119-126.

45. Alberta Association of Registered Nurses (AARN). *Client Status, Nursing Intervention and Client Outcome Taxonomies: A Background Paper*. Alberta: AARN; 1994.

46. Marek K, Lang N. Nursing sensitive outcomes. In: Canadian Nurses Association (CNA), ed. *Papers from the Nursing Minimum Data Set Conference*. Ontario: CNA; 1993:100-120.

47. O'Brien-Pallas L, Giovannetti P. Nursing intensity. In: Canadian Nurses Association (CNA), ed. *Papers from the Nursing Minimum Data Set Conference*. Ontario: CNA; 1993:68-76.

48. McGee M. Response to V. Saba's paper on Nursing Diagnostic Schemes. In: Canadian Nurses Association, editor. Papers from the Nursing Minimum Data Set Conference. Ottawa: Canadian Nurses Association; 1993. p. 64-67.

Ursula Hübner

Diversity of European National Healthcare Systems

The adoption and use of information technology (IT) in health care is influenced by many factors and depends on legal and cultural constraints prevailing in a country. While Europe is constantly coalescing on a political basis, health care is a sector still dominated by national legislation. Consequently, different types of national health care systems have existed throughout Europe for decades which now build the framework for the use of information and communication technology (ICT) by health care provider organizations.

The following paragraphs will, therefore, provide a concise overview of the different types of national health care systems in Europe and will characterize the countries with regard to key indicators.

Pursuant to a classification scheme for national health care systems used by the OECD,[1] the following three types of models will be described and discussed:

1. Public integrated model
2. Public contract model
3. Private insurance model

The public integrated health care systems are organized and operated like any government department. This department covers both the function of health care provision and that of health care insurance. The system is financed by taxation and is thus entirely controlled by the government which allows health care costs to be contained more easily than in other health care models. Health care providers are either public sector employees or private contractors to the health authority. Ensuring complete population coverage is easily realized under this scheme. The National Health Service (NHS) in the UK used to be an example of a public integrated health care system before it underwent major reconstruction in 2000 and has come closer to a public contract model. Variations of public integrated health care systems exist in the Scandinavian countries, Italy, Greece, and Portugal.[1]

U. Hübner
University of Applied Sciences Osnabrück, Caprivistr. 30A, 49080 Osnabrück, Germany
e-mail: u.huebner@fh-osnabrueck.de

M.J. Ball et al. (eds.), *Nursing Informatics*,
DOI: 10.1007/978-1-84996-278-0_23, © Springer-Verlag London Limited 2011

In the public contract model, the system is based on contracts between public payers and the health care providers. Typically, the public payers are social security funds, but can also be a state agency. There are variations of the model pertaining to whether there is a single payer or a competition among multiple payers. Cost containment is said to be more difficult and it often requires the government to take appropriate action. Health care systems in many Continental European countries are close to the public contract model, e.g., in Germany and France.[1]

The private insurance model provides for private insurance companies contracting with health care providers. In Europe, this model is realized in Switzerland[1] and in the Netherlands.[2] In contrast to the United States, private health insurance is mandatory for all citizens in Switzerland and the Netherlands. Like under the public contract scheme, special cost-containment activities are necessary to keep health care costs at bay.

Private health insurance is also employed in many countries to cover health services not paid for under the public scheme, to absorb out-of-pocket payments, or to increase the choice of health care providers and the timeliness of treatment.[1]

Irrespective of the type of model prevalent, all European countries achieved complete or nearly complete population coverage of health insurance.

Recent health care reforms in all European countries led to severe changes due to a series of measures[3] including

- Price regulations, e.g., hospital financing based on Diagnosis Related Group (DRG) systems[4]
- Improvement of the information base for decision making, e.g., implementing health technology assessment (HTA)[5]
- Budget setting, e.g., capping of budgets and supply limitations
- Cost sharing with households
- Special market incentives
- Measures addressing the delivery of care, e.g., management of waiting lists.

Measures which directly require an extended usage of clinical and financial information, particularly the introduction of DRG-based financing, have a strong influence on the need to use electronic information systems, e.g., electronic medical record systems.[6]

A country's health care systems and national peculiarities have a strong impact on the work of nurses and there is a considerable variation among European countries in terms of number of nurses (Table 23.1), their education and training, and their responsibilities. Table 23.1 shows a list of various countries in Europe ranked by the relative number of nurses. For comparison, it also shows the number of practicing physicians and total health expenditure. In contrast to the number of physicians per 1,000 inhabitants, which is relatively constant across the countries, the number of nurses varies widely between the countries with Norway having by far the most nurses per 1,000 inhabitants. Total health expenditure as a percentage of gross domestic product (GDP) also differs significantly. Countries with public integrated systems tend to spend less money in health care than countries with public contract or private insurance systems which face more challenges keeping their health care costs stable. However, the number of nurses does not change systematically with total health expenditure. The aging population and infant mortality

Table 23.1 Health care indicators of selected European countries (source: OECD[140]): number of practicing nurses and physicians, total health expenditure as percentage of gross domestic product (GDP), population 65 years old and over, infant mortality – sorted by number of practicing nurses (data for the USA and Japan included for comparison)

	Number of practicing nurses (total) per 1,000 population	Number of practicing physicians per 1,000 population	Health expenditure as % of GDP	Population 65 years old and over % of total population	Infant mortality per 1,000 life births
Norway	31.6	3.7	8.7	14.7	3.2
Ireland	15.4	2.9	7.5	11.1	3.7
Belgium	14.8	4.0	10.3	17.2	3.7
Switzerland	14.1	3.8	11.3	16.1	4.4
UK	11.9	2.5	8.4	16.0	5.0
Sweden	10.7	3.5	9.2	17.3	2.8
Germany	9.8	3.5	10.6	19.7	3.8
Netherlands	8.6	3.8	9.5	14.4	4.4
Finland	8.3	2.7	8.2	16.3	2.8
France	7.6	3.4	11.0	16.4	3.8
Czech Republic	7.5	3.6	6.8	14.2	3.3
Spain	7.3	3.6	8.2	16.7	3.8
Italy	7.1	3.7	8.7	19.6	3.9
Austria	6.1	3.6	10.1	16.7	3.6
Poland	5.1	2.2	6.2	13.4	6.0
Portugal	4.6	3.4	10.2	17.3	3.3
Greece	3.3	5.0	9.1	18.5	3.7
USA	10.5	2.4	15.3	12.4	6.9
Japan	9.3	2.1	8.1	20.8	2.6

indicate particular challenges of a national health care system that strongly affect the work of nurses. These challenges are stronger in some countries than in others as Table 23.1 shows.

Not only does the number of nurses vary between the countries, but also does their role in providing patient care within the system. There are European countries where nurses traditionally may operate independently in a variety of settings and make professionally autonomous decisions for which they are accountable, such as in the UK, the Netherlands, and the Scandinavian countries.[7] Expanding the role of nurses, in general, is discussed in many countries. It is known from many studies that replacing general practitioners (GP) with nursing practitioners for taking care of patients with common complaints leads to at least the same level of care.[8] This has been shown, for example, by a British randomized controlled trial (RCT) some years ago[9] and was recently replicated by a Dutch RCT study.[10] The physician shortage and the need for better care in rural areas have also become driving forces to redefine the role of nurses in providing care in other European countries, e.g., in Germany.[11]

Education is another driving force, and in fact, the key factor for reshaping the work of nurses.[12] There is a huge diversity among Western European countries with regard to raising general nursing education from the diploma to the graduate level, yet many countries that have embarked on transforming nursing education are facing similar problems, e.g., faculty members, role of graduate nurses, and curriculum.[13] Eventually, it is the "Bologna Process" that fosters harmonization in education – also for nurses. So, named after a declaration signed by a great number of European countries in Bologna, Italy, in 1999, the "Bologna Process" aims to achieve convergence in higher education across the European Union.[14] It is the most incisive and far-reaching political measure for reforming European universities which has taken place in decades and possesses a high potential for revolutionizing nursing education toward an all-graduate level.[15]

Finally, nursing informatics (NI) and the use of electronic resources in health care are powerful change agents that help to reshape the profile of nurses and their daily work for the sake of better and safer patient care. In the following section, initiatives, research projects, and well-established use of health care IT within the European nursing informatics arena are presented and discussed. The contribution of informatics nurses toward closing information gaps, enhancing interprofessional communication, providing continuity of care, making better clinical decisions, and equipping nurse leaders with facts is illustrated.

Informatics Supporting Patient Care

eHealth Initiatives in Europe

Since the late 1980s, the European Union has promoted research, evaluation, and use of ICT in health care through its various Framework Programmes. Research conducted within these Programmes has contributed to making health telematics applications widely known throughout Europe. The term "health telematics" denotes the convergence of telecommunication and information technologies applied to patient care and is used as "Telematik" in German, "télématique" in French, and "telematics" in English. Because there is considerable overlap with the meaning of "eHealth," both terms are used as synonyms. Based on the wealth of experience from the vast number of research and development projects, the European Commission adopted an eHealth action plan[16] in 2004 which sets out a series of short and middle-term targets including

- Providing recommendations for interoperability of systems
- Encouraging the member states to define a national or regional eHealth roadmap, to leverage investments, and to develop a legal framework for eHealth

- Implementation of pilots (access to public health information use of health insurance cards and setting up health information networks)
- Disseminating best practice examples

The deployment of interoperable electronic health record (EHR) systems is given special attention. While implementing eHealth solutions within one country may already become a challenging effort, the next step, to ensure cross-border interoperability between EHR systems, is even more demanding. The epSOS project (European patient Smart Open Services) is a large-scale undertaking that aims at developing an ICT framework and infrastructure for exchanging patient data across countries with patient summaries/emergency data sets and medication record/ePrescription as pilot applications.[17]

Apart from initiatives at the European level, there are national eHealth and health telematics programmes,[18] some at a more advanced stage, others in their beginnings. The programmes also differ with regard to the primary technological approach: some strongly focus on the use of smartcards as a medium for storing basic data (Germany), others pursue the approach of interconnected databases (UK). Applications prioritized within the eHealth programme can also vary; however ePrescriptions and medication records, patient summary information and emergency data sets, referral letters, information managed by the patients themselves, and finally EHR systems or parts of it are the most common target applications. The definition of access policies and rules and the implementation of a dedicated security infrastructure for accessing, managing, communicating, and storing the data is a major part in all national eHealth programmes, and smartcards are often the method of choice for governing authorized access.

As early as 1995, Denmark began a nationwide programme (MedCom) for establishing EDI message-based communication between the different health care providers such as hospitals, GPs, pharmacies, laboratories, diagnostic imaging departments, physiotherapists, psychologists, chiropractors, and health visitors. Messages include, among others, referral and discharge letters, test orders, prescriptions, and laboratory and radiological results. Starting as a project in the early phases, MedCom was permanently established in 2000 and has been further developed in different phases. Since its beginning, the number of messages has increased exponentially, demonstrating the acceptance and use of the system.[19] A health portal for citizens and health care professionals is available at www.sundhet.dk. It provides EHR functions for health care professionals in a secured area of the portal.

Other Scandinavian eHealth strategies include one in Finland where local health IT systems are integrated via Health Level 7 (HL7) messaging for more than 10 years,[20] in Sweden,[21] and in Norway.[22] One of the pilots in Norway is the drug chart project based on a core EHR.[23] In the Netherlands, the National IT Institute for Healthcare in the Netherlands (NICTIZ) is in charge of managing general IT issues, e.g., secure infrastructure, national health care information hub, as well as clinically oriented projects, e.g., breast cancer screening and stroke, and administrative services, e.g., expense claims.[24]

In 2002, England's Department of Health launched the National Programme for IT (NPfIT), an initiative for stimulating the use of IT systems in the NHS to improve quality of patient care.[25] The programme is managed by "NHS Connecting for Health," a directorate of the Department of Health, which came into operation in 2005. A clinical patient record that is electronically available throughout the NHS is the core element of the

Fig. 23.1 Newborns receive a unique identifier from the NHS. (Photo reprinted with kind permission by Lydia Margerdt / pixelo.de)

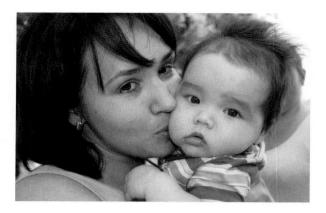

vision expressed in the NPfIT. In order to achieve this goal, a secure broadband network (N3) was set up which completely replaces NHSnet, the precursor of N3, since 2007. Applications of the NPfIT, which are currently developed and deployed, comprise electronic prescriptions, a summary care record system, an electronic referral service for patients, and reporting and statistics services. Deployment takes place in two stages, the early adoption phase (installation at selected sites) and the national roll-out phase.[26] In order for patients to be linked to their record, the NHS issues a unique identifier at birth, the NHS number (Fig. 23.1).

Since 2000, the NHS offers nationwide 24 h health services via telephone through NHS Direct. The service was enhanced via a website (www.nhsdirect.nhs.uk) in 2001. NHS Direct provides expert advice and information on a variety of common complaints and conditions.[27]

In Germany, the national concept for implementing eHealth strongly concentrates on the electronic Health Card (elektronische Gesundheitskarte – eGK), a smartcard, which is used both for authentication and storage of basic patient data. The initial motivation for using a card was to give patients as much control over the data as possible. Access to the data on the eGK as well as to data on servers is enabled by health professional cards (HPC). Both cards make up the core elements of the German Health Telematics Infrastructure, which connects the information systems of the health care providers to the virtual private networks (VPNs) of the infrastructure and provides security services. The foundation of the eGK and the HPC was laid by the Statutory Health Insurance Modernization Act (GKV Modernisierungsgesetz), which came into force in 2004. Besides administrative data, the initial concept of the health card included, among others, the electronic prescription, the medication record, the emergency data set, medical discharge letters, and the electronic patient record.[28] The initial concept has been repeatedly changed and current developments focus on the medical discharge summary, electronic prescriptions, and the emergency data set. Various tests and the roll out of the cards are managed and supervised by the gematik, an organization run by the health care self-government which consists of professional associations, the sickness funds, the private health insurers, and the German hospital association.[29]

Similar to Germany, the eHealth strategy in France embraces the implementation of smartcards, i.e., the health professional card and the health insurance card which complement each other. Since 1998, France has developed major experience in rolling out smartcards successfully on a countrywide basis in health care. The cards are essential elements within the SESAM Vitale Programme for transmitting health insurance certificates electronically. All insured persons older than 16 are issued a health insurance card and nearly 250,000 health care professionals are connected to the health insurance system via SESAM Vitale. SESAM Vitale 2 includes a new card with more memory and additional functions such as electronic signature and access to the EHR, the "dossier médical personnel."[30] HPCs are issued to all health professionals and other health care-related staff.[31]

Another country utilizing cards is Austria which had successfully issued the Austrian eCard to all citizens and physician offices by 2005. The eCard is a citizen's card capable of producing digital signatures, which is used as a social security card. It entitles its holder and family to utilize health services. It furthermore identifies physician offices. The concept for an Austrian-wide lifelong electronic health record (ELGA) is currently discussed.[32] In Slovenia where citizens use an electronic health insurance card since 2000, a new version of the card is rolled out. It allows for applications such as electronic prescriptions and the electronic patient record.[33] In Portugal, the new eID card, a citizen's card, replaces several cards including the health system card;[34]).

The full spectrum of national eHealth initiatives in European countries, including those in Italy and Spain, is summarized by the eHealth ERA report.[18]

Not all national eHealth initiatives have received unreserved support from the public, and in particular, not from physicians and their associations. In the light of criticism – which was also partly triggered by misinformation – programme directors and politicians are seeking to better inform the public and to involve clinicians for achieving consensus about which eHealth applications are actually realized.[35-37] These "unplanned reactions" toward eHealth implementations highlight the importance of respecting the human factor and of well-managed information policy. It also calls for better cooperation and cohesion among European countries in order to be able to avoid mistakes already made and to learn from the success of others.

The way national eHealth programmes include nurses strongly depends on the role and profiles of the nurses in that national health care system. In Sweden, for example, the Society of Nurses participated in developing the programme.[21] The Norwegian programme explicitly addresses the need to extend electronic interactions to all cooperating partners in the sector including nurses,[22] and the Finnish eHealth Roadmap refers to the electronic nursing summaries as a particular strength.[20] In Denmark, home care nurses and nursing homes are integrated into the electronic flow of information between the health care providers.[19] In England, over a third of the NHS Direct staff is made up of nurses.[38] Case studies of NHS pilot sites describe nurses accessing the data electronically in much the same way as physicians do.[26]

However, not all countries using eHealth to optimize the interprofessional flow of information include nursing information. In Germany, nurses are not allowed to use the health data on the card – only when being supervised by a physician. Omitting nurses and other health professionals, e.g., physiotherapists, may easily lead to detrimental consequences such as disrupted continuity of care and compromised patient safety.[39] The health

Fig. 23.2 The health professional card (HPC) for nurses in Germany – exemplary layout (Photo reprinted with kind permission by Nicole Egbert)

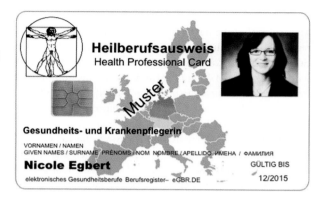

professional card for nurses is the first major step taken in Germany for overcoming this barrier. Nurses and other health professionals (except physicians and pharmacists who are registered at their professional association) will be electronically registered and will be equipped with an electronic health professional card (Fig. 23.2) that is needed for data access.[40] Further, Germany allows nurses to sign digital documents with a qualified electronic signature. This feature makes HPCs in general very valuable – even outside the German Health Telematics Infrastructure.

eHealth Standards

Standards and interoperability between systems are necessary to be able to participate in electronic communication networks and to have access to patient data necessary for treatment and care. This is the reason for standards to be of utmost importance in eHealth. Standards relevant for system (and also human) interoperability comprise syntactical and semantic standards.

Goossen and colleagues have demonstrated that the linkage between nursing domain information and the HL7s reference information model (RIM) is possible.[41] Various approaches were made to model clinical and nursing information with standards from the HL7 suite of standards in the Netherlands, e.g., for perinatology,[42] stroke patients,[43] clinical pathways in cardiology, and the Barthel Index.[44] In Finland, where there is considerable experience of using HL7 messaging to achieve integration among different health care providers, HL7s Clinical Document Architecture (CDA) was chosen as the Finnish national standard for the EHR.[45] The record also includes nursing information, in particular the nursing minimum data set (NMDS) containing nursing process information, intensity, and the discharge summary.[46] The German HL7 CDA-based standard for the nursing summary is the corresponding document to the medical summary with a nearly identical header and a highly structured body which is subdivided into the seven sections: nursing process, home care status, biographical information, social information, reference to legal documents, vital signs, and medication.[47]

Drawing on experience in Scotland, clinical templates have been proposed that allow clinical end users to develop tools for their own clinical use beyond complex technical standards and archetypes. Furthermore, templates are reusable for various clinical applications, which is an additional advantage besides clinical ownership.[48]

Another pillar of eHealth applications are terminology standards. These standards have attracted much attention in the context of developing a professional nursing language as well as from a nursing science point of view. In Europe, work on terminologies was strongly stimulated by the advent of the International Classification of Nursing Practice (ICNP). EU-funded projects contributed to making early stages of the ICNP (alpha and beta versions) known in many European countries and helped with translating the English version into a variety of European languages.[49] With the many different languages which are spoken in Europe, translations of the ICNP are of paramount importance for its acceptance. As experience shows, the translation process may become a project of its own.[50] In order for translators to collaborate over the web and to communicate with external experts for validating the translations, Schrader and colleagues developed a web-based tool. This tool assisted German, Swiss, and Austrian nurses in translating ICNP Version 1.[51] Research on and focused use of the ICNP take place in many European countries, e.g., Rumania,[52] Italy,[53] Poland,[54] and Greece.[55] Much of the early work was devoted to validating the ICNP terms in selected environments and to cross-mapping ICNP with other classifications.[56-59] The ICNP is a tool that goes beyond the question of finding a standardized term for an entity; it is a vehicle for promoting nurses' visibility,[60] a tool used in education[54] and research.[61] Due to its complexity, the raw version of the ICNP does not lend itself for use in clinical settings. Thus, further work is needed to extract and compile relevant information from the ICNP and to build subsets for clinically focused topics, e.g., oncology.[62]

Although well known and widely discussed, the ICNP is not the only terminology that plays an important role in Europe. Another international classification that gains attention is the International Classification of Functioning, Disability and Health (ICF). It was evaluated for applicability in nursing[63] and is used among other countries in the Netherlands.[64] It was chosen as the primary coding system in Switzerland for the Swiss Nursing Minimum Data Set.[65] Also, North American classifications and taxonomies have been translated into European languages and have been adopted in selected countries as prevalent terminology, e.g., NANDA taxonomy in Austria,[66] and Clinical Care Classification (CCC) in a modified version in Finland.[46] The Nursing Intervention Classification (NIC) and the Nursing Outcome Classification (NOC) were translated into French, German, Dutch, Spanish, and Portuguese and the linkage between NANDA, NIC, and NOC into German, Spanish, and Portuguese.[67] In addition, NIC was translated also into Icelandish.[68] In the UK, the Systematized Nomenclature of Medicine – Clinical Terms (SNOMED-CT), which is the result of a merger of two terminologies (Systematized Nomenclature of Medicine – Reference Terminology (SNOMED-RT) and Clinical Terms Version 3) from a collaboration between the College of American Pathologists and the NHS, has replaced NHS Clinical Terms Version 3, formerly known as Read Codes. The merger made further work necessary to ensure consistency, also in the area of nursing.[69] Since 2007, SNOMED-CT is managed and further developed by the International Health Terminology Standards Development Organization (IHTSDO), which was founded by nine nations: Australia,

Canada, Denmark, Lithuania, the Netherlands, New Zealand, Sweden, the United States of America, and the UK.[26]

There are many more clinical and nursing terminologies in use – in particular at local level or at individual sites; not all of them can be listed here. In addition to the international and North American terminologies already mentioned above, two developments originating from Europe are presented in more detail: VIPS from Sweden and LEP (Leistungserfassung in der Pflege) from Switzerland. Both have gained attention outside of the country where they were developed.

Initially published in 1991, VIPS (the acronym stands for the Swedish terms for well-being, integrity, prevention, and safety) was designed to systematize and improve nursing documentation by providing a documentation structure and a terminology. It completely supports the nursing process addressing nursing history, nursing status, nursing diagnoses, goals, interventions, and outcomes. In addition, it includes the nursing discharge note. The VIPS model was tested for reliability and validity.[70] VIPS underwent several modifications over the years and is now used in all Scandinavian and some Baltic countries (Estonia, Latvia).[71]

Another European terminology is LEP (Leistungserfassung in der Pflege = measuring nursing interventions), which was developed in Switzerland. It was designed for describing nursing interventions and incorporates a time value for each intervention. LEP is delivered in two versions, one which allows documentation at an abstract level (LEP 2) and one at a more detailed clinical level (LEP 3). With regard to the integrated time values, it is more than a terminology – a system that enables nurse leaders to perform workload analysis and planning of staff. LEP is widely used in Swiss health provider organizations and has been successfully introduced in German and Austrian hospitals.[72]

The above summary of terminologies implemented in Europe shows that a plethora of standards is in use, common enough within one country. Current developments do not suggest a quick harmonization, but rather indicate a coexistence of various terminologies mapped to each other.

From eHealth to Nursing Documentation Systems

Many eHealth programmes in Europe aim at the implementation of an EHR, as shown above. But as there is a huge variation in what EHRs actually mean, what technical subsystems they embrace, and what clinical functions they cover, there is no well-defined common goal across Europe. EHRs may support clinicians in primary, secondary, or tertiary care. They may be implemented in one department, throughout an organization, or span several institutions or even a region/country. EHRs may also vary in terms of who controls data management: health care professionals or the patients themselves. In advanced versions, EHRs support users from different professions and incorporate nursing information such as daily charting, medication administration, physical assessments, admission nursing notes, and nursing care plans.[73]

Based on the EHR definition of the Healthcare Information and Management Systems Society,[74] Austrian and German nurse leaders were asked about the benefit of EHR systems. The majority of respondents in both countries rated availability of data, data quality, and quality assurance as the three most important issues of the EHR that yielded benefit to

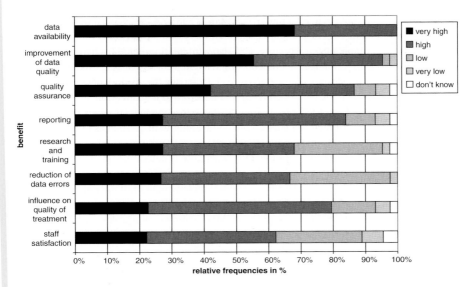

Fig. 23.3 Benefit of EHR systems rated by Austrian nurse leaders (source: own data)

the work of nurses (Fig. 23.3). The study also illustrates the knowledge of nurse leaders about the opportunities of EHR systems and reflects a widespread positive attitude toward them in the two countries.[66]

Whereas there were, by and large, identical installation rates of EHRs in Austrian and German hospitals, significant differences exist with regard to the prevalence of IT systems in nursing: Nearly 67% of the Austrian hospitals had nursing documentation systems in comparison to about 27% of the German hospitals. Also, other subsystems for nurses such as intensive care records and rostering/staff scheduling systems were more frequently installed in Austrian than in German hospitals. Besides many factors that influence IT-adoption, country size and a greater flexibility that may result from a smaller size can be key issues at the macrolevel.[66]

At the level of teams and individuals, other factors are discussed to play an important role in the adoption of nursing documentation systems such as the fit between user, task, and technology[75] and the familiarity with computers and acceptance of the nursing process.[76] Experience gained from introducing nursing terminologies suggested that terminologies facilitate the transition from manual to computerized record keeping.[77] A systematic review that covered European and international studies[78] confirmed this conception: Standardization of documentation was fostered by the use of structured terminologies as a series of studies demonstrated.

The review also revealed that factors promoting the use of standardized documentation may themselves in turn be positively affected by its use, e.g., nursing process and the use of terminologies are promoted by implementing electronic nursing documentation. Quality of content and time savings are other effects of computerized nursing records that are discussed in the literature, but with mixed results.[78] The Heidelberg study is one of the studies demonstrating that electronic nursing documentation systems may have a positive impact on the quantity and quality of the record content.[79] A similar result was found for nursing discharge notes: completeness, structure, and also content of nursing discharge notes were improved as compared to paper documents when standardized templates within the electronic patient record system were employed.[80] Referring to wound documentation, a Swedish group showed that computerized standardized documentation was needed in order to meet all legal requirements.[81] Some of the consequences of using IT in nursing may not be directly attributed to IT itself, but come along with IT such as clinical reasoning that was found to be strongly stimulated by the use of terminologies.[77]

The integration of an IT tool into the daily workflow is determined by the general attitude of that nurse toward IT. Positive as well as negative feelings were reported: A study in Dublin found positive expectations prior to the implementation of the nursing information system, in particular improved multidisciplinary working, improved nurses' work environment, improved and more legible nursing documentation, improved information for patient care, and more time for direct patient care.[82] On the other hand, IT could provoke the feeling of "being controlled by technology" among nurses.[83] Although this attitude seems to be dwindling with the computer evolving from representative of technology to being a regular part of our culture, criticism needs to be taken seriously.

Integrated into clinical pathway documentation, nursing records are becoming part of an overall multiprofessional documentation as in the case of the Piedmont region in Italy.[84] Clinical pathways in their role of governing quality of care and optimizing care processes incorporate clinical guidelines and evidence-based practice,[85] which makes them an attractive approach for supporting patient care. Experience[86] and concepts[87,88] exist to guide how to integrate clinical pathways into EHRs.

Multiprofessional systems, however, need to be designed properly. Not all systems presently available and in use support the multiprofessional dialog as has been demonstrated by a Dutch group studying the physician–nurse interaction mediated by a computerized provider order entry (CPOE) system. The authors argue that the findings are not only due to the specific system in the study, but are related to the idiosyncrasies of the workflow when administering a drug and monitoring its effects.[89] The findings are in line with previous work of a French group who came to the conclusion that asynchronous work of physicians and nurses in medication-related tasks, as it is implicated by CPOE systems, impaired the communication between physicians and nurses and led to less participation of nurses in the decision-making process and a lower understanding of the clinical case.[90] These studies underpin the need for systems that smoothly fit the clinical workflow. They also demonstrated that electronic systems cannot replace verbal interactions and coordination at a personal level.

Informatics Supporting Nursing Management, Leadership, and Policy

IT has a long tradition of being used in administration for automating routine processes – also in health care. This phenomenon can still be observed in health care organizations where IT systems for administrative tasks still outnumber those for clinical tasks, despite the tremendous increase in clinical systems over the last few years.[91] This result is also reflected in nursing where systems for staff scheduling are more frequently implemented than those for nursing documentation. In Germany, about 77% of all hospitals reported utilizing an electronic system for rostering and staff scheduling – as compared to 27% that said they were using a nursing documentation system. In Austria, 91% of the hospitals were found to use a rostering and staff scheduling system and 67 % to use a nursing documentation system.[66] Rostering is a time-consuming task that requires a high level of experience with integrating the many input variables and intrinsic knowledge about legal and organizational constraints. It is performed on a regular basis (usually 4–6 weeks with daily revisions) in uniform way. Rostering thus lends itself for automation or semiautomation.

Essential parameters for staff scheduling are optimal staff level and skill mix per nursing unit. Staff level needed to perform the work in a given environment is typically calculated on the basis of workload measures which provide time values for that specific environment. Nursing work is composed of patient-related and nonpatient-related tasks and workload measures should therefore reflect both parts of the work as has been pointed out by Morris et al.[92] from Dublin. As the time needed to accomplish patient-related tasks is influenced by patient characteristics such as patient dependency/acuity, workload can be predicted by levels of patient dependency. The Dependency/Acuity Tool of the Association of UK University Hospitals (AUKUH) is an example of such an instrument. It helps classifying patients into four resource categories of care (level 0–3). For each level, there is a multiplier that allows calculating the working time equivalent for a unit.[93]

From a conceptual point of view, instruments measuring workload may be subdivided into the two groups: task-oriented types, where nurses are required to record their tasks, and criterion-oriented types, where a criterion such as patient dependency is gauged to group patients into resource classes of a patient classification system. Both types of measures are used in Europe. In Switzerland the task-oriented tools PRN (Projet de Recherche en Nursing) and LEP are widely used.[94] In the UK, criterion type instruments such as the AUKUH tool, which was described above, are utilized.

The LEP workload concept comprises patient-related tasks, the variable component, and nonpatient-related tasks, the fixed component. Whereas patient-related tasks are documented by nurses on a daily basis to capture the periodic variability, nonpatient-related tasks are subsumed by a lump sum, the so called C-value (Fig. 23.4). Terms for patient-related tasks are derived from the LEP terminology.[95]

Staff levels are an issue not only in hospitals, but throughout different care settings. In nursing homes, the Resident Assessment Instrument (RAI) including the Resource Utilization Groups (RUGs), which was developed in the USA, is implemented in various European countries. It serves both quality assurance and resource calculation. RAI translations are currently tested for reliability and validity in an EU-funded project with participation of Italy, Czech Republic, Germany, Finland, France, Israel, the Netherlands, and the UK. The aim is to provide a standardized and common instrument that can be used across Europe to assess quality of care, resource utilization, and patient outcomes.[96]

PLAISIR is another example of a system that was developed outside Europe, namely in Canada, and that has been tested and introduced in European nursing homes.[97]

Measuring or predicting the caseload of community nurses is a particular challenge in countries with broad community nursing services as an Irish study demonstrates. The

Fig. 23.4 C-value concept of the Swiss LEP System (LEP AG n.y.)

$$\text{C-value} = 100 \left(1 - \frac{\text{patient related tasks (all)}}{\text{total hours of work (all)}}\right)$$

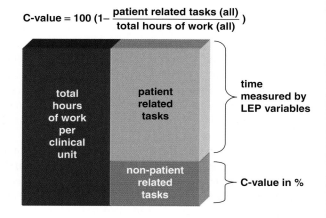

Community Client Need Classification System was found to be a valid and reliable tool for predicting workload (time) of community nurses' service for older people.[98]

In times of nursing shortage and scarce health care resources, benchmarking nursing staff levels within a country and at the international level gives insight into regional differences and helps nurse leaders and politicians in decision making. In Finland, benchmarking was performed for 14 hospitals utilizing the Finnish patient classification system RAFAELA, which allows nursing care intensity (NCI) to be measured, and among others, costs per NCI point and NCI per nurse to be calculated.[99] Benchmarking in a national context requires nursing staff levels to be available countrywide for different hospitals and units.

NMDS when collected uniformly across a country on a regular basis are excellent data pools for any statistical analysis at an aggregated level. The Belgian NMDS (B-NMDS) is the most famous one in Europe and one of the most widely known worldwide. Established by law in 1988, it initially contained information about the institution and the nursing unit, demographic patient data, 23 nursing intervention variables, and activities of daily living (ADL) data. Since 2000, there is a link to the medical hospital discharge data set which permits the combined analysis of nursing and medical data.[100] In 2005 a revised data set was proposed that comprises 37 core data and several supplementary data sets for special care programmes.[101] The data are recorded four times a year in all Belgian acute hospitals. The B-NMDS had been used for a series of statistical analyses. Most recently, it could be demonstrated that the B-NMDS provides a valid measure for nursing intensity, a multidimensional concept that includes, among others, patient dependency, severity of illness, and complexity of care.[100] Nursing intensity-adjusted staffing levels were benchmarked for Belgian hospitals[102] and staffing levels were correlated with patient outcomes.[103]

In Switzerland, work on the Swiss Nursing Minimum Data Set (CH-NMDS) was completed and published in 2005. The goal was to develop an instrument for describing nursing in all care settings. The CH-NMDS is subdivided into two categories, the first describing the environment in which the care of the patient took place (institutional data including data on the nurses in that institution), the second describing the case (medical diagnoses and nursing phenomena), the nursing interventions, economic data such as nursing intensity and nursing need category, and finally demographic data and the unit where the care took place. A list of reference terms derived from ICF and ICNP complements the data set.[104,105] Due to the fact that Switzerland is multilingual, the data set is available in German, French, and Italian. Other NMDSs exist for the Netherlands,[106] Finland,[107] Ireland,[108] Sweden, and Portugal (mentioned in[109]). In fact, the problem for NMDS does not seem to be its development, but rather its enforcement as a large-scale instrument for providing data on a regular basis at a national level.

NMDS and workload measurement systems may both contribute to providing the necessary data for the integration of nursing into hospital financial systems. Most European countries adopted DRG-based hospital financial systems[4] but only a few of these systems make use of nursing data.[109] In Belgium, the B-NMDS yields data for calculating variable nursing costs depending on the clinical case for special hospital departments. For all other departments, fixed values are assumed. This approach results in 6.5% of the total hospital budget to be allocated due to specific information retrieved from nursing. In Luxemburg, which has not embarked on DRG-based financing, retrospective nursing workload information for a hospital is utilized to calculate the staff budget which is allocated to that hospital. Workload information is derived from the Canadian PRN system.[109] DRG systems that are in development possess the greatest opportunity for incorporating information that has been neglected by other systems. In Switzerland, which is currently devising the Swiss-DRG system based on the German DRG system, nursing representatives have been included into the development process almost from the outset. They are proposing the implementation of a nationwide reporting system for nursing information that provides data for calculating the relative cost weights per DRG. As many Swiss hospitals are already collecting workload data with LEP and PRN, there is an excellent point of departure for including nursing data at the DRG level.[94]

As has been illustrated above, staff issues, be it in terms of staff scheduling, measurements of workload and nursing intensity, and budgeting, are traditional domains of nurse management. However, there are other areas where the knowledge of nurses becomes important. One of these areas is the supply chain which embraces all processes from requisitioning medical supplies to administering these products with patients or using these products in the care process. The large group of medical supplies comprises medical–surgical products, e.g., sutures and syringes, medical devices, e.g., blood pressure meters and wheel chairs, and pharmaceutical products. Supply chain management (SCM) is the systematic methodology for providing the right item at the right time to the right patient. SCM procedures manage the flow of materials, information, and money. When performed by nurses, the tasks of requisitioning and ordering supplies are considered as administrative duties, either as patient-related nondirect or nonpatient-related tasks. With the advent of eProcurement system and electronic product catalogs, ordering and logistics processes are more and more systematized and automated. The nurses' role in that process has hereby been revitalized and changed from an administrator to a decision maker. Due to more systematic approaches to purchasing that are pursued by materials management in recent years, a growing number of hospitals around the globe is establishing clinical product evaluation committees, very often multiprofessional teams, whose members decide which products from which suppliers are listed on the hospital's catalog of preferred products. Decision making in these teams is based on a good mixture of personal experience in testing and using products and of results derived from HTA studies. This process, which is also referred to as evidence-based purchasing, ultimately relies on patient data (clinical procedures and patient outcomes) of the electronic patient/health record and on knowledge management systems in which personal experience and scientific findings are accrued. The different levels of electronically supported procurement from transaction-oriented processes (e.g., ordering) to decision making were described in the eBusiness model of SCM. The model demonstrates how administrative and clinical processes converge, which makes a better integration of management and clinical information systems a prerequisite.[110]

Nursing Informatics in Education and Training

Nursing Informatics in the Pre- and Postregistration Phase of Nurses

Nurses' lack of computer skills and information competency has been documented for some time and is still an issue. Although preregistration curricula in nursing include some IT skills, there is a large variability among the programmes and NI as such is rarely addressed.[111]

However, the curriculum alone does not determine whether a computer is used. Recent work supports the concept that the nursing students' belief in their own computer skills and a supportive clinical environment that encouraged them to actually use the computer for patient care both impacted the degree of usage on placement. These findings demonstrate that the entire system, into which nursing education is embedded, may inhibit or facilitate its uptake – with the nurse educators' expertise in NI playing an important role.[112] What has been described for the UK could be observed in other European countries too.[113] Deficits in information retrieval skills are particularly serious when evidence-based methods are to be employed for improving patient care.[114]

In order to enhance basic IT skills for nurses in the pre- and postregistration phase, the European Computer Drivers Licence (ECDL) standard has been adopted by nursing schools and health care organizations. The ECDL, also known outside Europe as the International Computer Driving Licence (ICDL), is an end-user computer skills certification programme. It is managed by national hubs in the member country – presently 148 countries worldwide. The ECDL Foundation located in Dublin, Ireland, is the international governing body which acts as an umbrella organization and is in charge of setting ECDL standards and developing guidelines, licensing, auditing, and reviewing with the goal of ensuring a high level of quality. The ECDL programme consists of seven modules which cover competencies and knowledge in (1) basic concepts of ICT, (2) using the computer and managing files, (3) word processing, (4) spreadsheets, (5) using database, (6) presentation, and (7) web browsing and communication.[115] The ECDL is also used among other sectors in health care to enhance computer and information literacy among health professionals, including nurses.[116] To accommodate for the particular nature of health care delivery in different countries, local certifications were developed for Italy, UK, and Finland.[115]

Nursing and health informatics at postregistration and postgraduate level are well established in Europe. These courses are either addressing nurses only,[117-119] or are offered in the context of interprofessional education.[120-124] The list of examples given is not exhaustive and is not meant to be a reference list.

In addition to entire academic programmes, there is a range of NI courses in the continuing education domain. Often these courses make use of electronic resources themselves, e.g., the web, such as in the case of a NI course in Croatia provided by the Croatian Nursing Informatics Association on an open source learning management system.[125] One of the earliest clusters of electronic NI courses had been developed in the EU-funded project NIGHTINGALE.[126]

eLearning/Blended Learning

eLearning and blended learning scenarios are not restricted to NI, but cover many areas within nursing and are exploited in a variety of learning settings, such as pre- and postregistration level, continuing education and training to acquire new qualifications at one's work. However, the studies that are presented here are from the academic field as this is typically the environment in which systems and evaluation results are published. Many of the papers were published outside the classical informatics realm, in nursing or nursing education journals, which hints at the acceptance of using electronic media for education and training by a broader community within nursing.

More recent examples of eLearning applications embrace courses for the classification of ulcers;[127] critical care scenarios;[128,129] clinical skills using devices for measuring physiological parameters;[130] urethral catheterization;[131] social inclusion, i.e., learning to respect the diversity of patients and their background;[132] mental health services;[133] children's pain management;[134] research methods;[135] evidence-based practice methods;[136] independent, extended, and supplementary prescribing;[137] and genetics for health care professionals including nurses and midwives.[138] These examples made use of a wide spectrum of eLearning technology such as simulator devices controlled by hard- and software, interactive web-based modules, online quizzes, discussion forums, link to other resources (e.g., research articles, web sites), online-videos, and animated material, often integrated into a learning management system. However, in none of these studies technology was the primary focus, but it was rather the didactic aim pursued by employing eLearning which was in the center of attention. In the case of critical care, the electronic scenario provided a safe environment when clinically wrong decisions were made and to demonstrate possible consequences.[129] eLearning proved to be an appropriate means to support problem-based learning with its focus on student-centered learning, exploration, and the development of skills in critical thinking, decision making, and team work.[128,132] In another study, a moderated online discussion forum was utilized to bring together clients of mental health services and students in the attempt to develop empathetic understanding among the students for the special needs of these clients. This approach was integrated into an enquiry-based learning framework.[133]

The examples presented illustrate a specific goal-oriented approach to eLearning beyond mere technological interests and beyond a general motivation for flexible learning on the part of the educationalists and the teachers. The studies demonstrated a positive response to electronically supported learning on the part of the students.

Summary and Outlook

This account was compiled with a focus on the current practice of NI in Europe and on sustainable developments which have or will have an impact on the daily life of nurses and their work.

Many European countries have adopted eHealth and/or the EHR as a major political goal and have launched national initiatives in this area. Considerable experience, success as well as failure stories, has been made over the last 5–10 years, in some countries even longer. Denmark, for example, is looking back at 15 years of experience in connecting health care providers in different care settings. Slovenia has successfully implemented an electronic health card. In many of these countries nurses contributed to the success, e.g., in Finland.

Installation numbers of electronic nursing records as part or precursors of the EHR are increasing and there is a mutual stimulation between electronic nursing documentation and the use of standardized terminologies. The Swedish VIPS model for nursing documentation is practically used throughout Sweden and has been exported to a number of other European countries. In Switzerland LEP is utilized countrywide for the documentation of nursing interventions and workload measurement and is installed in hospitals within and outside Switzerland, e.g., in Germany and Austria.

With the implementation of rigorous documentation at various levels, data for nursing management have become available. The most famous NMDS is the one in Belgium which is collected on a regular basis since more than 20 years. The Swiss work on developing a NMDS has gained great attention in other European countries as a potential model for their own country.

Many of these countries, in which IT and organizational innovation in health care were adopted countrywide, belong to the smaller European countries with less population. It seems as if the number of stakeholders and end users is smaller and better manageable national consensus is within reach.

Interoperability between various systems in European countries, however, remains a challenge and is an issue on the agenda of the European Union.

Even though many European countries have embarked on DRG-based financing systems, the integration of nursing service and costs into the DRG system is still an open question.

The integration of NI into nursing education at pre- and postregistration levels varies largely and there is still much to do to increase IT skills of those entering the nursing workforce and of those who have been working as a registered nurse. Due to large differences in nursing education among the European countries, there is still a great potential for harmonization. The Bologna process contributes to raising nursing education to the level of higher education and to making degrees comparable. The strive for evidence-based practice, the development and use of nursing guidelines, and clinical pathways reflect a research-based approach to nursing which characterizes higher education. Together, they can pave the way toward better exploitation of information and technology in nursing.

Europe's diversity is one of its strengths. It provides different test beds and environments for implementing ICT in health care and hereby shows how these systems can be utilized under different conditions. Diversity without synchronization, however, is a weakness. National health care systems with their peculiarities may impede the synchronization needed. This is why harmonization in health IT that is mediated and fostered by the European Union is so important for Europe – as well as for nurses.

Major target areas for ongoing and future standardization in NI are:

- Structured nursing records as part of an overall EHR system
- Nursing discharge notes and other transfer documents
- Nursing minimum data sets
- Electronic HPC with digital signatures

Cross-mappings of the various nursing terminologies seem to be the method of choice rather than aiming at one standardized vocabulary. In Europe, the ICNP has the potential for becoming the reference terminology in nursing that helps systematizing these cross-mappings.

In terms of nursing education and training, much is being achieved in the wake of the Bologna process. However, special actions need to be taken to include those skills needed for exploiting information in a digital world. These actions should address the development of essential analytical competencies in nurse students combined with practical technical skills. Basically this means

- Helping to make nurses understand the power of data, information, and knowledge
- Helping to establish methods and tools for exploiting data, information, and knowledge for use in patient care, care management, and health care politics
- Helping to make use of data, information, and knowledge for the optimization of clinical workflows and communication among health care providers, for improved decision making with a foundation in evidence-based practice, and for leading organizations and advanced governance

It is desirable to coordinate these activities at European level.

This finally addresses the question raised by Strachan and colleagues of where the professional home of NI is[139] and of who is in charge of initiating these actions: the nursing associations or informatics/computer science societies? With the nursing associations being in charge, there is the advantage of reaching a large group – maybe even the large majority – of nurses. With informatics societies being in charge, NI is integrated into health and medical informatics and into the computer science arena. It is hard to answer the question conclusively because there are areas that have to be tackled by nursing associations, such as education and training in nursing, whereas other areas such as establishing multiprofessional electronic records require a close dialog with other medical and health informatics specialists which is stimulated in the context of an informatics/computer science society. One fact is clear, however, that as eHealth applications are increasingly pervading patient care and eHealth is raised to the level of national politics, nursing associations are forced to grapple with NI and to integrate it into their program. In the light of these developments, the national eHealth initiatives in Europe definitely contribute to a greater awareness of NI among nurses.

Appendix A: Some Nursing Informatics Workings Groups in European Countries

Croatia	Croatian Nursing Informatics Association
Europe	European Federation for Medical Informatics WG Nursing Informatics http://www.nicecomputing.ch/nieurope/
Germany	Deutsche Gesellschaft für Medizinische Informatik, Biometrie und Epidemiologie (GMDS) AG Informationsverarbeitung in der Pflege http://www.nursing-informatics.de
Ireland	Healthcare Informatics Society Ireland (HISI) nursing http://www.hisi.ie/html/nursing.htm
Spain	Sociedad Espanola de Enfermeria Informatica e Internet http://www.seei.es/
Switzerland	Schweizerische IG Pflegeinformatik (IGPI) CIG Informatique dans les soins infirmiers (GICI) http://www.swissnurse.ch
UK	British Computer Society Nursing Specialist Group http://www.bcs.org/server.php?show=nav.10013

Appendix B: Major European Conferences in the Nursing Informatics Domain

Medical Informatics Europe (MIE) Conference	Annual medical and health informatics conference of the European Federation of Medical Informatics (EFMI) with track/sessions or presentations in nursing informaticswww.efmi.org
Association for Common European Nursing Diagnoses, Interventions and Outcomes (ACENDIO) conference	Annual conference of ACENDIO with focus on nursing terminologies for diagnoses, interventions, and outcomeswww.acendio.net/
European Nursing Informatics (ENI) conference	Annual conference on nursing informatics hold in German speaking countries, i.e., Germany, Austria, and Switzerland, with keynote speakers from other European countries. Organized in cooperation with the scientific journal "Pflegewissenschaft"www.printernet.info

References

1. Docteur E, Oxley H. Health-Care Systems: Lessons from the Reform Experience. OECD Economics Department Working Papers, No. 374. OECD Publishing; 2003. doi:10.1787/884504747522.
2. Dutch Ministry of Health, Welfare and Sport. Health insurance system. http://www.minvws.nl/en/themes/health-insurance-system/; 2008. Accessed 16.05.09.

3. Rapoport J, Jonsson E, Jacobs P. Introduction and summary. In: Rapoport J, Jacobs P, Jonsson E, eds. *Cost Containment and Efficiency in National Health Systems: A Global Comparison*. Weinheim: Wiley-VCH; 2009:1-14.

4. European Hospital and Healthcare Federation – HOPE. DRGs as a financing tool. www.hope. be/05eventsandpublications/docpublications/77_drg_report/77_drg_report_2006.pdf;   2006. Accessed 16.05.09.

5. Sorensen C. The role of HTA in coverage and pricing decisions: a cross-country comparison. *Euro Obs*. 2009;11:1-4.

6. Müller ML, Bürkle T, Irsp S, et al. The diagnosis related groups enhanced electronic medical record. *Int J Med Inform*. 2003;70:221-228.

7. Goodyear R, Sheer B. Nurse practitioner/advanced practice nursing network: nurse practitioners respond with practice, policy, and regulation. http://www.medscape.com/viewarticle/446221_2; 2002. Accessed 16.05.09.

8. Horrocks S, Anderson S, Salisbury C. Systematic review of whether nurse practitioners working in primary care can provide equivalent care as doctors. *BMJ*. 2002;324:819-823.

9. Kinnersley P, Anderson E, Parry K, et al. Randomised controlled trial of nurse practitioner versus general practitioner care for patients requesting "same day" consultations in primary care. *BMJ*. 2000;320(7241):1043-1048.

10. Dierick van Daele AT, Metsemakers JF, Derckx EW, et al. Nurse practitioners substituting for general practitioners: randomized controlled trial. *J Adv Nurs*. 2009;65(2):391-401.

11. Bundesministerium Verkehr, Bau, Stadtentwicklung – BMVBS. Modellprojekt Schwester "AGnES".http://www.bmvbs.de/beauftragter/Gesellschaft-staerken-,1686.1057075/Modellprojekt-Schwester-AGnES.htm; n.d. Accessed 16.05.09.

12. European Federation of Nurses – EFN. Position paper on synergy between Directive 36, Bologna and European qualifications framework. www.efnweb.org; n.d. Accessed 16.05.09.

13. Spitzer A, Perrenoud B. Reforms in nursing education across Western Europe: from agenda to practice. *J Prof Nurs*. 2006;22(3):150-161.

14. European Union – EU. About the Bologna process. www.ond.vlaanderen.be/hogeronderwijs/bologna/about/; 2009. Accessed 20.05.09.

15. Davies R. The Bologna process: the quiet revolution in nursing higher education. *Nurse Educ Today*. 2008;28(8):935-942.

16. Commission of the European Communities – CEC. e-Health – making healthcare better for European citizens: an action plan for a European e-Health Area. eur-lex.europa.eu/LexUriServ/LexUriServ.do?uri=COM:2004:0356:FIN:EN:PDF; 2004. Accessed 20.05.09.

17. European patient Smart Open Services – EPSOS. www.epsos.eu/epsos-home.html; n.d. Accessed 20.05.09.

18. European Communities – EC. eHealth priorities and strategies in European countries. Luxembourg. ec.europa.eu/information_society/newsroom/cf/itemdetail.cfm?item_id=3346; 2007. Accessed 23.05.09.

19. MedCom. www.medcom.dk/wm109991; n.d. Accessed 23.05.09.

20. Finnish Ministry of Social Affairs and Health. eHealth roadmap – Finland. Helsinki. www. stm.fi/en/publications/publication/_julkaisu/1056833; 2007. Accessed 23.05.09.

21. Swedish Ministry of Health and Social Affairs, et al. Swedish strategy of eHealth – Status report 2008. Stockholm. www.sweden.gov.se/content/1/c6/11/48/75/39097860.pdf; 2008. Accessed 23.05.09.

22. The Directorate for Health and Social Affairs Norway. Te@mwork 2007 – electronic interaction in the health and social sector. Oslo. http://www.helsedirektoratet.no/english/publications/te_mwork_2007___implementation_plan_2007_47004; 2006. Accessed 23.05.09.

23. Heimly V, Berentsen KE. Consent-based access to core EHR information. *Methods Inf Med*. 2009;48:144-148.

24. National IT Institute for Healthcare in the Netherlands – NICTIZ. www.nictiz.nl; 2006. Accessed 27.05.09.
25. HC Committee of Public Accounts. Department of Health – the National Programme for IT in the NHS. London: The Stationery Office Limited. www.parliament.the-stationery-office.com/pa/cm200607/cmselect/cmpubacc/390/390.pdf; 2007. Accessed 22.05.09.
26. NHS Connecting for Health – NHS CfH. www.connectingforhealth.nhs.uk; 2009. Accessed 22.05.09.
27. NHS Direct. History of NHS Direct. www.nhsdirect.nhs.uk/article.aspx?name=HistoryOfNHS Direct; n.d. Accessed 23.05.09.
28. Bales S. [The introduction of the electronic health card in Germany]. *Bundesgesundheitsblatt Gesundheitsforschung Gesundheitsschutz*. 2005;48(7):727-731 [Article in German].
29. Gematik. Die elektronische Gesundheitskarte. www.gematik.de; 2009. Accessed 22.05.09.
30. GIE SESAM Vitale. Rapport Annuel 2007. www.sesam-vitale.fr/programme/programme.asp; 2007. Accessed 01.06.09.
31. GIP CPS. La CPS, carte d'identité électronique des professionnels de santé. http://www.gip-cps.fr; n.d. Accessed 01.06.09.
32. Dorda W, Duftschmid G, Gerhold L, et al. Austria's path toward nationwide electronic health records. *Methods Inf Med*. 2008;47(2):117-123.
33. eHealth Europe. Slovenia rolls out e-health card. www.ehealtheurope.net/news/4860/slovenia_rolls_out_e-health_card; 2009. Accessed 23.05.09.
34. IDABC – European eGovernment Services. eID Interoperability for PEGS – National Profile Portugal. epractice.eu/files/media/media2080.pdf; 2007. Accessed 23.05.09.
35. Thick M, Davies M, Eccles S, et al. Connecting for health. *Br J Gen Pract*. 2008;58(548):204-205.
36. Klar R, Pelikan E. [Telemedicine in Germany: status, chances and limits]. *Bundesgesundheitsblatt Gesundheitsforschung Gesundheitsschutz*. 2009;52(3):263-269 [Article in German].
37. Pfeiffer KP, Auer CM. [Challenges in the implementation of electronic health care records and patient cards in Austria]. *Bundesgesundheitsblatt Gesundheitsforschung Gesundheitsschutz*. 2009;52(3):324-329 [Article in German].
38. NHS Direct. Facts. www.nhsdirect.nhs.uk; n.d. Accessed 23.05.09.
39. Hübner U. Telematik und Pflege – Gewährleistet die elektronische Gesundheitskarte (eGK) eine verbesserte Versorgung für pflegebedürftige Bürgerinnen und Bürger? *GMS Med Inform Biom Epidemiol*. 2006;2(1):DOC01/20060221.
40. Gesundheitsministerkonferenz – GMK. Elektronisches Gesundheitsberuferegister. www.gmkonline.de/?&nav=beschluesse_80&id=80_05.09; 2007. Accessed 24.05.09.
41. Goossen WT, Ozbolt JG, Coenen A, et al. Development of a provisional domain model for the nursing process for use within the Health Level 7 reference information model. *J Am Med Inform Assoc*. 2004;11(3):186-194.
42. Goossen WT, Jonker MJ, Heitmann KU, et al. Electronic patient records: domain message information model perinatology. *Int J Med Inform*. 2003;70(2-3):265-276.
43. Goossen WT. Intelligent semantic interoperability: integrating knowledge, terminology and information models to support stroke care. *Stud Health Technol Inform*. 2006;122:435-439.
44. Goossen WT. The Netherlands: getting nursing evidence, terminology and data in the development of EHRs. In: Weaver CA, Delaney CW, Weber P, et al., eds. *Nursing and Informatics for the 21st Century*. 1st ed. Chicago: Health Information and Management Systems Society; 2006:399-405.
45. HL7 Finland. The Brochure of HL7 Finland. www.hl7.fi; 2009. Accessed 24.05.09.
46. Häyrinen K, Saranto K. The nursing minimum data set in the multidisciplinary electronic health record. *Stud Health Technol Inform*. 2006;122:325-328.
47. Hübner U, Flemming D, et al. Standardizing the electronic nursing summary: methods and results. In: Weaver C, Delaney C, Weber P, Carr R, eds. Nursing and Nursing Informatics for the 21st century: An International Look at Practice, Trends and the Future. 2nd ed. Chicago: Health Information and Management Systems Society Press; 2010:pp. 193-199.

48. Hoy D, Hardiker NR, McNicoll IT, et al. Collaborative development of clinical templates as a national resource. *Int J Med Inform*. 2009;78(suppl 1):S95-S100.
49. Mortensen RA, ed. *ICNP and Telematics Applications for Nurses in Europe – The Telenurse Experience*. Amsterdam: IOS Press; 1999.
50. Ehnfors M, Coenen A, Marin HF, et al. Translating the International Classification for Nursing Practice (ICNP) – an experience from two countries. *Stud Health Technol Inform*. 2004;107(pt 1):502-505.
51. Schrader U, Tackenberg P, Widmer R, et al. The ICNP-BaT – a multilingual web-based tool to support the collaborative translation of the International Classification for Nursing Practice (ICNP). *Stud Health Technol Inform*. 2007;129(pt 1):751-754.
52. Alecu CS, Jitaru E, Moisil I. Integrated internet based tools for learning and evaluating the International Classification of Nursing Practice. *Stud Health Technol Inform*. 2000;77:583-587.
53. Rognoni C, Mazzoleni MC, Quaglini S, et al. Using ICNP for nurse electronic charts and protocols in rehabilitation divisions. *Stud Health Technol Inform*. 2002;90:798-803.
54. Zarzycka D, Górajek-Jówik J. Nursing diagnosis with the ICNP in the teaching context. *Int Nurs Rev*. 2002;51:240-249.
55. Liaskos J, Mantas J. Measuring the user acceptance of a web-based nursing documentation system. *Methods Inf Med*. 2006;45:116-120.
56. Ruland CM. Evaluating the Beta version of the International Classification for Nursing Practice for domain completeness, applicability of its axial structure and utility in clinical practice: a Norwegian project. *Int Nurs Rev*. 2001;48:9-16.
57. Hardiker NR, Rector AL. Structural validation of nursing terminologies. *J Am Med Inform Assoc*. 2001;8:212-221.
58. Ehnfors M, Florin A, Ehrenberg A. Applicability of the International Classification of Nursing Practice (ICNP) in the areas of nutrition and skin care. *Int J Nurs Terminol Classif*. 2003;14(1):5-18.
59. Giehoff C, Hübner U, Berekoven B, et al. The Interaction of NANDA and ICNP coded nursing diagnoses: an application driven perspective. *Medinfo*. 2004;2004:1615.
60. Sansoni J, Giustini M. More than terminology: using ICNP to enhance nursing's visibility in Italy. *Int Nurs Rev*. 2006;53(1):21-27.
61. Saranto K. A controlled vocabulary for nursing practice and research. *Stud Health Technol Inform*. 2002;90:416-419.
62. König P, Siller M. Building a subset of ICNP terms for oncological patients. *Stud Health Technol Inform*. 2006;122:900-901.
63. Heinen MM, van Achterberg T, Roodbol G, et al. Applying ICF in nursing practice: classifying elements of nursing diagnoses. *Int Nurs Rev*. 2005;52(4):304-312.
64. van Grunsven A, Bindels R, Coenen C, de Bel E. Developing an integrated electronic nursing record based on standards. *Stud Health Technol Inform*. 2006;122:294-297.
65. Berthou A. The Swiss Nursing Minimum Data Set. www.isesuisse.ch/nursingdata/en/index.htm; 2005. Accessed 25.05.09.
66. Hübner U, Ammenwerth E, Flemming D, et al. IT adoption of clinical information systems in Austrian and German hospitals: results of a comparative survey with a focus on nursing. BMC Med Inform Decis Mak. 2010, 10:8.
67. University of Iowa. Current and pending translations. www.nursing.uiowa.edu/excellence/nursing_knowledge/clinical_effectiveness/TRANSLATIONS.pdf; n.y. Accessed 01.06.09.
68. Thoroddsen A. Applicability of the Nursing Interventions Classification to describe nursing. *Scand J Caring Sci*. 2005;19(2):128-139.
69. Casey A, Spisla C, Konicek D, et al. Practical definition of SNOMED CT concepts: the case of education, advice and counselling. *Stud Health Technol Inform*. 2006;122:742-745.
70. Ehrenberg A, Ehnfors M, Thorell-Ekstrand. Nursing documentation in patient records: experience with the use of the VIPS model. *J Adv Nurs*. 1996;24:853-867.

71. Ehnfors M, Ehrenberg A. Development of electronic health records to support nursing care in Sweden. In: Weaver CA, Delaney CW, Weber P, et al., eds. *Nursing and Informatics for the 21st Century*. 1st ed. Chicago: Health Information and Management Systems Society; 2006:393-398.

72. LEP AG. What is LEP? www.lep.ch/index.php/en; n.d. Accessed 25.05.09.

73. Häyrinen K, Saranto K, Nykännen P. Definition, structure, content, use and impacts of electronic health records: a review of the research literature. *Int J Med Inform*. 2007;77:291-307.

74. Healthcare Information and Management Systems Society – HIMSS. 19th Annual HIMSS leadership survey. http://www.himss.org; 2008. Accessed 23.05.09.

75. Ammenwerth E, Iller C, Mahler C. IT-adoption and the interaction of task, technology and individuals: a fit framework and a case study. *BMC Med Inform Decis Mak*. 2006;6:3.

76. Ammenwerth E, Mansmann U, Iller C, et al. Factors affecting and affected by user acceptance of computer-based nursing documentation: results of a two-year study. *J Am Med Inform Assoc*. 2003;10:69-84.

77. Müller-Staub M, Needham I, Odenbreit M, et al. Implementing nursing diagnostics effectively: cluster randomized trial. *J Adv Nurs*. 2008;63(3):291-301.

78. Saranto K, Kinnunen UM. Evaluating nursing documentation – research designs and methods: systematic review. *J Adv Nurs*. 2009;65(3):464-476.

79. Mahler C, Ammenwerth E, Wagner A, et al. Effects of a computer-based nursing documentation system on the quality of nursing documentation. *J Med Syst*. 2007;31(4):274-282.

80. Hellesø R. Information handling in the nursing discharge note. *J Clin Nurs*. 2006;15:11-21.

81. Törnvall E, Wahren LK, Wilhelmsson S. Advancing nursing documentation: an intervention study using patients with leg ulcer as an example. *Int J Med Inform*. 2009. doi:10.1016/j.ijmedinf.2009.04.002.

82. Murnane R. Empowering nurses: improving care nurses' response to the new Health Services Reform Programme in Ireland. *Int J Med Inform*. 2005;74:861-868.

83. Børmark SR, Moen A. Information technology and nursing; Emancipation versus control? *Stud Health Technol Inform*. 2006;122:591-595.

84. Marchisio S, Vanetti M, Valsesia R, et al. Effect of introducing a care pathway to standardize treatment and nursing of schizophrenia. *Community Ment Health J*. 2009. doi:10.1007/s10597-009-9198-3.

85. Manning B, Benton S. The safe implementation of research into healthcare practice. *Stud Health Technol Inform*. 2008;137:199-209.

86. Bürkle T, Baur T, Höss N. Clinical pathways development and computer support in the EPR: lessons learned. *Stud Health Technol Inform*. 2006;124:1025-1030.

87. Devlies J, De Clercq E, Van Casteren V, et al. The use of a compliant EHR when providing clinical pathway driven care to a subset of diabetic patients: recommendation from a Working Group. *Stud Health Technol Inform*. 2008;141:149-161.

88. Bernstein K, Andersen U. Managing care pathways combining SNOMED CT, archetypes and an electronic guideline system. *Stud Health Technol Inform*. 2008;136:353-358.

89. Pirnejad H, Niazkhani Z, van der Sijs H, et al. Evaluation of the impact of a CPOE system on nurse-physician communication – a mixed method study. *Methods Inf Med*. 2009;48(4):350-360.

90. Beuscart-Zéphir MC, Pelayo S, Anceaux F, et al. Cognitive analysis of physicians and nurses cooperation in the medication ordering and administration process. *Int J Med Inform*. 2007;76(suppl 1):S65-S77.

91. Hübner U, Sellemann B. Current and future use of ICT for patient care and management in German acute hospitals: a comparison between the nursing and the hospital managers' perspectives. *Methods Inf Med*. 2005;44:528-536.

92. Morris R, MacNeela P, Scott A, et al. Reconsidering the conceptualization of nursing workload: literature review. *J Adv Nurs*. 2007;57(5):463-471.

93. Association of UK University Hospitals – AUKUH. Patient care portfolio AUKUH acuity/dependency tool implementation resource pack. www.aukuh.org.uk; n.d. Accessed 28.05.09.

94. Kuster B, Baumberger D, et al. Reporting der Pflege in SwissDRG. Version 1.0. St. Gallen. www.lep.ch; 2009. Accessed 31.05.09.
95. Brosziewski A, Brügger U. [Scientific basis of measuring instruments in public health: on the example of LEP progress in the achievements of nursing]. *Pflege.* 2001;14(1):59-66 [Article in German].
96. interRAI. European Union funds large interRAI LTCF study. www.interrai.org; 2008. Accessed 29.05.09.
97. EROS. Produits. http://www.erosinfo.com/; n.d. Accessed 29.05.09.
98. Byrne G, Brady AM, Horan P, et al. Assessment of dependency levels of older people in the community and measurement of nursing workload. *J Adv Nurs.* 2007;60(1):39-49.
99. Fagerström L, Rauhala A. Benchmarking in nursing care by the RAFAELA patient classification system: a possibility for nurse managers. *J Nurs Manag.* 2007;15:683-692.
100. Sermeus W, Delesie L, Van Den Heede K, et al. Measuring the intensity of nursing care: making use of the Belgian Nursing Minimal Data Set. *Int J Nurs Stud.* 2008;45:1011-1021.
101. Sermeus W, van den Heede K, Michiels D, et al. Revising the Belgian Nursing Minimum Dataset: from concept to implementation. *Int J Med Inform.* 2005;74(11–12):946-951.
102. Van Den Heede K, Diya L, Lesaffre E, Vleugels A, Sermeus W. Benchmarking nurse staffing levels: the development of a nationwide feedback tool. *J Adv Nurs.* 2008;63(6):607-618.
103. Van den Heede K, Sermeus W, Diya L, et al. Nurse staffing and patient outcomes in Belgian acute hospitals: cross-sectional analysis of administrative data. *Int J Nurs Stud.* 2009; 46(7):928-39
104. Junger A, Berthou A. Why and how a nursing minimum dataset in Switzerland. In: Marin HF, Marques EP, Hovenga E, et al., eds. *Proceedings of the 8th International Congress in Nursing Informatics, E-Health for all: Designing Nursing Agenda for the Future.* Rio de Janeiro; 2003:469–475.
105. Berthou A, Junger A, Kossaibati S. Test du Nursing Minimum Data Set suisse (CH-NMDS) – Rapport final. Lausanne. www.isesuisse.ch/nursingdata/fr/travaux/test02_rapport_ final_0602-f.pdf; 2005. Accessed 30.05.09.
106. Goossen WT, Epping PJ, van den Heuvel WJ, et al. Development of the Nursing Minimum Data Set for the Netherlands (NMDSN): identification of categories and items. *J Adv Nurs.* 2000;31(3):536-547.
107. Turtiainen AM, Kinnunen J, Sermeus W, Nyberg T. The cross-cultural adaptation of the Belgium Nursing Minimum Data Set to Finnish nursing. *J Nurs Manag.* 2000;8:281-290.
108. Henry P, Mac Neela P, Clinton G, et al. Developing a data dictionary for the Irish nursing minimum dataset. *Stud Health Technol Inform.* 2006;122:510-513.
109. Laport N, Sermeus W, Vanden Boer G, et al. Adjusting for nursing care case mix in hospital reimbursement: a review of international practice. *Policy Polit Nurs Pract.* 2008;9(2):94-102.
110. Hübner U. The supply chain model of eBusiness in healthcare. In: Hübner U, Elmhorst MA, eds. *eBusiness in Healthcare – From eProcurement to Supply Chain Management.* London: Springer; 2008:297-318.
111. Bond CS, Procter PM. Prescription for nursing informatics in pre-registration nurse education. *Health Informatics J.* 2009;15(1):55-64.
112. Bond CS. Nurses, computers and pre-registration education. *Nurse Educ Today.* 2009. doi:10.1016/j.nedt.2009.02.014.
113. Ragneskog H, Gerdner L. Competence in nursing informatics among nursing students and staff at a nursing institute in Sweden. *Health Info Libr J.* 2006;23(2):126-132.
114. Koivunen M, Välimäki M, Hätönen H. Nurses' information retrieval skills in psychiatric hospitals: are the requirements for evidence-based practice fulfilled? *Nurse Educ Pract.* 2009. doi:10.1016/j.nepr.2009.03.004.
115. EDCL Foundation. ECDL/ICDL introduction. www.ecdl.org; n.d. Accessed 01.06.09.
116. Cole IK, Kelsey A. Computer and information literacy in post-qualifying education. *Nurse Educ Pract.* 2004;4:190-199.
117. Private Universität für Gesundheitswissenschaften, Medizinische Informatik und Technik – UMIT. Das Studienangebot der UMIT. http://www.umit.at/upload/v08_211_ib_doc_ pflege_07_internet_rz_doktorat.pdf; n.d. Accessed 01.06.09.

118. Schrader U. Migrating a lecture in nursing informatics to a blended learning format – a bottom-up approach to implement an open-source web-based learning management system. *Stud Health Technol Inform.* 2006;122:559-562.

119. University of Salford. Postgraduate studies with the Nursing Informatics Research Group. http://www.research.salford.ac.uk/scnmcr/nirg/nipostgrad.htm; n.d. Accessed 01.06.09.

120. Goossen WT, Goossen-Baremans AT, Hofte L, et al. ROC van Twente: nursing education in care and technology. *Stud Health Technol Inform.* 2007;129(pt 2):1396-1400.

121. Mantas J, Diomidous M. Implementation and evaluation of the MSc course in health informatics in Greece. *Methods Inf Med.* 2007;46(1):90-92.

122. Hübner U. Gesundheitsinformatik an der Fachhochschule Osnabrück. *Forum der Medizin-Dokumentation und Medizin-Informatik.* 2008;4/2008:183–185.

123. Liaskos J, Frigas A, Antypas K, et al. Promoting interprofessional education in health sector within the European Interprofessional Education Network. *Int J Med Inform.* 2009;78:S43-S47.

124. University of Kuopio – Department of Health Policy and Management. Doctoral degree programme on Health and Human Services Informatics. http://www.uku.fi/tht/english/etieto-hallinto/postgraduate_studies.shtml; n.d. Accessed 01.06.09.

125. Radenovic A, Kalauz S. Long distance education for Croatian nurses with open source software. *Stud Health Technol Inform.* 2006;122:532-534.

126. Mantas J. Developing curriculum in nursing informatics in Europe. *Int J Med Inform.* 1998;58:123-132.

127. Beeckman D, Schoonhoven L, Boucqué H, et al. Pressure ulcers: e-learning to improve classification by nurses and nursing students. *J Clin Nurs.* 2008;17:1697-1707.

128. Docherty C, Hoy D, Topp H, et al. eLearning techniques supporting problem based learning in clinical simulation. *Int J Med Inform.* 2005;74:527-533.

129. Tait M, Tait D, Thornton F, Edwards M. Development and evaluation of a critical care e-Learning scenario. *Nurse Educ Today.* 2008;28:970-980.

130. Kelly M, Lyng C, McGrath M, et al. A multi-method study to determine the effectiveness of, and student attitudes to, online instructional videos for teaching clinical nursing skills. *Nurs Educ Today.* 2009;29:292-300.

131. Jöud A, Sandholm A, Alseby L, et al. Feasibility of a computerized male urethral catheterization simulator. *Nurse Educ Pract.* 2009. doi:10.1016/j.nepr.2009.03.017.

132. Beadle M, Santy J. The early benefits of a problem-based approach to teaching social inclusion using an online virtual town. *Nurse Educ Pract.* 2008;8:190-196.

133. Simpson A, Reynolds L, Light I, et al. Talking with the experts: evaluation of an online discussion forum involving mental health service users in the education of mental health nursing students. *Nurs Educ Today.* 2008;28:633-640.

134. Jonas D, Burns B. The transition to blended e-learning: changing the focus of educational delivery. *Nurse Educ Pract.* 2009. doi:10.1016/j.nepr.2009.01.015.

135. Campbell M, Will Gibson W, Hall A, et al. Online vs. face-to-face discussion in a web-based research methods course for postgraduate nursing students: a quasi-experimental study. *Int J Nurs Stud.* 2008;45:750-759.

136. Johnson N, List-Ivankovic J, Eboh WO, et al. Research and evidence based practice: using a blended approach to teaching and learning in undergraduate nurse education. *Nurse Educ Pract.* 2009. doi:10.1016/j.nepr.2009.03.012.

137. Betts H, Burgess J. A preliminary evaluation of the first e-learning nurse prescribing course in England. *Stud Health Technol Inform.* 2006;122:153-157.

138. Gresty K, Skirton H, Evenden A. Addressing the issue of e-learning and online genetics for health professionals. *Nurs Health Sci.* 2007;9:14-22.

139. Strachan H, Delaney CW, Sensmeier J. Looking to the future: informatics and nursing's opportunities. In: Weaver CA, Delaney CW, Weber P, et al., eds. *Nursing and Informatics for the 21st Century.* 1st ed. Chicago: Health Information and Management Systems Society; 2006:507-516.

140. Organization for Economic Cooperation and Development. OECD health data 2008. www.oecd.org/health/healthdata; 2008. Accessed 15.05.09.

Evolution: Nursing Informatics in Brazil

24

Heimar F. Marin, Denise T. Silveira, Grace Dal Sasso,
and Heloisa Helena C. Perez

> *Yesterday is gone. Tomorrow has not yet come. We have only
> today. Let us begin… Agnès Gonxha Bojaxhiu, Mother Teresa*

In today's healthcare environment, communication and information technologies have made the delivery of nursing care more challenging, diverse, and complex. Due to the economy, policies to protect consumers and users, emerging diseases, workforce shortage, care delivery models, and globalization, there are many considerable changes in the practice of nursing informatics. As forecast by Hannah and Ball in the 3rd Edition of *Where Caring and Technology Meet*, nurses have become primary users in information technology, and nurses have also taken a leading role in the development, implementation, and evaluation of healthcare systems.

Nurses depend on accurate and timely access to appropriate information to perform the variety of activities including patient care, administration, consulting, education, and training.[1] So the nursing profession has been in the business of processing information, even before computers were introduced into healthcare industry. However, the process of decision-making along with the control and evaluation of nursing care has been significantly altered since information and communication technologies (ICT) were included as a tool in the hospitals and healthcare facilities. As a result, identifying the essential data needed for decision-making on patient care, evaluating the technology that can be used to achieve nursing care objectives and the patient's needs, as well as processing information have become an integral feature of the nursing profession.

Interest in retrieval and maintenance of information related to the patient for support of nursing interventions and decision-making is frequently noted and has been considered as a teaching and research model for nursing schools. Consequently, nursing education encourages the importance of getting all information – and getting it in different care settings. Although there are different approaches to obtaining patient information, the natural flow, formal and informal, of information is more accessible to the nursing professionals.

Nurses today are even more aware that the health status of any individual is dependent on the interconnection of genetics, brain, and environment, as well as the effect that each of these paradigms has on the expression of the others. This interconnection means that we

H.F. Marin (✉)
Federal University of Sao Paulo, Sao Paulo, Brazil
e-mail: hfmarin@unifesp.br

M.J. Ball et al. (eds.), *Nursing Informatics*,
DOI: 10.1007/978-1-84996-278-0_24, © Springer-Verlag London Limited 2011

need new ways to measure, to model, and to visualize the interaction of data and information. Given globalization and the awareness that everything has to be documented to exist, nurses have dedicated more attention internationally to make visible their contribution to the health of population. It has also been important to consider strategies for storing and retrieving information in addition to the way health-related information can better characterize and build nursing knowledge. The resulting new scientific knowledge combined with related data and information about the individual, family, and community opens up the possibility to personalize care and promote safer healthcare delivery.

For the purposes of this chapter, nursing informatics is defined as "the integration of nursing, its information, and information management with information processing and communication technology to support the health of people worldwide (URL: http://www. imiani.org)." Nursing informatics also plays an essential role to facilitate the evolution of nursing as science and profession in the global village.

Evolution of Nursing Informatics in Brazil

Brazil, the largest country in South America and the fifth largest in the world with its 8,514,876 km^2, covers almost half (47.3%) of the South American continent. The population of approximately 200 million inhabitants is very culturally, socially, economically, meteorologically, and geographically diverse. As a result, there are many different scenarios and contexts that contribute to the development and utilization of the information and communication resources.

The first initiatives in the informatics field began around 1975 in São Paulo with the first Brazilian Symposium in computer applications in medical hospitals. Early records related to nursing informatics date back to 1985, when faculty of nursing from Federal University of Rio Grande do Sul (UFRGS) presented their experience in the use of computers to teach nursing activities in home care.[2] Subsequently based on this interest in the contributions of technology resources in the healthcare, the Brazilian Society of Health Informatics was founded in 1986 when the First Congress in Health Informatics was held in city of Campinas.

In 1990, the third Congress of the Brazilian Health Informatics Society was held in the city of Gramado, Rio Grande do Sul. At this congress, a dedicated session for nursing informatics was organized by some of the national pioneers in the field, including Beatriz Lara dos Santos and Lia Funcke (UFRGS), Marli Theoto Rocha (Nursing School, University of São Paulo), Evanise Arone (SENAC), and Heimar de Fatima Marin (Federal University of São Paulo). At this meeting, for the first time, the keynote address was given by an internationally known nursing informatics leader, Dr. Kathryn Hannah from Canada.

During the same year, the Nursing Informatics Group at the Federal University of São Paulo (NIEn/UNIFESP) was established through the guidance of Prof. Daniel Sigulem. He was the president of the Brazilian Health Informatics Society (SBIS) and the chair of the Department of Health Informatics at the same university at that time. In 1991, the group hosted the Inter-American Symposium in Nursing Informatics with over 200 participants.

At this seminar, Brazil became a member of the International Medical Informatics Association, Nursing Informatics, Special Interest Group (IMIA, NI SIG).[3]

Currently, similar groups at universities across the country and several schools of nursing have established nursing informatics as a discipline in the nursing curriculum and have organized nursing informatics research groups. A retrospective search was conducted in the electronic directory of the Brazilian Research Council for Science and Technology (CNPq) of Brazil, between 1922 and 2008. This search revealed that there are 16 nursing informatics research groups that have been established in Brazil. However, among the total number of 323 research groups of all types included in this directory, approximately 28 groups (42%) had developed some type of study and research in ICT.

The pioneer research group registered is the Nursing Informatics Research Group at the Federal University of São Paulo (NIEn-UNIFESP). However, a growing research movement in this field can be observed with several groups having been established in the last 7 years across the country. Two such groups are the Research Group in Technology, Information, Health and Nursing Informatics, which is located at the Federal University of Santa Catarina (UFSC), led by Dra Grace dal Sasso, and the Research Group in Information Technology and Nursing Work Process at the Nursing School at São Paulo University led by Dr. Heloisa Peres.[4]

In 2002, the SBIS granted the creation of the Nursing Informatics Working Group (SBIS-NI), integrating nurses from several states within the country such as Rio Grande do Sul, Santa Catarina, Rio de Janeiro, and São Paulo. Established goals of the SBIS-NI were to: (1) develop a national strategy for NI education, research, management, and clinical practice, (2) determine priorities for implementing nursing informatics educational programs, (3) develop by consensus a definition of nursing informatics according to Brazilian education and professional regulations, (4) recommend NI competencies for clinical nurses, managers, faculty, and researchers, (5) develop innovative care models and standards balanced by human and technological resources, and (6) promote development of next generation electronic health records to facilitate patient-centric care at bedside, clinical research, and public health.

In November 2003, the SBIS-NI founded the TeleNursing Department at the CBTMS – Brazilian Telemedicine and Telehealth Council. The main goals established by this group were to: (1) increase and promote the use of telecommunications for distance learning education, (2) use telemedicine technologies to provide care to the minorities, (3) increase access to medical and nursing care centers, decreasing healthcare costs, (4) provide continuous education programs for nurses and nursing students to enhance public healthcare in rural and urban communities, and (5) promote the development and usage of telenursing strategies with advanced electronic representation of nursing and biomedical knowledge.

Over the last 10 years, nursing informatics and telenursing have advanced considerably in the Brazilian healthcare environment, following global trends. However, despite significant possibilities and outcomes, there are challenges and difficulties being faced as leaders try to demonstrate what has been achieved currently and identify what is needed in the future. Also some of the strategies defined by the nursing informatics groups continue to make contributions to the health of Brazilian populations. The primary focus of those strategies is to develop a safer healthcare environment and to stimulate research regarding redesign of professional practice according to the new technological trends.

Since 2006, an important ICT project named RUTE network has been deployed in the country.[5] The infrastructure was developed by the University Network of Telemedicine and Telehealth Care of the Science and Technology Ministry (MCT), which is coordinated by the National Network of Teaching and Research[6] and the National Program of Telehealth Care for primary healthcare. The RUTE project integrates teaching hospitals and the basic healthcare networks.[7,8] Currently, the RUTE network integrates approximately 57 health-care institutes throughout the country and hundreds of basic healthcare units in their respective states, covering all Brazilian states. In addition, RUTE handles the multi-professional integration in the healthcare of the community, and this infrastructure has improved access to healthcare and health information for the populations that live in regions that are remote and difficult to reach.

The RUTE project also opened an ongoing channel for the development of research studies and interchange of specialized health knowledge. This has resulted in the growth of scientific collaboration, increased enrollment in healthcare training courses, and improved access to continuing education with the introduction of the e-learning, m-learning, and the integrated evolution of telenursing procedures on a national level.

Key words in nursing informatics and telenursing are *networking* and *integration*. It is important to utilize all available, dedicated resources to develop, deploy, and evaluate the impact of ICT on nursing practice, administration, research, and education. With ICT resources, systems can be created that could provide strong support for nursing practice. Systems can be developed to demonstrate our commitment to the healthcare of the population, and that could be used to analyze our efficiency and effectiveness. Additionally, systems analysis would identify and verify the modifications needed for changing or improving roles and responsibilities as providers, researchers, and educators.

Only through research using real, point of care data from nursing practice can the nurs-ing profession be evaluated and capabilities be enriched. Additionally, research can drive trends and political decisions in the nursing informatics area.

In Brazil, nurse informaticists have historically faced many challenges, and most of them have been useful in enhancing the discipline. Caring for ill or injured people will still be an essential part of nursing. However, a new perspective should be considered by nurses in which patient is a partner and not a passive recipient of care. With that perspective, nurses can assist people to help themselves stay healthy and functional. When nurses pro-vide care *with* the patients, not *to* the patients, then patients become more involved and more responsible for their own health conditions.[3]

Practice, Research, and Education in Nursing Informatics

Since the early stages of nursing informatics development in Brazil, research, education, and practices have developed considerably. Currently, it is impossible to practice or to communicate without the support of some technology resource. Great achievements have been reached by nurses across the country in incorporating technology in the daily prac-tice. Informatics resources support practice-based knowledge generation as a significant approach to measure effectiveness of nursing care.

The decision to plan and deliver nursing care is always based on the available information of resources, science and technological development, patient/client needs, and technical skills. Better care can be delivered to the patient when more specific information is accessed to support clinical decisions. Quality of care is related to the scope of knowledge and information that providers can access to underpin the clinical decision-making processes. Technology drives the possibilities, and professionals are becoming even more aware of the necessity to apply technology resources to perform daily activities in taking care of patients/clients.[9]

Brazilian nursing practice and computerized systems are being developed based on the nursing process. In general, an important aspect that deserves to be highlighted is the usability of the system. If users are not able to explore all functionalities, then what value does a system bring? Usability refers to how well users can learn and use a product to achieve their goal and how satisfied they are with the process. The best way to achieve human-centered system design is with the active involvement of future users of the system.[9] Although this makes common sense and the importance of this is frequently stated by developers, in general, the systems deployed are not yet designed that are particularly user-friendly or human-centered.

Interoperability is also an important aspect needing emphasis in healthcare information systems development. In Brazil, several systems were developed by different facilities, either in-house or by vendors. The Department of Informatics of the National Health System (www.datasus.gov.br) developed the HOSPUB system, a hospital information system distributed to the public hospitals throughout the country. Today, the system is implemented in 156 health facilities in 14 states. However, some alterations have been made to promote customization, and as a consequence, interoperability has not been maintained as a primary objective.

Since interoperability was a fundamental attribute to be considered by developers, in 2002, an important project to assure interoperability was initiated by the Brazilian Society of Health Informatics and the Brazilian Medical Council. The main objective of the project was to provide system certification for any healthcare software so that systems would meet defined nationally standardized requirements (www.sbis.org.br).

Regarding the nursing aspects of the Brazilian electronic health record, it can be stated that many systems developed and implemented do not yet attend to nurses needs for documentation. However, systems are not yet standardized or structured in accordance with the needs of the respective facilities. Consequently, nurses are working to drive the process and to develop nursing care systems to support documentation, research, and education. There is a clear trend toward the use of standardized terminologies in the computerization of health records. Any nursing terminology should of course be appropriate for the domain or for particular subspecialties of the nursing profession. However, the language used or generated should be readily understandable to users, and it should accurately reflect nursing practice.[10] Terminologies also include the translation. For international communication purposes, terminologies need to be translated. However, the word-by-word translation is not the best method since the context is very important and drives how nursing care should be documented.

In Brazil, several terminologies were translated and have been applied in the development of computerized systems. The North American Nursing Diagnosis Association

(NANDA) is one of the most used terminologies, and it was the first to be translated into Brazilian Portuguese. Other translations include Nursing Interventions Classification (NIC), Nursing Outcomes Classification (NOC), Clinical Care Components (CCC), and International Classification for Nursing Practice (ICNP). Some states in the country such Alagoas and Parana decided to adopt ICNP as the basic terminology for nursing documentation.

Brazilian nurses are also discussing and developing some studies to identify the essential data for a national nursing data set. Once a consensus is reached about what kind of nursing data is essential to guarantee nursing care, several actions must be taken such as: (1) educating nurses to ensure the quality of nursing data and information in a documentation system; (2) creating mechanisms to evaluate the content of minimum data sets in a fast and easy way; (3) disseminating the idea of minimum data set nationally and internationally as a resource to compare nursing intervention and outcomes; and (4) using the results of minimum data-set analyses to influence decision of policy makers.[10]

In the last 5 years, public teaching hospitals have intensified the development of the EHR, and nurses have more actively participated in this process. Nurses must play key roles in the development and deployment of information systems to assure quality and safety of care. It is important that Brazilian nurses understand the need for development and implementation of computerized systems that remain patient-focused with all data captured at the point of care. This is particularly relevant to emerging activities such as the development of personal health records (PHRs).

In the research dimension, nursing informatics has been one of the priorities. The studies have been focused on the development and the appraisals of technologies that can meet the needs of the professional practice and the nursing education. For this purpose, the research on nursing informatics is configured within the contexts of the research groups linked to the universities. Each of the 16 research groups mentioned before is conducting several studies at their respective universities in accordance with the needs of their regions as well as those of the national priorities and guidelines of the graduate programs. Integrated through the Brazilian Health Informatics Society – Nursing Informatics Special Group, research groups of the universities are working together to define the priorities in the area.

Most of these research groups follow the targets proposed by the American Medical Informatics Association (AMIA) Nursing Informatics Working Group for nursing informatics research. These targets include the following: assessment and improvement of healthcare and health outcomes; strategies to reduce disparities in healthcare for minorities; and the building of data infrastructures to support quality evaluation, while protecting patient privacy and security.[11]

Due to the national political tendencies to develop telemedicine and telehealth in the country, nursing professionals are taking advantage of the built infrastructure to develop several resources needed to deliver nursing care to distant patients through the use of telecommunications technologies. It should be emphasized that the use of telecommunications technologies is not necessarily about nursing informatics science. Telenursing is more frequently understood as related to the use of telecommunications instruments, but it does not necessarily mean that users are making specific contributions to the knowledge of nursing informatics. However, the use of these instruments can improve nursing care and can provide care for patients located in distant regions where access to caring is difficult. Activities such as consultation, monitoring diseases and continuous education short course programs are being conducted at health care units and public and private hospitals integrated to the RUTE network. These units are gradually being structured as they are considered as isolated cases in some regions of Brazil, and consequently, the performance needs to be evaluated.[4] Studies can be conducted to measure the impact of the resources on the health of population and on the enhancement of nursing care plans. These studies will provide the scientific evidence to support the use of telenursing in the delivery of nursing care.

To establish and maintain their leadership, researchers must emphasize the investigation of potential applications of emerging technologies to nursing practice. Additionally, researchers in nursing informatics and telenursing began to conduct studies in persuasive technology, such as mobile phone systems as a strategy to change people's attitudes or behaviors. Persuasion strategies differ depending on the role being played by the computer that can be a tool, a medium, or a social actor.[12] These strategies can be applied in education and care systems to help people achieve their own goals. Intervening at the right time and place via network and mobile technology increases the chances of getting better results in healthcare. The learning process can happen anywhere and anytime, and the technology can be used not only as a support for learning but as a procedure in healthcare delivery.[13]

In 2001, some priorities for research were stated by Marin et al,[10] and some of the topics listed are still mandatory and in progress. This extensive list includes the following:

- Nursing information requirements analysis and system specifications.
- System functionalities and modeling, formalization of nursing vocabularies.
- Design and management of databases for nursing information.
- Telecommunications and interactive communications technologies applications.
- Direct-care patient applications.
- Patient use of information technologies, patient use of information technology in the environment of care.
- Evaluation of feasibility, appropriateness, and the impact of nursing information systems into the practice.

Education in nursing informatics was the preliminary activity in Brazil. The development of nursing informatics coincides with the establishment of nursing education programs with nursing informatics in the curriculum and the research. The pioneers of nursing informatics in the country were faculty, and the first product of nursing informatics research was a teaching tool to document nursing data in home care.

The nursing education focus has been at both the undergraduate and the graduate levels. At the undergraduate level, most schools of nursing (629 in the country) integrated nursing informatics content into the curriculum. There are also several graduate programs at the Master's and Doctorate levels. These specialized level programs focused on training nurses as users, developers, educators, and researchers in nursing informatics. Courses in these programs aim to train professionals in order to improve the quality and safety of patient care along with improved outcomes through the development, implementation, and evaluation of information and telecommunication tools at different levels of education.

More specifically, the graduate programs in Brazil have been focused on training leaders in the conceptualization, design, and research of computer-based systems in the healthcare organizations. Applications on evidence-based learning and problem-based learning have been included. Universities and nursing schools that have devoted more efforts to the education of nurses for the development and the implementation of the ICT in the country comprise the Federal University of Sao Paulo (UNIFESP), (the pioneer in the country since 1990); the Nursing School of the State University of Sao Paulo (EEUSP); the Nursing School of Ribeirão Preto (EERP-USP); the Nursing School at UFSC; and the Nursing School of the UFRGS. It is also important to note that the Open University of Brazil, a common program of distance learning provided by UNIFESP, offers a specialized degree program on healthcare informatics for 500 professionals at ten different centers spread throughout Brazil.

Lessons Learned

Over the last years, since the pioneering initiatives in nursing informatics began, several important accomplishments have been achieved to drive the profession and developments in support of practice and education. It is clear, however, that technology is the means but not the final product of accomplishing nursing care. Examples of specific remarks and concerns are provided below from nursing informatics expert and users presentations at symposiums and meetings:

- Nurses are not involved since the beginning in the development and evaluation of electronic patient record systems.
- We believe that nurse participation is a key factor for the success. There is no sense to develop a system that will be used by nurses without nursing active participation.
- The Patient Health Record is a process and not a product that can be deployed at the point of care.
- Clinical documentation in nursing care is not well integrated and included in the electronic health record.
- Without integration, we have no adequate system to document nursing data. Without integration, nursing data will not become nursing information to be used to plan and manage nursing care.
- When documentation is not standardized, records are duplicated, and data are collected but not necessarily used as information in the point of care.
- The need for multiple records and the lack of quality in nursing data do not reflect patient needs. In addition, the amount of information to be documented in nursing care is a challenge to the systems and users developers that can compromise the efficiency and efficacy of the nursing records.
- Nursing informatics is not completely integrated into the nursing curriculum, and the nursing informatics competencies are not established at national level.
- Nursing information systems do not support decision-making in clinical and management areas.
- Researchers and evaluation methods must be developed to provide evidence and guideline applications.

Future Directions

Since the initial activities in nursing informatics in Brazil, nurses have faced many challenges. Most of these challenges have helped nursing professionals enhance their determination to promote the field of nursing informatics. Leading members of the Brazilian Health Informatics Nursing Informatics Group consider the strategic plan developed by the IMIA NI SIG, their guide to drive national activities. They are working to establish a national plan that includes the (1) definition of nursing informatics competencies and the integration of nursing informatics into the nursing curriculum; (2) development of links with the nursing associations; (3) seeking of participations from nurses across country; (4) promotion of conferences to serve as a forum where experiences in nursing informatics can be shared; (5) expansion of users of interest to develop interdisciplinary and multicentric researches; (6) development of a full range of nursing practice tools; (7) study of strategies and methods linking genomic data to genetic information, and then to the patient record and placed into the patient's hands; (8) promotion of new technologies to empower patients and their caregivers for collaborative knowledge development; and (9) encouragement of innovative methodologies in education, research, and care delivery congregating human–computer interaction, organizational context, and the needs of the society.

To stimulate the participation of nurses, in February 2009, the first social web network was created on nursing informatics and telenursing with the purpose of being an ongoing source for nurses and other professionals to share information and innovations of knowledge as well as to gather specialists for the development of nursing profession. Since its creation, 90 participants have become involved in seven different working groups (http://infotelen.ning.com/).

By making nursing informatics more visible in the country of Brazil, nurses can influence policy makers to establish a national nursing informatics agenda. This national research agenda would focus on the evidence and benefits of information technology and communication, the design of nursing education programs focused on nursing informatics, and the promotion of safety and quality of patient care through the use of informatics and technology.

References

1. Marin HF. Nursing informatics: current issues around the world. *Int J Med Inform*. 2005;74 (11–12):857-860.
2. Marin HF. *Informática em Enfermagem*. Sao Paulo: EPU; 1995:3-20.
3. Marin HF. Nursing Informatics in Brazil: a Brazilian experience. *Comput Nurs*. 1998;16:327-332.
4. Sasso GT, Silveira DT, Peres HHC, Marin HF. The Americas: Case Study 14H: Brazil. In: Weaver CA, Delaney CW, Weber P, Carr R. *Nursing and Informatics for the 21st Century, 2nd edition, HIMSS*. 2010;337-342.
5. Rede Universitária de Telemedicina e Telesaúde. RUTE. http://www.rute.br. Accessed 2.03.09.
6. Rede Nacional de Ensino e Pesquisa. RNP. htttp://www.rnp.br/index.php. Accessed 2.03.09.
7. Brasil. Ministério da Saúde. Programa Nacional de Telesaúde. Portaria, 35 de 4 de Janeiro de 2007. Brasília. http://portal.saude.gov.br/portal/arquivos/pdf/portaria35jan07telessaude.pdf; 2007. Accessed 10.04.09.

8. Programa Nacional de Telessaúde. Programa de Atenção Primária. http://www.telessaudebra-sil.org.br/php/index.php. Accessed 2.03.09.

9. Marin HF. Nursing informatics: advances and trends to improve health care quality. *Int J Med Inform*. 2007;76S:S267-S269.

10. Marin HF, Rodrigues RJ, Delaney C, et al. *Building Standard-Based Nursing Information Systems*. Washington: PAHO, WHO; 2001:27-45.

11. McCormick KA, Delaney CJ, Brennan PF, et al. Guideposts to the future – an agenda for nursing informatics. *J Am Med Inform Assoc*. 2007;14:19-24.

12. Fogg BJ. *Persuasive Technology: Using Computers to Change What We Think and Do*. San Francisco: Elsevier; 2003.

13. Sasso GTMD, Phelps C. Mobile learning object on cardiopulmonary resuscitation (CPR): a collaborative, simulated and constructive proposal on health and nursing. In: *Advances in Teaching & Learning Regional Conference*. Houston; 2008:5-12.

14. INFOTELEN. Brazil's Nursing and Telenursing Network. http://www.infotelen.ning.com. Accessed 2.06.09.

Taiwan Model: Nursing Informatics Training
25

Polun Chang and Ming-Chuan Kuo

More than Computer Competency

The competency of using personal productive software, such as spreadsheets, word processing and presentation, has become the fundamental skill requirement for health care professionals to become information literate. For example, the advanced module of European Computer Driving License (ECDL) and the International Computer Driving License (ICDL) clearly identify these skills as core components in enhancing end-users' computer proficiency to expert levels.[1] This design has been recommended by the TIGER initiative[2] as part of the educational resources of the minimum set of informatics competencies for all nurses to practice today.

The potential value of personal productive software is not limited to the "use" of information tools but far beyond that. Often users are familiar with only very limited functionality of productive software and don't realize the great capabilities of its built-in advanced functionalities. It is called a "competency miss" when we have a great tool at hand but do not know its exact limits. Within the computer skills recommended by the ECDL/ICDL Advanced, it is emphasized that the use of a macro can automate and simplify the information processing procedures to a simple click of button on a toolbar.[3]

There is a "record macro" option in almost all personal productive software under the Tool/Macro menu. However, behind the "record" option of the Tool/Macro menu is a wonderland which can lead end-users to "design" very creative and innovative applications for professional information management purposes that in the past could only be done by specialized programmers. It is the macro "editor" that can be used with the productive software to serve very professional purposes. In this chapter, we discuss the importance of the macro editor in NI and the development of nursing informatics systems (NIS) under the concept of End-User Computing (EUC). We will recommend a learning map based on our successful experiences and demonstrate two creative and innovative applications done by nurses, which are even beyond the imagination of IT professionals.

P. Chang (✉)
Institute of BioMedical Informatics, National Yang-Ming University,
Taipei, Taiwan, Republic of China
e-mail: polunchang@gmail.com

M.J. Ball et al. (eds.), *Nursing Informatics*,
DOI: 10.1007/978-1-84996-278-0_25, © Springer-Verlag London Limited 2011

As a matter of fact, training in the use of EUC tools can enhance the individual nurse's computer competency and at the same time serve as a cost-effective strategy to promote nursing informatics on a national scale. Since 2003, this strategy has been used in Taiwan to promote nursing informatics nationwide. It has been enhanced through a series of Excel VBA Training Programs specifically targeted to nurses.[4] The IT competency in Taiwan has been very good throughout Asia. In one report published by the Economist Intelligent Unit about the global competitiveness of IT industry, the most competitive country is the United States of America and the second one is Taiwan.[5]

Hundreds of EUC-trained nurses from various institutes organized to establish the Taiwan Nursing Informatics Association (TNIA) in 2006, immediately following the International Nursing Informatics Symposium held in Korea.[6] Since then, the TNIA have held one or two national symposiums every year and invited internationally distinguished NI experts to attend, and support many local NI activities. Their efforts have made NI well recognized in many local medical centers and created numerous formal NI positions.

This accomplishment can be supported by observing Taiwan's growing active participation in the international NI activities. In Asia, whereby more than 60% of the worldwide population resides, there are currently 13 IMIA national members, including two of the most populated countries, China and India.[7] At NI 2009 in Finland, there were 30 presentations from Taiwan, compared to only one at the NI 2003 in Brazil, which is a very significant improvement. The other submissions from other Asian countries were 26 from Japan, 11 from Korea, and two from Israel. No submission was presented from other Asian nation members, including Singapore, Hong Kong and Malaysia, which were the sites for HIMSS AsiaPac in the years since 2007.

Evolving NI Need and Acting with Leading Role

Though there are fundamental and theoretical backgrounds in NI, the value of NI comes from its potential and capability of enabling nurses to realize their professional responsibilities of caring for people. This enabling process brings both an attitude and a technical challenge in order to make the NI useful for clinical nurses. The attitude challenge is the definition of the nurse's role in developing the NIS. Though the NI is regarded as a nursing specialty, some nurses and their leaders still take a passive and conservative role in NI and developing the NIS. They regard themselves as pure users of NIS and expect and depend on organizations and IT departments to provide support for their information needs.

When organizational IT resources are abundant, the information needs of nurses have a better chance of being served and the NIS can be implemented faster. However, most of the time, the IT needs of nurses are ranked low in the organizational IT priority list and suffer from a lack of resources. More importantly, the majority of HIS or NIS projects are a one-time shot. No matter the scale of systems, large or small, the hospital administrators usually consider that the investment of implementing the HIS or NIS should not occur very often. Once a system is built, it will not be expected to be replaced or reinforced in a short time. Therefore, the model of just being a pure user of a NIS will be very risky for the nursing department to have a quality NIS. This constraint might only be improved after nurses and their leaders are willing to take a more active role in becoming powerful users and lead the development of NIS during the entire life cycle of system development.

There are challenges requiring nurses to act more aggresively to lead the development of NIS. The first challenge is that the information needs of nursing care are evolving, which are dynamic, locally differential, and of long-term investment. Caring is never a static task and will always evolve with the accumulation of nursing evidences, knowledge and practices. There will be always new information needs once a system is first established. This is also true of the evolving of IT technologies. For example, the advancing of network and communication technologies have made point-of-care and telehealth more promising in proving quality care at the place it is needed and at the right time. This evolution brings up the issue of the dynamic feature of information systems in health care. Unlike the information systems of bank and telecommunication businesses, in which the information needs and processing are quite stable over time, functions, components, and contexts change frequently and sometimes even abruptly in health care. (Consider, for example, the impact in the United States of regulations introduced under the Health Insurance Portability and Accountability Act, or HIPAA.) This dynamic nature of the system makes the maintenance of NIS difficult and expensive. Furthermore, nursing care and processes are not universally the same all of the time across various institutes and even in different wards of the same hospital. For this reason, it is not easy to balance the customization vs. standardization of information systems. This localization issue makes the building of a system that can meet all kinds of information needs for every nurse almost impossible and impractical. Summing up the above realities, there is no wonder that the development of NIS is a long-term project and needs continuous investment to maintain it and keep it effective and efficient.

The second challenge is creating a model that can better connect the nurses and IT professionals and allow for the development of useful IT tools for nurses. The communication difficulties between these two professionals have long been noticed and have become part of the reason why medical informatics became an important specialty within medical professions. The best and most effective strategy is for IT people to build the right solutions given what the users can explain about their needs in a way the system developers can easily understand. Therefore, if health care professionals can better understand the languages used in the IT world, both sides will benefit. Furthermore, considering the limited IT resources in many health care institutes, it becomes difficult to expect that the IT department will satisfy all information needs for nurses in time.

A model of giving nurses a leadership role and more autonomy in designing and creating quality IT applications to cost-effectively meet their information needs is worth trying without any doubt. One such a candidate model is the EUC. As information technology becomes more popular, the applications become even easier to use, learn and develop not only by IT professionals but also by end users. The EUC model[8-10] is composed of a set of activities or techniques that allow people who are nonprofessional software developers to create or modify the software themselves.

Among many useful techniques, Microsoft Excel with its built-in Visual Basic for Applications (VBA) is the best tool to serve as EUC tools. VBA can not only be used to automate information management and processing, but it can also be used to design very interesting and powerful personal IT solutions. It has become a very standardized built-in component in productive software for automation and integration. Our studies[6,11] show high acceptance of learning Excel with built-in VBA by nurses, findings consistent with the literature.[12,13] We found that (1) nurses have been using Excel for their information management needs so they feel comfortable and confident (though they did not know many advanced and valuable Excel techniques); (2) all of their home, office, or station computers have already been installed with the Microsoft Office, so Excel was very accessible; (3) nurses do not prefer the database tools, such as Access, since it is more complex to learn the skills and the data are more difficult to be seen and maneuvered than those in Excel; (4) nurses perceive Excel is fun to learn and play with; (5) technically, the built-in VBA, which is hidden in the Tools/Macro, is easy to learn and understand and many training materials are available; and (6) most importantly, successful projects done by nurses using Excel VBA have been observed.[14]

Guiding Learning Map

There is a learning map that can be used to assist users in learning how to use VBA to automate Excel jobs and to provide a friendly interface to simplify the work in NI.[4] To date, this map has been used to train more than 400 nurses and other health care professionals in learning the concepts of medical informatics, designing practical solutions for clinical documentation and information management, providing a communication tool among clinical nurses and IT people, and creating innovative and stylish personal solutions.

A 6-day learning course is designed by following the learning map, as shown in Fig. 25.1. The learning map was designed from lots of experiences and is still under modification. The learning course is composed of 6 days for 6 h per day. To reduce the load of learning programming tools for clinical professionals who have never had IT training and also maintain the momentum of learning, these 6 days are grouped into three 2-day sessions. The first two 2-day sessions are 1 week apart and the last session is 2 weeks after the second one. The special training materials are organized based on the learning road map and includes one very educational textbook, with many great, clear examples that is partially used for the reference.[15]

There are five stages to go through. The first stage decides the Work Need in the first morning section. This stage covers the general ideas in NI and shows how to prepare a good request for proposal (RFP) for a project. Stage I combines the perspectives of ITs, information management and nursing professional objectives. Stage II, entitled EUC with Excel VBA, is scheduled during the first day afternoon section. This stage discusses the various active roles nurses could take during the development of any application. Although nurses do not need to be good programmers to lead the NIS projects, they could benefit a lot from hands-on training in programming simple applications with VBA in Excel. It is emphasized that the key points for a successful IT projects are actually those of how to really understand the professional needs and to express it in ways that the IT staff could understand. The following list is mentioned as the important but

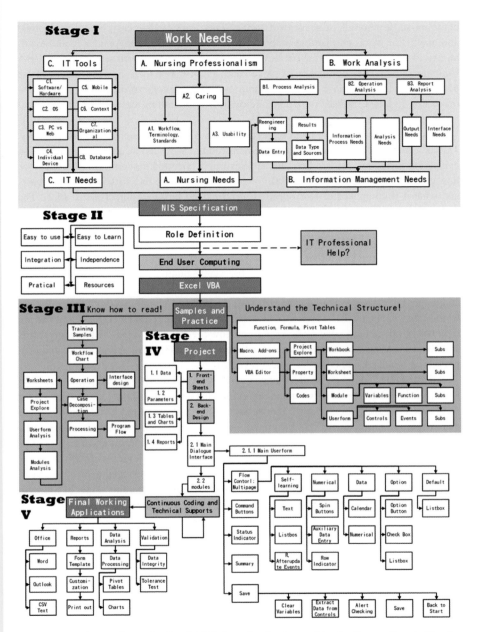

Fig. 25.1 Learning road map for Excel VBA (permitted to be used by the Perspectives in *Nursing Science*)

common-sense features of successful applications: easy to use, easy to learn, practical and useful for work, compatible with current systems, project independence and availability of minimum resources. All key concepts are enhanced with simple Excel VBA samples. The first day could then be closed with a quick introduction of the advanced use of Excel and the potential of VBA in automation. The strategy of case study and hands-on coding to assist trainees in understanding how applications are developed is used to assure learning effectiveness.

Stage III, Samples and Practice, occurs in the morning session of the second day. Trainees are asked to personally run a demonstrating case, such as a training satisfaction evaluation form, and explain how this application is operated in a concept of work flow, how data are collected through the form interface and saved to the worksheets as database, and what it is composed of worksheets, userforms and modules objects (Fig. 25.2). The entire morning session is designed to have the trainees "play" the sample inside-out and "understand how to read" its structures in the VBA development environment.

In the afternoon session, the technical parts of applications and those codes of subs and functions of one representative userform are explained and all trainees are required to do the coding line by line for some simple subs. Representative components and programming concepts of subs, such as variables declaration, value assignment, simple looping and judgmental statement, are explained. Trainees are encouraged to modify the codes and to see what happens. They are not expected to write correct codes at this stage but are required to understand what goes wrong and how the bugs are fixed. The second day is slow because almost all trainees are not yet familiar with the VBA environment and programming languages and they have never written codes before.

After the first 2-day section, the trainees' homework is to read introductory materials on Excel VBA and to a prepare two-page report on what applications they plan to design for their projects before the second 2-day session. They are suggested to attempt a simple documentation project instead of a complex one. The second session is the most exhausting period and when key programming knowledge and skills will be taught. This is a critical moment for the trainees because it covers the materials and logics with which nurses are unfamiliar and which they have never been taught before. They need to be encouraged to believe that programming is not difficult and that they can survive this stage. In addition, training materials are given and well designed processes are utilized.

During the entire 4 days of Stage IV, entitled Project, the core strategy is to cover only one sample, which is completed in functions and meaningful to nurses, such as nursing evaluation documentation, patient satisfaction evaluation or nursing scheduling. This demonstrating sample needs to be designed to meet nurses' work needs with minimum use of programming modules and skills. It is expected that nurses can develop their own applications by modifying examples to fit into their individual or departmental needs. It is not a good idea to ask nurses to develop applications from scratch.

For example, in a satisfaction evaluation sample (Fig. 25.2), a case of only nine basic modules is used, which could then be "copied" and "modified" to design any satisfaction evaluation questionnaire with as many as 5-point Likert-scale questions. Another nurse scheduling example is shown in Figs. 25.3–25.5. The operation flow (Fig. 25.3) and the corresponding interfaces (Fig. 25.4) of the application are illustrated step by step. The sample is decomposed from the userforms (1 of Fig. 25.5), through the way users

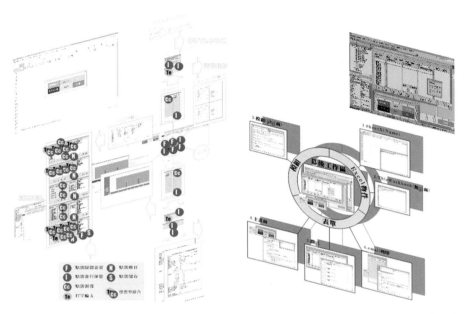

Fig. 25.2 The operating flow (*left*) and the technical components (*right*) of a Excel VBA-based training satisfaction evaluation form (permitted to be used by the *Perspectives in Nursing Science*)

interacted with the system (2 of Fig. 25.5) to the exact codes (6 of Fig. 25.5). Understanding the connection of codes to the ways users would interact with the system, and then the entire design of system, nurses could better learn how the application could be developed from their needs to the codes.

Trainees need to decide how to organize the worksheets first before the coding. Worksheets are used to store data and key parameter values such as items of disease history, display the analytical charts and tables, and create the paper-form-like display for print out by combining form templates and data. These are the information management needs for the project of nursing work. One feature of Excel worksheet is its representation and organization of data in columns and rows of cells and in theoretically unlimited numbers of worksheets.

Stage IV is separated into two 2-day sessions. In the first day, cases of codes from the minimum components of the sample are used to teach trainees programming fundamentals such as variable, looping and judgmental logics (6 of Fig. 25.5). All trainees are required to write all codes so they can really complete an application development project at the end of training and go through the details at each programming process. In the second day, trainees are taught how a userform interface is designed by arranging various control items, such as textbox and command button, and maneuvering their property values to change color, font size, etc. Each of the data they plan to collect for the work needs to have corresponding control items for users to respond to. It is emphasized that all control items need to be assigned a meaningful but nonreluctant name before starting to write the codes.

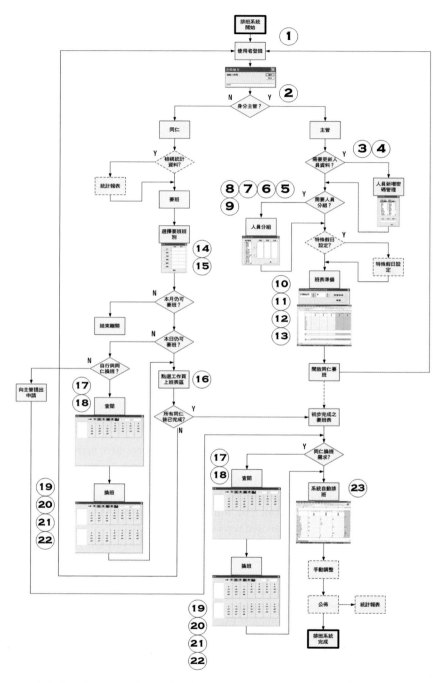

Fig. 25.3 The function map and operating flow of a concise nurse scheduling support system (permitted to be used by the *Perspectives in Nursing Science*)

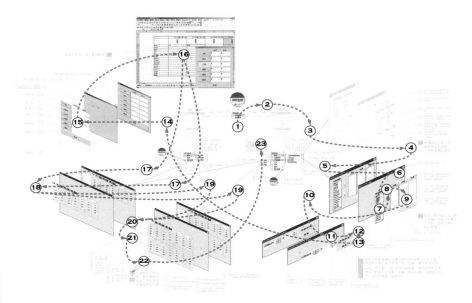

Fig. 25.4 The decomposition map of interfaces of a concise nursing scheduling support system (permitted to be used by the *Perspectives in Nursing Science*)

There is also an issue of interface efficiency. For example, the pull-down combo-box design may save space for the layout, but the users will need to do two taps to finish one data entry work. Using a list-box design takes more space, but the users can easily see the selections and can enter data with only one tap. The ease of use and prevention of errors are the criteria to decide the final design.

The homework for the second 2-day session is for trainees to design the main userform interface for their project. Trainees should first examine the original paper form to decide what data will be collected and think about their workflow so the interface can be easy to use. All trainees will find the benefits of learning programming at this moment. They will realize that it is not easy to communicate with IT people because while nurses care about the practical purposes of information system, IT people are thinking about the computer codes and data items in a different language. They will also find that the design of userform interfaces can help them think about the issues of usability and workflow. Also, the user-forms could be used as a supporting tool for them to express their needs and better communicate with IT people in the future. Most interestingly, the userform interface design is so easy and no special programming knowledge and skills are prerequired. To allow trainees to have time to work on the homework and rest after their first time programming training, the last 2-day session occurs 2 weeks later.

The entire fifth day is used to teach subs and functions of the minimum components of sample with two important concepts: event-driven programming and separation of parameters from computer codes. Both concepts are common in programming but sometimes even IT people fail to perform them correctly. The event-driven concept asks the programmers to consider how users will interact with systems and core codes will be saved to the

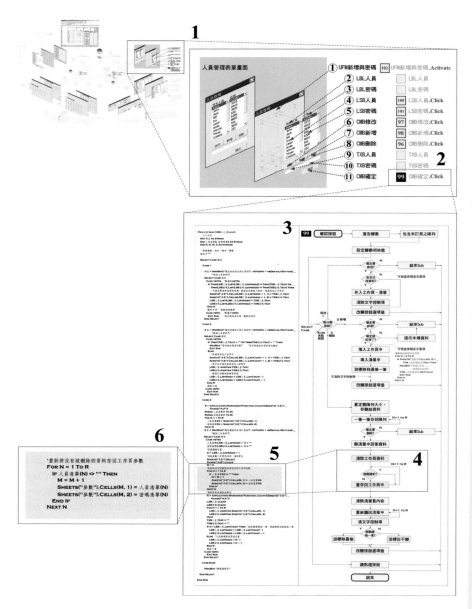

Fig. 25.5 The drilling-down of programming from interface design (*1*), through events which users interact with system (*2*), to flow-chart of codes (*3*–*6*) (permitted to be used by the *Perspectives in Nursing Science*)

corresponding methods of control items. The separation of parameters from the codes emphasizes the flexibility and maintenance of codes. For example, if the parameter values of disease history are stored in the worksheet and there is modification of the items, we only need to change the list items in worksheet without worrying about finding and changing the codes every time.

The last day will summarize all codes of minimum components and discuss how to extend to complete the entire sample. Other advanced skills of programming are partially illustrated with other cases such as importing data from exterior database, customizing the menu and toolbox, and interchanging with other office applications. Stage V begins right after the last day when nurses already have a basic capability of programming knowledge and skills. The trainees are encouraged to work on their projects and other supplementary training courses would be offered if needed. So far, we have observed the development of many successful and interesting projects. Some projects have been successfully implemented for years, such as an Automatic Nursing Shift Scheduling Support System[16] which won the Nursing Innovation Award in Taiwan in 2009. Other projects have been implemented, but they are mainly used for educational and promotional purposes. These are highlighted in the two case studies we discuss in the next section.

Great Solutions: Two Stories

New Design for the Touchscreen-Based Interface Future

Computer products with a touchscreen LCD have become more and more popular. The variety of products includes an all-in-one PC with a single-touch 24-in. touchscreen LCD to a smart phone with a multi-touch 3.5 touch screen LCD. The affordable prices of these products implies a very different interface design for future NIS because touch, as well as voice, have been perceived as the most friendly interfaces by nurses. However, most of the current NISs are still designed with the mouse and keyboard interface and the displays are full of many information control items that are too small to be easily touched. Therefore, it will be very important for the NIS designers to keep this in mind so that applications can be good for the traditional mouse-and-keyboard interface as well as to the touch one. The following case was developed to realize this trend.

The Excel-and-evidence-based applicaion was developed by following the procedure designed in association with the Coloplast Global Advisory Board.[17] This procedure evaluates the condition of the peristomal skin at the time of consultation and can be used to quantify the improvement or degradation of the skin over the time between consultations. This procedure can cut down the amount of time required by a nurse to evaluate a disorder and assists nurses in registering the occurrence, defining the severity, and provide the treatment regimen in time and to monitor the healing process and provide evidence-based clinical data. This procedure was designed on a sheet of paper and guides the nurse with baseline pictures coordinating with colors, scores, sizes, and frames to make users easily follow the instruction and evaluate the condition accurately. The peristomal skin is evaluated in terms of its discolouration, erosion, and tissue overgrowth. The result is represented with a DET score. Each problem is scaled from 0 to 5 to present the area affected and its severity. The evaluation process is shown in Fig. 25.6. The process is numbered and some representative screen shots with the corresponding process are shown in Figs. 25.7–25.10.

New Tool for Meeting Unlimited Documentation Needs

Documentation has been one of the very important tasks for clinical nurses not only for clinical caring but also for administrative purposes. The introduction of a new documentation form occurs quite frequently. Due to the mobility need of nurses, the solution of documentation installed in a mobile device can make the documentation much easier. However, the design needs to consider usability issues. The display size of mobile devices is often small and sometimes documentation will be very complex such as the assessment for long-term care residents. The following case shows how a general documentation design editor with data analysis capability was designed under a set of interface usability design principles to be able to design a documentation application consisting of more than 250 assessment questions.

This is an Excel-based point-of-care development tool support system. It was developed by an informatics nurse to assist users to easily design handheld-based documentation applications on their own, based on a set of interface design principles. It is also beneficial as it resolves the difficulty of the small screen display common to handheld devices.[18] The tools also will utilize the built-in data processing capability of Excel for database management, statistical analysis, and chart making to simplify the information management effort after the results are synchronized.

The support system is composed of four components: the Excel-based Form Designer, the PDA Template, the Data Transferring and the Excel-based Data Management. The PDA Template is precoded with a set of usability-engineered interface design principles, which is called as 3+ Hierarchical Grid Interface Design Principles,19 and is capable of transferring the assessment information synchronized from a Palm-based database generated from Excel on a personal computer to a PDA documentation application. The Form Designer, Data Transferring and Data Management components were all PC applications and programmed in Excel VBA. These three components were used mainly for designing the PDA documentation application, transferring data between the PDA devices and desktop, and data management and analysis.

Screen shots of the system and application are shown in Fig. 25.11–25.14.

Summary

The purpose of informatics competency is to assist users to simplify their information processing responsibility and to achieve better outcomes by the use of better information and communication techniques. As the capability of tools is evolving, the contents of informatics competency should evolve too. Many personal productivity software are

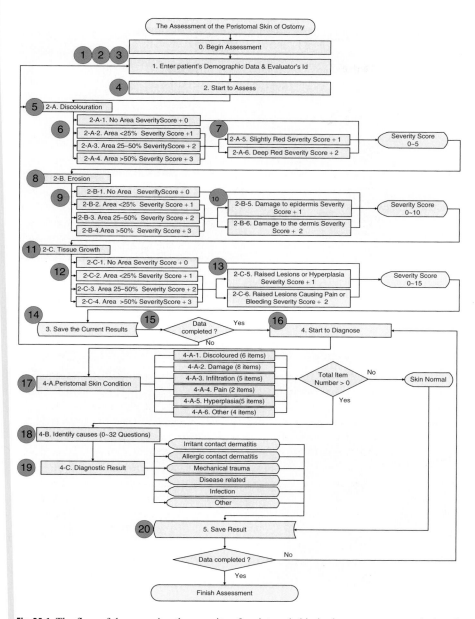

Fig. 25.6 The flow of the assessing the severity of peristomal skin in the support system designed with Excel VBA. The numbers inside the flowchart symbols stands for the category and structure of assessment results and those in *green circle* represents the procedural steps taken by nurses

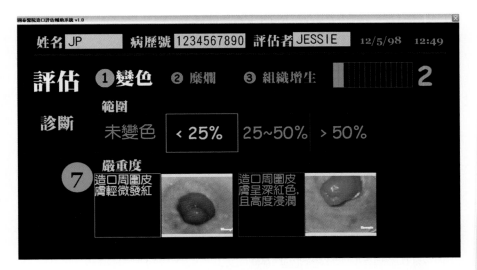

Fig. 25.7 Screen shot of step 7: end of evaluating the colors of skin, turning to blue by touching the 2-A-5/6 screen. During the assessment process, the severity score was shown at *right*, which is 2 for this case

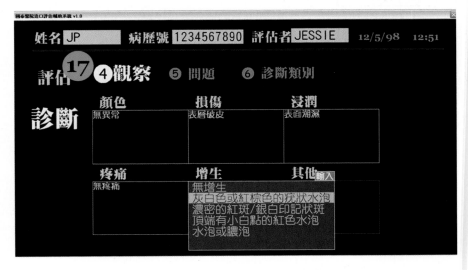

Fig. 25.8 Screen Shot of Step 17: Assessment of Skin Problems in the 4-A screen

indeed equipped with very powerful tools which can highly extend the limit of the competency level. We have introduced and discussed how a better use of built-in VBA in Excel, as an example, can make nurses design and create simple, effective and affordable information support solutions for their nursing needs. Competency can assist nurses to be more than power users but also creative information solutions designers and leaders.

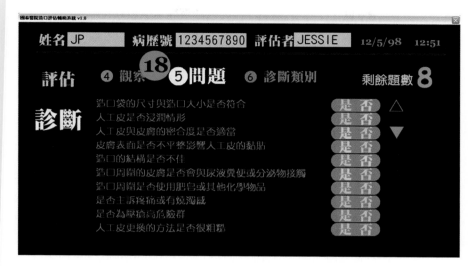

Fig. 25.9 Screen shot of step 18: 9 yes–no questions for patients to answer for latter diagnose in screen 4-B

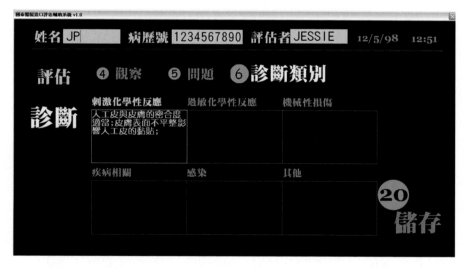

Fig. 25.10 Screen shot of step 20: accomplishment of assessment with diagnosis. Nurse then touch the big save button to save the result

Programming can be thought of manipulating machines/computers to do what we expect them to do with a language which can be understood. Learning a new language is not easy and it takes time. The built-in VBA in personal productivity software is quite easy to learn and to use. To this end, there are many text books and training materials available at a very reasonable price. Once the nurses can master the language, they will suddenly find the doorway to master more ICT techniques and then better understand how to collaborate information technology personnel for larger HIS projects.

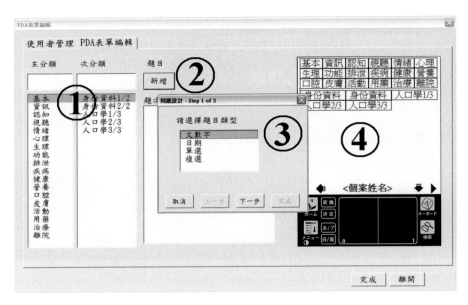

Fig. 25.11 The left-hand side of the form design interface shows (1) the category of questions, (2) adding new questions, and (3) the question information. The *right-hand side* is the preview on PDA

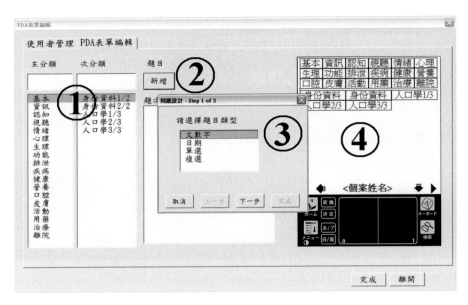

Fig. 25.12 All data about the documentation form are stored in an Excel worksheet which will be saved to a PDA data file in a designated directory awaiting synchronization to PDA

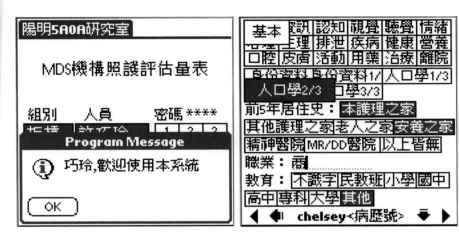

Fig. 25.13 Screen shot of logon and assessment pages on PDA after the documentation data are synchronized from the PC

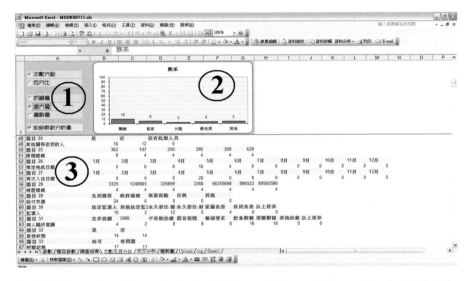

Fig. 25.14 Screen shot of data analysis after the documentation results are synchronized back to the PC. Users can then decide (1) what kind of charts to make and the Excel application will then show (2) the chart with (3) the corresponding results

Nurses as well as other health care professionals could really explore the possibilities and potentials within any personal productive software he or she has mastered. Mastering the programming tools' built in software will certainly make health care professionals better able to control the machine and thus achieve better outcomes which are readily needed.

Acknowledgments   We deeply appreciate Miss Chiao-Ling Hsu, MS, RN, Informatics Nurse at the Taipei Municipal Wan-Fang Hospital, on her support to share her application with us in this chapter and Joan Kiel, PhD, CHPS, Associate Professor, Department of Health Management Systems, University Compliance Officer – HIPAA, on her valuable comments and helpful editing.

References

1. ECDL/ICDL Advanced.http://www.ecdl.org/products/index.jsp?b=0-102&pID=102&nID=109; 2009. Accessed 27.06.09.
2. TIGER. Collaborative executive summary report. http://www.tigersummit.com/uploads/ TIGER_Collaborative_Exec_Summary_040509.pdf; 2009. Accessed 27.06.09.
3. ECDL/ICDL Advanced Spreadsheets, Module AM4. http://www.ecdl.org/products/index. jsp?b=0-102&pID=109&nID=124; 2009. Accessed 27.06.09.
4. Chang P, Hsu CL, Hou IC, Tu MH, Liu CW. The end user computing strategy of using Excel VBA in promoting nursing informatics in Taiwan. *Perspect Nurs Sci.* 2008;5(1):45-58.
5. Economist Intelligent Unit. How technology sectors grow? Benchmarking IT industry competitiveness. http://graphics.eiu.com/upload/BSA_2008.pdf; 2008. Accessed 10.07.09.
6. Liu SC. Attitudes of nurses toward end-user development. In: Hyeoun-Ae Park (Chair) *Nursing Informatics Conference, Seoul, Korea*; 2006.
7. IMIA National Member Societies. http://www.imia.org/members/national_list.lasso; 2009. Accessed 10.07.09.
8. Clark TD. Corporate systems management: an overview and research perspective. *Commun ACM.* 1992;35(2):60-75.
9. Guimaraes T, Igbaria M. Exploring the relationship between EUC problems and success. *Inf Resour Manage J.* 1996;9(2):5-15.
10. Mclean E, Kappelman L, Thompson J. Converging end-user and corporate computing. *Commun ACM.* 1993;36(12):79-92.
11. Hou IC, Chang P, Liu SC. Applying advanced Excel techniques in nursing. *J Taiwan Assoc Medical Inform.* 2006;15(3):69-80.
12. Igbaria M, Parasuraman S, Pavri FN. A path analytic study of the determinants of microcomputer usage. *J Manage Syst.* 1990;2(2):1-14.
13. Zinatelli N. A case study and survey of factors affecting EUC success in small firms in new zealand. Unpublished doctoral dissertation, New Zealand: University of Canterbury; 1994.
14. Hou IC, Chang P. A feasible strategy of promoting nursing informatics by end user computing. *AMIA.* 2005;2005:P985.
15. Walkenbach J. *Excel 2003 power programming with VBA.* Indianapolis: Wiley; 2004.
16. Cheng ST, Wung SH, Chang P. The development of a heuristic-based excel scheduling support system for nurses. In: The Ninth International Congress on Nursing Informatics (NI2006), Seoul, Korea; 2006:792.
17. Coloplast. The ostomy skin tool: a peristomal skin assessment tool. http://www.coloplast. com/ostomycare/topics/educationtools/theostomyskintool/about/pages/moreaboutthetool. aspx; 2009. Accessed 10.07.09.
18. Hsu CL, Chang P. Developing an SDK of usability-engineered handheld evaluation aid. *AMIA.* 2007;2007:P982.
19. Chang P, Hsu CL, Liou YM, Kuo YY, Lan CF. Design and development of interface design principles for complex documentation using PDAs. *CIN-Computers Informatics Nursing.* (in press)

Appendix

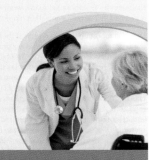

The TIGER Initiative

Collaborating to Integrate Evidence and Informatics into Nursing Practice and Education: *An Executive Summary*

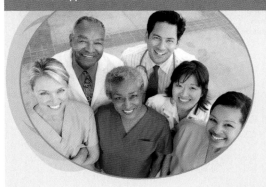

Technology Informatics Guiding Education Reform (TIGER)
www.tigersummit.com

M.J. Ball et al. (eds.), *Nursing Informatics*,
DOI: 10.1007/978-1-84996-278-0, © Springer-Verlag London Limited 2011

EXECUTIVE SUMMARY

The TIGER Initiative, an acronym for **T**echnology **I**nformatics **G**uiding **E**ducation **R**eform, was formed in 2004 to bring together nursing stakeholders to develop a shared vision, strategies, and specific actions for improving nursing practice, education, and the delivery of patient care through the use of health information technology (IT). In 2006, the TIGER Initiative convened a summit of nursing stakeholders to develop, publish, and commit to carrying out the action steps defined within this plan. The Summary Report titled *Evidence and Informatics Transforming Nursing: 3-Year Action Steps toward a 10-Year Vision* is available on the website at www.tigersummit.com.

A COLLABORATIVE APPROACH

Since 2007, hundreds of volunteers have joined the TIGER Initiative to continue the action steps defined at the Summit. Collaborative teams were formed to accelerate the action plan within nine key topic areas.

Each collaborative team researched their subject with the perspective of "What does every practicing nurse need to know about this topic?" The teams identified resources, references, gaps, and areas that need further development, and provide recommendations for the industry to accelerate the adoption of IT for nursing. The TIGER Initiative builds upon and recognizes the work of organizations, programs, research, and related initiatives in the academic, practice, and government sector, and references this work within the "references" and "resources" sections of the nine individual collaborative reports. Areas that need further action steps are listed in the "recommendations" section of each collaborative report.

SUMMARY REPORT

This report provides an executive summary of the TIGER activities through 2008, as well as a brief synopsis of each of the findings and recommendations of the nine collaborative teams. The comprehensive report from each of the nine collaborative teams will be available on the TIGER website at www.tigersummit.com.

COLLABORATIVE TEAMS

1. **Standards & Interoperability (p. 10)**

2. **National Health Information Technology (IT) Agenda (p. 12)**

3. **Informatics Competencies (p. 14)**

4. **Education & Faculty Development (p. 17)**

5. **Staff Development (p. 19)**

6. **Usability & Clinical Application Design (p.23)**

7. **Virtual Demonstration Center (p. 26)**

8. **Leadership Development (p. 21)**

9. **Consumer Empowerment & Personal Health Record (p. 28)**

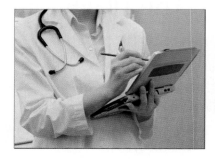

EXECUTIVE SUMMARY

The TIGER Initiative focused on raising awareness with nursing stakeholders in three areas:

1. **Develop a U.S. nursing workforce capable of using electronic health records to improve the delivery of healthcare.**

   In 2004, President Bush mandated that all Americans will be using electronic health records by the year 2014. As reported in *Building the Workforce for Health Information Transformation*[1], "A work force capable of innovating, implementing, and using health communications and information technology (HIT) will be critical to healthcare's success." President Obama continued this momentum when he took office in 2009, proposing to "Let us be the generation that reshapes healthcare to compete in the digital age." Less than 30 days after taking office, President Obama signed the American Recovery and Reinvestment Act, earmarking $19 billion to develop an electronic health information technology infrastructure that will improve the efficiency and access of healthcare to all Americans. In addition to the substantial investment in capital, technology and resources, the success of delivering an electronic healthcare platform will require an investment in people—to build an informatics-aware healthcare workforce.

   This has accelerated the need to ensure that healthcare providers obtain competencies needed to work with electronic records, including basic computer skills, information literacy, and an understanding of informatics and information management capabilities. A comprehensive approach to education reform is necessary to reach the current workforce of nearly 3 million practicing nurses. The average age of a practicing nurse in the U.S. is 47 years. These individuals are "digital immigrants[2]," as they grew up without digital technology, had to adopt it later, and some may not have had the opportunity to be educated on its use or be comfortable with technology. This is opposed to "digital natives": younger individuals that have

grown up with digital technology such as computers, the Internet, mobile phones, and MP3. There are a number of digital immigrants in the nursing workforce who have not mastered basic computer competencies, let alone information literacy and how to use HIT effectively and efficiently to enhance nursing practice.

Five of the TIGER collaborative teams developed recommendations focused on how to prepare nurses to practice in this digital era. The **TIGER Informatics Competencies Collaborative (TICC)** team helped develop a minimum set of informatics competencies that all nurses need to have to practice today.

> **Five Collaborative Teams Focused on Workforce Development:**
>
> 1. Informatics Competencies
>
> 2. Education and Faculty Development
>
> 3. Staff Development
>
> 4. Leadership Development
>
> 5. Virtual Demonstration Center

The **TIGER Education and Faculty Development Collaborative** team focused on engaging stakeholders that influence and deliver nursing education and licensing, including academic institutions representing all levels of nursing education, educationally-focused professional organizations, federal organizations that fund nursing education, and state boards of nursing.

There was widespread support of this effort from all of the key stakeholders. Most notably, both the American Association of Colleges of Nursing (AACN) and the National League for Nursing (NLN) have

---

[1] AHIMA/FORE and AMIA, (2006). *Building the workforce*. Available online at www.ahima.org/emerging_issues/.
[2] Prensky, M. (2001, October). Digital natives, digital immigrants. *On the Horizon*. Available online at www.marcprensky.com/writing/.

EXECUTIVE SUMMARY

supported the inclusion of informatics competencies in all nursing curricula moving forward.

The Health Resources and Services Administration (HRSA) has recognized the critical need for faculty development efforts related to informatics education and has made federal funds available for related projects under the Integrated Technology into Nursing Education and Practice Initiative (ITNEP).

To address the educational needs of the existing nursing workforce, the **TIGER Staff Development Collaborative** team focused on practical approaches to professional development that meet the minimum informatics competencies defined by TICC.

The **TIGER Leadership Development Collaborative** team expanded on the model developed by TICC to include additional competencies that nursing leaders need to accelerate successful adoption of electronic health records. Professional organizations focused on nursing leaders such as the American Nurses Association (ANA), American Organization of Nurse Executives (AONE), American Academy of Nursing (AAN), Sigma Theta Tau International (STTI), and American Nurses Credentialing Center (ANCC) Magnet™ Program helped disseminate the TIGER agenda to their members and provided suggestions on how to integrate health IT into their practice.

Finally, one of the barriers to improving informatics education for nurses remains the limited access to information systems and technology that could improve healthcare delivery. Nursing schools frequently rely on the clinical practicum site to provide access to and education on electronic health records. In any given practice environment, exposure to technology is limited to the systems that are currently deployed.   Yet this is inadequate to understand the capabilities that health IT can offer nurses. One TIGER collaborative team, the **Virtual Demonstration Center**, developed a virtual learning center supported by the Healthcare Information and Management Systems Society

(HIMSS) in order to provide exposure and education to nurses on a variety of technologies and information systems available today and in the future. The TIGER Initiative recommends further exploration into virtual learning platforms to improve access to information technology education.

2. **Engage more nurses in the development of a national healthcare information technology (NHIT) infrastructure.**

The TIGER Initiative focused on engaging nursing stakeholders from various practice settings by working with nursing professional organizations. Nurses comprise more than 55% of the current healthcare workforce in the U.S., and they can contribute to the redesign of the information flow of healthcare to be more efficient, patient-centered, equitable, accessible, and safe. Nurses are often at the center of care coordination for the patient and are well versed on the workflow and information flow critical to minimizing shortfalls with communication handoffs in the delivery of healthcare. Some practice specialty areas in nursing have been historically underrepresented in the development of use cases, technical infrastructure, and development of standards. This leaves a gap in creating interoperable electronic health records that cover the continuum of healthcare delivery through different practice environments. Two TIGER collaborative teams focused on engaging more nurses in the development of the NHIT infrastructure—the **Standards and Interoperability** team and the **National Health IT Agenda** team. Both of these teams recruited nurses from various practice settings to participate in use case discussions and standards organizations, and to provide their expertise with organizations representing the Office of the National Coordinator such as the Healthcare Information Technology Standards Panel (HITSP), American Health Information Community (AHIC), and Certification Commission for Healthcare Information Technology (CCHIT). Both teams also developed an inventory of standards and National Health IT activities relevant to nurses, as well as tutorials to assist in educating nurses about the urgency of these activities. Much work remains as the national and regional effort to develop and demonstrate health IT infrastructure is just getting

EXECUTIVE SUMMARY

started, so the effort to engage nurses from all practice and educational settings needs to remain a high priority.

> **Two Collaborative Teams Focused on National Health IT Initiatives:**
>
> 1. Standards and Interoperability
>
> 2. National Health IT Agenda

3. **Accelerate adoption of smart, standards-based, interoperable technology that will make healthcare delivery safer, more efficient, timely, accessible, and patient-centered.**

Studies have demonstrated that the current information systems and technology in practice do not meet the workflow and information flow requirements of nurses, and this has hampered adoption of electronic health records. Nurses and their interdisciplinary colleagues need innovative technology to simplify their work and provide them clinical guidance for the safety of their patients. Additional nursing input into the design and implementation process can improve technology solutions to be more usable, accessible, timely, interoperable, patient-centered, and improve the safety and efficiency of nursing care.

Three collaborative teams—**Usability, Consumer Empowerment/Personal Health Records,** and **Standards and Interoperability**—have developed an inventory of resources and guidelines to enable nurses to participate in the design process for both provider and patient-centered applications. The recommendations of these three collaborative teams

build upon the efforts of organizations that are focused on the development and adoption of standards, usability, and personal health records, including the vendors that develop technology solutions. All teams advocate for broader participation of nurses in all of these interrelated efforts.

> **Three Collaborative Teams Focused on Improving Technology Solutions:**
>
> 1. Usability and Clinical Application Design
>
> 2. Consumer Empowerment and Personal Health Records
>
> 3. Standards and Interoperability

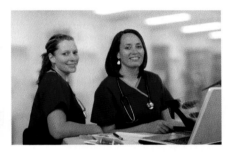

BACKGROUND

National attention on health IT has accelerated since 2004 when President Bush announced plans to support adoption of electronic health records for all Americans. In January 2005, a small group of nursing leaders and advocates met and resolved to **strengthen the voice of the nursing profession** in the transformation of healthcare for the 21st century. This group organized the Technology Informatics Guiding Education Reform (TIGER) Initiative.

NURSING ENGAGEMENT

Nursing has embraced the opportunity to reform healthcare using technology as an enabler. In 2006, the TIGER Initiative held an interactive summit titled "*Evidence and Informatics Transforming Nursing.*" The summit gathered over 100 leaders from the nation's nursing administration, practice, education, informatics, technology organizations, government agencies, and other key stakeholders to create **a vision for the future of nursing that bridges the quality chasm with information technology, enabling nurses to use informatics in practice and education to provide safer, higher-quality patient care.** While many of the statements resonate with a wide range of interdisciplinary health professions, the initial focus of the agenda was nurses and the nursing profession.

THE VISION

The vision focuses on seven components defined and ranked by the summit attendees using a wireless audience response system. Attendees concurred that essential components are interdependent and that culture is essential

to all other six areas. Together, all seven components act as pillars for the TIGER vision and provide the framework for TIGER's action plan.

TIGER VISION

Allow informatics tools, principles, theories and practices to be used by nurses to make healthcare safer, effective, efficient, patient-centered, timely and equitable.

Interweave enabling technologies transparently into nursing practice and education, making information technology the stethoscope for the 21st century.

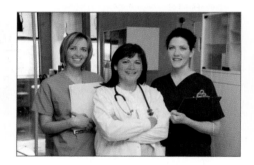

BACKGROUND

With the seven pillars as the framework, the TIGER Summit attendees developed an action plan to identify steps that the nursing profession must take over the next three years to achieve the TIGER vision.

Each of the organizations participating in the TIGER Initiative agreed that nursing must integrate informatics technology into education and practice. Each has pledged to incorporate the TIGER vision and action steps into their organization's strategic plans. Each fulfilled a critical role by distributing the TIGER Summit Summary Report within their network to engage additional support for this agenda. A list of the participating organizations is available on the TIGER website at www.tigersummit.com/participants.

From the TIGER Summit in 2006 until now, these organizations, together with hundreds of additional volunteers and industry experts, have collaborated to complete the action steps necessary towards achieving the TIGER vision. Articles and presentations at regional, national, and international conferences have brought TIGER activities to nursing colleagues. The TIGER Initiative remains focused on raising awareness of the need to engage nurses in the national effort to prepare the healthcare workforce towards *effective* adoption of **electronic health records**.

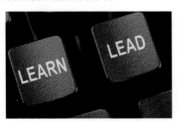

Seven Pillars of the TIGER Vision

1. **Management and Leadership:** Revolutionary leadership that drives, empowers, and executes the transformation of healthcare.

2. **Education:** Collaborative learning communities that maximize the possibilities of technology toward knowledge development and dissemination, driving rapid deployment, and implementation of best practices.

3. **Communication and Collaboration:** Standardized, person-centered, technology-enabled processes to facilitate teamwork and relationships across the continuum of care.

4. **Informatics Design:** Evidence-based, interoperable intelligence systems that support education and practice to foster quality care and safety.

5. **Information Technology:** Smart, people-centered, affordable technologies that are universal, useable, useful, and standards-based.

6. **Policy:** Consistent, incentives-based initiatives (organizational and governmental) that support advocacy and coalition-building, achieving and resourcing an ethical culture of safety.

7. **Culture:** A respectful, open system that leverages technology and informatics across multiple disciplines in an environment where all stakeholders trust each other to work together towards the goal of high quality and safety.

TIGER IMPACT

TIGER's mission of reaching the 3 million U.S. practicing nurses required widespread and rapid dissemination and support of the vision, action steps, and ongoing work with the collaborative teams. One of the challenges to reaching nurses is that there is no one professional organization representing all nurses. Instead, nurses are organized by professional associations that represent their role or specialty. As the timeframe for completing the action steps was 3 years, TIGER was intentionally structured as a program versus an organization. TIGER relied on the participating organizations to complete the action steps, recognizing that the organizations had the membership and existing mechanisms in place to organize activities and distribute information.

COLLABORATIVE APPROACH

By design, the TIGER Initiative was comprised of representatives from nursing specialty organizations that could work through the action plan *within their own organizations*. The support received from the practice specialties was timely and set a new industry precedent in raising awareness for TIGER in the broader nursing community.

To accelerate their progress, nine collaborative teams were developed to help increase the *collaboration across the participating organizations*. These teams were organized around strategic topics, and each was led by industry leaders and open to any interested participant. Over 400 individuals responded to the open call for participation on the collaborative teams.

Each of the nine collaborative teams developed their own wikis, similar to a website, to share information. The wikis were used as a project workspace and resource to communicate amongst the team, to other collaborative teams, and with the public. Most of the communication with the teams was done via webinars, or web meetings, teleconferences,

and email lists. A TIGER Advisory Council, comprised of the collaborative leaders and the program director, met monthly to coordinate activities and review progress. By the end of 2008, over 1,400 individuals had joined the TIGER effort and are helping to achieve the TIGER vision throughout the healthcare community. Most of this outreach was accomplished by the diverse communities that make up the TIGER Initiative, and a sampling of their activities is described in the following pages.

NURSING INFORMATICS COMMUNITY

Nursing informatics organizations provided numerous opportunities for TIGER presentations and meetings. The American Medical Informatics Association (AMIA) and Healthcare Information and Management Systems Society (HIMSS) organized TIGER presentations at several national, regional, and international conferences. The Alliance for Nursing Informatics (ANI), an umbrella organization for the nursing informatics community, provided financial and strategic support to TIGER for the collaborative teams. Nursing informatics organizations such as CARING, American Nursing Informatics Association (ANIA), Minnesota Nursing INformatics Group (MINING) and New England Nursing Informatics Consortium (NENIC) not only welcomed TIGER presentations at their meetings but were essential to distributing TIGER surveys and requests for information, and they were active participants on the collaborative workgroups.

PRACTICE SPECIALTY COMMUNITY

Several specialty organizations presented on TIGER at their regional and national conferences. For example, the Association of periOperative Registered Nurses (AORN), the National Association of Clinical Nurse Specialists (NACNS), and the Oncology Nursing Society (ONS) accepted TIGER presentations at their national conferences. Many participating organizations also presented on TIGER at

TIGER IMPACT

specialized conferences within their organizations, such as state chapter meetings or conferences focused on technology. Numerous articles were published in journals distributed to nurses, including **Nursing Outlook, CIN (Computers, Informatics, Nursing), Nursing Management,** and **Journal of Health Information Management.** Several organizations published articles in their member newsletters or journals, including the American Society of Peri-Anesthesia Nurses (ASPAN), Association of Women's Health, Obstetric and Neonatal Nurses (AWHONN), and the ONS. Ongoing work within the specialty organizations is planned. To name a few examples, the National Nursing Staff Development Organization (NNSDO) has plans to further develop the informatics competencies recommendations. The American Health Information Management Association (AHIMA) is planning a conference in late 2009 to engage allied health professionals in adopting informatics competencies.

NURSING LEADERSHIP COMMUNITY

Nursing leadership organizations provided critical support for TIGER, enhancing visibility and access to nursing executives. The American Nurses Association (ANA) supported TIGER on several committees and provided strategic support through the ANI. The American Nurses Credentialing Center, a division of ANA, scheduled a TIGER workshop at their National Magnet™ Conference, as did Sigma Theta Tau International (STTI). AONE provided access to nurse executives for the TIGER Leadership survey, and also facilitated TIGER presentations at both state and national conferences. Long term care nurse executives contributed numerous articles and presentations related to technology and the TIGER effort through their alliance with the National Association Directors of Nursing Administration in Long Term Care (NADONA/LTC). The American Academy of Nursing (AAN) publishes a monthly column on technology and devoted an entire issue of *Nursing Outlook* to nursing informatics.

EDUCATIONAL COMMUNITY

Nearly a fourth of the leaders and participants on the TIGER collaborative teams came from the academic community. As described in the TIGER Education and Faculty Development Collaborative report, all major stakeholders were active participants in the TIGER action plan. Numerous presentations to this community were done at national, state, and local levels. Comprehensive programs focused on nursing informatics are held annually at the University of Maryland through the Summer Institute in Nursing Informatics (SINI) and at the Rutgers International Nursing Computer and Technology Conference. Academic partnerships with industry are proliferating, and the National League for Nursing has plans to share resources on their website at www.nln.org.

STATE-WIDE COLLABORATION

Minnesota developed a state-wide approach to TIGER—bringing together stakeholders in an annual Minnesota TIGER conference. Other states have also brought together the key organizations to discuss issues related to technology adoption—including Massachusetts (Massachusetts Organization of Nurse Executives), North California, and California.

VENDOR COMMUNITY

Healthcare IT vendors that develop technology were active with TIGER in numerous ways. Many of the leaders of the TIGER collaborative teams were supported by the vendor community. The vendor sponsors of the TIGER Summit developed an interactive "Gallery Walk" to demonstrate technology capabilities to the attendees and supplied demonstrations and presentations to the TIGER Virtual Demonstration Center. Several vendors, such as GE Healthcare, McKesson, Cerner, CPM Resource Center and others, presented TIGER at their user group conferences or via webinars focused on their nursing community.

STANDARDS & INTEROPERABILITY COLLABORATIVE

One of the obstacles to widespread adoption of electronic health records is the lack of standardization of nursing-related data. The language that nurses use to describe their observations, actions, goals, and activities is important in communicating with other nurses as well as other healthcare professionals. The way that nursing data is organized is important to ensure consistent documentation and clear communication with other healthcare professions. If standardized across an organization, nursing data can be compared to identify practices that improve patient outcomes and those that do not. If nursing data is organized in a standard way, it can also be shared and compared across regional or national databases to identify trends, report outcomes, and research new opportunities to improve nursing practice. Consensus on the terms that are used to describe nursing problems, observations, actions, goals, outcomes and interventions is critical to aggregate, analyze and share nursing data with others. This process is called "standards harmonization," and requires the involvement of nurses representing different specialties, different environments, and different roles to be comprehensive and meaningful to all practicing nurses.

Interoperable systems will assist clinicians in delivering safe, effective, efficient and patient-centered care. Clinical data standards are the building blocks towards interoperable systems, including electronic health records (EHRs), electronic medical records (EMRs), and personal health records (PHRs). It is important that nurses understand these standards and their impact on care delivery.

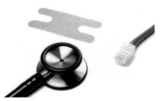

Standard - A definition or format that has been approved by a recognized standards organization or is accepted as a de facto standard by the industry. A standard specifies a well-defined approach that supports a business process and: (1) has been agreed upon by a group of experts; (2) has been publicly vetted; (3) provides rules, guidelines, or characteristics; (4) helps to ensure that materials, products, processes, and services are fit for their intended purpose; (5) is available in an accessible format; and (6) is subject to an ongoing review and revision process.

-    Dr. John Halamka, Chair of the Healthcare Information
     Technology Standards Panel (HITSP)

Interoperability - "Interoperability" means the ability to communicate and exchange data accurately, effectively, securely, and consistently with different information technology systems, software applications, and networks in various settings, and exchange data such that clinical or operational purpose and meaning of the data are preserved and unaltered.

-    President Bush, Executive Order (2006) to mandating the
     Federal Government use of interoperable standards

The benefits to nurses to adopt a standardized way of describing nursing practice and organizing nursing data are:

• Accurately describe the care delivered by nurses and facilitate communication among nurses and other healthcare providers.

• Enable the comparison of nursing data across clinical populations, practice settings, time, and geographic regions.

• Allow measurement of the impact of nursing interventions in relation to patient outcomes.

STANDARDS & INTEROPERABILITY COLLABORATIVE

- Provide timely access to evidence-based knowledge, especially during the delivery of patient care.

The TIGER Standards and Interoperability Collaborative team was formed to accelerate the following action steps identified at the TIGER Summit:

- Integrate industry standards for health IT interoperability with clinical standards for practice and education.
- Educate practice and education communities on health IT standards.
- Establish use of standards and set hard deadlines for adoption.

The TIGER Standards and Interoperability Collaborative team developed work groups to create tools and resources to promote health IT standards and interoperability. The first workgroup compiled a catalogue of nursing-related standards, standard organizations, and initiatives that are essential to building a national electronic health record framework. The standards in the catalogue are organized by what they describe: data exchange messages, terminologies, documents and assessment instruments, and technical infrastructure. The catalogue, titled the "Nursing Health IT Standards Catalogue" is available on the TIGER website at www.tigersummit.com/standards.

Another work group developed a series of web-based tutorials to educate nurses on the benefits of interoperable systems and the standards adoption process required to achieve interoperability in healthcare. These tutorials explain why technology and informatics are important to improve patient safety, describe the various types of standards and sources (authors) of standards, identify the nursing terminologies recognized by the American Nurses Association, and explain the role of standards to improve workflow and provide decision support at the point of care.

A third work group focused on the dissemination strategy of the work of the collaborative to the broader nursing audience. This work group is an awareness campaign designed to stress the importance of adopting standards to achieve interoperability for widespread health information exchange.

All stakeholders play a role in the standards harmonization and adoption process to achieve safer, higher-quality, more efficient, timely, and patient-centered healthcare. The successful adoption of standards requires consensus and adoption on a national scale, and to that end, more nursing input is needed in two ways:

- For the betterment of clinical practice and the profession, nurses must embrace collaboration and build a consensus agreement regarding standardization of nursing language.

- Nurses have a professional responsibility to be engaged in standards development, harmonization and implementation activities, including encouraging adoption of and patient engagement in personal health records and electronic health records.

These efforts will support the overarching effort of the TIGER Initiative to ensure that all nurses are educated in using informatics and thereby empowered to deliver safer, higher-quality patient care.

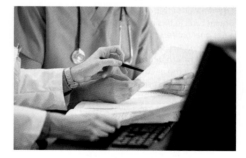

NATIONAL HEALTH IT AGENDA COLLABORATIVE

The escalating cost of the U.S. healthcare system and the need to improve patient safety and reduce medical errors, coupled with national disasters, terrorism, and other unsustainable healthcare trends, has necessitated major healthcare reform in the United States. Focusing on the adoption of electronic health records as a priority within the U.S. National Health IT Agenda is the key driver cited to achieving the transformation needed.

The series of U.S. healthcare reform reports published by Institute of Medicine (IOM), other agencies, and universities concluded that information technology was key to transforming the healthcare system to achieve the IOM aims of safety, effectiveness, patient family centeredness, timeliness, efficiency, and equity. President Bush led the charge by establishing the goal that most Americans would have an EHR by 2014. In April 2004, President Bush issued an Executive Order that established the position and Office of the National Coordinator for Health Information Technology (ONC) within the Department of Health and Human Services (HHS), "to provide leadership for the development and nationwide implementation of an interoperable health information technology infrastructure to improve the quality and efficiency of health care." Bush appointed Dr. David Brailer as the first Coordinator of this office. One of the first steps Brailer took in this new position was to convene a national conference to engage healthcare leaders in discussing the development of a "national health information infrastructure." Recognizing the need to ensure that the nursing profession's expertise is represented in the national HIT agenda and in EHRs, nurse informaticians and executives have advocated the need to transform nursing education and practice via the TIGER Initiative. The TIGER team's vision and strategic action plan was aligned with the ONC's strategic plan to ensure that the nursing profession's voice could be heard at the national level.

As a result of TIGER's strategic plan, the National Health IT Agenda Collaborative was formed. The purpose of this collaborative was to identify the most relevant health IT agenda and policies that are important to the TIGER and the nursing profession's mission and to assist in closing any representation gaps on said policy issues. The collaborative identified three areas where the nursing profession required greater visibility and where their contributions would enhance and promote the national HIT agenda and the transformation of health and care in the United States:

- In clinical, standards, and policy initiatives generated by the AHIC/National eHealth Collaborative (NeHC) and the ONC (such as participation in Workgroups and in Use Cases),

- In the standards harmonization and interoperability efforts of ANSI-HITSP (such as working on the Committees and developing the Interoperability Specifications), and

- In the certification process for HIT products (such as, volunteering for a Workgroup, and reviewing and commenting on the CCHIT Work products).

Since the passage of the American Recovery and Reinvestment Act of 2009, momentum and activities to-date in the areas of governance, policy, technology, and adoption have accelerated in both the federal and private sector. Nursing's involvement in the national HIT agenda, as the largest sector of the U.S. healthcare workforce, is even more urgent and critical today.

The TIGER National Health IT Agenda Collaborative has also developed tutorials (available on their website at www.tigersummit.com) to educate and encourage nurses to participate in HIT-related policy development, healthcare reform, and accelerate widespread HIT adoption by 2014.

NATIONAL HEALTH IT AGENDA COLLABORATIVE

> **National Health IT Organizations that Need Nursing Participation:**
>
> 1. National eHealth Collaborative
>
> 2. Healthcare Information Technology Standards Panel
>
> 3. Certification Commission for Healthcare Information Technology
>
> 4. HIT Policy Committee and HIT Standards Committee

How to Get Involved in the National Health IT Agenda

National eHealth Collaborative (NeHC)

www.nationalehealth.org

NeHC will have significant impact in setting the priorities for standards development and adoption. By participating in the development of these priorities into Value Cases, nurses and nursing informaticians can drive policies and HIT development that meet their needs and represent their practice. Nurses can:

- Become a member.

- Serve on the Board or committees.

- Stay abreast of the meetings and events.

Healthcare Information Technology Standards Panel (HITSP)

www.hitsp.org

The Panel's work is driven by a series of priorities, set by the AHIC/NeHC. Nurses can:

- Participate in the development of Use Cases

- Provide recommendations for Interoperability Specifications and related constructs in their related domain expertise.

- Serve on the Board, the Panel, or the Committees (i.e., Perspective, Domain, or Coordinating Committees).

Certification Commission for Healthcare Information Technology (CCHIT)

www.cchit.org

The best way for nurses to get involved with CCHIT is to

- Submit an application during calls for Commissioners' and Work Group Chairpersons' appointments.

- Volunteer to participate on one of their Work Groups that aligns most closely with the nurse's clinical specialty or expertise.

- Review draft materials and provide comments during Public Comment periods to ensure that nurses' voices are being heard.

- Attend Town Hall in-person meetings, Town Hall teleconference calls, and conference presentations.

- Monitor the Commission and Work Group activities through meeting minutes.

- Serve as a juror for CCHIT's commercial certification program.

HIT Policy Committee and the HIT Standards Committee

These two committees were formed to respond to the requirements outlined in the American Recovery and Reinvestment Act of 2009. They will facilitate the implementation of a nationwide health information technology.

INFORMATICS COMPETENCIES COLLABORATIVE

Nurses are expected to provide safe, competent, and compassionate care in an increasingly technical and digital environment. Yet technology has changed the role of the nurse and significantly altered the interactions between the nurse and patient and the nurse and healthcare provider. Nurses that do not have the basic skills to communicate within an electronic health record or other electronic medium will be significantly disadvantaged as we work to achieve 100% electronic health record adoption by 2014.

Nurses are directly engaged with information systems and technologies as the foundation for evidence-based practice, clinical-decision support tools, and the EHR. Nurses need to be equipped to integrate technology seamlessly within their workflow, and want better tools to work safer, more efficiently, and communicate more effectively with the patient and other healthcare providers. The American Nurses Association recognizes that nurses are "knowledge workers," and as a result, need to access information and apply knowledge appropriately to deliver high-quality nursing care.

As the Institute of Medicine reported in their 2006 report titled *Building the Workforce for Health Information Transformation*, "A work force capable of innovating, implementing, and using health communications and information technology (IT) will be critical to healthcare's success." This has accelerated the need to ensure that all nurses master a minimum set of competencies needed to work with electronic records, including basic computer skills, information literacy, and an understanding of informatics and information management capabilities including how to augment nursing practice.

The TIGER Informatics Competencies Collaborative (TICC) was formed to establish the minimum set of informatics competencies for *all* practicing nurses and graduating nursing students. The work of this team was

foundational to all TIGER work related to preparing the nursing workforce for EHRs, and preceded the work of the TIGER Education and Faculty Development, Staff Development, Leadership Development, and Virtual Demonstration Center Collaborative teams.

Nursing has historically provided leadership in the development and publication of informatics competencies in the healthcare industry. The recommendations of TICC built upon the informatics competencies work that had been previously published. In total, TICC collected over 1,000 informatics competencies from published literature and practice examples, then narrowed their focus for the scope of this project to describe the minimum set of competencies for practicing nurses and graduating nursing students. In addition, they established a model to organize the competencies that could be expanded upon by specialties and advanced practice roles.

Following a review of the literature and survey of nursing informatics education, research, and practice groups, the TIGER Nursing Informatics Competencies Model consists of three parts, detailed in the TICC Collaborative final report and summarized in this document:

(1) Basic Computer Competencies

(2) Information Literacy

(3) Information Management (including use of an electronic health record)

The model allowed the TICC to eliminate duplication and narrow down the specific competencies. Each of these categories is distinct enough to lend itself well to separate educational resources that can be completed in a modular fashion. There is also a logical progression to the order of mastering these categories. For example, basic computer competencies are necessary to easily search online sources of knowledge and information literacy competencies are essential to evaluate their appropriateness and applicability to

INFORMATICS COMPETENCIES COLLABORATIVE

support their practice. Finally, information management describes how a nurse interacts with an electronic or personal health record, and requires a mastery of computer skills and ability to find and apply knowledge to practice.

The team also identified that there is a component of "awareness," or professional consciousness and responsibility for learning, as a critical precursor to successful learning. Professional nursing practice can only advance as much as individual nurses are aware that a

knowledge gap exists in their practice, feel empowered to access further learning, and integrate evidence-based competencies into their professional practice to provide safe, effective, efficient, patient-centered, equitable care. This applies to achieving the minimum set of informatics competencies because until the nurse is aware of the need to master informatics and ready to learn new skills, the remaining competencies will be difficult to achieve.

TIGER Nursing Informatics Competencies Model

Component of the Model	Standard	Source (Standard-Setting Body)
Basic Computer Competencies	European Computer Driving License	European Computer Driving License Foundation
Information Literacy	Information Literacy Competency Standards	American Library Association
Information Management	Electronic Health Record Functional Model – Clinical Care Components	Health Level Seven (HL7)
	International Computer Driving License – Health	European Computer Driving License Foundation

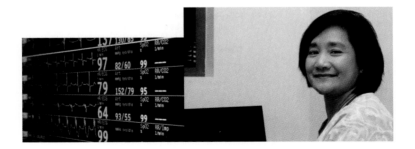

INFORMATICS COMPETENCIES COLLABORATIVE

Once the model was developed, each component was aligned with existing sets of competencies maintained by standard development organizations or *de facto* standards. The TICC found very good fits with the existing standards of the European Computer Driving License Foundation, the Health Level Seven's (HL7) Electronic Health Record Functional Specification for Clinical Care Components, and the American Library Association information literacy standards respectively. (See table describing the TIGER Informatics Competencies Model on the previous page.) All these sets of competencies are standards maintained by standard-setting bodies or organizations. Finding sets of competencies that are maintained by standard setting bodies allows the TIGER Informatics Competencies Collaborative (TICC) to recommend standards that are relevant to nurses and ones that will be sustainable as the standards evolve.

TICC outlined specific dates for adoption of the recommendations for each component of the model, and this information is available in the complete report on the TIGER website at www.tigersummit.com. In addition to the recommended adoption dates, TICC also identified a number of educational resources available today for each component. (See sidebar on this page.)

TICC established the informatics competencies framework needed to "scale" or expand to include specialty practices, different environments, and advanced degrees or practice such as leadership roles.

Informatics Competencies Educational Resources

European Computer Driving Licence (ECDL) Foundation http://ecdl.com
The ECDL syllabus is maintained and periodically updated by the not-for-profit ECDL Foundation.

CSPlacement www.csplacement.com
Offers CSP Basic, an e-learning course and a certification exam that is substantially equivalent to the TICC recommendation of a first and significant step towards basic computer competency.

Healthcare Information and Management Systems Society www.himss.org
Provides a certificate program called Health Informatics Training System (HITS) that is substantially equivalent to the TICC recommendation of a first and significant step towards basic computer competency.

American Library Association
http://www.ala.org/ala/mgrps/divs/acrl/standards/informationliteracycompetency.cfm
Defines competencies for information literacy as well as performance indicators and outcomes.

The Information Literacy in Technology
http://www.ilitassessment.com
The iLIT test assesses a student's ability to access, evaluate, incorporate, and use information.

HL7 EHR System Functional Model
http://www.hl7.org/EHR/
Information management competencies

ICDL-Health Syllabus http://www.ecdl.com
Provides the US-based the ICDL-Health syllabus.

Digital Patient Record Certification (DPRC)
http://dprcertification.com
An end-user EHR competency certificate program advised by U.S. informatics subject matter experts and endorsed by AMIA.

EDUCATION & FACULTY DEVELOPMENT COLLABORATIVE

Recognizing the demands of an increasingly electronic healthcare environment, nursing education must be redesigned to keep up with the rapidly changing technology environment. As federal initiatives push the adoption of EHRs throughout all healthcare institutions by 2014, it is imperative that nursing graduates are fluent in the use of these tools in order to practice safe and effective patient care.

The TIGER Education and Faculty Development Collaborative team engaged stakeholders that influence and deliver nursing education and licensing, including academic institutions representing all levels of nursing education, credentialing organizations, educationally-focused professional organizations, federal organizations that help fund faculty development, and state boards of nursing.

The TIGER Summit identified numerous objectives related to the education of nurses and the respective development of faculty, which are listed below. Emphasis was placed on the need for more nursing informatics specialists. These issues were raised in a variety of venues, including HRSA meetings and conferences. Based on the TIGER Summit Summary Report, the following specific objectives were set for the TIGER Education and Faculty Development collaborative:

- Use the informatics competencies, theories, research and practice examples throughout nursing curriculums.

- Create programs and resources to develop faculty with informatics knowledge, skill and ability and measure the baseline and changes in informatics knowledge among nurse educators and nursing students.

- Develop a task force to examine the integration of informatics throughout the curriculum.

- Develop strategies to recruit, retain, and educate current and future nurses in the areas

of informatics education, practice, and research.

- Improve and expand existing Nursing/Clinical/Health Informatics education programs.

- Encourage existing Health Services Resources Administration Division of Nursing to continue and expand their support for informatics specialty programs and faculty development.

- Encourage foundations to start programs that provide funding for curriculum development, research, and practice in nursing informatics and IT adoption.

- Collaborate with industry and service partners to support faculty creativity in the adoption of informatics technology and offer informatics tools within the curriculum.

To address these objectives, the TIGER Education Collaborative established several work groups to address the specific issues relevant to each stakeholder.

Focus of Work Groups – Key Stakeholders:

1. Nursing school accrediting bodies
2. Health Resources and Services Administration
3. State-wide informatics initiatives
4. State boards of nursing
5. Associate degree nursing programs
6. Other nursing specialty organizations
7. Academic partnerships with industry

TIGER was effective in influencing the accrediting agencies to include informatics education be incorporated into nursing curriculum. Both the **National League for Nursing** and the **American Association of Colleges of Nursing** addressed this position in 2008. The National League for Nursing Board of Governors approved a position

EDUCATION & FACULTY DEVELOPMENT COLLABORATIVE

statement, titled *Preparing the Next Generation of Nurses to Practice in a Technology-Rich Environment: An Informatics Agenda*[3]. The position statement outlined 23 recommendations for nursing school administrators, faculty and for the organization itself. In late 2008 at their national conference, the **American Academy of Nursing** unanimously endorsed the NLN's Position Statement, adding more momentum to this transition.

The **American Association of Colleges of Nursing** took the lead incorporating informatics as an essential element of Baccalaureate and the Doctor of Nursing Practice Education. This document, *Essentials of Baccalaureate Education for Professional Practice*[4], is an important step as the Essentials document serves as a framework for the preparation of nurses for professional practice in the 21st century. One of the nine essentials focuses on Information Management and Application of Patient Care Technology. For each essential element, a rationale is provided, and expected competencies and sample content are provided. It is the expectation that all baccalaureate education programs will incorporate the new essentials into their curriculum.

Both the associate degree nursing programs and the state boards of nursing were surveyed for their current inclusion of informatics competencies and related topics into their curricula or licensing criteria respectively. The surveys provided an opportunity to raise awareness of the mission of the TIGER Initiative as well as the changes occurring in the accrediting requirements. The detailed results of the survey are available in the TIGER Education and Faculty Development Collaborative report, available on the TIGER website at www.tigersummit.com.

Four states were identified that had either initiatives focused on informatics or had the infrastructure in place to begin informatics initiatives. Leading the state-wide effort, Minnesota formed their own TIGER Initiative, and has held two annual conferences. In Massachusetts, a State Initiatives committee brought together two additional states (North Carolina and California) to examine current and potential work in the area of informatics. Both Massachusetts and California had state-wide initiatives for faculty related to teaching with technology, in particular using simulations in nursing education. Both states have a readily available statewide infrastructure in place to begin a campaign to incorporate informatics into nursing education. These leading examples are models that can be replicated in other states as well.

The TIGER Initiative has worked closely with the Division of Nursing within HRSA to identify funding opportunities to advance informatics education. A successful outcome was the formulation of the Integrated Technology into Nursing Education and Practice Initiative (ITNEP). This initiative made funds available for projects to provide education in new technologies.

Finally, disseminating this information to faculty is critical. The TIGER Education and Faculty Development Collaborative held two webinars for educators on how schools of nursing have incorporated informatics into their curriculum and on three different approaches to forming partnerships to teach nurses about the electronic health record and clinical documentation.

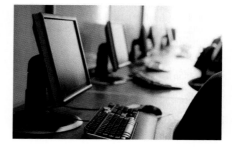

---

[3] Available online at NLN's website at
http://www.nln.org/aboutnln/PositionStatements/index.htm
[4] Available online at AACN's website at
http://www.aacn.nche.edu/Education/bacessn.htm

STAFF DEVELOPMENT COLLABORATIVE

Nurses need the knowledge, skills and resources to communicate and manage information effectively and efficiently in today's electronic environment. Studies are showing that technology correctly used by healthcare professionals can help improve patient safety. The user of the technology must first have an understanding and comfort with that technology. If technology is not used properly, it can have a negative effect on patient safety. Education targeting the practicing nurse is often the responsibility of the healthcare provider organization, and their educational resources in staff development. These resources can have a significant role in the adoption of new technology and improving patient safety.

The TIGER Staff Development Collaborative focused on three goals:

- Identify educational resources and affordable programs within the practice setting that foster IT innovation and adoption.

- Create competency-based, cost effective staff development and continuing education programs and training strategies specific for informatics knowledge, skills, and ability.

- Improve and expand existing nursing/clinical/health informatics education programs by collaborating with industry, service, and academic partners to support and enhance the use of technology and informatics in practice.

The team's first strategy was to better understand the current challenges to providing effective education to practicing nurses. They sent an electronic survey to TIGER participants requesting an evaluation of how prepared their nurses were in using electronic health records. A separate work group evaluated the recommendations of the TIGER Informatics Competencies team, and developed strategies for adoption by Staff Development resources. Another work group researched the literature for articles focused on learning methodologies and strategies related to informatics, and a fourth work group gathered and evaluated case studies or success and failure stories from practice.

WORKFORCE DEMOGRAPHICS

The demographics of the nursing workforce must be considered in order to develop a comprehensive strategy to educate nurses on the use of information technology. The average age of the nearly 3 million practicing nurses in the U.S. is 47. Practicing nurses often face more of an uphill battle than new graduates of colleges or universities in terms of computer literacy. Because of timing, the "average nurse" did not grow up with computer technology. Some nurses may have fear or anxiety related to using information technology, as they have not had the opportunity to learn basic computer skills. With the use of the electronic health record, nurses with higher levels of computer expertise are going to have more self-efficiency, or comfort and knowledge in being able to perform their work. Experienced nurses that have practice expertise may be disadvantaged if they have not developed computer expertise to keep up with the changing environment. A recent study[5] confirmed the finding that practicing nurses are not using evidence-based sources of information for decision making.

Unfortunately, these discrepancies may not be uncovered until the implementation of a new computer system for nurses. As the technology moves closer to the bedside, nurses become the largest group of clinical information systems users, and their attitudes will influence those of other works in the same area. Education on the new system is one of the largest costs to the implementation, and efforts to trim the costs mean limiting the education to *how to use the system* versus *how to use technology to deliver safer, more effective patient care*. Assessment of attitudes (such as fear or anxiety) or gaps in basic

---

[5] Pravikoff DS, Pierce ST, Tanner A. *Evidence-based practice readiness study supported by academy nursing informatics expert panel.* Nursing Outlook. 2005; 53: 49-50.

STAFF DEVELOPMENT COLLABORATIVE

computer skills must be addressed prior to system use or the success of even the most best-run projects is at risk.

STAFF DEVELOPMENT RESOURCES
Similar to the challenge with academic faculty, staff development personnel are often unfamiliar with the technology or do not have access to the system to master it. This often leaves the education to the vendor or consultants, or "super users," and the basic computer competency issue is never addressed. Even worse, the education does not address benefits of system or how to use to improve nursing practice.

INNOVATION IN PRACTICE
The TIGER Staff Development Collaborative gathered interesting case studies that could be replicated in other healthcare settings. This team identified six factors that lead to success:

- Addressing staff attitudes

- Improving access to technology

- Focusing on patient safety

- Using a variety of teaching methods

- Using Nursing Informatics specialists as resources

- Keeping the program competency-based

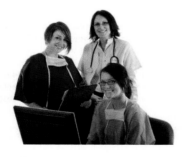

RECOMMENDATIONS
1. Adoption of technology may either be facilitated or impeded by attitudes towards technology. A strong association between attitudes and learning suggests that a first step in introducing new HIT should be an assessment of nurses' attitudes and basic computer skills.

2. The development of HIT-focused education should consider the multigenerational learning needs and styles, especially for nurses that entered practice before computers were integrated into educational curriculums.

3. Develop competency-based education that utilizes pre- and post-tests to demonstrate the effectiveness in meeting the competencies.

4. Staff Development resources must have adequate access and opportunities to develop their knowledge related to the use of technology.

National Nursing Staff Development Organization (NNSDO)

Many of the lessons learned can save an enormous amount of time and energy to eliminate the challenges and ensure success. The professional organization for staff development, the National Nursing Staff Development Organization (NNSDO), is taking the lead in organizing an effort to evaluate TICC's informatics-based competencies and provide further recommendations to the industry regarding strategies for practice-based education.

LEADERSHIP DEVELOPMENT COLLABORATIVE

Health information technology (HIT) has become a key focus of healthcare reform. Effective use of HIT will enable nurse executives to ensure nursing care that is safe, high quality, efficient, patient-centered, and help them deal with a looming workforce shortage. Today's leaders are required to transform their organization's values, beliefs, and behaviors. Technology is an underpinning to support the needed changes, but adoption of technology will not happen without leadership that is educated and prepared to lead future technology initiatives. This requires vision, influence, risk taking, clinical knowledge, and a strong expertise relating to professional nursing practice.

One of the highest priorities identified at the TIGER Summit was to develop *revolutionary leadership that drives, empowers and executes the transformation of healthcare*. Nursing leaders are often developed on the job, and the competencies defined by the TIGER Informatics Competencies Collaborative (TICC) are only the beginning of the informatics competencies necessary to lead an organization through the change that technology requires. This transformation requires nursing leadership to understand, promote, own, and measure the success of health IT.

The TIGER Leadership Development Collaborative team evaluated current nursing leadership development programs for the inclusion of informatics competencies. They built upon research that had been conducted by the American Organization of Nurse Executives (AONE) and developed a survey to identify the most urgent program development needs. The survey findings illustrated the need to ensure development of informatics competencies at the beginning management role, or the charge nurse. For example, the charge nurse needs to be competent in providing feedback regarding the use of technology that enhances the delivery of patient care, as well as mentor others, and become involved in system selection. Another key competency that all nurse managers need is the ability to evaluate outcomes from electronic clinical data. The informatics competencies for nurse executives require an expanded focus on budgetary, regulatory, safety, security and privacy policies related to the use of EHRs.

New implementations of EHRs put additional demands upon the nursing management team. As nurses are usually the largest group of clinical users of an HIT system, the nurse executive is expected to fully understand and articulate the goals and anticipated benefits of the technology implementation. Additionally, the nurse executive must remain engaged throughout the lifecycle of system selection, implementation and optimization.

Technology introduces change to many aspects of the role of the nurse, and nursing leadership is responsible for developing a culture that is innovative and ready to embrace change. Fortunately, a well-recognized professional model that engages nurses at all levels to incorporate change into their culture already exists. The TIGER Leadership Development Collaborative found significant alignment with the Magnet® Recognition Program, developed by the American Nurses Credentialing Center (ANCC). The Magnet Program exemplifies a model for change, and recognizes healthcare organizations that provide nursing excellence in the delivery of quality patient care, and demonstrates innovation in professional nursing practice.

As many HIT-savvy nurse leaders recommended correlating the Magnet Forces® to HIT success, the TIGER Leadership Development Collaborative collected dozens of examples of how organizations used HIT to demonstrate aspects of their Magnet Journey. These examples help to illustrate how technology can achieve each of the 14 forces of magnetism as well as transform the nursing organization to use technology for their benefit. The exemplars are meant to demonstrate the creativity and flexibility to

LEADERSHIP DEVELOPMENT COLLABORATIVE

transform the practice of healthcare delivery by rethinking current tools through gaining access to collective organizational experiences improved through fully automated integrated healthcare processes.

RECOMMENDATIONS

- Develop programs for nurse executives and faculty that stress the value of information technology and empower them to use HIT knowledgably.

- Expand and integrate informatics competencies into Nursing Leadership Development Programs.

- Promote sharing of best practices using HIT effectively to improve the delivery of nursing care.

- Promote alignment with the Magnet Recognition Program as a mechanism to demonstrate nursing excellence in using

technology to improve nursing practice and the delivery of safer, more effective patient care.

AONE's Technology Task Force Toolkit

One of the most promising efforts to equip nursing leaders with the necessary resources to promote health IT adoption is the Technology Toolkit that AONE's Technology Task Force is creating. This toolkit will focus on topics related to standards, IT contingency planning for disasters, wireless technology, return on investment, competencies for managers and executives, job descriptions, and share key learnings. (www.aone.org)

Criteria for Leadership Development

The critical need for leadership in nursing has accelerated faster than ever before – both to maintain knowledge of cutting edge practice and for management of clinical teams. The recommendations for leadership development include the following areas of focus:

- Evidence: Addresses improvement of quality, safety and value-added healthcare delivery professionals to identify care practices derived from scientific evidence

- Content: Builds evaluation of care practices for technical and content gaps

- Technology: Manages life-cycle change consistently to close the gaps with technology and knowledge resources found through evaluation

- Standards: Formal educational structured program, including Advisory Board Leadership Programs, AMIA 10 by 10 Program, AONE leadership programs or AACN accredited academic programs for nursing service administration.

USABILITY & CLINICAL APPLICATION DESIGN COLLABORATIVE

Current information systems and technology in practice today do not meet the workflow and information flow requirements of nurses. In fact, they can hamper widespread adoption of electronic health records. For one thing, much of this technology was not designed to support nursing work or thought processes. Products with good clinical design would support nurses every day in their practices. Often the current IT systems clinicians use were originally intended for finance, laboratory or other ancillary functions that do not support professional practice at the point-of-care. More important, a lack of *vision* and lack of *voice* is absent for what nurses need most. Information technology should provide evidence-based, patient-centric technology that allows interdisciplinary collaboration at the point-of-care. IT should be an enabler versus a barrier. To redefine reality, nurses must first understand the significance of usability and clinical application design that can shape the future of the products nurses use every day.

During the TIGER Summit, two critical and interdependent pillars to be further defined and acted on were:

1. **Informatics Design:** Evidence-based, interoperable intelligent systems that support education and practice to foster quality care and safety.
2. **Information Technology:** Smart, people-centered affordable technologies that are universal, usable, useful and standards-based.

These two critical components of informatics led to the development of the TIGER Usability and Clinical Application Design Collaborative to further define key concepts, patterns and trends and recommendations to health information technology (HIT) vendors and practitioners to assure useable clinical systems at the point of care.

> The Usability and Clinical Application Design Collaborative was ranked as the highest priority and had the greatest number of volunteers (53.5%) of all the TIGER Collaborative teams.

This speaks to the significance of the topic for practicing nurses and faculty today. Nurses who actively led and contributed to the collaborative cited reasons for their involvement to be: "*A good design can make the system easier to use and enhance clinical practice; Usability is a "make or break" part of a clinical informatics solution and "Many lessons from end-users as DESIGN is translated into PRACTICE. There is a definite need for standards and guidance.*"

The Usability and Clinical Application Design Collaborative recommends for the **TIGER Vision** to be fully realized, the nursing profession must educate itself on usability and key clinical application design principles. This education will determine how well evidence and informatics is integrated into day-to-day practice. The Usability and Clinical Application Design Collaborative organized their efforts to achieve the desired outcome of providing clear recommendations for good usability and clinical application design for technology.

USABILITY COLLABORATIVE OUTCOMES

- Synthesize a comprehensive literature review from nursing and other disciplines.
- Collect case studies and examples that illustrate usability/clinical application design – consisting of good examples to follow and bad examples to avoid.
- Develop recommendations for HIT vendors and practitioners to adopt sound principles of usability and clinical design for healthcare technology.

USABILITY & CLINICAL APPLICATION DESIGN COLLABORATIVE

The Collaborative established their goals and design principles for *Usability* and *Clinical Application Design*.

Usability Goals

1. An early and consistent focus on users of the product

2. Iterative design processes (multiple versions matched to users, tasks, and environments)

3. Systematic product evaluations (with product users and metrics)

Clinical Application Design

Clinical Application Design addresses how we integrate usability principles with evidence-based practice, interdisciplinary collaboration and knowledge discovery within a systems-thinking design (Figure 3, *adapted with permission from the CPM Resource Center, 2008).* In essence, we are *applying* usability and other design factors that are critical to making information technology the stethoscope of the 21st century.

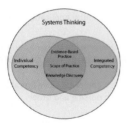

Figure 1 - Clinical Application Design Essentials

Literature Analysis

The Collaborative completed a comprehensive literature search, collected case studies, and synthesized material into a framework comprised of four areas:

- Determining Clinical Information Requirements
- Safe and Usable Clinical Design
- Usability Evaluations
- Human Factors Foundations

Each area includes a description of the topic, its significance for nursing, key points about the subject and recommendations for Health Information Technology vendors and point-of-care practitioners.

Case Studies

The Collaborative collected case studies that illustrated usability and clinical application design. These examples were intended to demonstrate best practice exemplars as well as challenging cases. Over 30 case studies were received.

Two key factors emerged. The first key factor was the *involvement of end users throughout the life of the project. A second key factor for end-user acceptance is integration with existing systems. This affects:*

- User acceptance and system adoption
- Accuracy (fewer transcription errors, avoids duplicate documentation)
- Patient safety due to synchronized, accurate information
- Timeliness of information collection, reporting and use

A second key factor for end-user acceptance is integration with existing systems. This affects:

- User acceptance and system adoption
- Accuracy (fewer transcription errors, avoids duplicate documentation)
- Patient safety due to synchronized, accurate information
- Timeliness of information collection, reporting and use

USABILITY & CLINICAL APPLICATION DESIGN COLLABORATIVE

Recommendations

Usability is the fit between system users, their work and environments. Imperatives include engaging the users early and often in the clinical systems lifecycle; understanding users, their tasks and their environments, conducting usability testing and redesigning before implementation. These steps better assure smooth implementations and user adoption of complex clinical systems. Clinical application design needs systems-thinking requirements that are critical to the complex health care environments. Contemporary designs include evidence-based practice, interdisciplinary collaboration and knowledge-discovery.

Good usability and clinical application design is no longer a choice but a mandate to support safe, effective decision-making. ALL nurses including practitioners, researchers, educators, and leaders should become aware of these principles and give voice to them at every venue where it impacts end-users and patient care. Nursing informatics specialists can help educate nurses about usability. Together nurses and nursing informatics specialists can assure that excellent clinical application design meets point-of-care practice needs for the 21st century.

DETERMINING CLINICAL INFORMATION REQUIREMENTS

An example of recommendations for vendors:

- Consider the requirements of different skill levels of practitioners. A novice nurse may need prompts and guidance more than an experienced nurse. Allow nurses to choose their own level of support.

- Clinician representation on vendor development teams is critical. Recommend clinicians as vendor product managers to assure understanding of clinical needs and to develop efficient and effective requirements.

An example of recommendations for practitioners:

- The requirements process should be owned by clinicians, not the information technology (IT) department or the vendor.

- Complete a workflow analysis for each user/department touching an electronic health record.

American Academy of Nursing Calls for the Thoughtful Development of Health IT

The AAN, in collaboration with the Robert Wood Johnson Foundation and other nursing organizations, has been instrumental in supporting efforts to improve how technology is developed and deployed in order to achieve an increase in the amount of time nurses and other providers spend with patients. The Academy's Workforce Commission started work on their Technology Targets Project in 2005. One component of the project is a process called Technology Drill Down (TD2), and provides medical/surgical units the opportunity to develop and improve their process and workflow inefficiencies by identifying technological solutions. This program has made available resources for others to follow, including a guide to replicating their process, available online at the Academy's website: www.aannet.org/files/public/facilitator_manual.pdf.

VIRTUAL DEMONSTRATION CENTER COLLABORATIVE

One of the recognized barriers to improving informatics education for all nurses remains the limited access to information systems and technology that could improve healthcare delivery. Often times, access is limited to the systems that are currently deployed in a given location. Nursing schools often rely on the clinical practicum site to provide access and education on EHRs. Nurses in practice are limited to the currently-deployed technology solutions at their organization, and have limited exposure to new technologies that could be applied in innovative ways to their environment to improve healthcare delivery.

The TIGER Virtual Demonstration Center (VDC) Collaborative team was created to develop a dynamic Internet and possibly a physical destination to demonstrate highly effective and efficient, technology-enabled, solutions of exemplary healthcare delivery systems of the next three to ten years. One of their primary goals was to encourage innovative and disruptive approaches to improving healthcare delivery with the use of technology. A key requirement was to allow access to the Center from anywhere the Internet is available. A secondary requirement was to expand current thinking about what healthcare is, by engaging visitors to the demonstration lab in potential healthcare futures that demonstrate innovative, high-quality, and maximally efficient care scenarios in compelling ways. To create this future vision we built on what is known today, but also conceptualized what could be possible.

Two virtual conferences, held in April and November of 2008, were supported by the TIGER VDC team in conjunction with partners and colleagues. All TIGER participants were invited to attend the conference and share their feedback on the experience.

The VDC was intended to provide a virtual "Gallery Walk" to all nurses, nursing faculty and nursing students via web access to nurse-focused technology applications. The VDC provided exemplars of best practice for technology utilization, contact resources and virtual networking opportunities. Guidelines and example scenarios were developed for vendors to ensure that the demonstrations would be based on the Integrating the Healthcare Enterprise (IHE) framework. Interoperability and security were among the principles highlighted in all demonstrations. The first conference had approximately 150 visitors provided feedback in a brief exit survey. Feedback was generally positive, but indicated that an "interactive experience" was most desirable by the attendees. The feedback was used to enhance the offerings in the second conference to more real-time presentations, interactive displays, and videos.

Virtual Demonstration Center Goals

Through these efforts, the TIGER VDC achieved the following goals:

- Provided visibility to the vision of IT-enabled nursing practice and education to the broader healthcare audience.

- Demonstrated future IT resources that will be in use by nurses to enhance their practice and educational environments.

- Demonstrated collaboration between industry, healthcare organizations, academic institutions, and professional organizations to create educational modules for nurses that were based upon informatics competencies.

- Provided universal accessibility to this demonstration for all nursing stakeholder groups.

- Used practice examples from different practice environments to demonstrate best practices, results of research, case studies and lessons learned by partnering with nursing professional organizations.

- Demonstrated how integrated IT systems impact nurses and the quality and safety of patient care.

VIRTUAL DEMONSTRATION CENTER COLLABORATIVE

Benefits and Virtual Demonstration Center Outcomes for 2008

Specific benefits and outcomes of the TVDC are intended to support nursing professionals as they adopt IT in their practice environments and also to support nursing education as curricula change to prepare nurses for the future. These benefits and outcomes are:

1. Nurses who can visualize the benefits of an IT-enabled future will be more likely to fully engage in the electronic health record within their practice setting.

2. Most exposure to IT capabilities are site-specific, the exception is nursing informatics resources, which are being increasingly woven throughout the practice environment.

3. Most academic institutions have very limited accessibility to IT demonstration resources to use within their curricula. The VDC provided a vision of how to partner with colleagues to widen the availability of resources.

4. Most IT education occurs in a specific field setting when a new system is implemented and focuses on system mechanics vs. user benefits and impact on patient care. The VDC provided an example of how education can be made more widely available through virtual resources and environments.

5. Universal adoption of informatics competencies for all nurses will require access to informatics resources at anytime from any site. The goal of the DVC was to support this outcome through innovative examples.

Future Opportunities

The Tiger VDC team would like to develop a virtual environment in order to extend the opportunity for clinical IT education via tools such as Second Life®. Virtual technology is being used by insurance companies, some schools of nursing and even the Centers for Disease Control and Prevention for educational purposes. The virtual world provides 3D interactive "avatars" that allow the participant to interact with the program to increase their knowledge and familiarity with current and future technology. Social networks and virtual technology have proven to support behavior change and sustain that change over time. There are hundreds of nursing academic centers across the country, and for that matter the world, that need access to IT solution in order to educate nurses. The cost and growing demand for health IT educational tools demand a virtual solution that can be accessed by nurses from various locations. As part of the TIGER legacy, the goal is to secure funding to help build out a virtual island that will support the TIGER mission of educating nurses about the possibility and benefits of IT with the goal of improving patient care and outcomes.

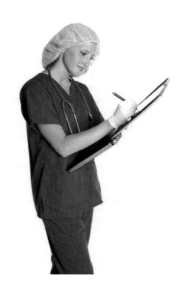

CONSUMER EMPOWERMENT & PERSONAL HEALTH RECORDS COLLABORATIVE

Healthcare consumers are only too aware of the fragmentation of the current healthcare system. According to one poll, "only one third (33%) of adults are very confident in their physicians and other healthcare providers having a complete and accurate picture of their medical history"[6]. In fact, many errors occur because individual professionals are not fully aware of all the therapies that the patient is receiving or has received[7]. There is ample evidence of the need for consumers to take a more active role in their healthcare, starting with a comprehensive personal health record controlled and maintained by the consumer. The Personal Health Record (PHR) is an Internet-based set of tools that allows people to access and coordinate their lifelong health information and make appropriate parts of it available to those who need it.[8]

If the PHR is a tool that promotes patient empowerment and supports the patient's engagement in their own healthcare, then nurses as healthcare professionals and patient advocates are obligated to become familiar with the technology and to promote its use when the technology is available and the patient is amenable. Education in the health professions for all disciplines should include information about PHRs as well as methods for teaching patients how to use them[9]. One of the primary objectives of TIGER's Consumer Empowerment and Personal Health Records Collaborative team was to make information available to nurses

about PHRs and to encourage inclusion of this content into nursing curricula.

This collaborative team identified several ways that nurses can impact the adoption and use of consumer empowerment strategies such as the PHR. First, PHRs must be easy to use and accessible to consumers. Applications do not always take into account the needs of consumers, who may suffer from disabilities, lack of computer expertise, and poor health literacy. To address this concern, the collaborative developed an inventory of usability principles for patient-focused applications.

Another barrier to adoption of PHRs is the lack of interoperability with other systems. If the PHR is to be an aggregation of health information, it would be most useful to be able to interact with other systems to share information. National Health IT activities have focused on identifying and supporting the adoption of standards for PHRs. As with the other National Health IT Agenda items, more nursing input is critically needed to ensure that safer nursing practice is enabled with the use of this technology.

President Obama is supporting greater use of technology in healthcare and has included significant funds in the economic stimulus package to increase adoption of PHRs. The environment has never been more promising for the prospect of achieving PHRs that are complete, accessible, affordable, easy-to-use, feature-rich, interoperable and secure.

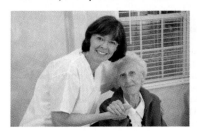

---

[6] Harris Interactive (2007). *U.S. Adults Not Very Confident that Physicians have the Complete Picture*. Available online at http://www.harrisinteractive.com/news/printerfriend/index.asp?NewsID=1264.

[7] Ghandi TK, Weingart SN, Borus J, et al (2003). *Adverse Drug Events in Ambulatory Care*. N Engl J Med. 348:1556-64.

[8] Markle Foundation/Connecting for Health. *The Personal Health Working Group Final Report*. (July, 2003). Available online at http://www.connectingforhealth.org/resources/final_phwg_report 1.pdf

[9] Tang P, Ash J, Bates DW, Overhage JM, Sands DZ (2006). *Personal Health Records: Definitions, Benefits, and Strategies for Overcoming Barriers to Adoption*. Journal of the American Medical Informatics Association, Vol 13 No 2: 121-126.

ACKNOWLEDGEMENTS

The TIGER Initiative would like to acknowledge and extend its thanks to the hundreds of volunteers and nursing professional organizations who lent their leadership, expertise, and support to the development of the *TIGER Initiative Collaborative Reports*.

TIGER Initiative's Advisory Council was led by Program Director, Donna DuLong, the author of this report. Leadership support was provided through the Alliance for Nursing Informatics co-chairs Carole Gassert, Joyce Sensmeier, Karen Greenwood, and Christel Anderson. The TIGER Advisory Council comprised of the Nine Collaborative Committee Co-Chairs, who are listed below, provided strategic oversight and guidance to the entire effort and lent their expertise, experiences, review, and hands-on support to the effort. Special thanks are also in order to the numerous work group leaders, listed within each of the collaborative reports, who provided significant leadership and contributions to the various sub-components of the final report for each collaborative team.

TIGER ADVISORY COUNCIL

Dana Alexander, RN, MSN, MBA
Chief Nurse Officer
GE Healthcare Integrated IT Solutions

Christel Anderson
Senior Manager, Clinical Informatics
Healthcare Information and Management
Systems Society

Marion J. Ball, EdD, FHIMSS, FCHIME, FAAN
IBM Research, Fellow, Center for Healthcare
Management, Professor Emerita
Johns Hopkins University School of Nursing

Connie White Delaney, PhD, RN, FAAN, FACMI
Professor and Dean, School of Nursing
University of Minnesota

Donna DuLong, RN, BSN
Program Director
TIGER Initiative

Carole A. Gassert, RN, PhD, FACMI, FAAN

Karen Greenwood
Executive Vice President
American Medical Informatics Association

Brian Gugerty DNS, RN
Clinical Informatician
Principal Consultant
Gugerty Consulting, LLC

Elizabeth C. Halley, RN MBA
The MITRE Corporation

Patricia Hinton Walker, PhD, RN, FAAN
Vice President
University of Uniformed Services Health Science
Center

Elizabeth O. Johnson, MSN, BSN, RN, FHIMSS,
Vice President of Clinical Informatics
Tenet Health System

Joan M. Kiel, PhD, CHPS
Chairman, University HIPAA Compliance
Associate Professor
Duquesne University, Pittsburgh, PA

Teresa McCasky, RN, MBA
Chief Nursing Strategist
McKesson

CDR Alicia Morton MS, RN-BC
Department of Health and Human Services
Office of the National Coordinator for Health IT

Judy Murphy, RN, FACMI, FHIMSS
Vice President, Information Services
Aurora Health Care, Milwaukee, WI

Carolyn Padovano, PhD, RN

ACKNOWLEDGEMENTS

Mary Anne Rizzolo, EdD, RN, FAAN
Interim Chief Program Officer
National League for Nursing

Joyce Sensmeier, MS, RN-BC, CPHIMS, FHIMSS,
VP, Informatics
Healthcare Information and Management
Systems Society

Diane J. Skiba, PhD, FAAN, FACMI
Professor
UCDHSC and Chair, Task Force Faculty
Development related to informatics
National League for Nursing

Nancy Staggers, PhD, RN, FAAN
Professor, Informatics, College of Nursing
University of Utah

Michelle Troseth, MSN, RN
Executive VP and Chief Professional Practice
Officer
CPM Resource Center
Elsevier/Mosby/MC Strategies

Charlotte Weaver RN, PhD
Senior VP and Chief Clinical Officer
Gentiva Health Services

Bonnie Westra, PhD, RN
Assistant Professor and Co-Director ICNP Center
University of Minnesota, School of Nursing

Rita D. Zielstorff, RN MS, FACMI

This project has been funded in part with funds from the Alliance for Nursing Informatics (ANI), a joint sponsorship between the American Medical Informatics Association (AMIA) and Healthcare Information and Management Systems Society (HIMSS). The ANI is a collaboration of organizations, representing a unified voice for nursing informatics. This project has also been funded in part with federal funds from the National Library of Medicine, National Institutes of Health, Department of Health and Human Services, under Contract No. N01-LM-6-3505. This project has also been supported by grants from the Robert Wood Johnson Foundation and the Agency for Healthcare Research and Quality.

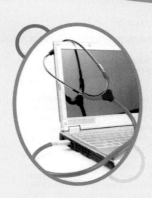

For additional information, please contact:

Donna DuLong

TIGER Initiative

donna@tigersummit.com

www.tigersummit.com

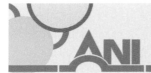

**Alliance for Nursing Informatics comments on the preliminary definition of
"Meaningful Use," as presented to the HIT Policy Committee on June 16, 2009**

Background

The Alliance for Nursing Informatics (ANI) is a collaboration of organizations that enables a
unified voice for nursing informatics. ANI represents more than 5,000 nurse informaticists and
brings together over 25 distinct nursing informatics groups in the United States. ANI crosses
academia, practice, industry, and nursing specialty boundaries and works in collaboration with
the nearly 3 million nurses in practice today. A full listing of the ANI membership organizations
is available at: http://www.allianceni.org/members.asp

Nurses constitute the largest single group of healthcare professionals and serve as the providers
and coordinators of care. In their front-line roles, nurses have a profound impact on the quality
and effectiveness of healthcare and thus must be supported by electronic health records (EHR)
that adequately enable their knowledge work. In this role, nurses are key leaders in the effective
use of information technology to impact the quality and efficiency of healthcare services, and are
familiar with roles requiring the inclusion and engagement of patients, families and care
providers to promote health and advocate an environment of patient centric care. In that spirit
we offer the following comments on the preliminary definition of "Meaningful Use," as
presented to the HIT Policy Committee on June 16, 2009. ANI supports the ultimate vision of
the Healthcare Information Technology (HIT) Policy Committee to realize improvements in
population health through a transformed healthcare delivery system, enabled through the use of
information technology.

Summary Recommendations

* Expand the definition of healthcare provider to include nursing and all other healthcare
  professionals to accurately reflect the continuum of care and include patient-centered
  documentation from all disciplines within the definition of the meaningful use objectives and
  measures;
* The patient is the "center of the (healthcare) universe" and as such is also potentially a
  meaningful user and participant in the planning of their care.
* Incorporate valid measures of continuity of care that include evidence that key information is
  available in the EHR and evidence that members of the patient's care team are aware of and
  utilize to deliver care.
* Patient data must be ubiquitous, and privacy and security concerns must be appropriately
  handled – It should be made available whenever and wherever needed, to those with a right
  to use it, and in a format that assists the user in distilling the information for use in decision
  making.
* Use existing initiatives such as the Healthcare Information Technology Standards Panel
  (HITSP) and Integrating the Healthcare Enterprise (IHE) to guide standards use including the
  use of standardized terminology within all systems that record, transmit, collect, and share
  information for care delivery.

Alliance for Nursing Informatics www.allianceni.org
c/o HIMSS c/o Christel Anderson
230 East Ohio, Suite 500 Chicago, IL 60611

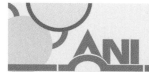

- Expand 2011 objectives related to reporting of quality measures by using processes and infrastructure defined by HITSP; initially focus on a subset of existing National Quality Forum (NQF)-endorsed measures, and include the 15 nursing sensitive measures.
- Expand the policy priorities, objectives, and measures to encompass support of registered nurses (RNs) and advanced practice registered nurses (APRNs), and all healthcare professionals.
- Recognize the importance of a workforce capable of providing technologies that meet "meaningful use" criteria.
- Each measure of meaningful use should be justified: include the purpose of the measure, intended value, method of data capture, and at least one successful study or evaluation to demonstrate the value of the measure; preferably there should be convincing evidence that the measure brings the intended value.

Discussion
Improve Quality, Safety, Efficiency and Reduce Health Disparities
ANI supports the electronic capture and reporting of coded patient information for purposes of care delivery, decision support, and outcomes analysis. Nurses have a profound impact on the quality and effectiveness of healthcare and are large contributors to patient information contained within EHRs. Standardized clinical performance measures that are adapted to consider unique complexities of various environments of care should be collected as a byproduct of care delivery and clinician documentation. ANI believes that measures as defined by the HIT Policy Committee may not be applicable to every care environment. The American Recovery & Reinvestment Act (ARRA) provides a robust definition of "Health Care Provider" which accurately reflects the continuum of care and demonstrates the complexity of the care delivery environment. It is our opinion that adaptation and further development of measures to address unique attributes of care environments will be needed. The above serves two important national goals: a) clinical decision support and trending in patient outcomes for real-time decision support and intervention at the point of care delivery, and b) the ability to aggregate enterprise-wide performance evaluation. We recommend that a subset of existing NQF endorsed measures are incorporated for acute and post acute care settings, including the 15 NQF identified nursing sensitive measures and HITSP standards that can enhance decision support and clinical measure reporting.

Engage Patients and Families
In order to effectively achieve outcome improvements patients and families will need access to their health information along with health education delivered in a patient-appropriate learning environment and format. The 2011 objectives to provide patients with access to data, knowledge, and tools to make informed decisions about their health, requires the development of resources equivalent with existing literacy, culture and language levels among other attributes. EHR systems should provide an integrated view of the patient /family learning needs assessment and education provided, and facilitates access to condition specific, credible education material. Nurses have an extensive knowledge base in patient education methods. We strongly

Alliance for Nursing Informatics www.allianceni.org
c/o HIMSS c/o Christel Anderson
230 East Ohio, Suite 500 Chicago, IL 60611

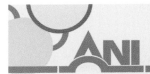

recommend that this body of knowledge be leveraged to facilitate the definition of achievable objectives in this area of health literacy.

Improve Care Coordination
ANI recognizes that patient care invariably requires collaborative interactions among multiple clinicians from a broad array of specialties, often in different locations. As such, "meaningful use" should strive for nothing less than an integrated healthcare community, including the healthcare consumer as an enabled active participant and "center of the (care delivery) universe", where enabling technologies promote usable, efficient and seamless information flow. Including information-rich, patient documentation within the definition of "meaningful use" can enhance cross-continuum communication, thereby enabling improved safety, quality, and processes of care delivery. ANI recommends a more explicit inclusion of RNs and APRNs, who are instrumental in coordinating care across the continuum. In this coordinating role, nurses are often the focal point for connecting acute, ambulatory, long-term, community-based, home care, and public health based settings ensuring that data necessary for managing specific patients and these populations is not only shared but translated into action. To this extent, ANI recommends taking a broader perspective utilizing documentation from all members of the clinical team; specifically nursing plans of care and progress notes must be incorporated into the EHR for "meaningful use." To meet this need, EHR systems should integrate patient care information from the patient and all healthcare professionals into the person's health record, including the exchange of patient summary data after each transition of care. This integrated approach sets the foundation for evolutionary growth providing the building blocks for health information exchange between disparate HIT systems. Valid measures of continuity of care must include evidence that key information is available in the EHR and evidence that members of the patient's care team are aware of and utilize it to deliver care.

Care Coordination Recommendations for 2013
We recommend that by 2013 the coordination of care measures of "meaningful use" be focused on ensuring that a well tested continuity of care summary is included in the EHR and that the process of use is specified and utilized. The summary and process selected must facilitate both inter and intra disciplinary communication about care that transfers key patient care information to all health professionals at handoffs and transitions within and across settings. The long term goal is for this summary and process is to become consistent within and across EHRs and settings enabling all clinicians involved in a patient's care to quickly and easily understand key care information. The patient summary contains a core data set of the most relevant administrative, demographic, and clinical information facts about a patient's healthcare, covering one or more healthcare encounters. The eventual use of a common summary in turn will provide the means to directly assess the coordination of care and the impact on safety, quality, and efficiency through EHR generated measures.

Alliance for Nursing Informatics www.allianceni.org
c/o HIMSS c/o Christel Anderson
230 East Ohio, Suite 500 Chicago, IL 60611

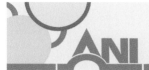

Continuity of care summary measures:
- Current valid list of clinical priority problems, general interventions, clinical outcomes being followed and status of clinical outcomes (nursing sensitive measures) (medical, nursing and other collaborative problems)

And provides:
- User interface and database that captures the linkages among medical diagnoses, clinical problems, interventions, and outcomes
- Historical continuity of care summary provides a view for current and past episodes of care

Process of use measures:
Evidence that an organization:
- Has a formalized process for keeping the continuity of care summary updated and current; use in handoff communication; provides training in update, use and validation.

Standardized Infrastructure within the EHR

ANI endorses the use of standards integrated across systems that record, transmit, collect, and share information that is clear, concise, and unambiguous in all settings of healthcare services. Meaningfully adopted health information must be available whenever and wherever it is needed and must be in a format that is usable and reusable. Healthcare professionals as knowledge workers must not only have access to information but the enabling technologies needed to help distill the information so that it provides value in any clinical setting. Education of an informatics workforce capable of meeting these needs and achieving value through technology should also be considered as part of the "meaningful use" discussion.

Furthermore, ANI believes that an infrastructure using standardized terminologies supports data sharing, aggregation, identification, use of evidenced based practices, and development and integration of new evidence derived from clinical research. This terminology core is necessary and a prerequisite for supporting the Health Outcomes Policy matrix objectives of decision support, discovery of disparities, reporting, maintaining accurate lists of problems and medications, and the general use and re-use of information needed for quality, safety, and efficiency.

Lastly, harmonized standards and related guidance from HITSP and IHE should be utilized to provide further recommendations for standards use. Systems must enable the sharing of integrated information while maintaining patient privacy and allowing for de-identification of subjects involved in clinical research to generate new knowledge about health and healthcare services. Assure patients and providers that privacy and security concerns are strictly and appropriately handled to ensure confidence in the technology through accuracy and security of information. This information can be accomplished in a phased approach as the nation moves towards fully interoperable EHRs. ANI supports clear regulation and incentives to increase participation in the adoption and harmonization of documentation standards, thereby promoting

Alliance for Nursing Informatics www.allianceni.org
c/o HIMSS c/o Christel Anderson
230 East Ohio, Suite 500 Chicago, IL 60611

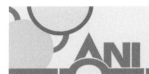

interoperability of patient data gathered by healthcare professionals when utilizing EHRs across the care continuum.

Conclusion
In closing, nurses hold a critical role as organizations continue to expand their focus on "meaningful use" by leveraging the data and information contained in electronic health records. With the passage of the ARRA, the nursing profession will continue to perform an instrumental role in the key areas of patient safety, change management, design, and usability of systems as evidenced by quality outcomes, enhanced workflow, and user acceptance. These areas highlight the value of these knowledge workers and their role in the adoption of health information technologies with greater integration across systems to deliver higher quality clinical applications in healthcare organizations. ANI's position is that "meaningful use" of health information technology, when combined with best practice and evidence based care delivery, will result in improved healthcare for all Americans. The membership organizations of ANI are well positioned to assist with future develop efforts and we welcome the opportunity to collaborate with HIT Policy Committee on this important endeavor.

Alliance for Nursing Informatics www.allianceni.org
c/o HIMSS c/o Christel Anderson
230 East Ohio, Suite 500 Chicago, IL 60611

**T.I.G.E.R. comments on the preliminary definition of
"Meaningful Use," as presented to the HIT Policy Committee on June 16, 2009**

Background
The TIGER Initiative, an acronym for Technology Informatics Guiding Education Reform, was formed in 2004 to bring together nursing stakeholders to develop a shared vision, strategies, and specific actions for improving nursing practice, education, and the delivery of patient care through the use if health information technology (HIT). In 2006, the TIGER Initiative convened a summit of nursing stakeholders to develop and execute a plan to move nursing into action steps to adopt evidence and informatics into their daily practice. Since then, hundreds of volunteers across the nation have joined the TIGER Initiative to engage in the action steps defined at the Summit. Nine collaborative teams were formed in 2007 to address key areas identified as most critical for nurses to focus on to accelerate the adoption of HIT for nursing. It is with this increased knowledge and recommendations around these critical areas that TIGER makes comments to the Health Information Policy (HIT) Policy Committee on the preliminary definition of "Meaningful Use" that were presented on June 16, 2009.   TIGER supports the ultimate vision of the HIT Policy Committee to enable improvements in population health through a transformed healthcare delivery system, enabled through the use of information technology. A listing of TIGER members and sponsors, along with published reports are available at: http://www.tigersummit.com.

With over 3 million nurses who make up 55% of the healthcare workforce in the nation, the TIGER efforts and comments are important for the HIT Policy Committee to consider. As the largest single group of healthcare professionals who serve as the providers and coordinators of care, having a strategy to ensure that the practicing nurse is supported by electronic health record (EHR) and HIT "meaningful use" is critical to achieving the HIT Policy Committee's goals as outlined in the American Recovery and Reinvestment Act (ARRA). TIGER also brings a strong voice and action recommendations to the investment in people – to build an informatics-aware healthcare workforce requiring health professions education reform as well.

The following TIGER recommendations represent the voice of the largest constituent of nurses in the nation committed to integrating evidence and informatics into practice and education:

Recommendations to the Health Outcomes Policy Priorities
- Engage nurses in future workgroups and HIT Policy Committee review activities related to "meaningful use" definitions and recommendations;
- Include patient-centered integrated interdisciplinary clinical documentation within the definition of the meaningful use objectives and measures;

- Assure standards harmonization efforts accurately supports nursing data in different specialties, environments and roles within the EHR so it is comprehensive and meaningful to all practicing nurses;
- Expand the collection of standardized clinical performance measures and terminologies as a byproduct of care delivery and clinician documentation;
- Address the significance of usability and clinical application design as it relates to clinical documentation, evidence-based practice, clinical decision support and adoption by clinicians. If clinical documentation and clinical summaries are not designed well with good usability they will not be adopted;
- Consider a virtual demonstration center to showcase "best practices" today for clinicians to visualize the benefits of "meaningful use: criteria;
- Recognize the critical role nurses and advanced practice nurses (APNs) will have in the role of engaging patients in accessing and updating their Personal Health Record (PHR). Nurses are also significant contributors to the patient's family medical history and are critical in guiding interoperability as it relates to patient health data as coordinators of care;
- Develop requirements for academia's accountability to workforce development by integrating meaningful use expectations into their curriculums and encourage partnerships between education and practice;
- Address the need for a minimum set of informatics competencies for clinicians to master the role of HIT in their education and practice settings.

Recommendations to the 2011, 2013 and 2015 Timelines:

- Move the following criteria from 2013 to 2011:
  - o Clinical documentation recorded in EHR[IP]
  - o CDS at the point-of-care [OP, IP]
  - o Manage chronic conditions using patient lists and decision support [OP, IP]
  - o Documentation of family medical history [OP, IP]

Most HIT vendor software has the ability to perform clinical documentation today. By waiting until 2013 to require nurses and their interdisciplinary colleagues to document their professional services delivered will significantly impact the ability to deliver quality, safe and efficient care on a timelier basis. Nurses are in need of evidence-based information at their fingertips when delivering care and leveraging technology to access clinical decision support in their workflow is a high priority as evidenced by the TIGER Summit. Nurses also play a critical role in managing patients with chronic conditions and preventing common complications they are at risk for so to have the ability to manage chronic conditions using patient lists and decision support would add value to the contributions of nurses as they coordinate care and collaborate with other health team members. Lastly, nurses are frequently the first discipline to document a patient's family medical history as part of their professional practice and clinical documentation; therefore, requiring an interdisciplinary approach to document this information as part of clinical documentation in the EHR would decrease duplication and fragmentation as well as improve care coordination.

Conclusion

In closing, nurses are critical in the success of the nation's agenda on achieving "meaningful use" by leveraging health information technology to transform the delivery of health care services. Nursing has demonstrated amazing leadership and vision through the TIGER Initiative which was initiated as a result of President Bush's mandate that all Americans will be using electronic health records by the year 2014. We recognized the sense of urgency to raise awareness of nursing stakeholders to:

1. Develop a U.S. nursing workforce capable of using electronic health records to improve the delivery of healthcare
2. Engage more nurses in the development of a national healthcare information technology infrastructure; and
3. Accelerate adoption of smart, standards-based, interoperable technology that will make healthcare delivery safer, more efficient, timely, accessible, and patient-centered.

With the passage of ARRA under President Obama, nurses are poised and ready to make significant contributions to defining "meaningful use" criteria and shaping the policies to support the ultimate vision of a transformed health care delivery system enabled by health information technology. The TIGER Initiative Advisory Council, our sponsors and affiliated national nursing organizations, are well positioned to assist with future development efforts of the HIT Policy Committee on this very important endeavor.

Index

A

AACN. *See* American Association of Colleges of Nursing
AAN. *See* American Academy of Nurses
Academic programs, NI
  attributes
    credentialing members, 95
    educational programs, 95
    focal points, 94–95
    organizations, 95
  competencies
    definition, 97
    practice and professional performance, 98
    Work Group's designation level, 97–98
  definition of, 94
  education
    continuing, 99–100
    courses, 100
    doctoral specialization, 103–104
    master's programs, 103
    models, 99
    opportunities Web page, 98
    postgraduate fellowships, 104–105
    programs, 105
    specialization, master, 100–103
  informatics nurse specialist (INS) role, 97
  practice
    activities, 96–97
    arenas, 96
    INs, 96
    nursing administration educational, 96
  preparation, 93
AGREE tool. *See* Appraisal of guidelines for research & evaluation
AHIMA. *See* American Health Information Management Association
Alliance for nursing informatics (ANI), 189

American Academy of Nurses (AAN), 114, 308
American Association of Colleges of Nursing (AACN)
  doctor of nursing practice (DNP), 108
  education and faculty development, 60
  information and health care technology, 114
  NLN and, 30
American Health Information Management Association (AHIMA)
  allied health professionals, 46
  HIT, 200
  PHR definition, 274, 284
American Medical Informatics Association (AMIA)
  and HIMSS, 45
  informatics community, 3, 54
  mentorship program benefits, 52
  US, 107
  Web page, educational opportunities, 98–99
American Nurses Association (ANA)
  NI
    certification process, 95
    definition, 94, 106
    educational sessions, 99
    Principles for Documentation, 307
    recognized nursing languages, 175
    terminologies, clinical practice, 367
American Nursing Informatics Association (ANIA), 45, 54
American Recovery and Reinvestment Act (ARRA)
  CER, 331, 337
  EHR, 113
  HIT, 2, 5, 207
  innovative technology, funding, 260
  policy committee, 284

AMIA. *See* American Medical Informatics
        Association
AONE's Technology Task Force, 152
Appraisal of guidelines for research &
        evaluation (AGREE) tool, 253–254
Attribution theory, 25

B
Baccalaureate nursing (BSN) program
    assessment
        classmates and laboratory partners, 173
        "hands-on" mistakes, 173
        point of care *vs.* mobile decision
            support systems, 174
    clinical practice model resource center
        (CPMRC), 173
    knowledge-based charting (KBC)
        module, 173
"Bologna Process", 378
Boston Home, 315
Bridging technology, academe and industry
    BSN nursing program
        assessment, 173–174
        curriculum, 173
        knowledge-based charting (KBC)
            module, 173
    CIS, simulations
        EHR, 177
        JHUSON and Eclipsys Corporation,
            178–186
    diagnosis, languages
        ANA recognized, 175
        nursing classification system, 174–175
    healthcare informatics
        automation use, 171
        description, 170
        educational directive
            transformation, 171
        TIGER, 171–172
        tools, 170
    implementation
        evaluation, 176–177
        Micro Sim cases, 176
        second life, 176
        simulations, 175
    nursing education, informatics
        and simulation
        airline industry, 172–173
        competencies, 172
        computing, 172
    nursing implications
        practice environments, 187
        simulation activities, 187

"preparation-practice gap", 167
    simulations
        advantages and challenges,
            curricula, 168
        CIS, 170
        defined, 168
        framework, 169–170
        implementing and testing, 168–169

C
California HealthCare Foundation (CHCF)
    consumerism, 267
    Deloitte survey, 266
    tools, health, 266–267
Canadian Health Outcomes for Better
        Information and Care (C-HOBIC),
        368–369
Care transformation
    comparative effectiveness
        research, 336–338
        stakeholders, 338
    HIT (*see* Health Information Technology)
    information technology and knowledge
        dissemination, 331
    personalized medicine
        description, 332–333
        genomic science, 334–335
        human genome, 333
        SACGHS, 333–334
        stakeholders, 335
        translation process, 332
Centers for disease control (CDC), 28, 333
CER. *See* Comparative effectiveness research
Certification commission for health
        information technology (CCHIT)
    commercial, 203
    criteria, 200–201
    EHR systems, 211
    HIT, 200
"Charting by Parameters", 183, 185
CHCF. *See* California HealthCare Foundation
Clinical application design
    EBP, 223
    essentials, 224
    interdisciplinary collaboration, 225
    safety, 224
Clinical information system (CIS)
    EBP
        documentation-based clinical decision
            support, 254–255
        framework, documentation, 255, 256
        knowledge integration, 254
        smart forms, 255

EHR, 177
JHUSON and Eclipsys Corporation
  EHR system implementation, 178
  faculty members and IT staff, 178
  health assessment, 182–185
  principles and applications, nursing,
    179–182
  technical challenges, 185–186
Clinical practice guidelines, EBP
  AGREE tool, 253–254
  description, 252
  development methods, 253
  recommendation, 254, 255
Commission on collegiate nursing education
  (CCNE), 72
Comparative effectiveness research (CER)
  Coordinating Council, 337–338
  evidence types, 337
  purpose, 336
  stakeholder, 338
Competencies
  approach and strategy
    TICC, 82
    TIGER, standards and standard-setting
      bodies, 83
  basic computer
    CSPlacement, 85
    "digital native" and "digital immigrant",
      83
    ECDL syllabus,
      83–85
    HIMSS, 85
  information literacy
    ALA, 86
    description, 85
    implementation, 85
    recommendation, 86
    TICC, 85–86, 89
  information management
    data-information-knowledge
      continuum, 86
    definition, 87
    DPRC and HITS, 89
    ECDL health, 87–88
    EHRS, 87, 89–91
    recommendation, 88
  nurses, 81–82
Consumer health informatics, defined, 284
Continuing education and staff development
  academic health center
    and library personnel, 119
    objectives, 118–119
  Cleveland clinic
    training, 119

"trial and error" information
  technology, 119–120
computer skills assessment, 126
electronic documentation, U.S.
  nurses, 117
LGH
  implementation process, 120
  phases, 120
  physicians, 120–121
National Nursing Organization
  AACN and AONE, 114
  IOM, 114–115
  NLN and AAN, 114
quality of care, patient safety and
  operational issues
  clinical systems training approaches,
    129–130
  information technology, 129
  recommendations, 128–129
St. Vincent Mercy Medical Center
  computer-based training, 124–125
  educators, 125
  HER, 124
  improvements needed, 124
  medication administration records
    (MARs), 123–124
success criteria, 128
Summa health system
  achievement, 122
  Allied Health classes, 122
  chief medical information officer
    (CMIO), 121
  clinical information systems staff and
    consultants, 122
  computerized physician order entry
    system (CPOE), 121
  "maintenance" training, 123
  "Super Users", 122–123
THC, training
  plan, 126
  team, 125
TIGER survey
  computer literacy, training and skills,
    115
  facility, bed count, 116
  in-house training, 116–117
  practice environment, 116
  role, organization, 115
  staff nurses, computer literacy, 116
training
  delivery methods, 127
  schedules, 127
  super user, 127–128
  team, 126

WINI conference, 118
Cultural change strategies. *See also* Culture
  bioinformatic technology, 30
  "caring" and "holism", 31
  caring and technology
    comparison, 17–18
    description, 17
    EMRs, EHRs and PHRs, 18
    issues, 18
    IT, 18
    patient, 17
    personal, 17
  education
    description, 20
    Master's education programs, 21
    nurses and health care professionals,
      20–21
    TIGER initiative, 21
    TIGER Phase II Report, 21–22
  health care provider, 29–30
  nursing's history, 30–31
  organizational change
    definition, 22
    hardware/software development
      and business processes, 22–23
    high velocity, 23
    informatics and technology, 22
    leadership, 24
    patient safety, 23–24
    social-technical implications, 23
    United Kingdom, 23
  personal health, 29
  social, innovation and disruption
    catalytic innovators, qualities, 25–26
    "e-patients", 28
    health care, 28–29
    IndivoHealth, 26
    media, 27–28
    "neuro-chip", 27
    PHR, 26, 27
    Project Health Design, 26–27
    "shaping strategies", 26
  theoretical models
    implementation, 25
    innovation diffusion, 25
    social cognitive theory, 24
    sociotechnical systems theory, 25
    TAM, 24–25
  TIGER initiative
    description, 18–19
    model, 19–20
    opinion leaders and communication
      channels, 19
    phase II, 20

    planning stages, 19
    Roger's diffusion of innovation
      theory, 19
    summit, impact actions, 13–14
Culture
  definition, 15
  industrial age, 16
  information age, 16–17
  internet and HIT, 16
  "socioculture", 15–16
Curriculum development centers, 204

D
Department of Health and Human Services
    (DHHS), 5
Disruptive innovation, point of care
  health care success model
    business units, 296
    Medical Home, 297–298
  health IT systems, 292
  information technology, future
    human–computer interaction, 296
    Internet, 295
    software products, 295–296
  Medical Home
    CER, 301–302
    functions and data requirements,
      299–300
    implementation phases, 300–301
    recommendations, 299
  smart point of care (POC) system
    analyses, informed decisions, 295
    attributes, 294
    components, 294–295
    conceptual architecture, 294
    improved quality of care, 293
    nursing support, 292–293
  TIGER initiative, 291
Dragon Medical® speech-recognition
    software, 304

E
Educational technology and information
    management advisory council
    (ETIMAC)
  faculty development, 70
  informatics competencies, 68
Education and faculty development
    collaborative
  AACN
    health care improvement and
      transformation, 72

patient care technology, 71–72
    TIGER, 71
accreditation bodies, 72
articles, 65–66
Associate Degree Nursing Committee
    EMRs, 73–74
    National Organization for Associate
        Degree Nursing (N-OADN), 73
    PDAs, 73
HRSA
    IT, 78
    ITNEP, 76–77
    National Advisory Council on Nurse
        Education and Practice
        (NACNEP), 77
    TIGER Summit, 76
innovators
    electronic documentation and health
        records, 78–79
    nursing curriculum, 78
IOM and IT, 66
NLN
    deans/directors/chairs, 69
    ETIMAC, 68, 70–71
    nurse faculty, 69
state boards of nursing
    current practice, 74–75
    online survey, 74
    survey questions, 74
state initiatives
    California, 76
    Massachusetts, 76
    Minnesota TIGER, 75
    North Carolina, 75–76
TIGER initiative
    collaborative teams, 67
    objectives, 67–68
    seven pillars, 66
Education, NI
    concentrations and minors, master's
        program, 103
    continuing
        HIMSS, 99
        professional development, 99
        summer institute, 100
        universities, 100
    courses, 100
    doctoral specialization
        informatics researchers, 104
        information management and
            technology, 104
        interdisciplinary approach, 104
        scientist preparation, 103–104
        state-of-the-art technology, 104

master's specialization
    computer competencies, 101
    curriculum and programs, 101
    information systems management/
        biomedical computing, 101
    New York University, 103
    nursing science, 100–101
    practicum sites, 101
    Saint Louis University, 103
    specialty courses credit hours, 101–102
    state-of-the-art technology, 101
    University of Maryland, Baltimore, 102
    University of Utah, 102
models, 98–99
postgraduate fellowships
    Douglas Porter Fellowship, 104–105
    Massachusetts general hospital
        (MGH), 104
    programs, 105
eHealth, Eurpoe
    initiatives
        action plan, 378–379
        EHR systems, 379
        electronic health card, 380–381
        France and Austria, 381
        Germany, 381–382
        health telematics, 378
        NPfIT, 379–380
    to nursing documentation systems
        EHRs, 384–385
        Heidelberg study, 385–386
        multiprofessional systems, 386
        terminologies, 385
    standards
        and interoperability, 382
        terminology standards, 383
        VIPS and LEP, 384
EHRs. See Electronic health records
Electronic health records (EHRs)
    access, 338
    benefits, 384–385
    CIS, 177
    clinical document architecture (CDA), 382
    course flowsheets, nursing, 180
    eHealth programmes, Europe, 384
    evolution, 274
    Google, 272
    Health Level 7 (HL7), 144
    implementation factors, 178
    information management, 87
    interoperable, 379
    Knowledge-Based Charting (KBC)
        module, 173
    nurses, levels of, 172

nursing skills class, 179
pilot test, 181
public teaching hospitals, 406
sharing, 362
St. Vincent Mercy Medical Center, 124
use, 87
Electronic medical records (EMRs)
adoption rates, 292
care quality improvement, 324–326
documentation, 73–74
implementation, 23, 323
software, 74
speech recognition, 304
use, hospitals and agencies, 73
Electronic personal health records (ePHRs)
barriers, use and acceptance
awareness, lack of, 280
interoperability and portability lack, 281
privacy and security concerns, 280
required features, 281
costs, consumer, 279
empowering technology, 277
innovations
"conversational assistant", 281
electronic account, 281–282
Shared Care Plan, 282
nurse, promoting use, 283
product types, 279
standards and usability principles
certification, 282–283
difficulty, usage, 282
use and usage, 280
EMRs. See Electronic medical records
ePHRs. See Electronic personal health records
Equity implementation theory, 25
Essentials of Doctoral Education for Advanced
Nursing Practice, 72
Evidence-based clinical decision support
EBP (see Evidence-based practice)
health quality initiatives and supporting
organizations
databases, 250
patient safety initiatives, 248–249
HIT advancement
guiding principles, 250
software functionality and features, 251
vendor systems, 250–251
nursing role
convergence, technology, 256
tool, 256–257
Evidence-based practice (EBP)
definition, 244
implementation models
adoption, 249

multifaceted approaches, 248
individual clinician practice
attitude, 247
skill level and readiness, 247
time constraints, 246–247
IOM, 246
organizational culture and infrastructure
barriers, 247–248
fragmented efforts, 248
priority, health care
omissions, 245–246
traditional approaches, 245
strength, hierarchy, 244
theory, 243
tools and technology use
clinical practice guidelines, 252–254
evidence retrieval systems, 252
information systems, 254–256
quality care movement, 251
website searches, 252, 253

H
Health Affairs, 8
Healthcare Informatics
CIO, 327, 328
DMC folks, 322
Healthcare information and management
systems society (HIMSS)
annual informatics conference, 99
certificate, 85
documents, 56
education, 54, 99
TIGER presentations, 45
usability, 222
voice-assisted care, 317
Health care transformation
consumerism, 194
disaster preparedness and planning, 194
emerging telehealth, 195
information and cost transparency, 195
nursing shortage, 194
unsustainable spending
costs, 194
medicare, 193–194
Health information technology (HIT)
EBP integration, 223, 224
enabler vs. barrier, care, 219
federal government's role
adoption, 200–201
governance, 198
Office of the National Coordinator
(ONC), 197–198
partners, 201

policy, 198–199
technology, 199–200
health reform and
health care delivery system, 5
investment, positive outcomes, 6
individualized healthcare delivery
system, 338
interoperability, 338–339
personalized medicine and comparative
effectiveness, 339
TIGER initiative
collaboratives, 11
EHR and PHR, 10
nurse-relevant data elements, 10
Phase I Summit Summary Report, 10
Health information technology standards
panel (HITSP)
framework, 213
interoperability, 212, 213
mission, 199–200
National Health IT Agenda and, 211
Health telematics Europe
diversity, national healthcare systems
education, 378
general practitioners (GP), 377–378
health care indicators, 377
measures, 376
public contract and private insurance
model, 376
public integrated model, 375
eLearning/blended learning
goal-oriented approach, 391–392
simulator devices, 391
informatics, patient care
eHealth initiatives, 378–382
eHealth standards, 382–384
nursing documentation systems,
384–386
nursing management, leadership and policy
C-value concept, 387–388
evidence-based purchasing, 390
NMDS, 388–389
rostering, 387
routine process, automation, 386–387
supply chain, 389
task-oriented and criterion-oriented,
workload measurement, 387
pre-and postregistration phase, nurse
ECDL programme, 390
electronic resources, 391
Heuristically programmed algorithmic (HAL)
computer system, 303
HFs. See Human factors
HIMSS. See Healthcare information

and management systems society
HIT. See Health information technology
HITSP. See Health information technology
standards panel
HL7 EHR system functional model, 87
Human factors (HFs)
foundations construction
description and significance, 234
points, 234–235
recommendations, 235–236
usability (see Usability)

I
Informatics competencies
basic computer skills
European Computer Driving License
(ECDL), 141
International Computer Driving License
(ICDL), 141
TIGER leadership development
workgroup, 141–142
education
"digital immigrants", 139–140
"digital natives", 140
HIT and TIGER, 140
practicing nurse age, 139
literacy
application framework, 143
levels of, 142
TIGER leadership development
collaborative, 143
management, 143–144
data, 143–144
electronic/personal health record, 143
TIGER informatics competencies
collaborative, 144
models
TIGER, 140–141
TNIC, 141
nurse leaders, 144–147
HIT, 146
policies, 147
TIGER Leadership Collaborative team,
144–146
nurses, 139
virtual communication tools, 142
Information technology (IT).
See also Disruptive innovation,
point of care; Technology
informatics guiding education
reform
caring and technology, 18
clinical leadership, 327–328

education and faculty development
    collaborative
        HRSA, 78
        IOM, 66
    health (*see* Health information
        technology)
    leadership
        adopters and laggards, 160
        current supported system
            components, 159
        impact, organizational changes, 162
        innovators, 160
        late majority, 160
        lifecycle, 159–160
        obsolescence, 160
        productivity, efficiency and job
            satisfaction, 160–161
        technology acquisition and utilization
            process, 162
    performance improvement methodologies,
        326–327
Institute of Medicine (IOM)
    CER, 301, 337–338
    evidence review report, 270
    impact, United States, 7
    information technology and informatics
        skills, 6–7
    literacy evidence reviews, 268
    "patient-centered care", 271
    report
        aims, 195–196
        recommendations level reforms, 196
    US healthcare system, 271
Integrating technology into nursing education
        and practice initiative (ITNEP),
        76–77
International Classification for Nursing
        Practice® (ICNP®)
    Beta 2 version, 368
    seven-axis model, 367
    version 1, 368
*International Journal for Quality in Health
        Care,* 7
International Medical Informatics Association
        (IMIA), 54
Invisibility to visibility
    controlled language types
        categorization level, 365–366
        classification system, 365
        clinical vocabularies, 365
        confusion, 366
        nomenclature, 364–365
        thesaurus, 366
    data standards

interpretability, 363
    language categories, 364
    nursing, 359
environmental forces, health information
        development
    data aggregation, 362
    influencing factors, 362
    terminologies, healthcare, 363
implications, nursing data
    databases, 370–371
    outcomes of care, 369–370
    professional compartmentalization
        and marginalization, 370
    issues, 369
nursing data determination
    conceptual model, 361–362
    contributions, healthcare, 360
    data standards, 362
    elements, 360–361
    NMDS, 361
nursing data standards determination
    C-HOBIC, 368–369
    ICNP®, 367–368
    i-NMDS, 366
    terminologies, clinical practice, 367
structured data, 359–360
IT. *See* Information technology

J
Johns Hopkins University School of
        Nursing (JHUSON) and Eclipsys
        Corporation
    EHR system, 178
    faculty members and IT staff, 178
    goals, 178
    health assessment, semester one
        assessment/intervention flowsheet,
            182, 184
        within defined limits (WDL)
            (*see* "Charting by Parameters")
        EHR system, 183, 185
    principles and applications,
        semester one
        computer workstations, 184
        EHR content, 181–183
        flowsheets, 179–180
        lab environment, 182
        multi-select list, 181, 182
        radio buttons, 181
        skills classes, 179
    technical challenges
        Laerdal SimMan, 186
        SCM system, 185–186

L

Lancaster general hospital (LGH),
    120–121
Leadership collaborative
    AONE's Technology Task Force, 152
    development needs, 152
    development programs
        academic graduate, informatics
            education, 137–138
        categories, 137
        health industry network, 138
        organizational fellowship, 138
        self-education opportunities, executives
            and managers, 139
        technology vendor-sponsored,
            138–139
    HIT, 133
    industry and national imperatives
        EHRs, 134
        HIT, 134–135
        Leapfrog Group, 134
        U.S. Department of Health and Human
            Services (DHHS), 134
    informatics competencies
        basic computer skills, 141–142
        education, 139–140
        information management,
            143–144
        literacy, information, 142–143
        models, 140–141
        nurse leaders, 144–147
        virtual communication tools, 142
    IT, 134
    magnet program collaboration
        model, 147
        TIGER, 147–148
    nurse leaders involvement, 135
    nursing survey
        director/manager role, 149
        methodology, 148
        recommendations, 149–151
        results, 148–149
    TIGER
        action steps, 136–137
        definition, 135
        issues, HIT, 136
Leadership status
    benefits, clinical system, 156
    chief nursing officers (CNOs), 155
    CNOs and IT, patient care
        competency lack, 157–158
        functionality discussions,
            156–157
        nursing executives, 156
        vendor companies, 157
    entrepreneurial mindset
        disparate systems, 165
        intellectual property (IP), 164
        IT, 163
        nursing executive dashboard (NID),
            164–165
        professional organizations and
            affiliate groups, 165
        profit commercialization, 163
    IT
        adopters and laggards, 160
        current supported system
            components, 159
        impact, organizational changes, 162
        innovators, 160
        late majority, 160
        lifecycle, 159–160
        obsolescence, 160
        productivity, efficiency and job
            satisfaction, 160–161
        technology acquisition and utilization
            process, 162
    nurse executives
        power inherent, relational databases,
            161
        research and operational analysis,
            161–162
    nursing-critical function, 155–156
    patient care
        nurse executives, 158
        "today's" practice, 158–159
    total cost of ownership (TCO)
        budgets, 163
        IT, 162–163
    universal approach, nursing, 158

M

Medical Home model
    definition, 297
    IT infrastructure
        CER, 301–302
        functions and data requirements,
            299–300
        implementation phases, 300–301
        recommendations, 299
    members, 298
    online access, 298
    private and public sectors, 297
Micro Sim cases, 176
Minnesota nursing informatics group
    (MINING), 45
Minnesota TIGER, 75

N

National Advisory Council on Nurse Education
    and Practice (NACNEP), 65, 77
National informatic landscapes
    federal momentum and activities
        executive order (EO), 197
        HIT, 197
        IOM, 196
    health care transformation
        and cost transparency, 195
        disaster preparedness and planning, 194
        emerging telehealth, 195
        growing health care consumerism, 194
        nursing shortage, 194
        unsustainable spending, 193–194
    HIT adoption, Federal government's role
        adoption, 200–201
        governance, 198
        national coordinator office, 197–198
        partners, 201
        policy, 198–199
        technology, 199–200
    opportunities, nurses
        Certification Commission for Health
            Information Technology
            (CCHIT), 203
        HIT Policy and Standards Committee,
            202–203
        National eHealth Collaborative
            (NeHC), 202
        Recovery Act, 2009, 203–205
        TIGER, 201–202
    technology adoption, priority
        IOM report, 195–196
        recommendation levels, 196
National Institutes of Health (NIH), 28,
    332–334
National League of Nursing (NLN)
    and AACN, 30–31
    accredited schools, 100
    position statement, 70
    trends, 114
Nationwide health information network
    (NHIN), 199
Networking
    conferences, 54
    electronic resources, 55
    history project, 55
    organizational resources, 51
    people resources
        AMIA mentorship program benefits, 52
        CARING, 52
        health care and nursing informatics,
            51, 53

informal programs, 51
TIGER
    daily e-news bulletins, 55
    informatics literature, 56
    web sites, 56
New England Nursing Informatics Consortium
    (NENIC), 45
Nursing informatics (NI) evolution, Brazil
    networking and integration, 404
    practice, research and education
        evidence-based and problem-based
            learning, 408
        incorporating technology, 404
        levels, program, 407
        public teaching hospitals, 406
        telenursing, 406–407
        terminologies, 405–406
        usability and interoperability, 405
    remarks and concerns, 408
    retrospective search, 403
    RUTE project, 404
    SBIS-NI goals, 403
    strategic plan, 409
    symposium, computer applications, 402
*Nursing Informatics: Where Technology
    and Caring Meet,* 11
Nursing leadership development programs
    academic graduate, informatics education
        life cycle and management, 138
        master's degree, 137–138
    categories, 137
    health industry network, 138
    organizational fellowship, 138
    self-education opportunities, executives
        and managers, 139
    technology vendor-sponsored, 138–139
Nursing leadership survey
    methodology, 148
    recommendations, role
        charge nurse, 149
        chief nurse executive and dean, 150
        director/manager, 149
        HIT competencies, 150–151
    results, 148–149
Nursing minimum data set (NMDS)
    Belgian NMDS (B-NMDS), 388, 389
    CH-NMDS, 388–389
    international nursing minimum data set
        (i-NMDS), 366–367
    purpose, 361
Nursing's contribution
    clinical informaticist
        skill sets and characteristics, 329
        transformation, 330

clinical information systems, 321
clinical-IT leadership link
    chief information officers (CIOs), 327
    patient safety and care quality, 328
    transparency, 327–328
EMR, care quality improvement
    central-line insertion, 324–325
    infection rates, 324
    medication administration errors, 326
    smart-pump technology, 325
industry trends converging,
        323–324
performance improvement
    advanced pharmacy systems, 323
    Detroit Medical Center (DMC), 322
    electronic medication administration
        record (eMAR), 322
    methodologies and IT, 326–327

P

Patient record and information system
        management (PRISM), 328
Personal digital assistants (PDAs)
    Associate Degree Nursing Committee, 73
    students, 178
    template, 422
Personal health records (PHRs)
    consumer empowerment and technology
        Consumer Reports, 265
        pervasive information availability, 266
        trends, behaviors and expectations,
            266–268
    consumer health informatics, 284
    definition
        AHIMA, 284
        consensus-based, 275
        Markle Foundation, 274
    emergence, health policy
        electronic record, 275
        Healthy People 2010 and Markle
            Foundation, 274
    ePHR (*see* Electronic personal health
        records)
    health literacy, U.S. population
        definition, 269–270
        literature resources and milestone
            contributors, 268–269
        policy, 270–272
    historical evolution
        advocacy, foundations and consumer
            groups, 276–277
        assistive reminders, 278
        communication and support services, 278

    education and decision support,
            277–278
    ePHRs, empowering technology, 277
    integration, EHR, 278–279
    patient safety, 277
National Library of Medicine (NLM)
    conference, 16, 26–27
    rural and remote communities, 30
Personalized medicine
    description, 332–333
    genomic science
        clinical utility, 334
        consumers, 335
        translational research process, 334
    human genome, 333
    SACGHS, 333–334
    stakeholders, 335
PHRs. *See* Personal health records
Program of assistance for university-based
        training, 205

R

Recovery Act of 2009
    funding, 203
    Health Information Technology for
            Economic and Clinical Health Act
            (HITECH)
        description, 203–204
        professionals, 204–205
        programs and regulations, 204
        training, 205
Regional extension centers program, 204
Robert Wood Johnson Foundation, 27
Roger's diffusion of innovation theory, 19
RUTE project, 404

S

Second Life, 176, 346, 352
Secretary's Advisory Committee on Genetics
        Health and Society (SACGHS),
        333–334
"Shared Care Plan", 282
Six Sigma methodology, 129, 130
Standards and interoperability
    action call
        EHR systems, 215
        TIGER collaborative, 215–216
    adoption process
        health IT, 211
        HITSP, 211–213
    benefits
        EHR, 214–215

TIGER health IT standards tutorials
    workgroup 2, 215
description, 210
health IT
    ANA, 208–209
    code sets, 209
    complexity, 210
    EHRs, 207
    HITSP, 208
    multidisciplinary terminologies, 209
    national agenda, 210–211
    nursing terminologies, 209
    standards, 209–210
involvement opportunities, 216–217
nursing role
    EHR, 213–214
    IT, 214
    TIGER standards and collaborative, 214
objectives, 215
State health information exchange cooperative
    agreement program, 204
Strategic health information technology
    advanced research projects
    (SHARP), 204
Summer institute in nursing informatics
    (SINI), 54

T
Taiwan model, training
    computer competency and
        "competency miss", 411
        end-user computing (EUC), 411–412
        TNIA, 412
    learning map
        codes summarization, 421
        course, 414
        drilling-down, programming, 420
        event-driven programming and
            parameter separation, 419, 421
        Excel VBA, 415
        interfaces, 419
        operation flow, concise nurse
            scheduling support system, 418
        stages, 414, 416
        training satisfaction evaluation form,
            416, 417
        userform interface design, 419
        worksheets, 417
    NI leading role
        attitude challenge, 412
        information needs and model
            creation, 413
        organizational IT resources, 412–413

Visual Basic for Applications (VBA),
    413–414
touchscreen-based interface future
    accomplishment, assessment, 425
    description, 421
    Excel-and-evidence-based application,
        421–422
    peristomal skin, evaluation, 423
    skin color evaluation, 424
    skin problems assessment, 424
    yes–no questions, patients, 425
unlimited documentation needs
    data, 426, 427
    form design interface, 426
    logon and assessment pages, 427
    mobility, nurses, 422
Taiwan Nursing Informatics Association
    (TNIA), 412
Technology acceptance model (TAM)
    engineering science, 2, 24
    literature, 25
    use and usefulness, 24
Technology Drill-Down (TD2),
    308, 309, 317
Technology informatics guiding education
    reform (TIGER). See also Cultural
    change strategies; TIGER usability
    and clinical application design
    collaborative
    actions, impact, 13–14
    collaborative team results
        activities, 44–45
        nursing stakeholders, 44
    communication and collaboration, 40
    continuing education and staff development
        computer literacy, training and skills,
            115
        facility, bed count, 116
        in-house training, 116–117
        practice environment, 116
        role, organization, 115
        staff nurses, computer literacy, 116
    definition, 35
    education, 40
    healthcare informatics, 171–172
    impact, communities
        educational, 46–47
        leadership, nursing, 46
        nursing informatics, 45
        practice specialty, 45–46
        vendor, 47
    informatics design, 41, 219
    initiative
        mission, 38

NOA, 38
initiative, education and faculty
development
collaborative teams, 67
objectives, 67–68
seven pillars, 66
intellectual capital
human and structural, 36
productivity and organization/
community, 35
IT, 41, 219
knowledge management and leadership
human capital, 37
informatics community, 37–38
social capital, 37
management and leadership
attendees, 39–40
social capital, 40
networking
daily e-news bulletins, 55
informatics literature, 56
web sites, 56
phase II
collaborative teams, 43–44
Summit Summary Report, 43
wikis, 44
phase III activities, 263
policy
HIT and PHR, 41
postsummit activities, 42
report, summit, 43
second symposium, 262
social capital
definitions, 36–37
description, 36
strategies, success, 47–49
summit, 39
Tenet healthcare (THC), 125–126
Theory of planned behavior (TBI), 24
Theory of reasoned action (TRA), 24
The Social Life of Health Information, 28
*The Social Transformation of American
Medicine,* 113
TIGER. *See* Technology informatics guiding
education reform
TIGER informatics competency collaborative
(TICC)
competencies, 60, 84
informatics recommendations, 82
TIGER usability and clinical application
design collaborative
case studies
challenging, factors, 237
exemplars, 236–237

imperatives, 238
implementations, 237–238
selection process, 238, 239
usability and outcomes, 238, 239
clinical information requirements
recommendation
description and significance, 227
points, 227–228
practitioners, 228–229
vendors, 228
conduct usability evaluations
description and significance, 231–232
points, 232
practitioners, 233–234
vendors, 233
design safe and usable clinical information
technology
description, 229
points, 230
significance, 230
vendors and practitioners, 230–231
foundations construction, human factors
description and significance, 234
points, 234–235
practitioners, 236
vendors, 235–236
literature review and analysis process
excel spreadsheets, 226
research databases, 225
usability terms, 226
recommendations, 220
TIGER Virtual Demonstration Center Pilot,
347
Transforming nursing
costs
documentation, 9
IT, 9
job dissatisfaction and burnout, 8–9
nursing hours, RNs, 8
practice environment impact, 9
health reform and HIT
health care delivery system, 5
investment positive outcomes, 6
HIT and TIGER initiative
collaboratives, 11
EHR and PHR, 10
nurse-relevant data elements, 10
Phase I Summit Summary Report, 10
IOM
impact, United States, 7
information technology and informatics
skills, 6–7
outcomes
hospital staff nursing and patient, 7

patient care quality, 7–8
RNs work hour, 7
safer care and adverse events, 8

U
Usability
　definitions
　　human–computer interaction (HCI),
　　　221–222
　　human factors (HFs), 221
　　products and, 222
　goals, 223
　origin and essence of, 220
　principles, 221
　products and systems, significance
　　goals, 222
　　principles incorporation, 223
　terms, 226

V
Virtual learning environment
　demonstrations, virtual
　　current technology, 351–352
　　future technology, 353
　　internet-based 3-D virtual world
　　　experience, 351
　　short-term future technology, 352
　Diffusion theory, 344
　exemplars
　　academic education solutions, 346
　　demonstrations, 344–345
　　observable, 345
　　simulation, 346
　　trialable, 345
　technology, nursing education
　　classroom setting, 348–349
　　clinical setting, 351
　　faculty, 348
　　simulation laboratory setting, 349–351
　　virtual setting, 349
　TIGER, 343–344
　TIGER Virtual Demonstration Center
　　Pilot, 347
Voice technology
　Boston Home, 315
　Butler Memorial Hospital, 316

drivers, 306
electronic records trend
　documentation, 306
　innovations, adoption, 309
　keyboard and voice-assisted entry, 307
　nurses, 307–309
governmental and regulatory demands
　catheter-associated urinary tract
　　infections (UTIs), decrease, 312
　falls/trauma, reduction, 312
　glycemic control, 311–312
　HACs, 310–311
　quality rating systems, 310
HAL (*see* Heuristically programmed
　algorithmic)
patient/consumer perception, health care
　connectivity and privacy, 314
　ergonomics and design considerations,
　　313
　form factor, 313
　improvement, need, 312–313
　recognition accuracy, 313
　standards and integration, 314
　workflow, 313–314
person-centered care and associated culture
　change
　aging and disability, 309
　LTC sector, 309–310
speech-based applications, health care
　documentation, information retrieval
　　and paging, 305
　EMRs and wireless call
　　systems, 304
　recognition, front-end and back-end,
　　304
St. John specialty care center
　"abundant life" model, 315
　acuity levels and staffing
　　requirements, 316
　care plans, 315–316
voice-assisted care
　acute care health systems, 306
　benefits, 305–306

W
Weekend Immersion In Nursing Informatics
　(WINI) Conference, 108, 118